Treatment and Rehabilitation of Fractures

Treatment and Rehabilitation of Fractures

Editors

Stanley Hoppenfeld, M.D.
Clinical Professor
Orthopaedic Surgery
Albert Einstein College of Medicine
Attending Physician
Jack D. Weiler Hospital of the Albert Einstein College of Medicine
Montefiore Medical Center and Our Lady of Mercy Medical Center
Bronx, New York
Associate Attending
Orthopaedic Institute of the Hospital for Joint Diseases
and Westchester County Medical Center

Vasantha L. Murthy, M.D.
Assistant Clinical Professor
Rehabilitation Medicine
Albert Einstein College of Medicine
Attending Physician
Montefiore Medical Center
Attending Physician
Our Lady of Mercy Medical Center
Bronx, New York

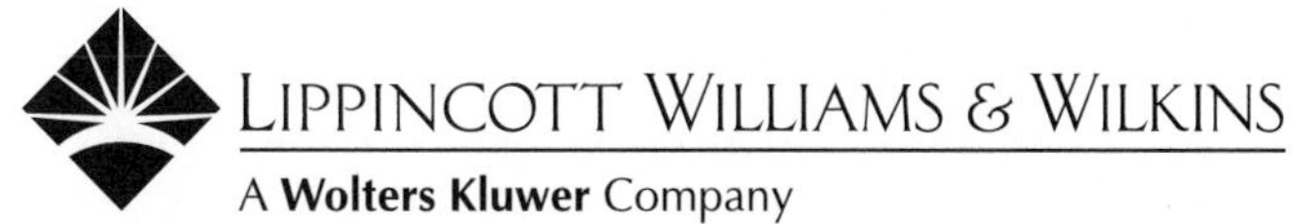
LIPPINCOTT WILLIAMS & WILKINS
A **Wolters Kluwer** Company
Philadelphia • Baltimore • New York • London
Buenos Aires • Hong Kong • Sydney • Tokyo

Acquisitions Editor: Stuart Freeman
Developmental Editor: Carol Field
Production Editor: Tony DeGeorge
Manufacturing Manager: Tim Reynolds
Cover Designer: Christina Jenny
Compositor: Lippincott Williams & Wilkins Desktop Division
Printer: Courier Westford

227 East Washington Square
Philadelphia, PA 19106-3780 USA
LWW.com

Printed in the USA

Library of Congress Cataloging-in-Publication Data
Treatment and rehabilitation of fractures / [edited by] Stanley Hoppenfeld, Vasantha L. Murthy.
p. cm.
Includes bibliographical references and index.
ISBN 0-7817-2197-0
1. Fractures—Treatment. 2. Wounds and injuries—Treatment. I. Hoppenfeld, Stanley, 1934– . II. Murthy, Vasantha L.
[DNLM: 1. Fractures—rehabilitation. 2. Fracture Fixation.
WE180 T784 1999
617.1'5—dc21
DNLM/DLC 99-16183
for Library of Congress CIP

Care has been taken to confirm the accuracy of the information presented and to describe generally accepted practices. However, the authors, editors, and publisher are not responsible for errors or omissions or for any consequences from application of the information in this book and make no warranty, expressed or implied, with respect to the currency, completeness, or accuracy of the contents of the publication. Application of this information in a particular situation remains the professional responsibility of the practitioner.

The authors, editors, and publisher have exerted every effort to ensure that drug selection and dosage set forth in this text are in accordance with current recommendations and practice at the time of publication. However, in view of ongoing research, changes in government regulations, and the constant flow of information relating to drug therapy and drug reactions, the reader is urged to check the package insert for each drug for any change in indications and dosage and for added warnings and precautions. This is particularly important when the recommended agent is a new or infrequently employed drug.

Some drugs and medical devices presented in this publication have Food and Drug Administration (FDA) clearance for limited use in restricted research settings. It is the responsibility of the health care provider to ascertain the FDA status of each drug or device planned for use in their clinical practice.

10 9 8 7 6 5 4 3 2 1

To my wife, Norma, for her unswerving support and love and to my children, Jon-David, Robert, and Stephen, who provided inspiration. To my parents, Agatha and David, for making it all possible.

Stanley Hoppenfeld, M.D.

To Sri Satya Sai Baba who gives me the inner strength and guidance always. To my family, my husband, Kris, and my children, Sai and Sumana, for their continued support and cooperation, and to my parents, Vardhani and Avadhani, who gave me the opportunity to become a physician.

Vasantha L. Murthy, M.D.

To all the physicians over many generations who have added to and expanded this body of knowledge and passed it on to a succeeding generation.

S.H., V.L.M.

Contents

Part IV: Spine Fractures

Contributing Authors

Ricardo F. Gaudinez, M.D. *Assistant Clinical Professor, Department of Orthopaedics and Rehabilitation, Yale University, New Haven, Connecticut; Attending Physician, Yale New Haven Hospital, New Haven, Connecticut; Office: Center for Orthopaedics, One Church Street, New Haven, Connecticut 06510*

Samuel A. Hoisington, M.D. *Attending Physician, Phelps Memorial Hospital Center, Sleepy Hollow, New York; Office: Hudson Valley Bone and Joint Surgeons, 239 North Broadway, Sleepy Hollow, New York 10591*

Stanley Hoppenfeld, M.D. *Clinical Professor, Orthopaedic Surgery, Albert Einstein College of Medicine, Bronx, New York; Attending Physician, Jack D. Weiler Hospital of the Albert Einstein College of Medicine, Montefiore Medical Center and Our Lady of Mercy Medical Center, Bronx, New York; Associate Attending, Orthopaedic Institute of the Hospital for Joint Diseases and Westchester County Medical Center, New York; Office: 1180 Morris Park Avenue, Bronx, New York 10461*

Derek A. Kram, M.D. *Attending Physician, Montgomery General Hospital, Olney, Maryland; Office: Greater Washington Orthopaedic Group, 2101 Medical Park Drive, Silver Spring, Maryland 20902*

Jonathan D. Lewin, M.D. *Assistant Professor, Orthopaedic Surgery, Albert Einstein College of Medicine, Bronx, New York; Attending Physician and Chief of Minimal Invasive Spine Surgery, Montefiore Medical Center, Bronx, New York*

Baron S. Lonner, M.D. *Assistant Professor of Orthopaedic Surgery, Albert Einstein College of Medicine, Chief of Spine and Scoliosis Surgery, Long Island Jewish Hospital, New Hyde Park, New York; Attending Physician, Montefiore/Einstein Hospitals and Our Lady of Mercy Medical Center, Bronx, New York; Office: 1180 Morris Park Avenue, Bronx, New York 10461*

Anne P. McCormack, M.D. *Clinical Associate Professor, Department of Orthopaedic Surgery, University of Washington School of Medicine, Seattle, Washington; Research Associate–Biomechanics Lab, Department of Orthopaedic Surgery, Harborview Medical Center, Seattle, Washington*

Vasantha L. Murthy, M.D. *Assistant Clinical Professor of Rehabilitation Medicine, Albert Einstein College of Medicine, Bronx, New York; Attending Physician, Montefiore Medical Center, Bronx, New York; Attending Physician, Our Lady of Mercy Medical Center, Bronx, New York; Office: 1180 Morris Park Avenue, Bronx, New York 10461*

Ashvin I. Patel, M.D. *Attending Physician, Sarasota Memorial Hospital, Sarasota, Florida; Consultant, Spinal Cord Injury Center, Health South Rehabilitation Hospital, Sarasota, Florida; Office: 1818 Hawthorne Street, Sarasota, Florida 34239*

Babak Sheikh, M.D. *Attending Physician, Westside Regional Medical Center, Plantation, Florida; Office: Total Orthopaedic Care, 4850 West Oakland Park Boulevard, Suite 201, Lauderdale Lakes, Florida 33313*

Lane D. Spero, M.D. *Clinical Instructor of Orthopaedic Surgery, New York Medical College, Valhalla, New York; Attending Physician and Chief of Spine Surgery, Sound Shore Medical Center, New Rochelle, New York; Office: 311 North Street, White Plains, New York 10605*

Robert Taffet, M.D. *Assistant Professor of Orthopaedic Surgery, Robert Wood Johnson Medical School, New Brunswick, New Jersey; Attending Physician, Cooper Hospital, Camden, New Jersey; Office: #3 Cooper Plaza, Camden, New Jersey 08103*

Kenneth W. Taylor, M.D. *Attending Physician, Memorial Regional Hospital, Hollywood, Florida; Office: Broward Institute of Orthopaedic Specialties, 4440 Sheridan Street, Hollywood, Florida 33021*

Bradley M. Thomas, M.D. *Resident Physician, Department of Orthopaedics, Montefiore Medical Center, Albert Einstein College of Medicine, Bronx, New York*

Mark A. Thomas, M.D. *Associate Chairman and Director, Residents Training, Department of Rehabilitation, Associate Professor of Clinical Rehabilitation Medicine, Albert Einstein College of Medicine, Bronx, New York; Office: Montefiore Hospital, 111 East 210th Street, Bronx, New York 10467*

Introduction

For optimal treatment of fractures, the fields of rehabilitation and orthopaedics need to be joined. Both disciplines deal with muscles, ligaments, and bones as well as human mobility and function, and cross-disciplining represents the ideal treatment of fracture problems. Creating a continuum encompassing orthopaedics and rehabilitation allows the most seamless and complete patient care, reduces recovery time, and provides patients with a secure feeling.

Treatment and Rehabilitation of Fractures serves to join the two fields by instructing the reader in providing sequential treatment of fractures. The book contains four sections: foundation chapters on fracture management, upper extremity fractures, lower extremity fractures, and spine fractures. Current medical terminology is used as much as possible.

The foundation chapters, which cover the fundamentals of fracture treatment, discuss the basic principles of bone healing, treatment modalities, biomechanics, assistive devices and adaptive equipment, gait, splints and braces, therapeutic exercise and range of motion, and determining when a fracture is healed. The chapters dealing with individual fractures are organized uniformly in order to provide a foundation for understanding the healing of fractures and the process of treating them. Once the reader is familiar with the introductory material, the book's contents may be read fracture by fracture on an as-needed basis.

Each chapter on an individual fracture is organized by weekly post-fracture time zones to provide a framework for managing follow-up care. Residents need guidance after the initial treatment of the fracture, and they have a natural fear of disrupting the fracture site. By emphasizing bone healing, biomechanics, and weight bearing at each stage of management, the information presented here will help the resident to develop confidence and understanding in treating fractures.

Although the rehabilitation protocols outlined here will allow patients to participate in sports, this book is not specifically concerned with sports medicine. We do not include fractures of the pelvis because of their special complexity.

The rehabilitation of a fracture depends upon the type of fracture and the fixation used; perfect prescriptions cannot be written because so many variables exist within any one diagnosis. Instead we provide guidelines for treatment on the basis of medical information, while recognizing the subtleties of each fracture and its variations.

The following outline is used in each chapter to show how the fracture is treated from both an orthopedic and a rehabilitation standpoint.

- I. Introduction
  - A. Definition
  - B. Mechanism of Injury
  - C. Treatment Goals
    - 1. Orthopaedic Objectives
    - 2. Rehabilitation Objectives
  - D. Expected Time of Bone Healing
  - E. Expected Duration of Rehabilitation

- F. Methods of Treatment
  - A. Cast
  - B. Internal Fixation
  - C. External Fixation
- G. Special Considerations of the Fracture
- H. Associated Injury
- I. Weight Bearing
- J. Gait

II. Treatment
- A. Rx: Early to Immediate (day of injury to one week)
- B. Rx: Two Weeks
- C. Rx: Four to Six Weeks
- D. Rx: Six to Eight Weeks
- E. Rx: Eight to Twelve Weeks

  Each treatment section time zone addresses the following issues:
  1. Bone Healing Box
  2. Orthopaedic and Rehabilitation Considerations
     - i. Physical Examination
     - ii. Dangers
     - iii. X-rays
     - iv. Weight Bearing
     - v. Range of Motion
     - vi. Strength
     - vii. Functional Activities
     - viii. Gait
     - ix. Methods of Treatment—Specific Aspects
     - x. Prescription Boxes

III. Long-Term Considerations and Problems

IV. Summary Box

Mechanism of Injury describes how the fracture occurs.

Treatment Goals are presented in terms of both orthopaedics and rehabilitation and include objectives for range of motion, strength, and functional activity.

Expected Time of Bone Healing explains when the fracture should be stable—crucial information as the patient progresses.

Expected Duration of Rehabilitation provides a time frame for the patient and the therapist to achieve the set goals.

Methods of Treatment, which may include casting, internal fixation, and external fixation, are presented in order of the frequency of their use. Specific treatment at each time marker is presented for each method, and the biomechanics, mode of bone healing, and indications for each method are outlined. Understanding the biomechanics helps the physician determine how well the fracture is fixed, whether the mode of bone healing is primary or secondary, and when the patient can bear weight on the fracture.

Special Considerations of the Fracture discusses the special problems and needs surrounding each fracture. These include the patient's age, osteoporosis, articular involvement, fracture pattern, compartment syndrome, and tendon and ligamentous injuries.

Associated Injury acknowledges that fractures do not occur in isolation and are usually accompanied by other injuries that also require ongoing care. These include nerve, vascular, ligament, and muscle injuries.

Weight Bearing has special importance because the main goal is for patients to bear weight through the fracture site without disturbing the fracture. The progress of weight bearing is discussed in relation to bone healing and stability at the fracture site. Certain types of fixation allow earlier weight bearing than others.

Gait presents the rehabilitation of the patient in terms of restoring a normal gait cycle.

The second section of each chapter deals with the specifics of treatment, divided into time zones. This gives the treating clinician confidence in providing care for the patient without fearing that the fracture site will be disturbed as it heals.

Under each time zone we present the following considerations: The discussion of Bone Healing provides a complete explanation of what is happening at the fracture site, so that the treating physician can correlate clinical healing, x-ray findings, and microscopic bone healing. Orthopaedic and Rehabilitation Considerations include Physical Examination; Dangers, particularly those that relate to the individual fracture; X-ray findings and how they relate to healing; Weight Bearing; Range of Motion; Strength; Functional Activities; and Gait. This is followed by Methods of Treatment—Specific Aspects. Each form of treatment is considered in its totality.

The last consideration in this area is writing a *Prescription* for a rehabilitation program. This gives the treating clinician a complete picture of what must be done to enable the patient to regain function during the various stages of fracture treatment.

The next section of each chapter is concerned with Long-Term Considerations and Problems. Perfect results cannot be guaranteed in the treatment of any fracture, and it is important to be aware of the long-term considerations for the patient.

The final section is the Summary Box, which provides a quick review of patient care for the particular fracture during each time zone.

Studying the material presented in the chapters will allow the reader to learn quickly from experienced practitioners in the field. Although a book cannot presume to replace the hands-on process of learning to treat a fracture under the guidance of a seasoned physician, *Treatment and Rehabilitation of Fractures* does present the basics of fracture management and subsequent rehabilitation in an organized format designed to enhance standard teaching programs and allow time for more in-depth learning.

Stanley Hoppenfeld, M.D.
Vasantha L. Murthy, M.D.

Acknowledgments

To my office staff: **Marie Capizzuto** (Manager), **Joan Hoppenfeld**, **Anita DeBiase**, **Donna Fennell**, **MaryLou Centrone**, **Joann Regno**, **Maryanne Becchetti**, **Yolanda Bucello**, **Maria DeSanctis**, **Debra Sullivan**, and **Kathy Langevin** for all of their help, loyalty, and support during the writing of this book.

James Capizzuto for his professional help in providing the artwork and translating the written word into illustrations.

Barbara Ferrari for her typing and retyping of the book--keeping us organized, reading and understanding our handwritten notes, making positive suggestions, and her good humor.

Roberta and **David Ozerkis**, my sister and brother-in-law, for their constant support and friendship.

A. Sudhakar Rao, M.D. and **Chandrasekhar Rao, M.D.**, my brothers, for guiding me and teaching me to be an understanding, caring, and responsible physician.

Jerry Sallis, M.D. in appreciation for his review of the foot and ankle chapters. His professional acumen was most helpful in making sure all of the important points were presented.

Roy Kulick, M.D. in appreciation for his help in reviewing Colles', forearm, wrist, and hand fractures. We appreciate his sharing his special knowledge with us on many occasions.

Neil Cobelli, M.D. in appreciation for his help in preparing the biomechanics area of the book, reviewing the femoral and tibial fractures, and sharing his specialized knowledge of trauma.

Uriel Adar, M.D. in appreciation for his help in reviewing the clavicular chapter and making positive suggestions.

Martin Levy, M.D. in appreciation for his review of the patellar chapter and keeping us updated.

David Hirsh, M.D. in appreciation for his reviewing fractures of the proximal end of the femur. Over these years he has been gracious in sharing his detailed knowledge of evaluation and treatment of these fractures.

Laurie Hirsh, M.D. in appreciation for reviewing many chapters of the book from a PGY 1 point of view. We appreciate her professional comments and thoughtfulness.

Mark Thomas, M.D. for reviewing and critiquing all of the chapters and adding an additional dimension to the book.

Dr. Aldo Perotto in appreciation for his sharing his knowledge of rehabilitation with us. His suggestions were appreciated and his specific professional thought during conference is respected.

Matei Roussan, M.D., former Chairman of the Department of Rehabilitation Medicine. I thank him for giving me the encouragement to write this book and pursue my career.

Tracy Davis: We appreciate her professional efforts in editing the text. Sentences were shortened, unnecessary words eliminated, making the book easier to read. We especially appreciate her ability to educate herself in the field of fractures, absorbing information and learning a new vocabulary.

Abraham Irvings for his friendship and guidance over these many years and keeping the accounts.

Dr. Nat and **Mimi Shore** for their inspiration, direction, and friendship. It has made a difference.

Stuart Remer, M.D. in appreciation for his help in reviewing the spine and humerus chapters. His advice was greatly appreciated.

Brad Thomas, M.D. in appreciation of his diligence in helping us obtain representative x-rays of the fractures, and helping with the captions. We appreciate his review of some of the chapters, presenting the resident's point of view.

Bonnie and **Danny Tish** in appreciation for providing the Jack D. Weiler Hospital of the Albert Einstein College of Medicine with the Michael Wolff Day Surgical Center where patients with fractures are admitted and cared for at this very special facility.

To the **members of the Department of Orthopaedics** at the Albert Einstein College of Medicine for their constant source of stimulation, new information and friendship: **Dr. Edward Habermann** (Chairman), **Dr. Leonard Seimon**, **Dr. David Shein**, **Dr. Monroe Szporn**, **Dr. Arthur Sadler**, **Dr. Lawrence Rosenberg**, **Dr. John Olsewski**, **Dr. Neil Macy**, **Dr. Cyril Kaplan**, **Dr. Joseph Marguiles**, **Dr. Benisse Lester**, **Dr. Howard Dorfman** (Pathology), **Dr. Cherise Dyal**, **Dr. Cathy Compito**, **Dr. Mel Adler**, **Dr. Arnold Wilson**, **Dr. Mel Manin**, **Dr. Dean Lorich**, **Dr. Kevin Plancher**, **Dr. Shelly Manspeizer**, **Dr. David Gonzales**, **Dr. Dominic Catanese**.

To my colleagues and the members of the **Department of Rehabilitation Medicine,** at Montefiore Medical Center and Jack D. Weiler Hospital of Albert Einstein College of Medicine (**Dr. Avital Fast**, Chairman) for their friendship and sharing their clinical knowledge with us.

The **Physical Therapy Department** at the Jack D. Weiler Hospital of Albert Einstein College of Medicine and Jacobi Medical Center. We appreciate the help the therapists gave us in reviewing the concepts of rehabilitation with regards to fractures and sharing their clinical knowledge with us.

The **Occupational Therapy Department** at the Jack D. Weiler Hospital of Albert Einstein College of Medicine and Jacobi Medical Center. We appreciate the help the therapists gave us in reviewing the upper extremity chapters and sharing their expertise with us.

Brian Rosenthal, M.D. in appreciation for his help in preparing some of the early writings of this book. His help is greatly appreciated.

Lori Laubich, Attorney-at-Law in appreciation for her advice, friendship, and review of contracts for this special project.

Herman Spater, M.D. in appreciation for his knowledge, insight, and wisdom.

Tony DeGeorge (Production Editor), **Diana Andrews** (Creative Director), **Diane Harnish** (Marketing Director), **Carol Field** (Developmental Editor), **William Wiebalck** (Editorial Assistant) and **Toni Ann Scaramuzzo** (Production Manager) for giving this book its final form, shape, and a quality look.

Stuart Freeman, Jr., my long-term editor and friend. Our relationship extends over 30 years, crisscrossing between Philadelphia and New York City.

CHAPTER *One*

Bone Healing

BABAK SHEIKH, MD

Events in fracture healing are responsible for débridement, stabilization, and, ultimately, remodeling of the fracture site. Healing can take place either primarily, in the presence of a rigid fixation, or secondarily in the absence of a rigid fixation.

Primary bone healing occurs with direct and intimate contact between the fracture fragments. The new bone grows directly across the compressed bone ends to unite the fracture. Primary cortical bone healing is very slow and cannot bridge fracture gaps. There is no radiographic evidence of a bridging callus with this mode of healing. It usually occurs approximately 2 weeks from the time of injury. This is the only method of fracture healing with rigid compression fixation of the fracture. Rigid fixation requires direct cortical contact and an intact intramedullary vasculature. The healing process depends primarily on osteoclastic resorption of bone followed by osteoblastic new bone formation (Figures 1-1 and 1-2).

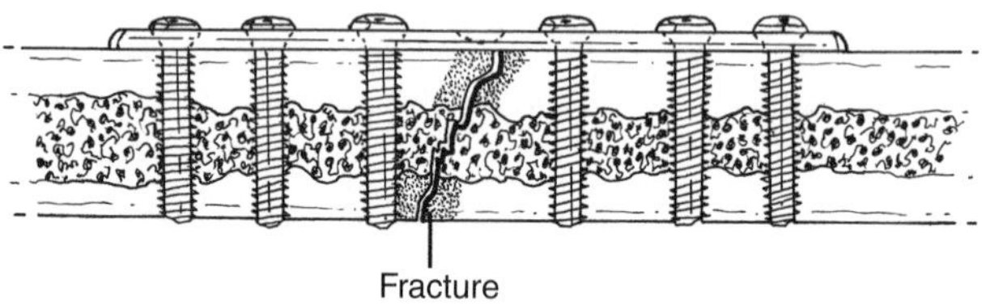

FIGURE 1-1 Rigid compression fixation of a fracture with a plate. There is direct cortical contact and an intact intramedullary vasculature, which allows primary bone healing. The new bone grows directly across the compressed bone ends to unite the fracture.

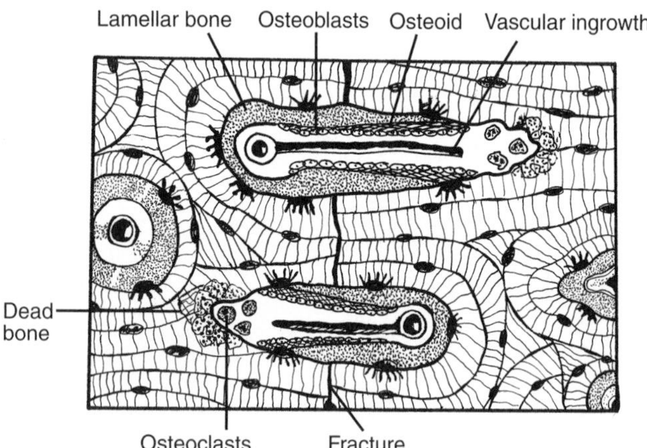

FIGURE 1-2 Microscopic view of primary bone healing. There is osteoclastic resorption of bone across the fracture site, followed by osteoblastic new bone formation. The new bone grows directly across the compressed bone ends. The absorption of bone is called *cutting cones*. This is followed by vascular ingrowth and osteoblastic new bone formation.

Secondary healing denotes mineralization and bony replacement of a cartilage matrix with a characteristic radiographic appearance of callus formation. The greater the motion at the fracture site, the greater will be the quantity of callus. This external bridging callus adds stability to the fracture site by increasing the bony width. This occurs with casting and external fixation as well as intramedullary rodding of the fracture. This is the most common type of bone healing.

The three main stages of fracture healing as described by Cruess and Dumont are (a) the inflammatory phase (10%), (b) the reparative phase (40%), and (c) the remodeling phase (70%). These phases overlap, and events that occur mainly in one phase may begin in an earlier phase.

The length of each stage varies depending on the location and severity of the fracture, associated injuries, and the age of the patient.

The *inflammatory phase* lasts approximately 1 to 2 weeks. Initially, a fracture incites an inflammatory reaction. The increased vascularity that encompasses a fracture allows for the formation of a fracture hematoma, which is soon invaded by inflammatory cells, including neutrophils, macrophages, and phagocytes. These cells, including the osteoclasts, function to clear necrotic tissue, preparing the ground for the reparative phase. Radiographically, the fracture line may become more visible as the necrotic material is removed (Figure 1-3).

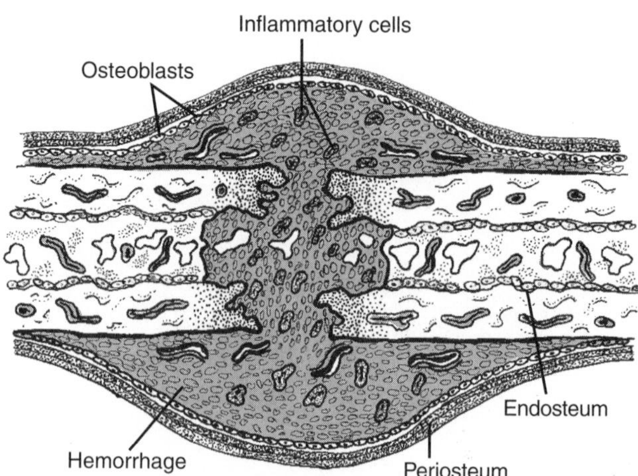

FIGURE 1-3 Inflammatory phase of secondary bone healing. A fracture hematoma has been invaded by inflammatory cells and the periosteum is elevated. Osteoblasts begin to absorb necrotic bone. This phase lasts for 1 to 2 weeks.

The *reparative phase* usually lasts several months. This phase is characterized by differentiation of pluripotential mesenchymal cells. The fracture hematoma is then invaded by chondroblasts and fibroblasts, which lay down the matrix for the callus. Initially, a soft callus is formed, composed mainly of fibrous tissue and cartilage with small amounts of bone. Osteoblasts are then responsible for the mineralization of this soft callus, converting it into a hard callus of woven bone and increasing the stability of the fracture. This type of bone is immature and weak in torque and therefore cannot be stressed. Delayed union and nonunion result from errors in this phase of bone healing. The completion of the reparative phase is indicated by fracture stability. Radiographically, the fracture line begins to disappear (Figures 1-4 and 1-5).

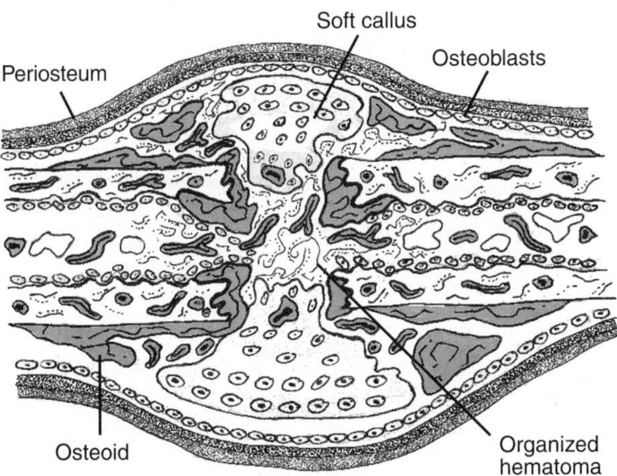

FIGURE 1-4 Soft callus formation of the reparative phase of bone healing. The hematoma begins to organize and is invaded by chondroblasts and fibroblasts that lay down the matrix for callus formation. The soft callus is composed mainly of fibrous tissue and cartilage with small amounts of bone.

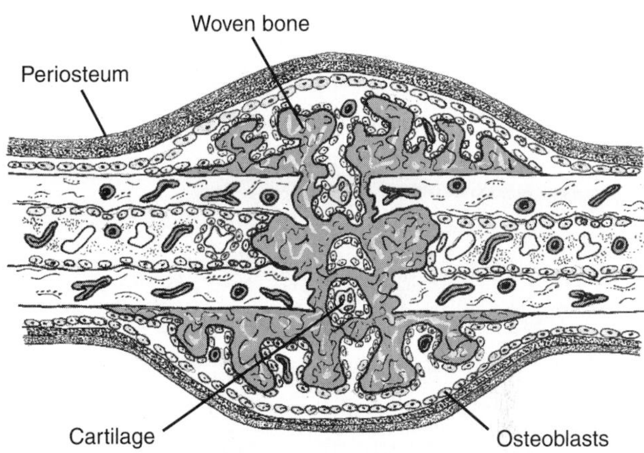

FIGURE 1-5 Hard callus formation, reparative phase. Osteoblasts are responsible for mineralization of the soft callus, converting it to hard callus, the woven bone. The soft callus is replaced by a mechanically more resistant one. This phase lasts for several months.

The *remodeling phase*, which requires months to years for completion, consists of osteoblastic and osteoclastic activities that result in replacement of the immature, disorganized woven bone with a mature, organized lamellar bone that adds further stability to the fracture site. Over time, the medullary canal gradually reforms. There is resorption of bone from the convex surfaces and new formation on the concave surfaces. This process allows for some correction of angular deformities but not rotational deformities. Radiographically, the fracture usually is no longer visualized (Figure 1-6 and Table 1-1).

The endosteum accounts for approximately two thirds of the blood supply to the bone; the remainder is provided by the periosteum. It is therefore not surprising that open or severely comminuted fractures with significant periosteal stripping have difficulties with bony union. Reaming of the medullary canal during the insertion of an intramedullary rod disrupts the endosteal blood supply, requiring weeks for its regeneration, if not longer.

Injuries to the soft tissue envelope deprive the fracture fragments of blood and alter bone healing. The soft tissue envelope surrounding the bone absorbs some of the

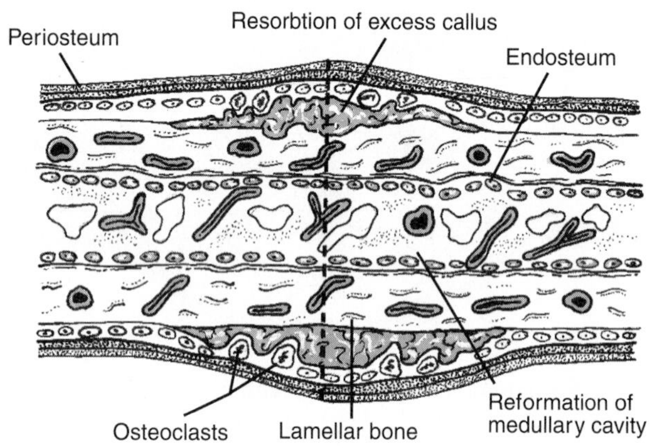

FIGURE 1-6 Remodeling phase. Excess callus is resorbed. Osteoblastic and osteoclastic activity result in replacement of immature, disorganized woven bone with more organized lamellar bone, adding stability to the fracture site. The medullary canal reforms. Remodeling requires months to years for completion.

TABLE 1-1 ***Phases of Bone Healing***

Phase	Time	Healing Phase	Percentage of Main Activity	Strength (0–4)*	Function
Inflammatory	Days	10%	Débridement of bone Inflammatory reaction and osteoclastic activity Release of growth factor Chemotaxis of blood vessels and bone cells	0	Totally restricted
Reparative	Weeks to months	40%	Soft callus Fibrous tissue Cartilage and small amounts of bone	1–2	Restricted
			Hard callus Woven bone Deformable tissue is replaced by mechanically more resistant one	3	Improved
Remodeling	Years	70%	Lamellar bone formation Resorption of excess callus Osteoblastic and osteoclastic activity Reformation of medullary canal	4	Near normal

*Strength 0–4, 4 being the strongest.

force transmitted to the bone during the initial insult. It also protects the bone from desiccation and provides a vascular supply for a healing fracture. The metaphyseal area of bone has no periosteal cambium layer. As a result, less exuberant callus formation is visualized radiographically in this region compared with the diaphyseal areas.

The method of fracture treatment used determines to some extent the mode of bone healing. In general, stress-sharing devices such as casts, intramedullary nails, and external fixators do not provide rigid fixation at the fracture site. Therefore, secondary bone healing with callus formation may be expected in those cases. With a statically locked intramedullary nail, more rigidity is achieved, and callus formation may not be as abundant. Stress-shielding devices such as compression plates result in rigid fixation at the fracture site in the absence of significant comminution. These devices lead to a primary mode of bone healing and a lack of radiographically visible callus.

BIBLIOGRAPHY

Anderson DA. Compression plate fixation and the effect of different types of internal fixation on fracture healing. *Instr Course Lect*, 42:3–18, 1993.

Baron R. Anatomy and ultrastructure of bone. In: *Primer on the Metabolic Bone Diseases and Disorders of Mineral Metabolism.* New York: Raven Press, 1993, pp. 3–9.

Bechtold EJ. Biomechanics of fracture fixation devices. In: Gustillo BR, et al, eds. *Fractures and Dislocations.* St. Louis, MO: Mosby, 1993, pp. 11–44.

Cornell NC, Lane MJ. Newest factors in fracture healing. *Clin Orthop*, 277:297–3111, 1992.

Einhorn AT. Enhancement of fracture healing. *Instr Course Lect*, 45:401–416, 1996.

Kasser RJ, ed. Bone healing and grafting. *Orthopaedic Knowledge Update*, 5:21–26, 1996.

Schenk RK, Biology of fracture repair. Schenk RK, ed. *Skeletal Trauma.* Philadelphia: W.B. Saunders, 1998, pp. 33–96.

Tencer FA, Johnson KD, Kyle RF, Fu FH. Biomechanics of fracture and fracture fixation. *Instr Course Lect*, 42:19–55, 1993.

Uhthoff KH. Fracture healing. In: Gustillo BR, *Fractures and Dislocations*. St. Louis, MO: Mosby, 1993, pp. 45–74.

CHAPTER Two

Determining When a Fracture Has Healed

BABAK SHEIKH, MD

How to assess when a fracture has sufficiently healed to withstand normal daily forces remains the fundamental question facing the clinician and the therapist. Clinical judgment, radiographic evaluation, and historical knowledge of how long each fracture takes to heal remain the mainstay for evaluating fracture healing. These methods have not substantially changed for many decades and are based on empirical information developed over the years.

The goal of fracture treatment is for the fracture to heal so that the mechanical function of the bone—its ability to withstand weight bearing and provide joint motion—is restored. The race is between fracture healing and negative sequelae such as loss of fracture reduction, tissue stiffness, and muscle wasting.

The clinical judgment that a fracture has healed is based on the combination of the patient's symptoms and physical findings over time, which usually are good indicators of the status of healing. The clinical history should focus on the presence, absence, or diminution of the patient's pain as well as the nature of that pain, especially as it relates to weight bearing, lifting, or range of motion. On examination, the clinician should evaluate the fracture site for tenderness and motion; the absence of pain, tenderness, and motion indicates a healed fracture. The absence of motion in the presence of tenderness indicates a healing fracture, whereas the presence of motion with or without tenderness indicates a fracture that has not healed. The patient must be assessed during functional activities, including weight bearing, to see if any pain, discomfort, or instability occurs. The patient may have local pain secondary to stiffness and disuse, despite a healed fracture.

Radiographic evaluation focuses on callus formation as well as the blurring or disappearance of the fracture line on subsequent x-ray films. A fracture is considered healed when there is progressive callus formation as occurs with secondary bone healing, with blurring and disappearance of the fracture line. These changes, along with the clinical findings, provide the clinician with sufficient information to assess the stability of the fracture in most patients (Figures 2-1, 2-2, 2-3, 2-4, 2-5, and 2-6; *see* Figures 12-10, 19-10D, 28-5, and 34-8).

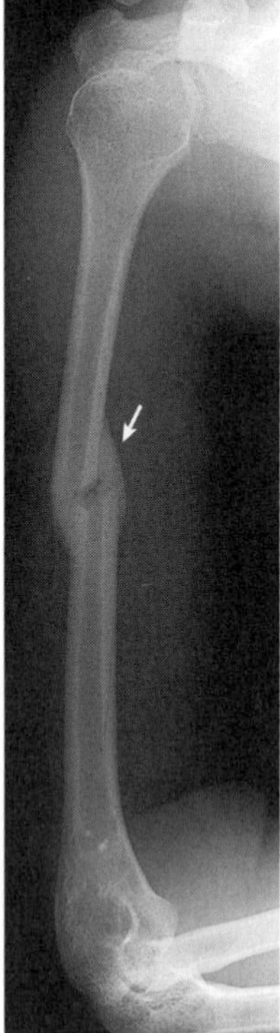

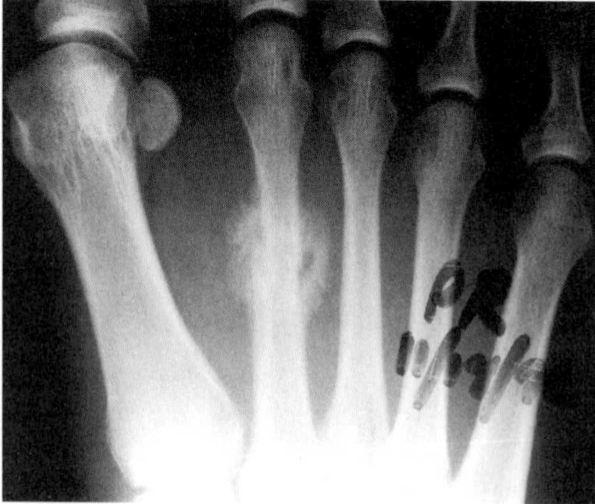

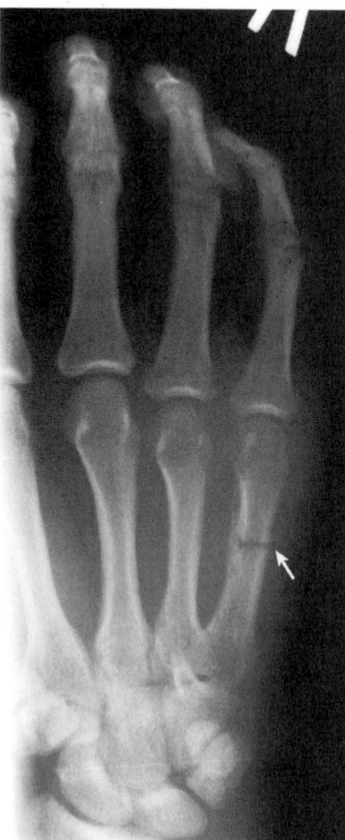

FIGURE 2-1 *(above, left)* Healed fracture of the humeral diaphysis. Bridging callus has obliterated most of the fracture line. The medullary canal and callus will remodel with time.

FIGURE 2-2 *(above, middle)* Healed fracture of the second metatarsal with large amounts of callus formation. The fracture is in the remodeling stage. The patient may bear weight.

FIGURE 2-3 *(above, right)* Fracture of the fifth metacarpal diaphysis with visible callus formation.

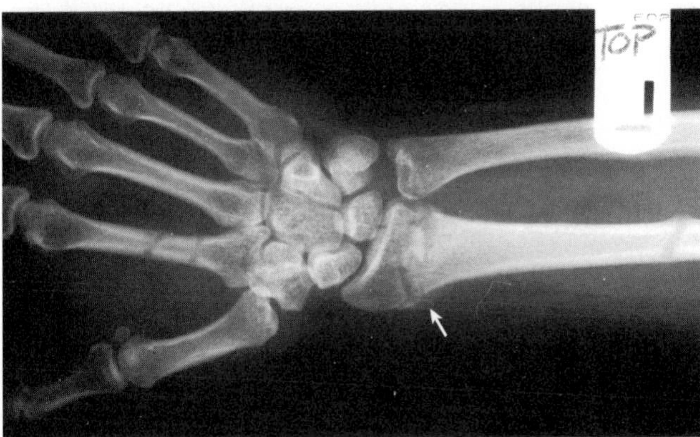

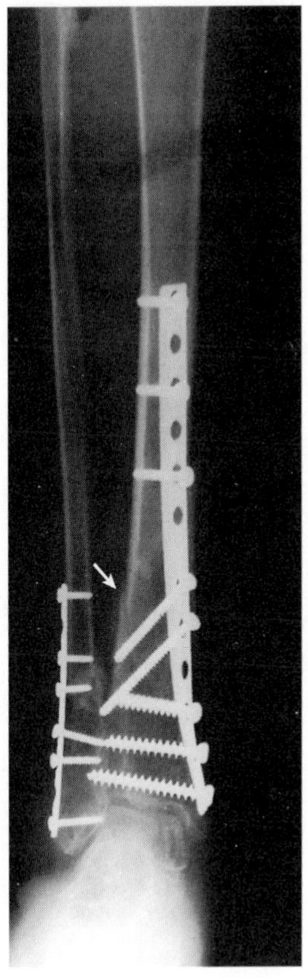

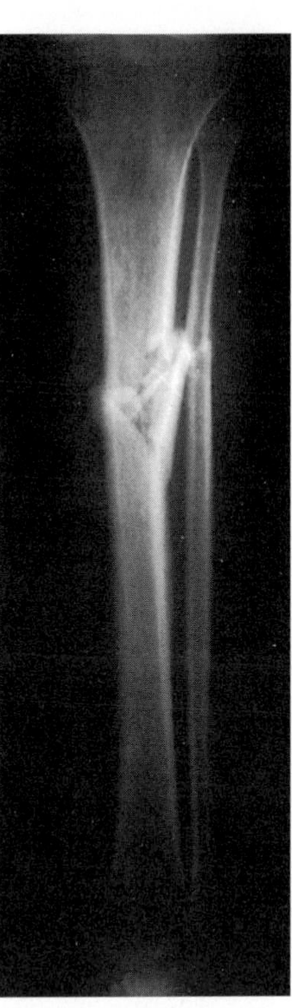

FIGURE 2-4 *(above)* Colles' fracture with callus formation.

FIGURE 2-5 *(right)* Fracture of the distal tibia and plafond with callus formation.

FIGURE 2-6 *(far, right)* Fracture of the tibial shaft with callus formation.

Historical knowledge plays a major role in fracture management. Each fracture has a general time line for healing and, with experience, a clinician can adequately assess the progression of the fracture. For example, a distal radius fracture is expected to heal within 6 to 8 weeks, whereas a mid-diaphyseal tibial fracture might require more than 3 months.

The location of the fracture also affects the type of bony union achieved and aids the physician in predicting the amount of callus response. Stable metaphyseal fractures tend to heal with little visible external callus because of stable interdigitation and impaction of the fracture fragments as well as minimal periosteal presence (*see* Figure 11-1). In contrast, diaphyseal fractures, if stabilized adequately, unite with external callus secondary to lack of impaction, the presence of a gap that is bridged by new bone formation, and the presence of adequate periosteal coverage (*see* Figure 2-1). Intracapsular fractures (e.g., fracture of femoral neck)—as opposed to extracapsular fractures (e.g., intertrochanteric fracture of femur)—tend to heal with less callus formation because of the lack of periosteum and the presence of synovial fluid (*see* Figures 21-4 and 22-5).

The type of fixation also affects fracture healing. Rigidly fixed fractures have less radiographic evidence of callus because they have less motion, which is necessary to induce callus formation (*see* Figure 16-6).

Another factor is the extent of overall trauma. The amount of comminution and soft tissue trauma, as well as open injuries, guide the clinician to expect an extended period of fracture healing. Age also plays a role in fracture union: fractures in older patients heal more slowly than those in children.

One difficult task is identifying a delayed union or nonunion. Only by knowing the type and severity of the fracture can the clinician truly assess if a fracture is healing in a timely fashion. Sometimes the patient's clinical findings do not correlate well with the radiographic findings. For example, a lack of pain or tenderness combined with the radiologic persistence of a fracture line is suggestive of a fibrous union. In such cases, the use of other modalities such as bone scans, plain and computed tomography, and magnetic resonance imaging might play a role in determining if a fracture has healed.

In most cases, the clinician can assess the fracture's healing progression simply by relying on good clinical judgment, sound radiographic evidence, and knowledge of fracture management.

CHAPTER *Three*

Biomechanical Principles of Fixation Devices

STANLEY HOPPENFELD, MD

CONTRIBUTIONS BY NEIL COBELLI, MD

Many types of devices are used for the fixation of fractures (Table 3-1). The biomechanics of fixation is based on either stress-sharing or stress-shielding devices.

A stress-sharing device permits partial transmission of load across the fracture site. When a fracture is treated with a stress-sharing device, micromotion at the fracture site induces secondary bone healing with callus formation. Casts, rods, and intramedullary nails are examples of stress-sharing devices.

A stress-shielding device shields the fracture site from stress by transferring stress to the device. The fractured ends of the bone are held under compression, and there is no motion at the fracture site. Stress-shielding devices result in primary bone healing without callus formation. Compression plating is an example of this type of treatment.

Bone healing in fractures that heal with callus formation (secondary bone healing) is relatively fast. Fractures that heal without callus formation (primary bone healing) heal more slowly. Thus, the amount of time that protected weight bearing is necessary varies not only with the location of the fracture but with the rate of bone healing.

TABLE 3-1 ***Principles of Fixation Devices***

	Cast	Rod	Plate	Pin, Screw, or Wire	External Fixator
Type of fixation	Short or long	Reamed or unreamed	Compression		Exoskeleton
Biomechanics	Stress sharing	Stress sharing	Stress shielding	Stress sharing	Stress sharing
Type of bone healing	Secondary (callus)	Secondary (callus)	Primary (no callus)	Secondary (callus)	Secondary (callus)
Rate of bone healing	Fast	Fast	Slow	Fast	Fast
Weight bearing	Early	Early	Late	Delayed	Early
Addendum	Most frequently used form of treatment	Reamed: most frequently used Unreamed: used in open fractures of the tibia	Requires secondary support	Frequently used with other fixation	Mainly used with associated soft tissue injuries

CASTS

A cast is a stress-sharing device. Stress sharing allows for callus formation and thus relatively rapid secondary bone healing. The joint above and the joint below the fracture are immobilized in the cast to prevent rotation and translation of the fracture fragments. Early weight bearing is allowed if the fracture pattern is stable, as in a transverse midshaft fracture of the tibia. Occasionally, weight bearing must be delayed until sufficient callus has developed to prevent displacement, as in an oblique midshaft fracture of the tibia (Figures 3-1, 3-2, and 3-2A).

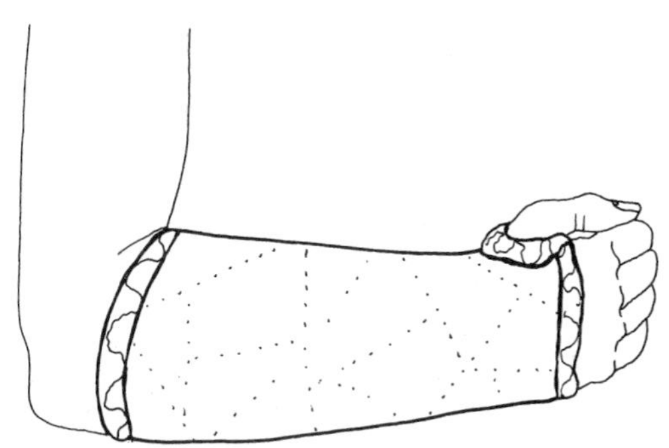

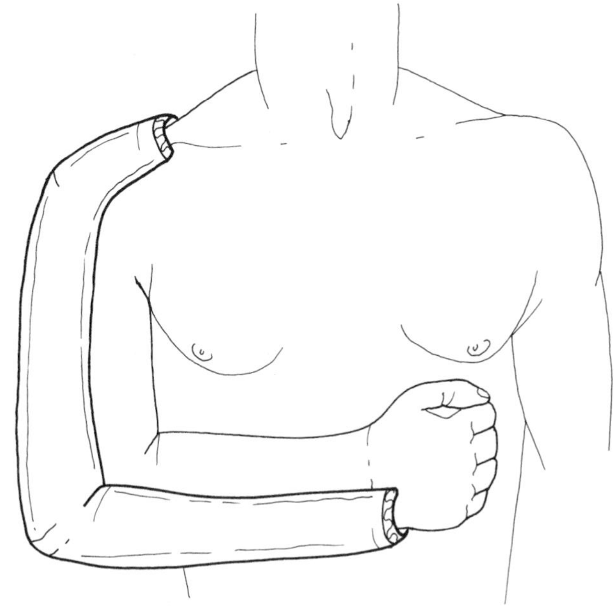

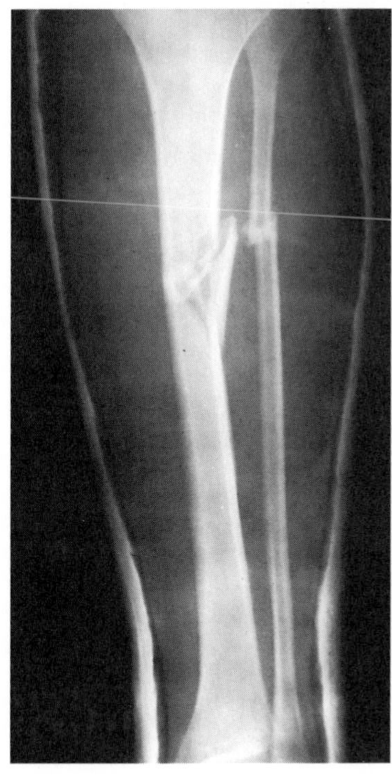

FIGURE 3-1 *(above, left)* Forearm cast; a stress-sharing device.

FIGURE 3-2 *(above)* Sugar tong splint/cast; a stress-sharing device.

FIGURE 3-2A *(left)* Cast treatment of a tibia fracture; a stress-sharing device.

INTRAMEDULLARY RODS AND NAILS

These are stress-sharing devices that allow for callus formation and fairly rapid secondary bone healing. An intramedullary rod or nail provides good fixation and allows the joints above and below the fracture to remain free for early mobilization. These devices are most frequently used in femoral shaft and tibial shaft fractures and occasionally in humeral shaft fractures.

Reamed nails have a large transverse diameter, making them very strong. However, reaming may disrupt the blood supply in the intramedullary canal, slowing endosteal bone healing. Reamed nails are frequently used in tibial and femoral shaft fractures. They may be statically locked by passing two screws transversely through both cortices of the bone and through the nail or rod, both proximally and distally. This rigid fixation prevents shortening and rotation at the fracture site, especially if the fracture is comminuted. Even statically locked nails allow for some early weight bearing. Once the fracture develops callus, the proximal or distal screw fixations may be removed to dynamize or create compression at the fracture site to further enhance bone healing. Weight bearing is allowed to create compression at the fracture site. Reamed nails are most frequently used in tibial and femoral shaft fractures (Figures 3-3, 3-4, and 3-5; *see* Figures 12-11, 12-13, 24-5, 28-6, 28-7, 28-8, 28-10, and 28-12).

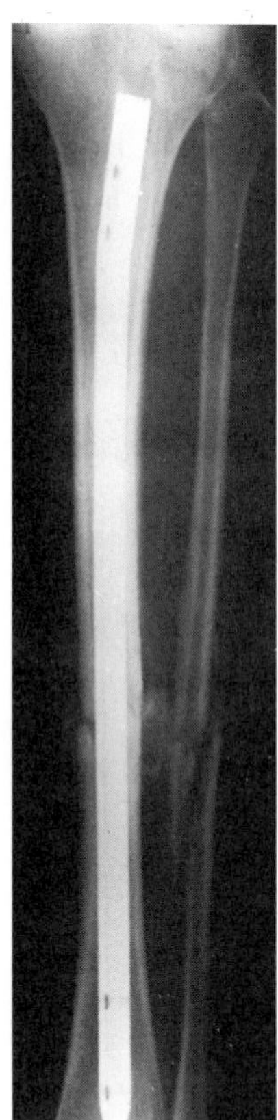

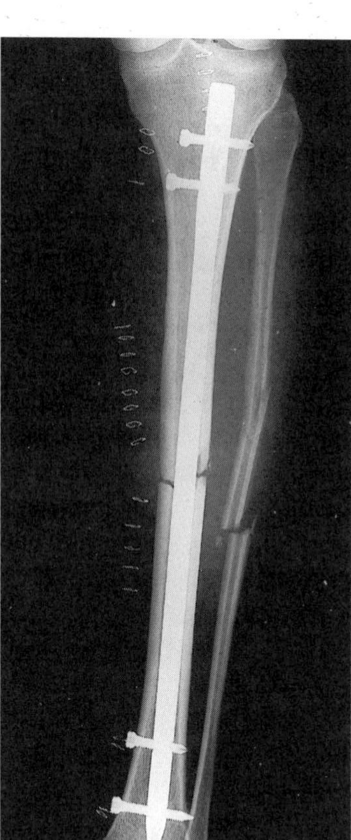

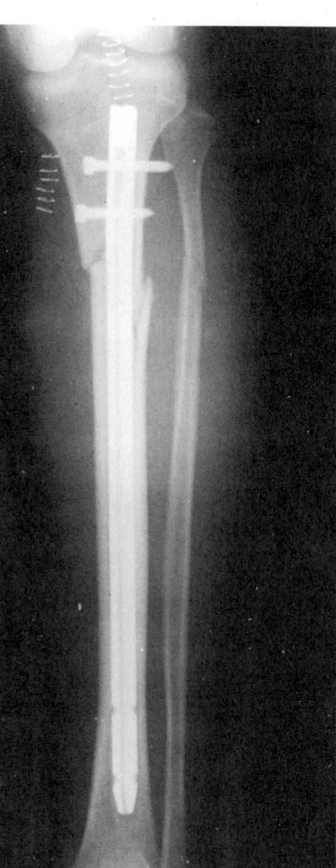

FIGURE 3-3 *(above, left)* Unlocked tibia nail; a stress-sharing device.

FIGURE 3-4 *(above, middle)* Statically locked nail; a stress-sharing device.

FIGURE 3-5 *(above, right)* Dynamically locked reamed tibia nail; a stress-sharing device.

Unreamed nails are smaller in diameter and therefore tend to have less strength, although they may maintain a better endosteal blood supply. Unreamed nails are most often used with open fractures. They may be used in a statically locked, dynamically locked, or unlocked position. They are used less frequently than reamed nails.

COMPRESSION PLATES

Compression plates are narrow, rectangular metal plates with curved surfaces that fit on the surface of the bone and are attached by screws in such a way as to create compression at the fracture site. They allow for anatomic reduction and fixation of the fracture (Figures 3-6, 3-7, and 3-8). These plates are stress-shielding devices because the area of the fracture under the plate is under diminished load. In time, the cortices of the bone under the plate may be thinned because they have been shielded from stress and have a reduced blood supply (*see* Figures 16-17 and 16-24). Compression plates are used most frequently in the upper extremity, particularly the radius and ulna.

Primary bone healing occurs because of the rigidity of the fixation, compression at the fracture site, and anatomic reduction. Because primary bone healing is a slow process, compression plate fixation requires a long period of nonweight bearing (3 months) to prevent hardware failure. Before fracture healing, all weight is borne by the hardware, which may not withstand early cyclical loading. Secondary support of the fracture site is usually needed, such as a cast or splint (Figure 3-9).

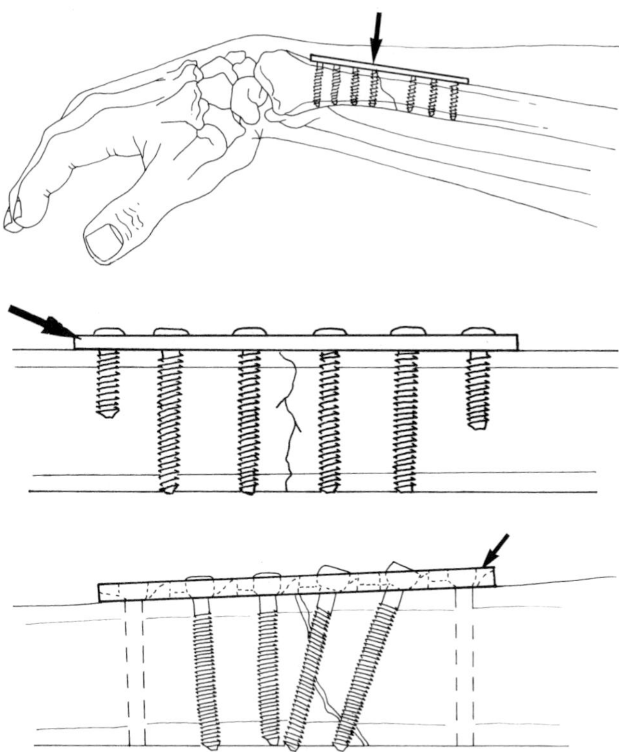

FIGURE 3-6 *(top)* Compression plating for diaphyseal forearm fractures; a stress-shielding device.

FIGURE 3-7 *(middle)* Tension band plating.

FIGURE 3-8 *(bottom)* Compression plate. Frequently used to treat forearm fractures, this is a stress-shielding device.

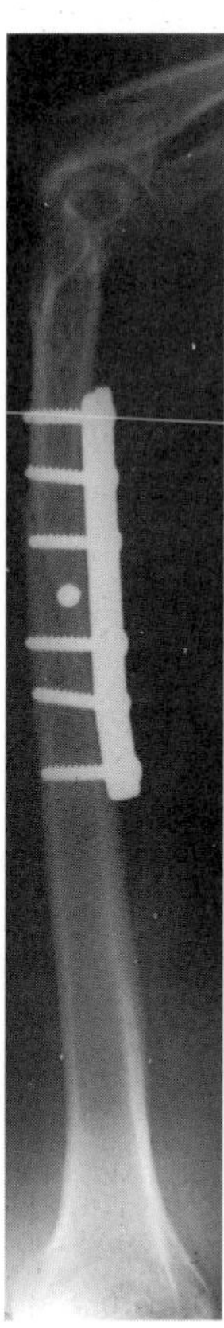

FIGURE 3-9 Compression plating of a humeral fracture. This is a stress-shielding device. If fixation is not rigid, it becomes a stress-sharing device.

BUTTRESS PLATES

These thin metal plates are used most frequently on the proximal tibia after tibial plateau fractures. They are used in conjunction with lag and wood screws to create anatomic reduction of the fracture. Buttress plates are stress-sharing devices. The patient is initially kept from weight bearing (Figure 3-10; *see* Figure 27-11).

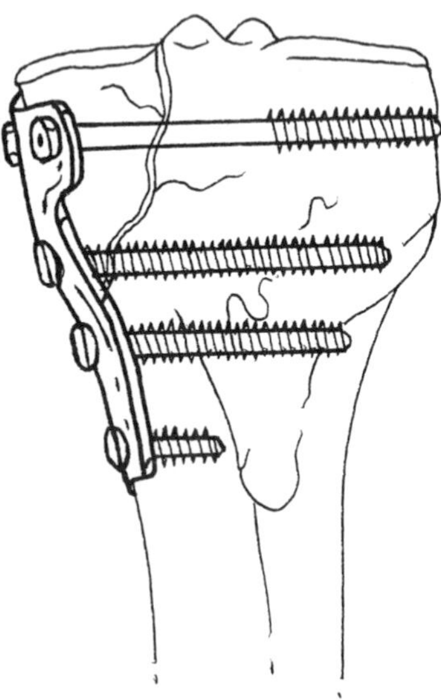

FIGURE 3-10 Buttress plate with screws creating a lag effect, and plain wood screws holding the plate to the bone.

PINS, WIRES, AND SCREWS

Kirschner wires (K-wires), pins, and screws are thin metal devices that provide partial immobilization at the fracture site; they may be threaded (screws) or nonthreaded (K-wires and pins). They are all stress-sharing devices that allow micromotion at the fracture site and therefore secondary bone healing. These devices may be used independently or with another type of fixation, such as a cast, to produce further immobilization. Weight bearing is usually delayed. Pins, K-wires, and screws are frequently removed after bone healing has occurred. These devices are often used in ankle, patellar, metacarpal, and olecranon fractures (Figure 3-11; *see* Figures 14-2, 14-7, 17-9B, 26-7, and 30-19).

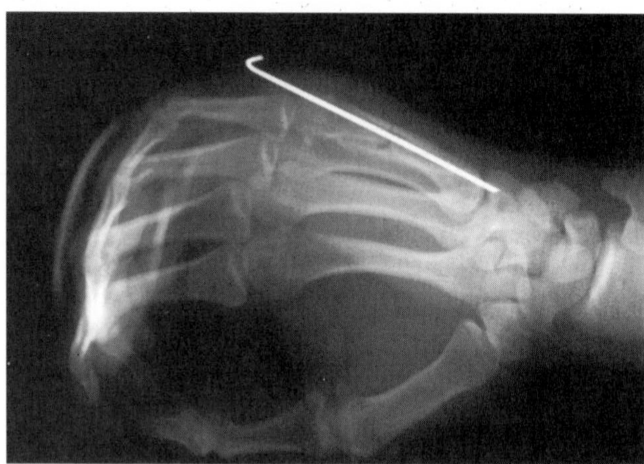

FIGURE 3-11 Metacarpal fracture treated with K-wire fixation; a stress-sharing device.

COMPRESSION SCREWS

Compression screws draw fragments of bone together. The smooth barrel of the screw crosses the fracture site, and the threaded portion extends into the distal or lateral part of the fracture. When the screw is tightened, the fragments are drawn together in what is known as the lag effect. This is a stress-sharing device, and therefore weight bearing is usually delayed (Figure 3-12).

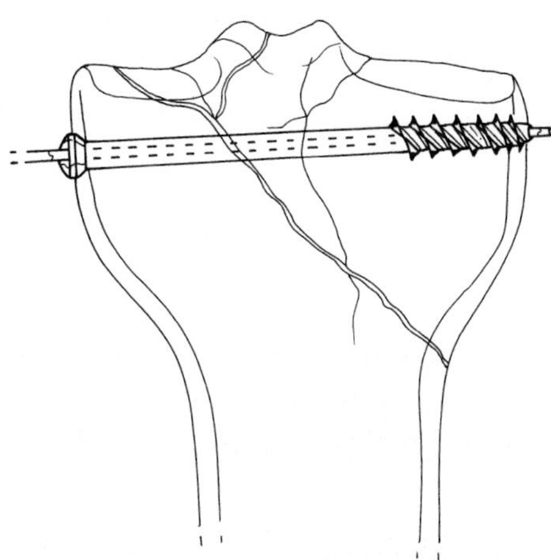

FIGURE 3-12 Cannulated screw with lag effect used to treat tibial plateau fractures.

SLIDING HIP SCREW AND PLATE

This is a special device used for fixation of fractures at the proximal end of the femur. A sliding hip screw is a stress-sharing device. It is most frequently used with intertrochanteric fractures of the femur. Because of the comminution at the fracture site, it is difficult to have the fracture rigidly fixed (Figure 3-13; *see* Figure 22-5). This device is also used to treat subcapital fractures of the femoral neck.

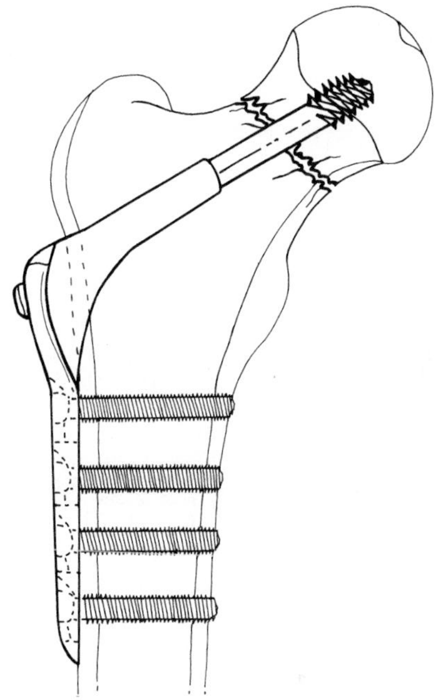

FIGURE 3-13 Sliding hip screw and plate used to treat a femoral neck fracture. This device is used most frequently for intertrochanteric fractures. It is usually a stress-sharing device, especially in comminuted fractures.

95-DEGREE CONDYLAR COMPRESSION PLATE

Fixation with the 95-degree condylar compression plate is frequently used for supracondylar fractures of the distal femur. This is a stress-sharing device because it is difficult to fix these fractures rigidly, but when a fracture is rigidly fixed, the 95-degree compression plate is a stress-shielding device (Figure 3-14; *see* Figure 25-8).

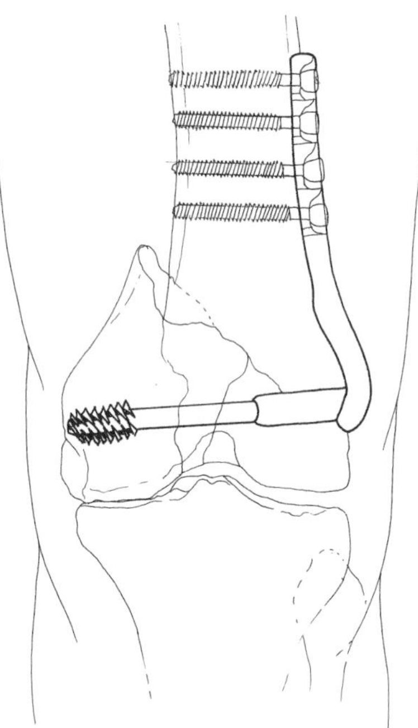

FIGURE 3-14 The 95-degree dynamic compression condylar plate used to treat supracondylar fractures of the femur. When rigidly fixed, this is a stress-shielding device, but it is usually a stress-sharing device.

EXTERNAL FIXATOR

The external splint, or exoskeleton, maintains fracture alignment and length and allows the patient to be mobile. Pins are placed above and below the fracture site and externally united to stabilize the fracture. Because this tends to be a stress-sharing device, secondary bone healing occurs through callus formation. External fixation is most often used with open fractures that are associated with massive soft tissue injuries. This allows the fracture to be fixed and the soft tissue injury to be accessible for wound checks and treatment. These proximally and distally placed pins eliminate the need to place metal at the fracture site and therefore do not increase trauma to the bone in the area of the fracture. The fixator also avoids excessive soft tissue dissection because the pins are placed percutaneously, away from the fracture site. However, the pins must traverse multiple soft tissue planes, which may result in further soft tissue problems, with loss of associated joint motion. Motion of the soft tissues may also loosen the pins, limiting their effectiveness in achieving bony union. The external fixator may be used on any of the long bones of the body (Figure 3-15; *see* Figures 12-19, 28-13, and 28-15).

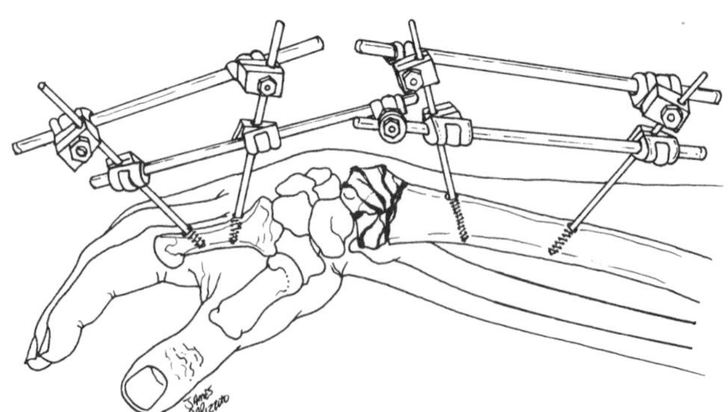

FIGURE 3-15 External fixator for treatment of a comminuted Colles' fracture; a stress-sharing device.

CHAPTER Four

Therapeutic Exercise and Range of Motion

MARK A. THOMAS, MD

CONTRIBUTIONS BY VASANTHA L. MURTHY, MD

The ultimate purpose of an exercise program is to restore function, performance, muscle strength, and endurance to pretrauma levels. Unused muscles atrophy and lose strength at rates from 5% per day to 8% per week. With immobilization, atrophy is found in both slow-twitch (type one) and fast-twitch (type two) muscle fibers. Fast-twitch fiber atrophy is first seen as a loss in strength, whereas atrophy of slow-twitch fibers is noted as a loss of endurance.

Muscle strength is basically the ability of the muscle to contract against resistance. The basic principle of strength training is to use resistance and repetitive contraction to promote recruitment of all muscle motor units; this is done each day at an intensity that does not overload the muscle. An example of this is the leg press exercise, where the quadriceps muscles are strengthened by extending the knee against progressively heavier weight. This is done until a sense of fatigue is experienced, but not to the point of pain or exhaustion.

Endurance is the ability to do the same movement repeatedly. This is achieved by repetitive exercise until the muscle fatigues (overload). Examples of endurance exercise include walking for increasing distances, repetitively contracting the gastrocnemius after a tibial fracture, or repetitively contracting the quadriceps after a femoral fracture. The best exercise to improve the performance of a task is the repeated performance of the task itself, such as walking or washing the hair. Exercise performed by the patient accomplishes the goals of maintaining range of motion and increasing strength and endurance. These are important to improve the patient's ability to perform a given function or task. The following types of exercises are most frequently prescribed for a comprehensive exercise program.

RANGE OF MOTION

The movement of a joint through partial or full excursion, range of motion is performed to maintain or increase the excursion of a joint. It is the most basic type of exercise prescribed in all phases of fracture rehabilitation. Range of motion may be full (anatomic) or functional (the movement required to perform a specific task).

Full Range of Motion

Full range of motion is the available range of motion of a given joint as defined by its anatomy. The restriction of movement by the bony configuration of the joint, as well as ligamentous checks, determines the possible joint excursion, or range of motion. For example, the knee has a range of motion of 0 to 120 degrees (full extension, 0 degrees, to full flexion, 120 degrees).

Functional Range of Motion

Functional range of motion is the movement required from a specific joint for the performance of activities of daily living or for any patient-specific task (e.g., pitching a baseball). To sit comfortably, for example, 90 degrees of flexion at the knee is desirable. A range of motion at the knee from full extension (0 degrees) to 90 degrees of flexion is not full, but it is functional for sitting.

Active Range of Motion

The patient is instructed to move the joint through full or partial available motion on his or her own volition. The purpose of active range of motion exercise is to prevent loss of available movement at the joint. These exercises are indicated in the early phase of bone healing when there is no or little stability at the fracture site. Direct patient sensory feedback helps to prevent motion that might increase pain or affect the stability of the fracture site.

Active Assistive Range of Motion

In this exercise, the patient is directed to use his or her own muscle contraction to move a joint, while the treating professional provides additional or assistive force. This is most commonly used in instances of weakness or inhibition of motion due to pain or fear, or to increase the available range of motion. Some stability at the fracture site, such as that provided by bone healing or fracture fixation, is required for this exercise.

Passive Range of Motion

These exercises consist of joint movement without patient muscle contractions. All motion is provided by the physician or therapist. The purpose of this exercise is to maintain or increase the available motion at a joint, depending on the force applied. These exercises are indicated when voluntary muscle contraction is impossible, undesirable, or not strong enough to overcome joint capsule contracture. Because of the decreased direct sensory feedback to the patient, passive range-of-motion exercises should not be prescribed when excessive joint movement might affect the stability of a healing fracture.

MUSCLE STRENGTH GRADING

Although uncomplicated fractures do not present neurologic problems, the muscles surrounding the site of fracture are weaker, usually secondary to direct trauma, immobilization, or reflex inhibition. Muscle testing is a useful guide for evaluating the improvement in muscle strength during the recovery period. This is not discussed separately in each chapter. Muscle strength is graded according to the following scale (Table 4-1):

TABLE 4-1 *Muscle Grading Chart*

Muscle Gradations	Description
5—Normal	Complete range of motion against gravity with full resistance
4—Good	Complete range of motion against gravity with some resistance
3—Fair	Complete range of motion against gravity
2—Poor	Complete range of motion with gravity eliminated
1—Trace	Evidence of slight contractility; no joint motion
0—Zero	No evidence of contractility

Grade V—Normal: The muscle has normal strength, is able to move a joint through a full range of motion despite full resistance by the examiner.

Grade IV—Good: Indicates that partial resistance by the examiner can be overcome as the muscle moves through the full range of motion.

Grade III—Fair: The muscle moves a joint through a full range of motion against gravity, but cannot overcome any degree of resistance by the examiner.

Grade II—Poor: The joint has a full active range of motion after gravity is eliminated. The muscle lacks sufficient strength to move a joint through the full range of motion against the force of gravity.

Grade I—Trace: The muscle cannot demonstrate movement, although some contraction of the muscle may be evident by palpation.

Grade 0—Zero: The muscle shows no evidence of contraction.

STRENGTHENING EXERCISES

Strengthening exercises increase the amount of force that a muscle can generate. These exercises improve the coordination of motor units innervating that muscle as well as the balance between muscle groups acting at a given joint. Strengthening exercise is geared to increase the potential tension that can be produced by contractile and static elements of the muscle–tendon unit. Strengthening exercises are of various types.

Basic Strengthening Exercises

Isometric Exercises

In isometric exercise, muscle fiber length is constant, so muscle contraction occurs without joint movement (Figure 4-1). Isometric exercise is very useful when the

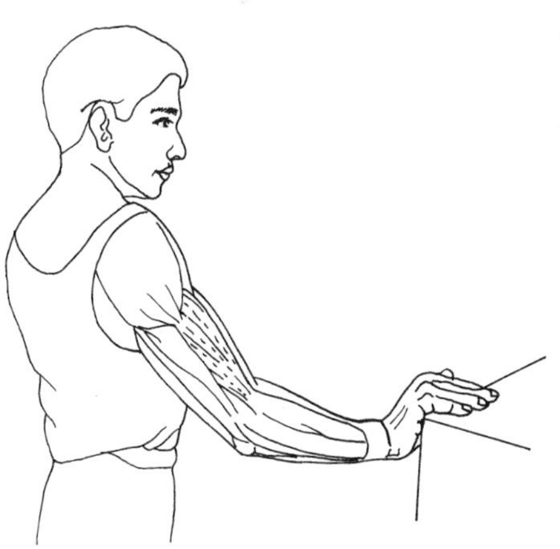

FIGURE 4-1 Isometric exercises. Muscle fiber length is constant, so muscle contraction occurs without joint movement. Isometric exercises are very useful when the strength of a muscle is to be maintained or increased but the movement of the joint is either contraindicated because of fracture instability or undesirable because of pain.

strength of a muscle is to be maintained or increased but the movement of a joint is either contraindicated because of fracture instability or undesirable because of pain. This is the earliest type of strengthening exercise to use after most fractures because it has the least chance of disturbing the stability of the fracture site. Examples include contracting the quadriceps muscle while the leg is in a long leg cast or the biceps muscle while the arm is in a long arm cast. These exercises are also referred to as *set exercises.*

Isotonic Exercise

Isotonic exercise is a dynamic exercise performed using a constant load or resistance, but uncontrolled speed of movement. Therefore, tension within a muscle fiber is relatively constant in these exercises. The muscle fiber lengthens and shortens, causing joint motion (Figure 4-2). Isotonic strengthening exercises are most frequently prescribed for increasing strength in the intermediate and late stages of fracture rehabilitation. Progressive resistive exercises are one example of isotonic exercise, such as biceps curls with increasing dumbbell weights, or leg presses. This type of exercise is not done when a cast is in place. Progressive resistive exercises result in greater strength.

Isokinetic Exercise

This exercise provides joint movement at a constant rate. To maintain a constant rate of motion, resistance is varied in response to the muscle force applied. The advantage of isokinetic exercise is that the muscle can be optimally strengthened throughout the joint's entire range of motion, which is not possible with either isometric or isotonic exercise. These exercises are prescribed in the late stage of rehabili-

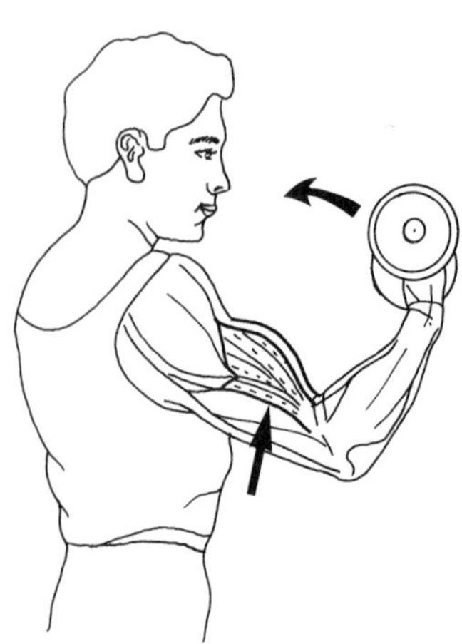

FIGURE 4-2 Isotonic exercise. This is a dynamic exercise form using a constant load or resistance but uncontrolled speed of movement. Therefore, tension in a muscle fiber is relatively constant during this exercise. These exercises are most frequently prescribed for increasing strength in intermediate and late stages of fracture rehabilitation.

tation, when there is good stability at the fracture site. The disadvantage of isokinetic exercise is that it requires the use of a machine, such as the Cybex, to vary resistance while maintaining a constant rate of motion (Table 4-2). For example, during the late stages of rehabilitation after a femoral fracture, the Cybex machine can be used to strengthen the quadriceps muscle (Figure 4-3).

High-Performance Strengthening Exercise

Closed-Chain Exercise

This type of exercise requires fixation of the proximal and distal portions of the body that are being moved during exercise. Closed-chain exercises are good for strengthening multiple muscle groups simultaneously and have the added value of enhancing func-

TABLE 4-2 *Strengthening Exercises after Fracture*

Effects of Exercise	Isometric	Isotonic	Isokinetic
Muscle length	No change	Shortens and lengthens	Shortens and lengthens
Joint motion	No	Yes	Yes—constant rate of motion
Muscle fiber tension	Increases	Increases initially, then there is constant tension throughout the range of motion	Increases
Strength gain	In one joint position	Throughout the range of motion; maximal gain at the ends of joint range	Equal gain throughout the range of motion
Effect on range of motion	No change	Maintains or increases	Maintains or increases
Timing of exercise	Early stage	Intermediate stage	Late stage
Example of strengthening exercise	Contracting the biceps while in a long arm cast	Biceps curl	Biceps curl performed on a machine that varies resistance to allow for a constant rate of motion

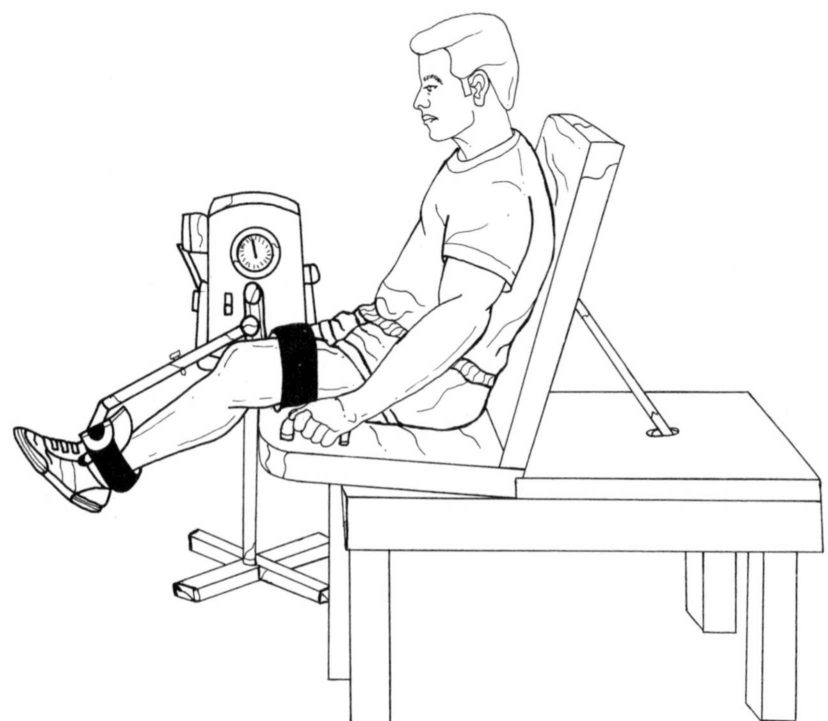

FIGURE 4-3 Isokinetic exercise. During this exercise, the joint moves at a constant rate, but the resistance applied is variable. The muscle can be optimally strengthened through the joint's entire range of motion. These exercises are prescribed in the late stage of rehabilitation when there is good stability at the fracture site.

tion, because most "real-life" movements occur in a closed kinetic chain. Examples of closed-chain exercise include wall slide exercises and squats, both of which strengthen all the major extensor muscle groups of the lower extremities (the closed kinetic chain includes the ankle, hip, and knee joints).

Open-Chain Exercise

In this exercise, there is no fixation of the distal limb. This type of strengthening exercise is more commonly prescribed after fracture. Examples include leg or biceps curls.

Plyometric Exercise

This exercise is performed by maximal muscle contraction after a quick stretch, such as jumping and hopping exercises. Because of the torque generated at a lower extremity fracture site, these exercises should be prescribed only in the late phase of rehabilitation to enhance the patient's strength and performance beyond that required for routine activities of daily living.

Open-chain, closed-chain, and plyometric exercises may be prescribed for specific tasks or levels of performance as part of the rehabilitation program after fracture. For example, closed-chain or plyometric exercises may be prescribed to achieve the strength required for athletic performance (jumping; strengthening the gluteal and quadriceps muscles after a femur fracture), or open-chain biceps curls prescribed for isolated strengthening of the biceps after humeral fracture.

FUNCTIONAL OR TASK-SPECIFIC EXERCISE

These exercises increase performance while increasing strength. In addition to muscle fiber hypertrophy, they improve neuromuscular coordination, agility, and strength. Examples of this type of exercise include stair climbing after femoral fracture or ball squeezing and turning door knobs after the removal of a cast for a Colles' fracture.

CONDITIONING EXERCISE

Conditioning exercises increase endurance. They are used to increase overall cardiopulmonary function rather than to treat deficits after a specific fracture. Conditioning exercises enhance peripheral oxygen utilization and muscular efficiency and result in aerobic muscle metabolism.

They are performed at an adequate target heart rate for more than 20 minutes. Common conditioning exercises include riding a stationary bicycle or using a treadmill.

TYPES OF MUSCLE CONTRACTION DURING EXERCISE

Muscles contract in various ways to allow smooth function of the joints. There is a "traditional" or shortening contraction that flexes the joint, an elongation contraction that allows the joint to extend in a controlled manner, and a contraction that produces no motion. Rehabilitation considerations for specifying the type of contraction by which a muscle is exercised are based on the stability of the fracture site, the effect of joint motion on the fracture site, the rapidity of muscle fatigue, and any selective muscle strengthening necessary to perform a specific task.

Concentric

In concentric contraction, the muscle fibers shorten as the muscle contracts and the insertions of the muscle move closer together. Muscles contracting in a concentric manner usually function to accelerate joint motion, such as contraction of the biceps to flex the elbow or contraction of the quadriceps to extend the knee to raise the body up a step (Table 4-3).

TABLE 4-3 *Types of Muscle Contraction*

	Concentric	Eccentric	Isometric
Fiber length	Shortens	Lengthens	No change
Joint motion	Accelerates	Decelerates	None
Force of contraction	Less	Greater	Great
Quadriceps muscle contraction	Knee extension	Progressive knee flexion—squatting	Stabilizes the knee in fixed flexion—squatting position

Eccentric

During eccentric contraction, the muscle fibers lengthen and the insertions of the muscle move farther apart. Functionally, eccentric contraction serves to brake joint motion in controlled deceleration. Eccentric contractions are capable of generating greater force than concentric contractions because the static elements of muscle (noncontractile proteins, tendons, and septa) are recruited into resisting a load. For example, using the quadriceps to control the knee as it flexes in a squat is an eccentric, or lengthening, contraction.

The biceps contracts concentrically while the triceps contracts eccentrically to provide smooth control of elbow flexion in a balanced manner.

Eccentric contractions generate greater heat as well as greater force. They carry a greater risk of postexercise myoedema and myalgia than do concentric or isometric contractions. When exercises are prescribed as part of a fracture rehabilitation program, eccentric exercises should be specified only when there is good stability at the fracture site, to prepare for functional activities, or in combination with concentric exercise to restore muscle balance.

Isometric

In isometric contractions, there is no change in muscle fiber length and no joint motion. The normal function of isometric contraction is to stabilize a joint. An example is use of the quadriceps to maintain the knee in fixed flexion, such as squatting.

Muscle contraction is not equivalent to muscle shortening. Muscle fibers shorten in concentric contraction, lengthen in eccentric contraction, and do not change length in isometric contraction.

BIBLIOGRAPHY

Borquist L, Lindelow G, Thorngren KG. Costs of hip fracture: rehabilitation of 180 patients in primary health care. *Acta Orthop Scand*, 62:39–48, 1991.

Braddom R. *Physical Medicine and Rehabilitation*. Philadelphia: W.B. Saunders, 1996.

Brotzman SB, ed. *Clinical Orthopaedic Rehabilitation*. St. Louis: Mosby, 1996.

Ceder L, Svensson K, Thorngren KG. Statistical prediction of rehabilitation in elderly patients with hip fractures. *Clin Orthop*, 152:185–90, 1980.

Delisa J. *Rehabilitation Medicine: Principles and Practice*. Philadelphia: J.B. Lippincott, 1988.

Grundes O, Reiker O. Effect of physical activity on muscle and bone blood flow after fracture: exercise and tenotomy studied in rats. *Acta Orthop Scand*, 62:67–69, 1991.

Hoppenfeld S. *Physical Examination of the Spine and Extremities*. Norwalk, CT: Appleton-Century-Crofts, 1976.

Mehta Arun JMB, ed. Rehabilitation of fractures. *State of the Art Reviews in Physical Medicine and Rehabilitation*, Vol. 9, No. 3. Philadelphia: Hanley & Belfus, 1995.

Norkin C, Levangie P. *Joint Structure and Function*, 2nd ed. Philadelphia: F.A. Davis, 1992.

Soderberg G. *Kinesiology: Application to Pathological Motion*. Baltimore: Williams & Wilkins, 1986.

CHAPTER *Five*

Modalities Used in the Treatment of Fractures

MARK A. THOMAS, MD

Physical therapeutic treatment modalities (i.e., heat and cold, hydrotherapy, fluidotherapy, and electrical stimulation) are frequently used after a fracture to reduce discomfort and enhance the effects of exercise (Table 5-1). Modalities all have a predictable biologic effect when externally applied. Just as with pharmacologic treatments, the rehabilitation prescription for these modalities must take into account indications, contraindications, and possible adverse reactions, as well as dosage and frequency of application. It is necessary to be familiar with the specific physiologic effects of the various modalities to use them properly.

THERAPEUTIC HEAT

Therapeutic heat increases local and regional circulation, reduces tissue viscosity, and improves collagen elasticity. It also reduces the firing rate of both muscle spindle and peripheral pain receptors (nociceptors). When properly prescribed and applied, heat is useful for pain reduction and muscle relaxation; it may also enhance healing by increasing the regional blood flow. Heat increases the metabolic rate and circulatory demand at the area to which it is applied and, when inappropriately applied, may cause burns and local or

TABLE 5-1 *Heat Modalities*

Modality	Tissues Heated	Indications	Contraindications	Frequency of Use
Superficial heat				
Hot packs,	Skin and subcutaneous	Pain and muscle tension	Burn or anesthetic area Peripheral vascular disease	Common
Paraffin bath;	Skin and subcutaneous	Pain and muscle tension Reduced range of motion	Burn or anesthetic area Peripheral vascular disease	Common
Fluidotherapy*	Skin and subcutaneous	Reduced range of motion Pain and muscle tension	Burn or anesthetic area Peripheral vascular disease Ischemic area Bleeding	Common
Deep heat				
Ultrasound	Bone/muscle	Contracture of muscle or joint capsule	Local fracture Metal implant	Occasional
Short-wave diathermy	Subcutaneous	Postoperative adhesion, superficial contracture	Metal implant Pacemaker Drug delivery system	Rare
Microwave diathermy	Muscle	Muscle contracture	Metal implant Pacemaker Drug delivery system	Rare

*Prolonged immersion may provide deep heat to small, superficial joints such as the digits.

regional ischemia. Because of this, it is contraindicated in areas that are burned, anesthetic, bleeding, ischemic, or have a tenuous vascular supply.

Heating may be applied directly using hot packs (thermal energy) or by converting ultrasound (acoustic energy), microwaves, or short waves (diathermy) into heat. Hot packs and ultrasound are the heating modalities most commonly used during postfracture rehabilitation.

Superficial Heat

This is the most common form of heat prescribed after fracture. *Hot packs* and radiant heat (heat lamps) are used to heat the skin and subcutaneous tissues. This allows for patient relaxation and free mobilization of skin and scar tissue. Superficial heating methods do not effectively reach muscle.

A *paraffin bath*, immersion in melted paraffin wax and glycerin, heats the skin and subcutaneous tissue, and, with prolonged immersion, the small joints and muscles of the hand. Indications for this modality include pain and loss of distal upper extremity (hand and wrist) range of motion after a fracture. It should not be used in the presence of significant edema or open wounds, and requires close supervision when the skin is anesthetic.

Like paraffin immersion, *fluidotherapy* heats by convection and conduction and is used for the distal upper extremity (hand and wrist) after fracture. With fluidotherapy, the patient inserts the distal forearm into a closed chamber in which particulate material (such as ground corn husks) is suspended by warm air. In addition to the thermal effects, fluidotherapy provides a gentle mechanical stimulation of the skin and subcutaneous tissue, allowing further relaxation. This modality is useful to help decrease pain and increase the range of motion of the wrist and hand after fracture.

Paraffin baths and fluidotherapy may provide either superficial or deep heat to the hand, depending on the treatment method and parameters. Although it is possible, these modalities usually are not used to treat the foot.

Deep Heat

Ultrasound, short-wave diathermy, and microwave diathermy are also used for rehabilitation after fracture to provide deeper heating. Short-wave and microwave diathermy are infrequently used because of limited availability of equipment and therapist expertise.

Ultrasound heats the bone–muscle interface. Indications for its use include postfracture muscle shortening and joint capsule contraction. The contraindications to the use of ultrasound are somewhat controversial, but ultrasound is usually not used over a fracture site or near implanted hardware because the heat concentration could lead to a burn or disruption of fracture healing.

Short-wave diathermy selectively heats subcutaneous tissue more effectively than superficial heat modalities. Indications for its use include treatment of postfracture contracture and subcutaneous adhesion. Short-wave diathermy is contraindicated when there is implanted metal or a pacemaker or drug delivery system because it may interrupt system electronics.

Microwave diathermy selectively heats muscle. Indications for its use are limited to postfracture muscle shortening. It is contraindicated when there is implanted metal or another type of implanted device.

THERAPEUTIC COLD

Cold, applied either by an ice pack or other type of cold pack, or by the use of a vapocoolant spray that cools by evaporation, is most often used very early in fracture rehabilitation for analgesia and control of edema immediately after injury. Cold produces its numbing effect by decreasing the firing rate in peripheral receptors, including pain receptors. In the later phases of rehabilitation, therapeutic cold is useful for reducing pain and muscle spasm, but is used less often than heat and hydrotherapy modalities. The use of cold versus heat for pain reduction is patient specific. The most effective modality for the individual patient is the one that should be used.

HYDROTHERAPY

Hydrotherapy may include whirlpool or therapeutic pool treatment, depending on the desired therapeutic effect. The benefits of therapeutic heat and exercise are often synergistic when applied in conjunction with hydrotherapy. The general uses of hydrotherapy are to:

- Improve range of motion, especially after cast removal
- Stimulate wound healing (by mechanical débridement and cleansing the skin of excess corneum collected under the cast)
- Improve circulation (depending on water temperature)
- Increase weight acceptance by a lower extremity

The degree of weight bearing, a product of buoyancy and gravity, can be varied by adjusting the height of the water. Treatment in a walk-tank or therapeutic pool is a good way to advance weight bearing.

ELECTRICAL MODALITIES

Electrical stimulation may be provided as part of a strengthening program after a fracture has healed, particularly when patient anxiety has led to the inhibition of contraction. In select instances, high-volt galvanic (direct current) stimulation may be useful to reduce muscle spasm, particularly when this is necessary to increase range of motion after cast removal (e.g., to stimulate the quadriceps after a distal femur fracture).

SPRAY AND STRETCH

Spray and stretch therapy consists of slow, unidirectional application of a vapocoolant (fluorimethane) followed by manual stretching. If there is persistent muscle spasm after fracture healing, especially of the cervical/scapular or lower back muscles, this can be useful to help stretch and relax the muscle, leading to reduced pain and improved range of motion.

BIBLIOGRAPHY

Braddom R. *Physical Medicine and Rehabilitation.* Philadelphia: W.B. Saunders, 1996.

Brotzman SB, ed. *Clinical Orthopaedic Rehabilitation.* St. Louis, Mosby, 1996.

Ceder L, Svensson K, Thorngren KG. Statistical prediction of rehabilitation in elderly patients with hip fractures. *Clin Orthop,* 152:185–90, 1980.

DeLisa J. *Rehabilitation Medicine: Principles and Practice.* Philadelphia: J.B. Lippincott, 1988.

Mehta Arun JMB, ed. Rehabilitation of fractures. *State of the Art Reviews in Physical Medicine and Rehabilitation,* Vol. 9, No. 3. Philadelphia: Hanley & Belfus, 1995.

CHAPTER *Six*

Gait

MARK A. THOMAS, MD

STANLEY HOPPENFELD, MD

VASANTHA L. MURTHY, MD

The purpose of the lower extremities is ambulation. After fracture of a lower extremity, this function is compromised. When the clinician evaluates the quality of ambulation, gait becomes a focus of concern. *Gait* is the manner in which a person ambulates. A careful assessment of gait identifies problems that result in inefficient or limited ambulation and allows for their treatment.

The goal of rehabilitation of lower extremity fractures is the restoration of normal gait to the preinjury level of function whenever possible. Therefore, it is essential for the practitioner to understand all aspects of normal gait.

THE GAIT CYCLE

The gait cycle describes the activity that occurs during ambulation. It is divided into two phases, the stance and the swing phase.

Stance Phase

The stance phase, representing 60% of the cycle (62%, to be exact), is divided into the following segments:

1. *Heel strike:* The heel of the foot touches the ground. At this point, the stance phase begins (Figure 6-1).

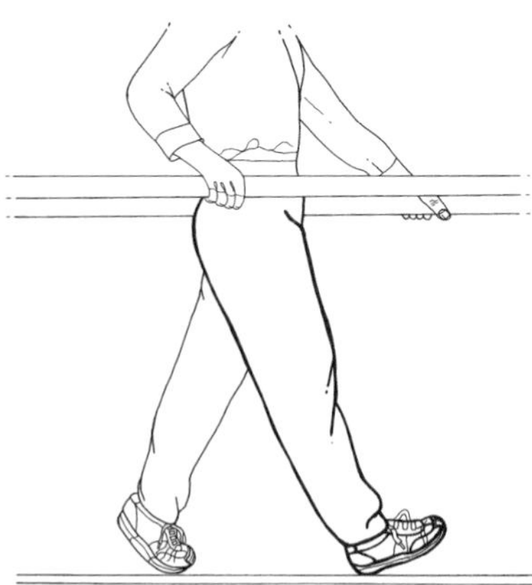

FIGURE 6-1 Heel strike: the heel of the foot touches the ground. At this point, the stance phase begins.

2. *Foot-flat:* As the body progresses forward, the midfoot and forefoot are lowered to the ground (Figure 6-2). Foot-flat occurs as the entire plantar surface of the foot comes into contact with the ground, but before the body's weight is directly over the foot.
3. *Mid-stance:* As the body continues to move anteriorly, the weight line passes directly over the foot at mid-stance (Figure 6-3).
   a. *Double stance:* Both feet are on the ground, weight bearing, approximately 20% of the time during double stance (*see* Figure 6-4).
4. *Push-off:* Push-off occurs as the weight-bearing limb is propelled forward and lifted off the ground. There are two components of push-off: (i) heel-off (the heel is lifted off the ground); and (ii) toe-off (after the heel is lifted, the toes are brought off the ground (Figures 6-4 and 6-5).

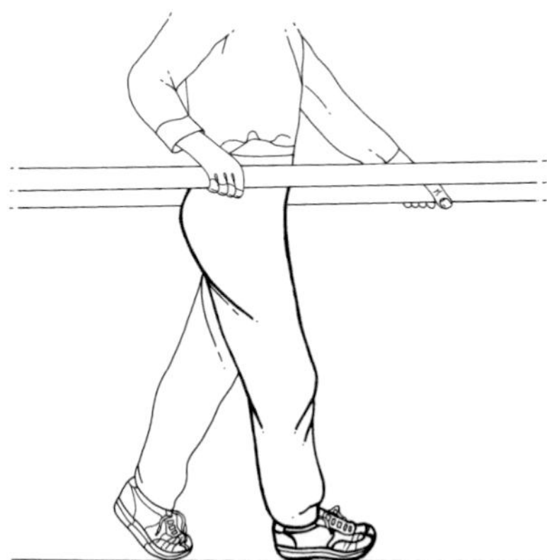

FIGURE 6-2 Foot-flat: the body progresses forward. The midfoot and forefoot are lowered to the ground. Foot-flat occurs as the entire plantar surface of the foot comes in contact with the ground, but before the body's weight is directly over the foot.

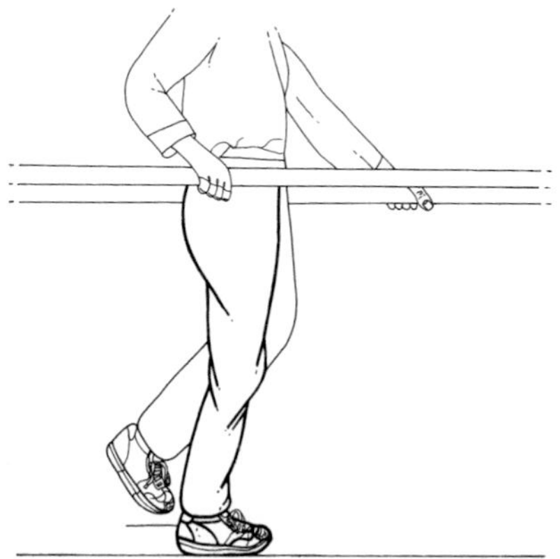

FIGURE 6-3 Mid-stance: as the body continues to move forward, the weight line passes directly over the foot at mid-stance.

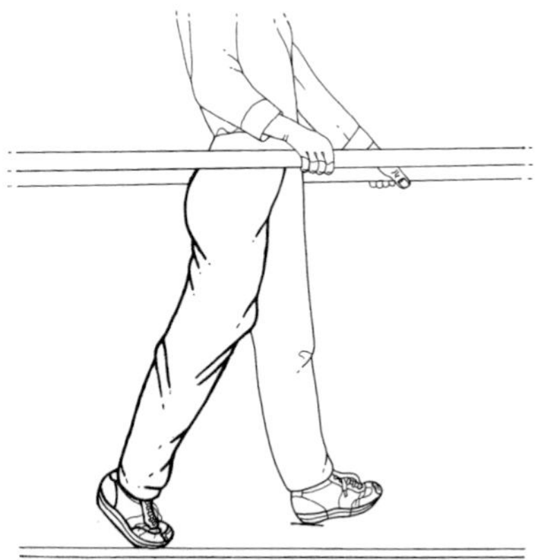

FIGURE 6-4 Push-off occurs as the body's weight is propelled forward and the limb is lifted off the ground. There are two components of push-off: (i) heel-off (the heel lifts off the ground), and (ii) toe-off.

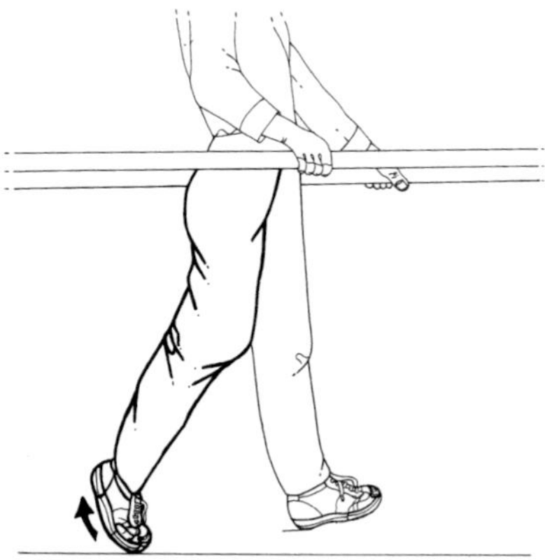

FIGURE 6-5 Toe-off. When the heel is lifted, the toes are brought off the ground.

Swing Phase

The swing phase, representing 40% of the cycle (38%, to be exact), is divided into the following segments:

1. *Acceleration:* Swing phase starts at the end of push-off when the toes lose contact with the ground. The first component of the swing phase is acceleration (Figure 6-6). During acceleration, the body is anterior to the limb. Gravity assists the extremity into a forward swing.
2. *Mid-swing:* At mid-swing, the limb is directly under the body and moving forward by momentum (Figure 6-7).

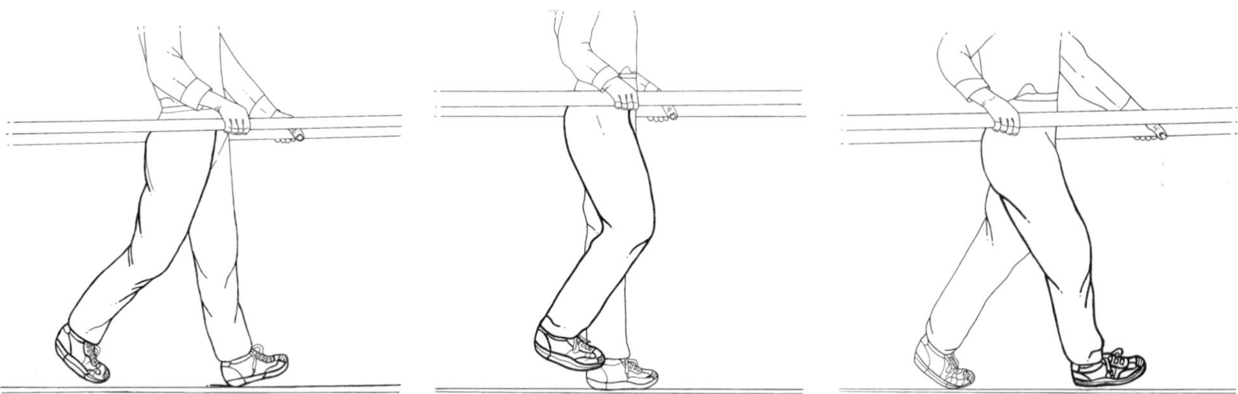

FIGURE 6-6 *(above, left)* Acceleration. Swing phase starts at the end of push-off as the toes lose contact with the ground. The first component of swing phase is acceleration. During acceleration, the body is anterior to the limb. Gravity assists the extremity in a forward swing.

FIGURE 6-7 *(above, middle)* Mid-swing. At mid-swing, the limb is directly under the body and moving forward by momentum.

FIGURE 6-8 *(above, right)* Deceleration. As the leg approaches the terminus of its arc of motion, deceleration of the limb prevents a terminal snap or heel thud and positions the extremity to accept weight as it approaches heel strike, thus completing the cycle.

3. *Deceleration:* As the leg approaches the terminus of its arc of motion, the deceleration of the distal limb prevents a terminal snap and positions the extremity to accept weight as it approaches heel-strike, thus completing the cycle (Figure 6-8 and Table 6-1).

TABLE 6-1 ***Components of the Gait Cycle***

Standard Classification	Alternate Classification[a]
Heel-strike	Initial contact
Foot-flat	Loading response
Mid-stance	Mid-stance
Heel-off	Terminal stance
Toe-off	Pre-swing
Acceleration	Initial swing
Mid-swing	Mid-swing
Deceleration	Terminal swing

[a]Perry J. *Gait Analysis: Normal and Pathological Function.* Thorofare, NJ: Slack, 1992.

Activity during the swing phase allows the limb to advance and clear the ground by limb shortening and lengthening. If normal flexion and pelvic movement do not allow this functional limb length change, compensatory mechanisms such as circumduction (abduction, flexion, then adduction of the leg while it advances), hip-hiking (lifting the hemipelvis so that the limb can clear the floor), or vaulting (raising the body over a plantar-flexed ankle) are brought into play.

Another classification of gait is sometimes used that offers the advantage of simultaneously describing bilateral lower extremity muscle functions and forces at different points in the gait cycle. Although this is extremely valuable, this book uses the more common nomenclature (*see* Table 6-1).

THE GAIT CYCLE IN FRACTURE REHABILITATION

The gait cycle is a blueprint for muscle activity during human walking. Clinically, we identify muscles that may affect the fracture, usually the muscles that cross the fracture site. Because the principal goal of rehabilitation after a fracture of the lower extremity is to restore normal ambulation, it is important to evaluate the patient's gait to identify the deficits that will require attention. Understanding the gait cycle facilitates the identification of gait abnormalities and treatment goals in the later stage of rehabilitation. The muscles that are the most active during each phase of the gait cycle are presented in Tables 6-2 and 6-3.

TABLE 6-2 ***Key Lower Extremity Muscle Activity during the Gait Cycle***

Phase	Muscle Contraction
Stance phase	
Heel strike	Hip: gluteus maximus Knee: quadriceps and hamstrings Ankle: tibialis anterior
Foot-flat	Hip: none Knee: quadriceps Ankle: tibialis anterior
Mid-stance	Hip: gluteus medius Knee: quadriceps Ankle: gastrocnemius-soleus
Heel-off	Hip: none Knee: quadriceps Ankle: gastrocnemius-soleus
Toe-off	Hip: none Knee: hamstrings Ankle: gastrocnemius-soleus
Swing phase	
Acceleration	Hip: iliopsoas Knee: quadriceps Ankle: tibialis anterior
Mid-swing	Hip: none Knee: quadriceps Ankle: tibialis anterior
Deceleration	Hip: gluteus maximus Knee: hamstrings Ankle: tibialis anterior

TABLE 6-3 *Concentric and Eccentric Activity during Normal Gait*

Phase	Eccentric Activity	Concentric Activity
Heel-strike to foot-flat	Tibialis anterior Quadriceps Gluteus maximus Hamstrings Extensor hallucis Extensor digitorum	
Foot-flat to mid-stance	Quadriceps	
Mid-stance to heel-off		Triceps surae
Heel-off to toe-off	Quadriceps Gluteus medius (contralateral)	Triceps surae Tibialis anterior Peroneus longus Flexor digitorum Flexor hallucis
Toe-off to acceleration	Gluteus medius (contralateral)	Triceps surae Tibialis anterior Hamstrings
Acceleration to mid-swing	Gluteus medius (contralateral)	Quadriceps Iliopsoas Tibialis anterior
Mid-swing through deceleration	Hamstrings Gluteus medius (contralateral)	Tibialis anterior

Many of the lower extremity muscles act in both concentric and eccentric fashion (*see* Table 6-3 and Chapter 4). Understanding of when and how muscles contract during normal gait helps us in writing a prescription to minimize gait deficits and restore a normal gait pattern. Table 6-2 summarizes the muscle activity frequently considered during gait retraining after fracture.

Most of the muscles involved are active at the beginning and the end of the stance and swing phases. During mid-stance and mid-swing, there is minimal muscle activity, although maximal weight bearing occurs at mid-stance. Also, muscles frequently contract in an eccentric rather than a concentric manner (*see* Table 6-3). This may be significant if the torque produced at a fracture site by an eccentric contraction is greater than that produced by a concentric contraction, as has been demonstrated for muscle contraction in uninjured people.

Parameters of Gait

The following parameters of gait—step angle, step width, step length, stride length, cadence, and speed (Table 6-4)—are the elements of static and dynamic function that are assessed during a quick check on the status of an ambulating person.

TABLE 6-4 *Gait Parameters*

Parameter	Normal Value
Step angle	6–7 degrees external rotation
Step width	3–4 in.
Step length	15–20 in.
Stride length	30–40 in.
Cadence	120 steps/min
Speed	2.5–3 miles/hr

Step Angle

The normal step angle is 0 to 7 degrees measured from the sagittal plane. Initially, the step angle is reduced after a lower extremity fracture to control torque at the fracture site. This is particularly important after hip fracture.

Step Width

Step width, or the distance between the medial borders of the feet, is normally 2 to 4 inches. It is widened until the late stage of rehabilitation to increase the base of support and stability after fracture (Figure 6-9).

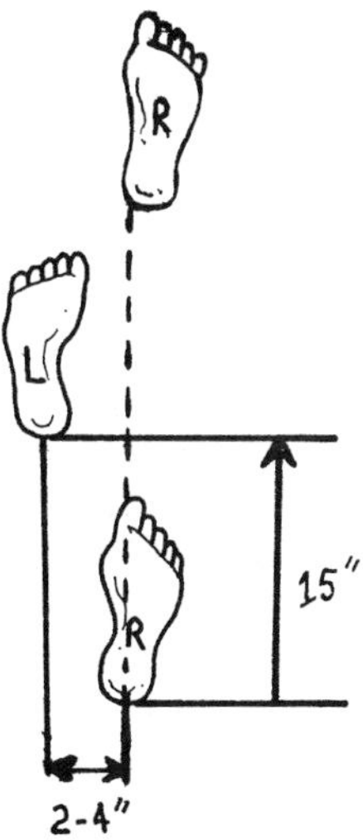

FIGURE 6-9 Step width (normal: 2 to 4 inches), or the distance between the medial borders of the feet, is widened until the late stage of rehabilitation to increase the base of support and stability following fracture. Step length (normal: 15 to 20 inches) is the distance measured from the heel strike of one foot to the heel strike of the other foot. Stride length is the distance measured from heel strike to heel strike of the same foot.

Step Length

Step length, normally approximately 15 to 20 inches, is the distance measured from the heel strike of one foot to the heel strike of the other foot (*see* Figure 6-9). After fracture, the step length shortens; this may be associated with a tentative, fearful gait or an antalgic gait. Step length is initially longer for the fractured limb and shorter for the uninvolved limb.

Stride Length

Stride length is the distance measured from heel strike to heel strike of the same foot. Two steps are equal to one stride (*see* Figure 6-9).

Cadence

Cadence, the rate of walking, is approximately 120 steps/minute. This decreases as a result of pain, fear of falling, or a sense of instability, which are commonly present in the early and intermediate stages of rehabilitation.

Speed

Normal walking speed is approximately 2.5 miles/hour. Speed slows with either reduced cadence or a decrease in the step or stride length.

Changes in the parameters of gait (step length, stride length, step width, cadence, speed, and step angle) are common because of the patient's fear of instability, refracture, or disturbance of the fracture site. After fracture, the normal functional change in lower extremity length is occasionally disrupted, leading to an unsightly gait that is inefficient and wastes energy. The parameters of gait must be normalized to restore cosmetic, energy-efficient, and safe ambulation.

The Determinants of Gait

The determinants of gait are the movements that improve efficiency, minimize the energy expended in walking, and provide a smooth gait by minimizing the excursion of the person's center of gravity in the sagittal and coronal planes. The determinants of gait include pelvic tilt, shift, and rotation; hip–knee–ankle movement; knee flexion in stance; and ankle movement. These movements can all be thought of as increasing or decreasing the functional length of a lower extremity, thereby reducing the amplitude of lateral and vertical (up-and-down motion) while walking.

These determinants fine-tune gait and in general are not perceived as major factors in gait retraining because the patient usually compensates for them. If there is severe leg length discrepancy and severe loss of range of motion, and the patient is unable to compensate, then these determinants must be addressed.

Pelvic Tilt

During gait, the limb is functionally lengthened or shortened by anterior or posterior pelvic tilt. In fractures of the lower lumbar spine, tilt is reduced because of pain and stiffness.

Pelvic Shift

Lateral movement of the pelvis over the leg in stance serves functionally to lengthen the extremity and shift the center of gravity closer to the long axis of the limb. This both decreases the vertical amplitude of movement and provides a mechanical advantage to the gluteus medius to prevent dropping the contralateral hemipelvis in swing. Hip fractures and hip surgery impair the normal mechanics of pelvic shift, particularly when the gluteus medius is compromised. Because of pain, the patient is unable to shift the pelvis laterally.

Pelvic Rotation

The pelvis rotates medially (anteriorly) as the swing phase ends and stance begins, lengthening the limb as it prepares to accept weight. The opposite rotation (lateral or posterior) occurs as the leg leaves the stance phase, with functional shortening by lateral rotation decreasing the height needed to clear the swing-phase limb. Fractures of the hip or lumbar spine impair or prevent normal pelvic rotation during gait.

Hip–Knee–Ankle Movement

Flexion at the hip and knee and dorsiflexion of the ankle serve functionally to shorten a limb, whereas extension or plantar flexion at the joints makes the leg functionally longer. The net effect of this is to decrease vertical movement and concomitant energy cost while walking. Fractures of the femur or tibia disrupt the normal mechanics of hip–knee–ankle movement during walking. Hip, knee, or ankle fractures may prevent limb shortening during swing because of reduced motion and or pain.

Knee Flexion in Stance

This limits the maximum height a person achieves during gait, which reduces the up–down amplitude of movement, as illustrated by the ability to walk fully erect through a tunnel slightly too low to allow standing fully erect. Knee flexion in stance is abnormal with patellar or intraarticular knee fractures, leading to a reduced vertical amplitude or up-and-down movement.

Ankle Movement

Ankle and subtalar motion reduces energy cost by reducing the amplitude of movement and smoothing the translation of movement. Ankle and foot fractures prevent normal ankle motion during gait. This may persist once a fracture has healed because of muscle or other soft tissue contracture.

Arm swing, rotation of the femur and tibia, and trunk bending may also be considered determinants of gait because they serve to smooth transitions in direction of motion, further conserving both momentum and energy.

An analysis of the determinants of gait becomes important in the late stage of rehabilitation after fracture, when more subtle deviations in the gait are identified so that normal ambulation may be restored as fully as possible. When actual shortening due to bone loss or functional shortening due to muscle shortening (e.g., inability fully to extend the hip or knee) occurs after a fracture, the determinants of gait are affected and must be corrected to restore normal ambulation.

Gait Deviations

Pathologic changes in gait after a lower extremity fracture occur as a consequence of shortening, weakness, pain, anxiety, or fear. A decrease in efficiency with reduced speed, increased energy cost, and loss of the normal cosmesis of gait result regardless of the specific abnormality.

If weakness or shortening persist, the initial pathologic gait changes as the body attempts to compensate for the problem. Although the gait remains abnormal in such an instance, the extra energy expended in ambulation is reduced. Once a fractured limb is fully weight bearing, the most common gait deviations are due to pain, weakness, or inefficiency of muscle contraction due to injury and pain, plantar flexion contracture, and lack of patient confidence.

Antalgic Gait

This painful gait is an attempt to avoid bearing weight on the fractured lower extremity. In an antalgic gait, there is prolonged stance on the unaffected lower extremity, reduced step length on the unaffected side, and a prolonged period of double support; the goal is to minimize the time spent on the fractured limb. This may result from pain or anxiety and almost invariably follows any fracture of the lower extremity.

Short-Step Gait

Step length is reduced after any fracture of the lower extremity. This may be due to pain, anxiety, weakness or poor endurance.

Short-Leg Gait

If shortening has occurred after a lower extremity fracture, the patient attempts to limit the vertical excursion during gait. The opposite "long" leg may be "shortened" by abducting the leg, flexing the hip and knee more than usual (steppage gait), circumducting the leg, or raising the hemipelvis (hip-hiking).

Vaulting Gait

The patient may plantar flex the short limb, thus "lengthening" it by remaining on tiptoe. The patient jumps or vaults over the shortened limb, and this is called a vaulting gait.

Gluteus Maximus Lurch

In the case of gluteus maximus weakness, such as may follow a subtrochanteric fracture, the patient may experience difficulty preventing flexion of the trunk at heel strike (salutation gait). This is the uncompensated gluteus maximus lurch. If gluteal weakness persists, the patient may use trunk extension before heel strike to maintain balance (compensated gluteal lurch; Figure 6-10).

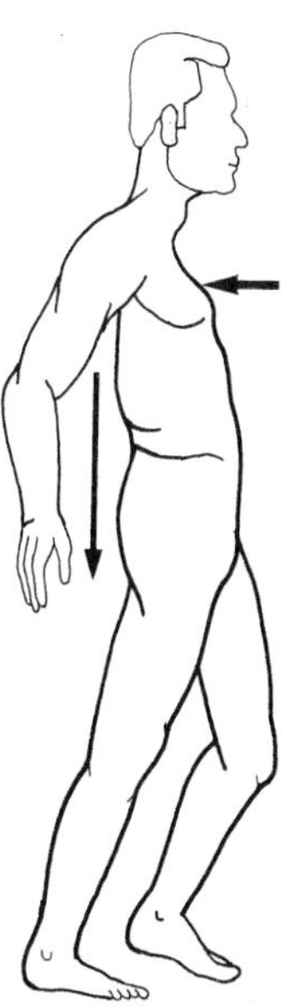

FIGURE 6-10 Gluteus maximus lurch. A patient with a weak gluteus maximus muscle may experience difficulty in preventing flexion of the trunk at heel strike and may use trunk extension (gluteus maximus lurch) just before heel strike to maintain balance.

Gluteus Medius Lurch

After a trochanteric fracture, the gluteus medius is initially ineffective in preventing the drop of the contralateral hemipelvis during the swing phase. This is the gluteus medius lurch, or uncompensated Trendelenburg gait. If this lurch persists, a patient begins to shift weight over the fractured leg to shift the center of gravity over the supporting limb. This throwing of the trunk to the side of the impaired gluteus medius (lateral list) is the compensated Trendelenburg gait (Figure 6-11).

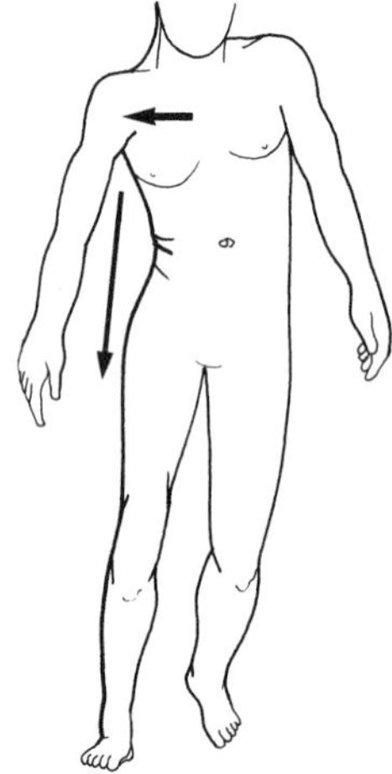

FIGURE 6-11 Gluteus medius lurch. A weak gluteus medius is ineffective in preventing the drop of the opposite hemipelvis during swing phase. To compensate, the patient shifts weight over the weak side to shift the center of gravity over the supporting limb. This throwing of the trunk to the side of the impaired gluteus medius is gluteus medius lurch.

Quadriceps Weakness

When there is weakness or inhibition of the quadriceps, such as after a patellar or distal femoral fracture, one of three basic compensations arise to prevent buckling at the knee. The limb may be externally rotated, to position the joint axis incongruent with the line of progression, thus preventing buckling. Alternatively, with a mild degree of weakness, hyperextension of the knee after heel strike prevents buckling; this is called *genu recurvatum*. Less frequently, the patient may manually assist the quadriceps by pushing backward on the thigh with the hands.

Steppage and Circumducted or Abducted Gait

This type of gait may result from peroneal nerve injury, from direct trauma, or from compartment syndrome after either soft tissue trauma or bleeding after a tibial fracture. To clear the foot during the swing phase, the patient may excessively flex the hip and knee to gain additional height (Figure 6-12).

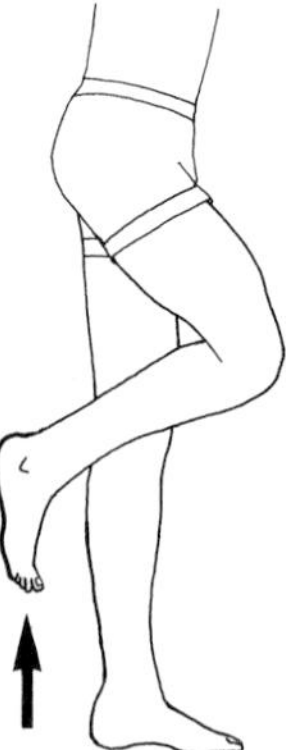

FIGURE 6-12 Steppage gait may occur from nerve or soft tissue trauma that leaves the patient unable to dorsiflex the foot in the swing phase. To clear the foot during swing phase, the patient may excessively flex the hip and knee to gain additional height.

Alternatively, the patient may exaggerate abduction or circumduction of the fractured limb during the swing phase.

Quick Heel Rise

If shortening of the triceps surae has occurred, such as with an os calcis fracture, loss of dorsiflexion results in rapid heel rise. This manifests itself during the stance phase with early heel-off and a longer period of stance taking place on the forefoot.

Gait Considerations with Lower Extremity Fracture

Weight-bearing status is defined as follows:

1. Non-weight bearing
2. Toe-touch weight bearing
3. Partial weight bearing; the degree of weight bearing is determined by the physician depending on the probable stability of the fracture at any given point
4. Weight bearing as tolerated
5. Full weight bearing

Gait Patterns after Fracture

Common gait patterns after fracture can be classified by the type of step taken (step-to, step-through), or by the number of contact points used to take a step (two-, three-, or four-point gait). Because weight bearing on the affected extremity is restricted, the patient may use various gait patterns with crutches or other assistive devices.

Step-to Gait

In the step-to gait, the fractured limb is advanced, and then the intact limb brought to the same position. When weight-bearing status is restricted to partial, toe-touch, or as tolerated, crutches or a walker are necessary and help the patient step to the fractured limb by pushing down with the upper extremities, thus transferring weight from the fractured limb to the assistive device.

Example: Partial weight bearing or toe-touch weight bearing after a tibial shaft fracture, using a two-point gait. In this case, the partially weight-bearing limb and crutches are advanced, and then the intact limb is advanced to the same position.

Step-through Gait

In the step-through gait, the intact leg is advanced, and then the fractured leg is advanced past it. With restricted weight bearing, crutches are used instead of the injured limb, and the patient steps past the crutches with the weight-bearing lower extremity; the gait assumes a two-point or three-point pattern.

Example: Oblique midshaft tibial fracture that is non-weight bearing; the intact leg is advanced past the crutches and then the fractured leg and crutches are advanced past the intact limb (Figures 6-13, 6-14, and 6-15).

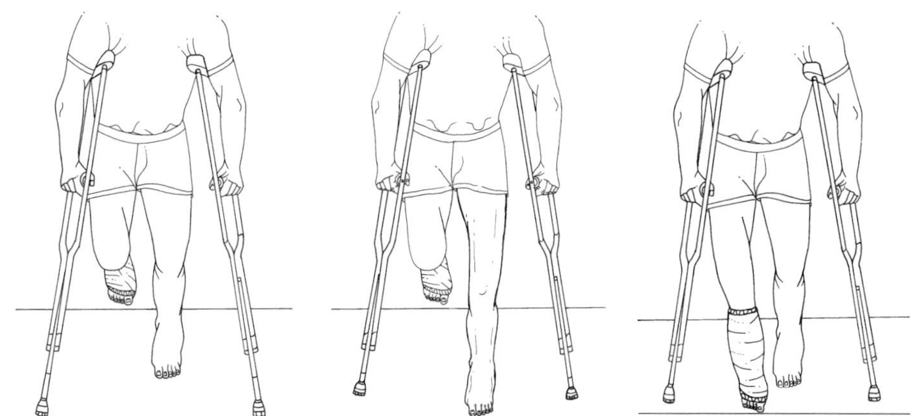

FIGURE 6-13 *(above, left)* Step-through gait starting position. With restricted weight bearing, crutches are used instead of the injured limb.

FIGURE 6-14 *(above, middle)* Step-through gait: the intact leg is advanced past the crutches.

FIGURE 6-15 *(above, right)* Step-through gait: the fractured leg and crutches are then advanced past the unaffected limb.

Gaits Used on Level Surfaces

Two-Point Gait

In a two-point gait (sometimes called hop-to gait), the crutches and the fractured leg are one point and the uninvolved leg is the other point. The crutches and fractured limb are advanced as one unit, and the uninvolved weight-bearing limb is brought forward to the crutches as the second unit (Figure 6-16).

Example: A non–weight-bearing fracture of the femur used in a step-to gait pattern where the crutches are brought forward with the fractured limb and the intact limb steps up to the crutches.

Three-Point Gait

In a three-point gait, the crutches serve as one point, the involved leg as the second point, and the uninvolved leg as the third point. Each crutch and the weight-bearing limb are advanced separately, with two of the three points maintaining contact with the floor at any given time (Figure 6-17).

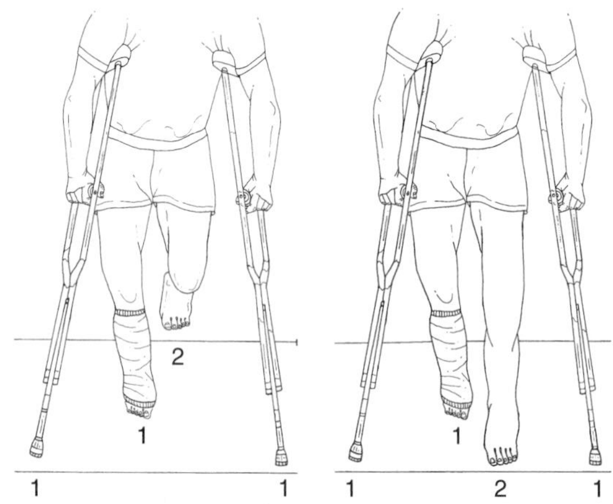

FIGURE 6-16 *(above, left)* Two-point gait (hop-to gait). *(above, right)* The crutches and fractured leg are one point and the uninvolved leg is the other point. The crutches and fractured limb are advanced as one unit and the uninvolved weight-bearing limb is brought forward to the crutches as the second unit.

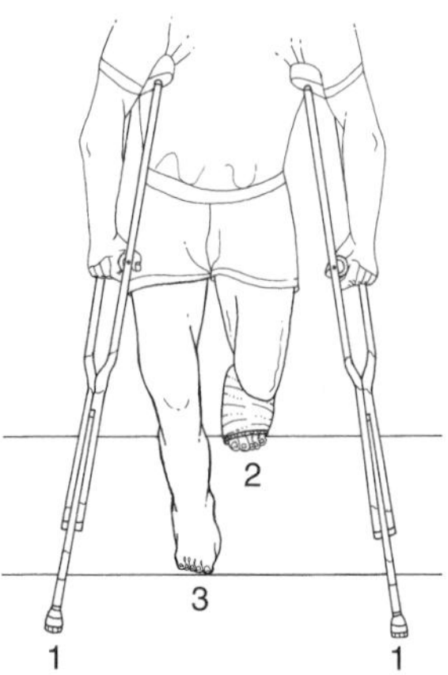

FIGURE 6-17 Three-point gait. The crutches serve as one point, the involved leg as the second point, and the uninvolved leg as the third point. Each crutch and weight-bearing limb is advanced separately, with two of the three points maintaining contact with the floor at any given time.

Example: A partially weight-bearing femoral neck fracture. In this instance, the crutches are advanced, the fractured limb is advanced next, and finally the intact limb is brought forward.

Four-Point Gait

In a four-point gait, point one is the crutch on the involved side, point two is the uninvolved leg, point three is the involved leg, and point four is the crutch on the uninvolved side (Figures 6-18 and 6-19). The crutches and limbs are advanced separately, with three of the four points on the ground and bearing weight any given time.

Example: A partially weight-bearing fracture with a secondary problem such as weakness, poor motor control, or anxiety. This type of gait is not efficient, but it does enhance stability or balance and may provide reassurance to an elderly patient experiencing significant fear or anxiety.

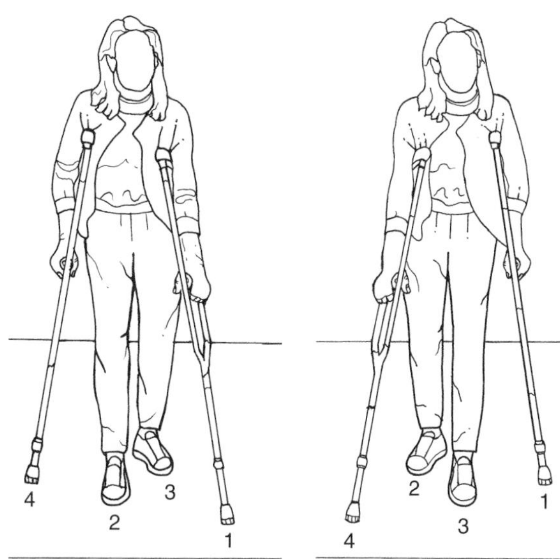

FIGURE 6-18 *(above, left)* Four-point gait. Point one is the crutch on the involved side, point two is the uninvolved leg, point three is the involved leg, and point four is the crutch on the uninvolved side.

FIGURE 6-19 *(above, right)* Four-point gait. The crutches and limbs are advanced separately, with three of the four points on the ground and bearing weight at any given time.

Gait Used on Uneven Surfaces

Patients with lower extremity fractures must also be taught how to negotiate uneven surfaces such as stairs and curbs. To reduce or eliminate weight bearing on the fractured extremity, the patient climbs stairs by ascending with the unaffected limb first and bringing the fractured limb up to meet it, either simultaneously with the crutches or by keeping the crutches on the step below until both feet are on the step above. The crutches are then brought up to the step (Figures 6-20, 6-21, and 6-22). The patient

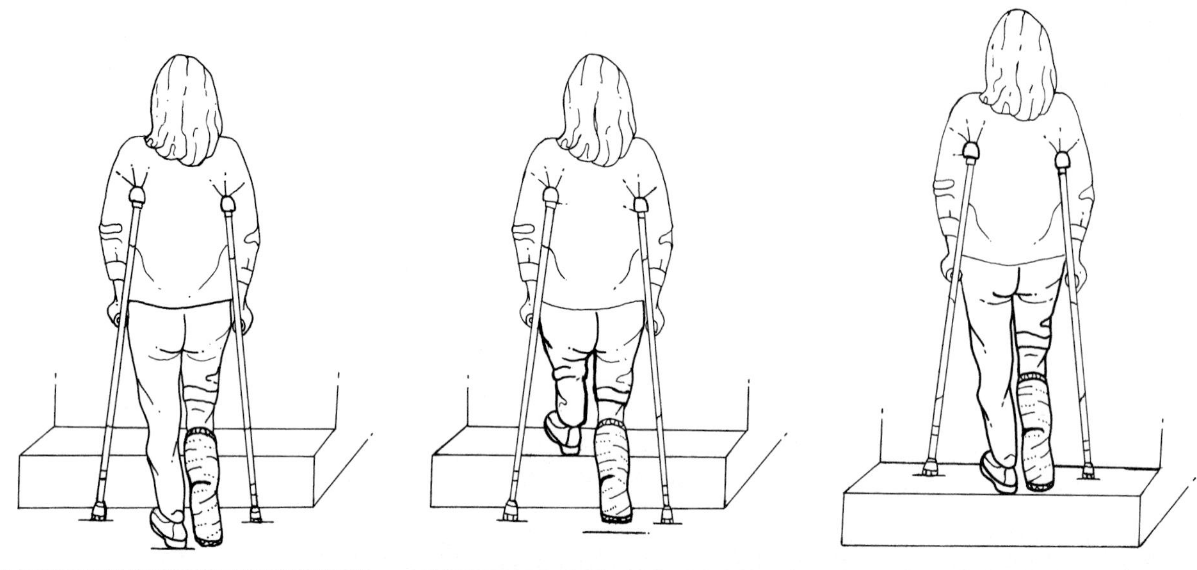

FIGURE 6-20 *(above, left)* Patients with lower extremity fractures must be taught how to negotiate uneven surfaces such as stairs and curbs.

FIGURE 6-21 *(above, middle)* To reduce or eliminate weight bearing on the fractured extremity, the patient climbs stairs by ascending with the unaffected limb first.

FIGURE 6-22 *(above, right)* After ascending with the unaffected limb first, the patient brings the fractured limb up to meet it, either simultaneously with the crutches or keeping the crutches on the step below until both feet are on the step above. The crutches are then brought up to the step.

descends stairs with the fractured limb first, bringing the unaffected limb down to meet it. The crutches are placed on the step below, and then the fractured limb is brought down a step and the unaffected limb is brought last (Figures 6-23, 6-24, and 6-25). An easy way to remember this approach is "the good go up to heaven and the bad go down to hell."

If a banister is present and the patient is non-weight bearing, the patient uses one or two crutches together on the uninvolved side and holds the banis-

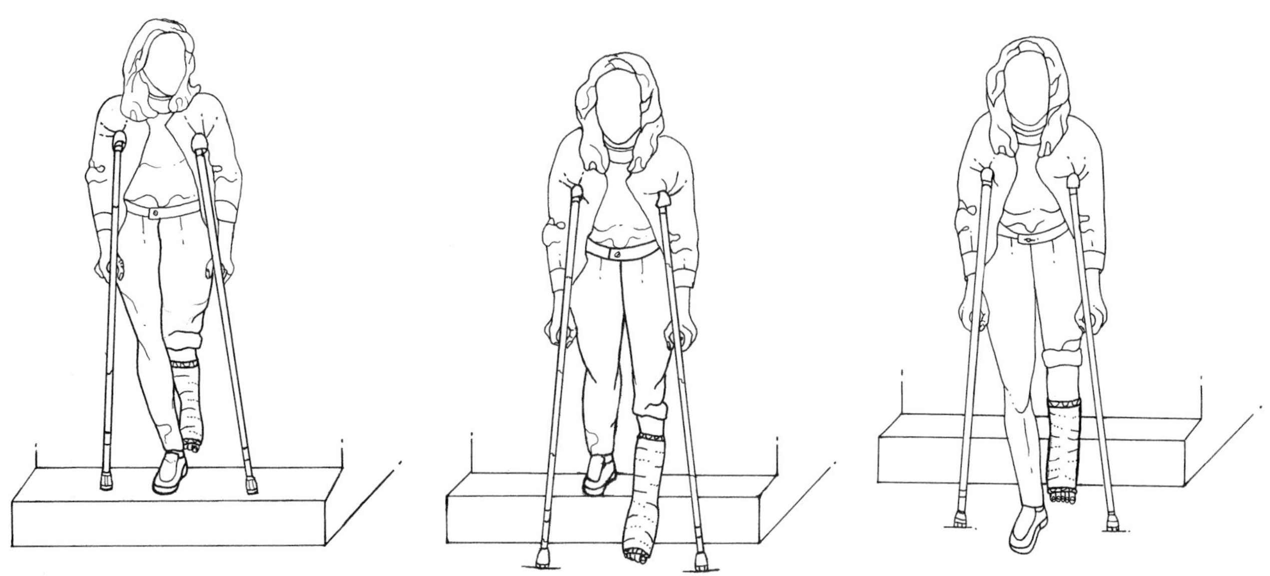

FIGURE 6-23 *(above, left)* The patient descends stairs with the fractured limb first, bringing the unaffected limb down to meet it.

FIGURE 6-24 *(above, middle)* The crutches are placed on the step below and then the fractured limb is brought down a step.

FIGURE 6-25 *(above, right)* The unaffected limb is brought down last.

ter with the hand on the same side as the fracture. The uninvolved extremity is placed on the step above, and while the patient pulls up on the banister, the fractured limb and crutches are advanced and brought up a step (Figures 6-26, 6-27, and 6-28). To descend stairs, the patient holds the banister with the hand on the same side as the fracture, and the fractured limb is placed on the step below concomitant with the crutches. The uninvolved extremity is then brought down to the step (Figures 6-29, 6-30, and 6-31). In

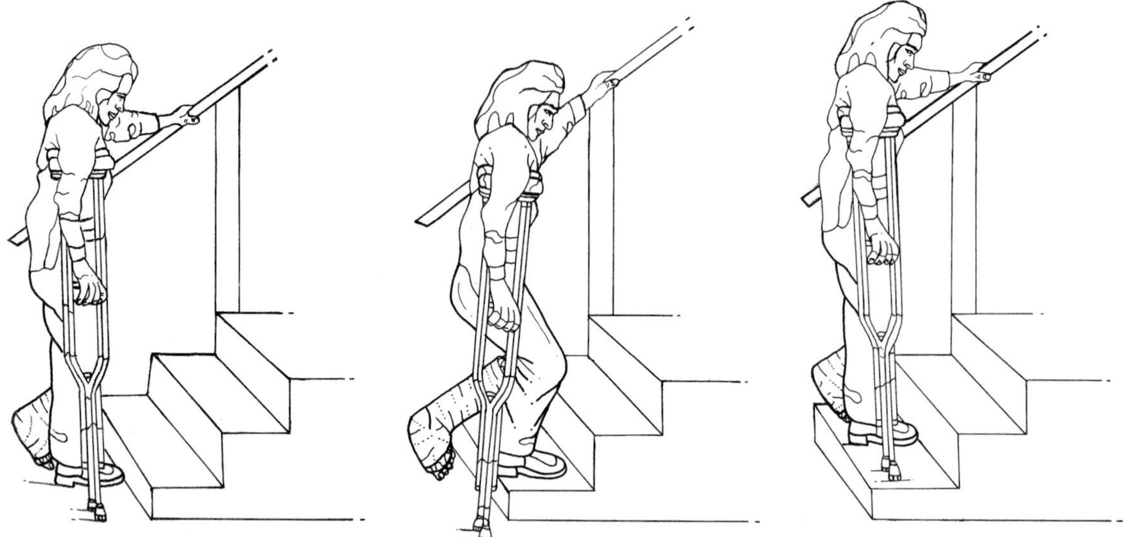

FIGURE 6-26 *(above, left)* Walking up stairs with a banister: If a banister is present and a patient is non-weight bearing, the patient uses one or two crutches together on the uninvolved side and holds the banister with the hand on the same side as the fracture.

FIGURE 6-27 *(above, middle)* The uninvolved extremity is placed on the step above while the patient pulls the body up using the banister.

FIGURE 6-28 *(above, right)* The fractured limb and crutches are then advanced and brought up a step.

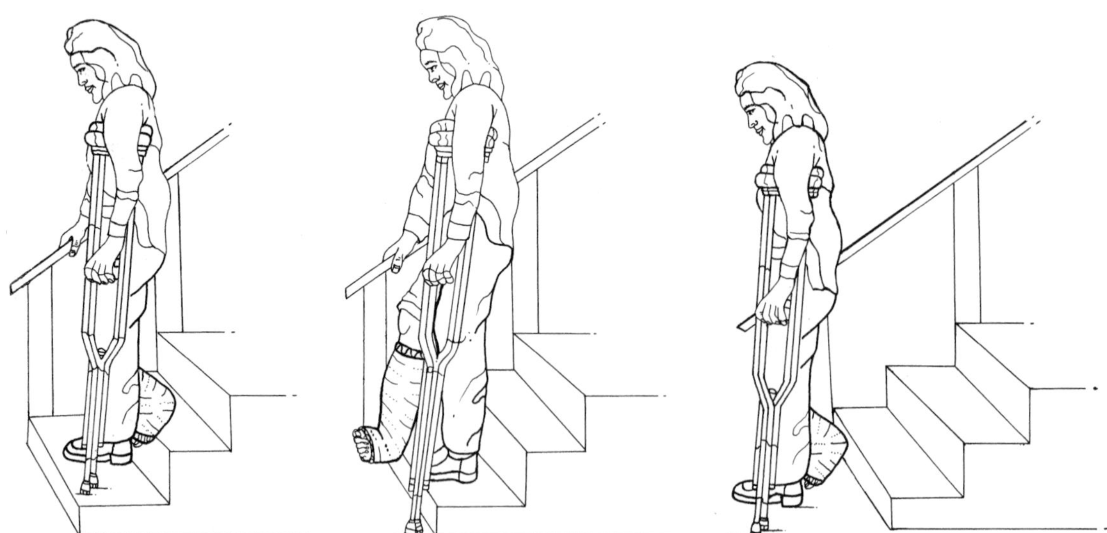

FIGURE 6-29 *(above, left)* Descending stairs using a banister. To descend stairs, the patient holds the banister with the hand on the same side as the fracture and uses one or two crutches together on the uninvolved side.

FIGURE 6-30 *(above, middle)* The crutches and the fractured limb are placed simultaneously on the step below.

FIGURE 6-31 *(above, right)* The uninvolved extremity is brought down to the step.

general, patients with good balance and coordination prefer using two crutches.

Transfers

The patient's weight-bearing status also affects transfers, or changes in position or location. Transfer techniques include stand-pivot, ambulatory, and seated transfers.

Stand-Pivot Transfers

A pivot transfer is designed to keep the fractured limb non-weight bearing to avoid transmitting a large amount of torque to the fracture site. The patient stands on the uninvolved lower extremity and pivots with the use of an assistive device (crutches or a walker) without bearing weight on the fractured limb.

Ambulatory Transfers

During ambulatory transfers, the patient is fully weight bearing on the uninvolved extremity and toe-touch or partially weight bearing on the fractured extremity. The patient does not pivot during transfer, but does require the use of an assistive device to bear partial weight on a fractured limb.

Seated Transfers

Seated transfers do not require lower extremity weight bearing. They are used when neither lower extremity is fully weight bearing. This occurs with bilateral lower extremity fractures or pelvic fractures after multiple trauma. To perform a seated transfer, the patient supports his or her body weight with the upper extremities, while sliding the buttocks from one surface (e.g., a bed) to another (e.g., a wheelchair).

BIBLIOGRAPHY

Borkan JM, Quirk M, Sullivan M. Finding meaning after the fall injury: injury narratives from elderly hip fracture patients. *Soc Sci Med*, 33:947–957, 1991.

Borquist L, Lindelow G, Thorngren KG. Costs of hip fracture: rehabilitation of 180 patients in primary health care. *Acta Orthop Scand*, 62:39–48, 1991.

Braddom R. *Physical Medicine and Rehabilitation*. Philadelphia: W.B. Saunders, 1996.

Brotzman SB, ed. *Clinical Orthopaedic Rehabilitation*. St. Louis: Mosby, 1996.

Ceder L, Svensson K, Thorngren KG. Statistical prediction of rehabilitation in elderly patients with hip fractures. *Clin Orthop*, 152:185–190, 1980.

Hoppenfeld S. *Physical Examination of the Spine and Extremities*. Norwalk, CT: Appleton-Century-Crofts, 1976.

Inman VT, Ralston TR, Todd F. *Human Walking*. Baltimore: Williams & Wilkins, 1981.

Mehta Arun JMB, ed. Rehabilitation of fractures. *State of the Art Reviews in Physical Medicine and Rehabilitation*, Vol. 9, No. 3. Philadelphia: Hanley & Belfus, 1995.

Norkin C, Levangie P. *Joint Structure and Function*, 2nd ed. Philadelphia: F.A. Davis, 1992.

Perry J. *Gait Analysis: Normal and Pathological Function*. Thorofare, NJ: Slack, 1992.

CHAPTER *Seven*

Assistive Devices and Adaptive Equipment for Activities of Daily Living (ADL)

MARK A. THOMAS, MD

CONTRIBUTIONS BY VASANTHA L. MURTHY

INTRODUCTION

Basic activities of daily living (ADL) include the fundamental tasks required for independent living such as dressing, bathing, grooming, toileting, and ambulating. An upper extremity fracture, particularly of the dominant side, significantly disrupts a patient's ability to perform basic ADL. Usually, patients quickly adapt by using the uninvolved upper extremity for most non–weight-bearing ADL, although they may still need to use assistive devices. Activities such as moving in bed or pushing up from a chair may also be problematic. Fracture of the lower extremity not only impairs normal ADL (e.g., dressing the lower extremities), but disrupts normal ambulation.

Instrumental ADL go beyond these fundamental tasks to include such things as using a telephone, shopping, and banking. Because the disability after a fracture is temporary, instrumental ADL usually are not addressed as part of postfracture rehabilitation.

In general, the goal of rehabilitation after an upper extremity fracture is the restitution of independent function, beginning with basic ADL. In the early phases of rehabilitation, enhancing the residual function of a fractured limb may require an assistive device. For the upper extremities, these devices aid in manipulative tasks, compensating for decreased range of motion and extent of reach. For the lower extremities, assistive devices include those used for ambulation as well as equipment that reduces the need for muscular activity or joint movement.

ASSISTIVE DEVICES FOR ACTIVITIES OF DAILY LIVING

Devices to Extend Reach

These devices extend reach without requiring the patient to bend, ambulate, or rise from sitting, and thus avoid or reduce stress across the fracture site. They are most commonly used by the uninjured upper extremity in the case of an upper extremity, spinal, or lower extremity fracture. A long-handled shoe horn, reacher or grabber, or long-handled bath sponge limits or avoids the need for arm/hand or trunk motion, eliminating torque at the fracture site (Figures 7-1 and 7-2).

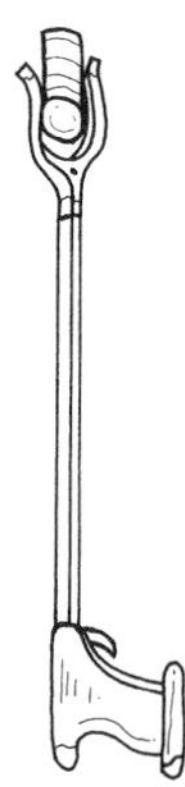

FIGURE 7-1 Long-handled grabber is used to extend the patient's reach.

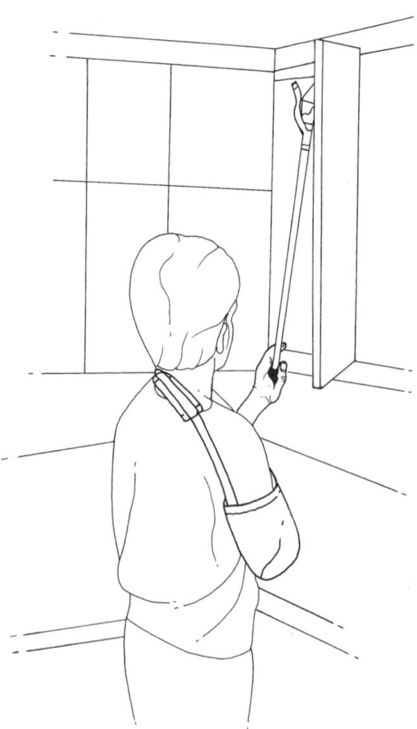

FIGURE 7-2 Reacher or grabber. The patient is able to extend the reach, particularly into cabinets.

Devices to Provide Grasp

Devices such as a reacher, grabber, or sock aid not only extend reach, but provide a limited ability to grasp (Figure 7-3). This is particularly important in lower extremity fractures when both extended reach and extended grasp are required, as in picking up a piece of clothing from the floor. These devices serve to reduce but not eliminate force across the fracture site in many ADL.

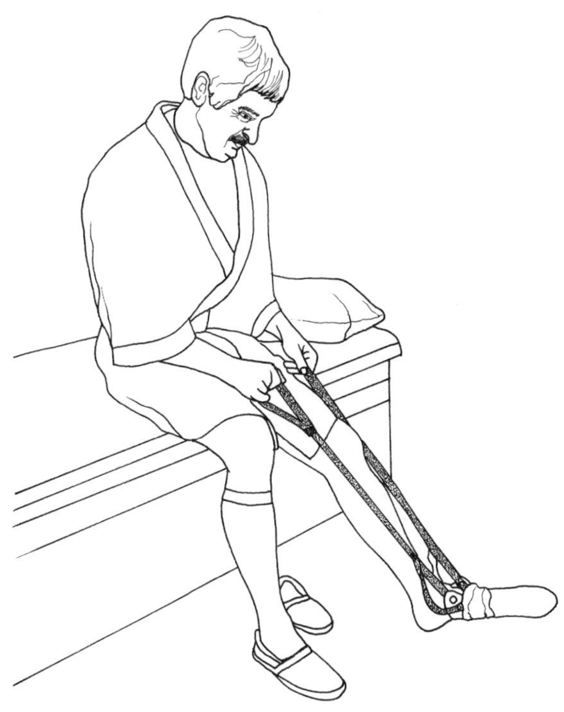

FIGURE 7-3 Sock aid helps the patient put on socks without bending the hip or knee joint. It extends reach to prevent stress on the joints and across the fracture site.

Devices to Reduce Torque or Force

Raised toilet seats, adjustable-height beds, firm seat cushions, chair arms, and built-up handles for door-knobs, utensils, or other tools may reduce torque by limiting the movement necessary to perform certain activities, thus reducing stress on the fracture site (Figure 7-4). For example, a raised toilet seat or adjustable-height bed or chair is useful for fractures of

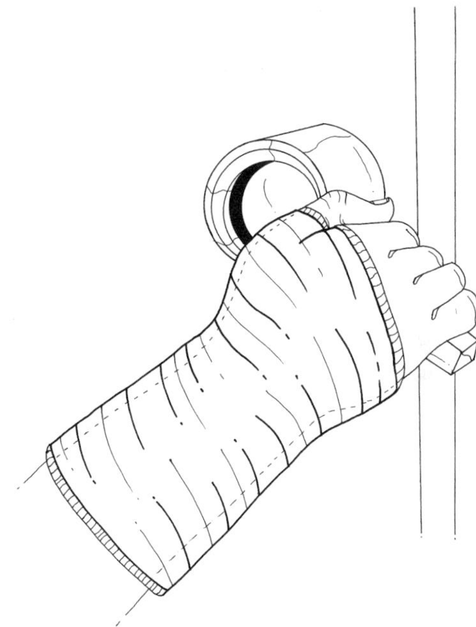

FIGURE 7-4 Built-up handle for door knobs reduces torque and stress of the fracture site, as in a Colles' fracture or both-bones forearm fracture.

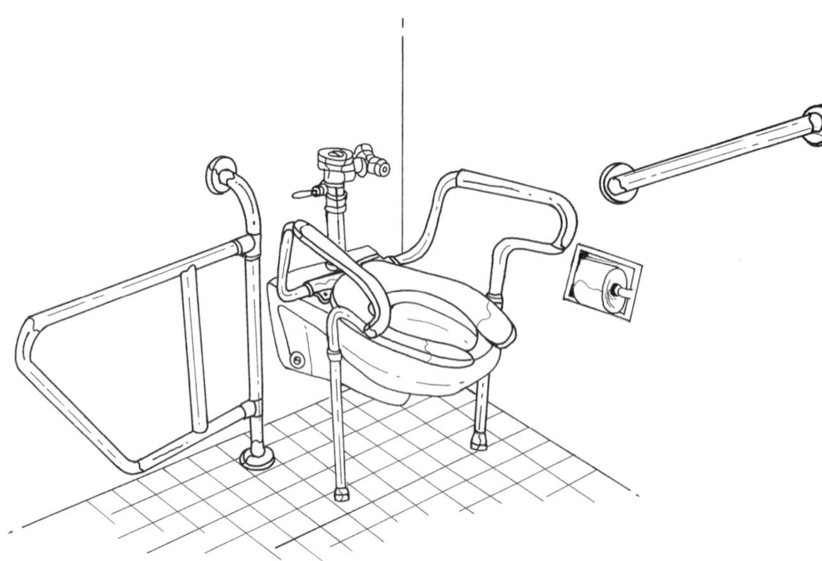

FIGURE 7-5 Raised toilet seats reduce the hip/trunk flexion necessary for sitting or standing. This reduces the force generated by the gluteus maximus muscle, which is most critical in hip and lumbar spine fractures. Grab bars are helpful to improve balance and safety when going from a sitting to an erect position in the bathroom.

the hip or lumbar spine (Figure 7-5). These devices reduce the necessary hip/trunk flexion for sitting down or standing, and this reduces the force generated by the gluteus maximus (the hip extensor), which is used both to sit and stand.

Building up the handles for various tools, utensils, grooming aids, or doorknobs decreases torque and general movement in the forearm, wrist, and digits and provides a mechanical advantage, resulting in less force across a distal upper extremity fracture.

A firm seat is helpful in cases of lower extremity or spinal fracture. A too-soft seat cushion requires greater hip flexion to sit on because the body sinks into the surface, and more hip extensor force to get up. Chair arms allow a patient to use upper extremity strength to reduce the force generated by the hip extensors across a proximal lower extremity fracture.

A hand-held shower may be useful if turning around or raising the arms produces stress at the fracture site.

Devices to Improve Safety

Grab bars, nonskid floor or tub surfaces, walkers (see later), and appropriate lighting improve balance and safety, thus reducing the risk of slipping or falling, which can potentially disrupt a healing fracture or result in a new injury (*see* Figure 7-5). After lower extremity fractures, stall showers are recommended over bathtubs because less torque is produced in the lower extremities when entering or exiting. A shower or tub chair may be useful for patients who are deconditioned or are partially or non-weight bearing on a lower extremity (Figure 7-6).

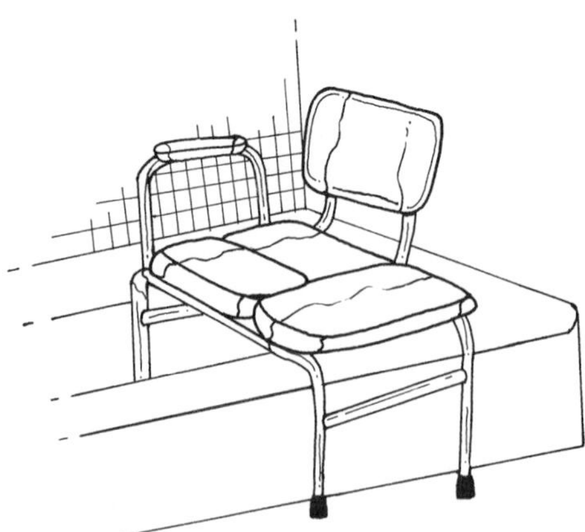

FIGURE 7-6 Tub chair. This is most helpful for patients who are non-weight bearing or deconditioned. The patient can slide into the chair and take a shower without having to bear weight.

Other Devices

Activities of daily living may also be facilitated by a variety of task-specific assistive devices. For example, a plate with a brim, a rocker knife, or another type of adapted utensil may allow a person with a fractured upper extremity to grasp a plate, cut food, and feed independently. A leg lifter, a shaft that ends in a loop, may allow a patient to dress independently when spinal movement is restricted or there is notable leg weakness after fracture. Many assistive devices designed for specific uses are commercially available, and it is often helpful to keep a catalog in the office as a resource for specific patients with unique or unusual needs.

AMBULATION ASSISTIVE DEVICES

Devices that assist ambulation are often required to eliminate or reduce weight bearing on a lower extremity after fracture. The amount of weight reduction depends on the type of device and the patient's training.

Canes

Canes come in various types, including straight canes and narrow- or wide-based quad canes, and have a variety of differing grips, design elements, and accessories (Figure 7-7). A cane unweights a fractured lower

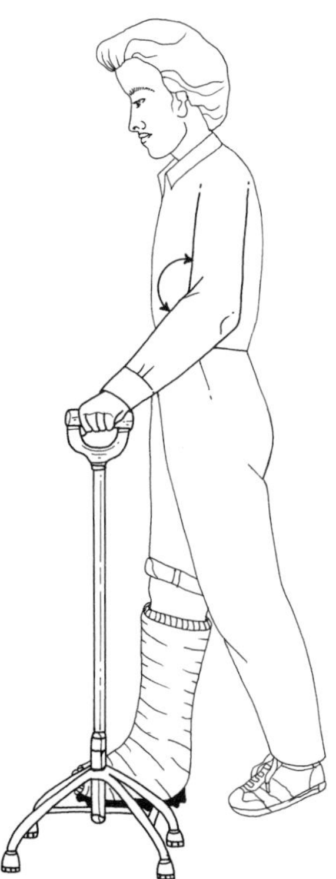

FIGURE 7-7 Wide-based cane helps to reduce postfracture weight bearing on a lower extremity because the weight is transferred through the cane to the upper extremity. Thirty degrees of elbow flexion is necessary for push-off and weight bearing against the cane.

extremity by between 0% and 20% of body weight depending on the design and the patient's training. The top of the cane should reach approximately the level of the greater trochanter to allow the 30 degrees of elbow flexion needed for push-off and weight bearing. The cane should be held in the hand opposite the fracture and advanced simultaneously with the fractured limb.

Crutches

Crutches may be either axillary or forearm (Canadian, Lofstrand) in design. When used correctly, crutches can completely eliminate weight bearing on a lower extremity during ambulation (Figures 7-8 and 7-9).

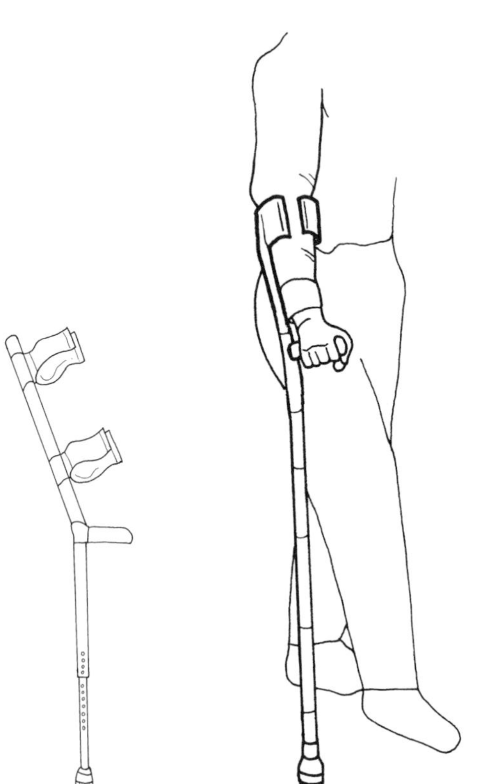

FIGURE 7-8 *(above, left)* Forearm crutch helps to reduce or eliminate weight bearing on a lower extremity.

FIGURE 7-9 *(above, right)* Forearm crutch eliminates axillary pressure. Most of the weight is taken on the hand and forearm.

After lower extremity fracture, the use of axillary crutches is the rule (Figure 7-10). Forearm crutches are used when open wounds or grafted skin on the arm preclude the use of axillary crutches.

If crutches are not used or sized appropriately, a variety of compression neuropathies may develop because of axillary, forearm, or carpal tunnel compression of the median nerve.

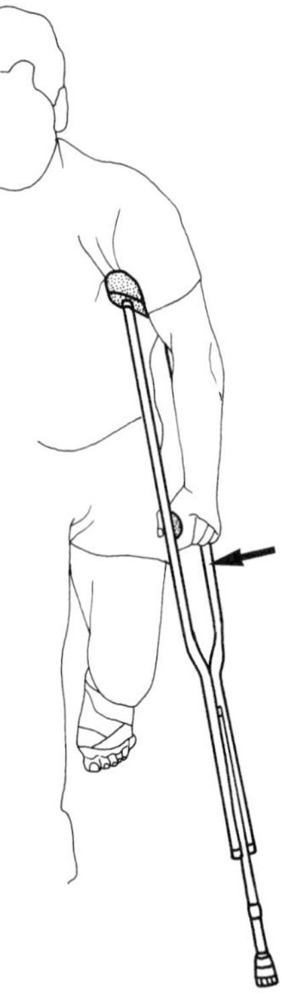

FIGURE 7-10 Axillary crutch, the most common crutch used, eliminates lower extremity weight bearing. Excessive force in the axilla must be avoided. The elbow is kept at 30 degrees of flexion to allow push-off and weight bearing on the upper extremity.

Walkers

A walker is an ambulation aid that consists of a light-weight frame that provides a large base of support and the ability to reduce lower extremity weight bearing by bearing weight through the upper extremities and the walker (Figure 7-11). The four legs of the walker may be equipped with rubber caps, metal caps (gliding walkers), or wheels (rolling walkers), selected for both the type of surface on which the patient will walk and the safety and stability of the patient when walking (Figures 7-12 and 7-13). Walkers unweight a

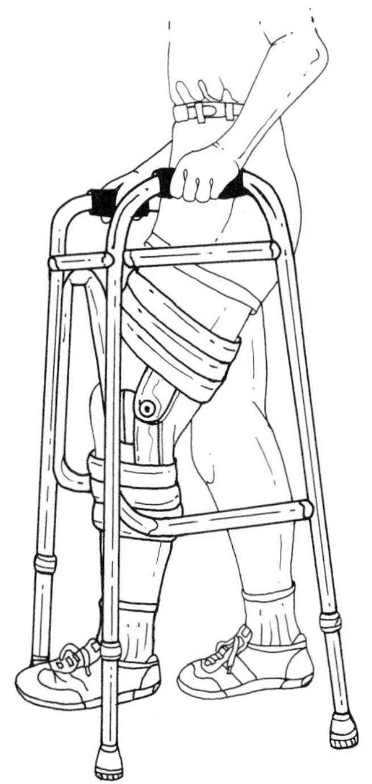

FIGURE 7-11 Standard walker provides a large base of support and helps reduce lower extremity weight bearing.

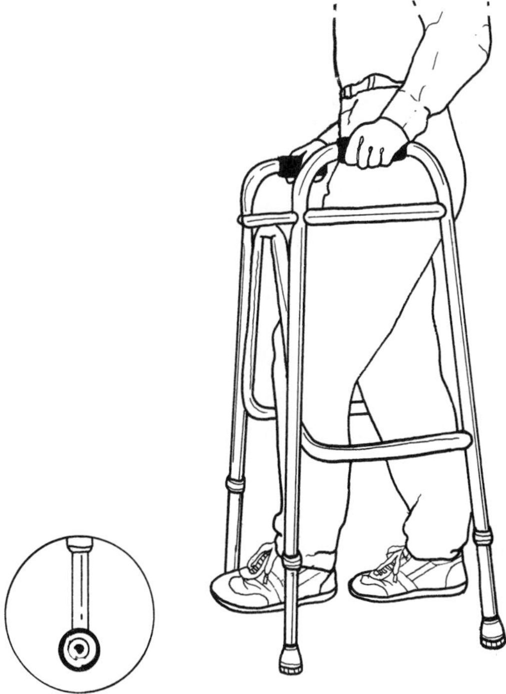

FIGURE 7-12 Standard walker with rolling wheel adaptation. The four legs of the walker are usually equipped with rubber caps or wheels (rolling walkers). This makes walking on different surfaces easier and makes it unnecessary to lift the walker to advance.

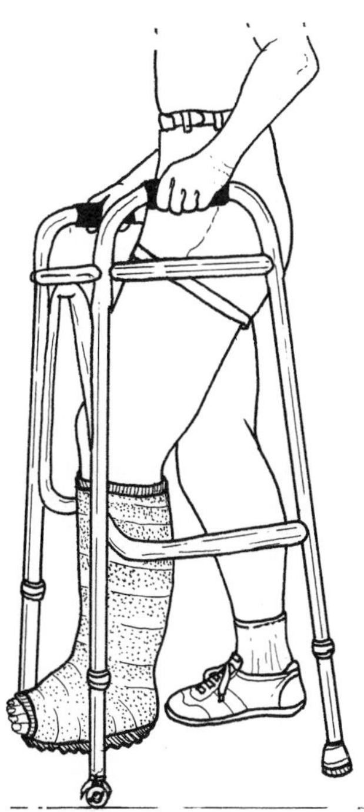

FIGURE 7-13 Rolling walker used to unweight a lower extremity or provide partial weight bearing. The standard walkers and rolling walkers are used mostly by elderly patients who require more stability to ambulate.

fractured limb by up to 100% depending on how they are used. A walker should be considered for a post-fracture patient who requires a large base of support because of impaired balance or motor control. This is frequently the case with elderly patients after hip or other lower extremity fractures.

Platform Walkers and Crutches

A platform device is a walker or crutch that is adapted to reduce or eliminate distal upper extremity weight bearing by the addition of a an expanded plate and modified grasp (Figure 7-14). These devices are useful for patients with multiple fractures in which weight bearing on one upper and one lower extremity is contraindicated, such as in a Colles' fracture with a concomitant femur fracture. With a platform device, the upper extremity weight is borne through the elbow and thus bypasses the hand, wrist, and part of the forearm (Table 7-1).

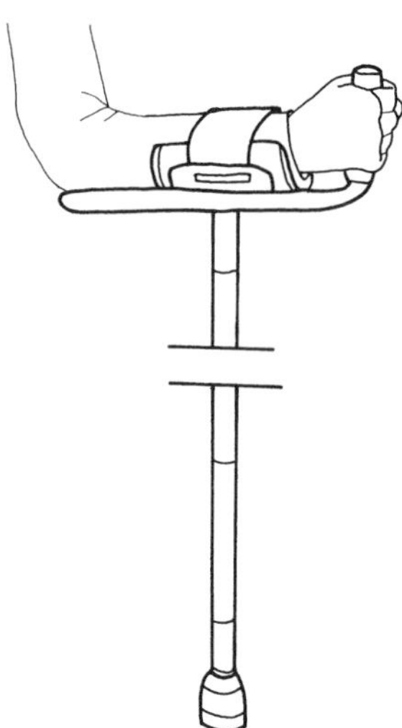

FIGURE 7-14 Platform crutch is used when weight bearing at the wrist must be avoided, as with a Colles' fracture. The weight is borne by the forearm and elbow. This is most frequently used with multiple extremity fractures.

TABLE 7-1 *Assistive Devices for Activities of Daily Living*

Fracture	Equipment	Mechanism of Action
Shoulder	Grooming aids Reacher	Extends reach
Elbow	Grooming aids Reacher	Extends reach
Forearm	Built-up door handles	Decreases torque
Wrist	Built-up door knobs and keys	Decreases torque
Hand	Built-up fork, spoon Rocker knife	Augments grasp Allows one-handed cutting
Spine	Reachers Grabbers Sock-aid Long-handled shoe horn	Extends reach Increases grasp and reach Extends reach Extends reach
Hip	Raised toilet seat Reacher Walker/crutches	Reduces torque/force Extends reach Reduces weight bearing
Knee	Crutches/cane Reacher Sock-aid	Reduces weight bearing Extends reach Extends reach
Tibia	Reacher Crutches/cane	Extends reach Reduces weight bearing
Foot and ankle	Reacher Crutches/cane	Extends reach Reduces weight bearing

BIBLIOGRAPHY

Braddom R. *Physical Medicine and Rehabilitation*. Philadelphia: W.B. Saunders, 1996.

Brotzman SB, ed. *Clinical Orthopaedic Rehabilitation*. St. Louis: Mosby, 1996.

Ceder L, Svensson K, Thorngren KG. Statistical prediction of rehabilitation in elderly patients with hip fractures. *Clin Orthop*, 152:185–190, 1980.

Goldstein FC, Strasser DC, Woodard JL, Roberts VJ. Functional outcome of cognitively impaired hip fracture patients on a geriatric rehabilitation unit. *J Am Geriatr Soc*, 45:35–42, 1997.

Mehta Arun JMB, ed. Rehabilitation of fractures. *State of the Art Reviews in Physical Medicine and Rehabilitation*, Vol.9, No. 3. Philadelphia: Hanley & Belfus, 1995.

CHAPTER *Eight*

Braces and Splints

MARK A. THOMAS, MD

STANLEY HOPPENFELD, MD

INTRODUCTION

Braces, or orthoses, are devices that stop or limit range of motion, facilitate movement, or guide a joint through an arc of motion. Splints are used to immobilize and position one or several joints. After fracture, splints and braces are prescribed to protect a partially healed fracture once weight bearing or movement is allowed. They may also be used to immobilize the fracture and to prevent pain that occurs with motion (Figure 8-1A).

CAST BRACES

Immobilizing the joint above and the joint below a fracture often leads to stiffening and the need for a prolonged period of rehabilitation. This can be minimized somewhat by the use of a cast brace, which provides partial immobilization while allowing some range of motion and weight bearing on a limb. Once a fracture has achieved some stability, as with callus formation, the cast is replaced in the form of a hinged splint or brace. This allows range of motion to the joints proximal and distal to the fracture without compromising support at the fracture site (*see* Figure 8-1)

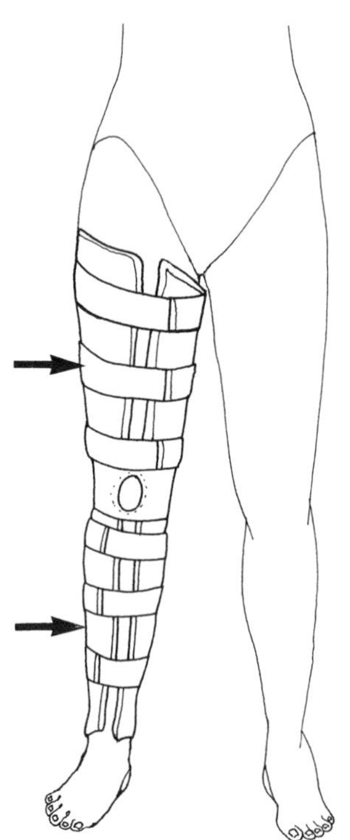

FIGURE 8-1A Long leg splint, used to immobilize the fracture and to prevent pain that occurs with motion.

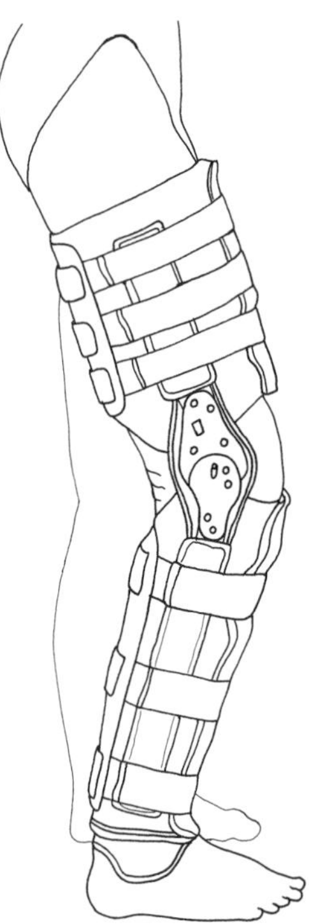

FIGURE 8-1 Hinged brace. Once a fracture has achieved some stability with callus formation, the cast may be replaced by a hinged splint or brace. Range of motion may be accomplished in the joints proximal and distal to the fracture.

For example, when a hip spica is applied to stabilize a femoral shaft fracture, the spica is cut and hinged at the joints above and below the fracture, when partial healing (stability) has occurred. In this way, early movement of the hip and knee can limit stiffness while the femur fracture is supported by the cast. This same principle applies to an upper extremity forearm fracture.

TURNBUCKLE AND DYNAMIC BRACES

A turnbuckle or dynamic brace is usually used after a fracture when there is a fixed joint contracture that is not responding to stretch. This type of brace is applied after the fracture is healed. Fractures of the humerus, elbow, radius, ulna, femur, knee, and tibia or fibula may result in elbow or knee contractures. In this instance, a turnbuckle brace provides progressive stretch to the joint capsule and soft tissues by a serial increase in the joint angle, which is set by the treating physician or therapist. A dynamic brace provides constant stretch through a spring mechanism. The patient is able to overcome this constant stretch by active movement. Both of these orthoses are used to increase range of motion; in general, they require prolonged use and are infrequently used.

SPINAL BRACES

A variety of brace designs and materials are available that provide differing degrees of spinal fixation after spinal fracture. Spinal braces usually restrict but do not completely prevent motion in the thoracic or lumbar region.

Thoracolumbosacral Orthoses

The most confining type of thoracolumbosacral orthosis (TLSO) is the rigid body jacket. An example of this is the Boston modular plastic shell, which provides fixation of individual vertebral bodies in relation to each other as well as fixation of the spine to the pelvis by containment of an adequate amount of the gluteal area. The iliac crest bumper prevents the brace from rotating. The Boston brace opens posteriorly and is customized to the individual patient, as are body jackets in general (Figures 8-2 and 8-3). The New York

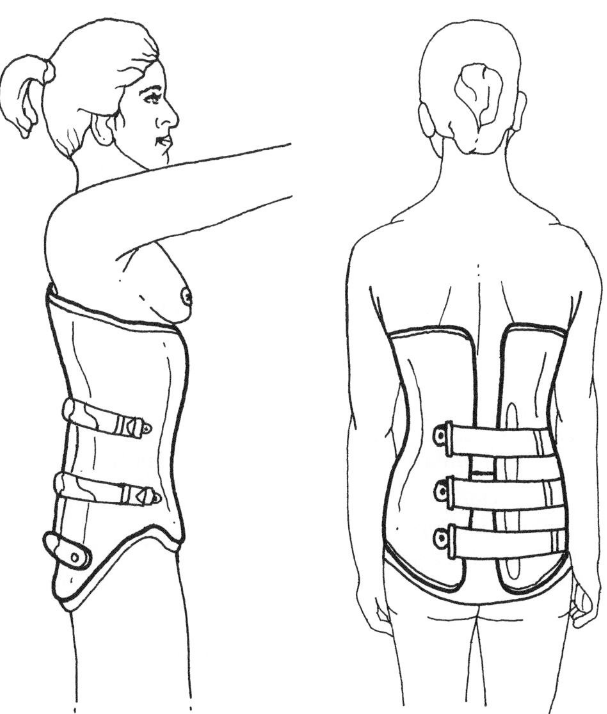

FIGURE 8-2 *(far left)* Boston model brace, a thoracolumbosacral orthosis, is a rigid body jacket and controls spinal motion in all planes.

FIGURE 8-3 *(left)* Boston model brace (posterior view) is posteriorly open as customized to the individual patient. Individual vertebral bodies are immobilized in relation to each other, and the spine is fixed to the pelvis.

brace is similar to the Boston brace, but has an anterior opening. This type of orthosis controls spinal movement in all planes. To provide firm fixation of the spine to the pelvis, a thigh extension piece is needed.

Other types of rigid spinal orthotics are not molded to the individual, but use specific support to control movement in one or two planes. These types of braces include the Jewett, Knight-Taylor, chair back, and cruciform design braces, which limit flexion and extension (Figures 8-4, 8-5, and 8-6). These braces may also be used with internal spinal instrumentation.

In general, the use of soft TLSOs, such as corsets, does not play a role in rehabilitation after fracture except when a fracture has healed and the TLSO is used with physical therapy to provide comfort, partially restrict trunk movement, and reduce patient anxiety (Table 8-1).

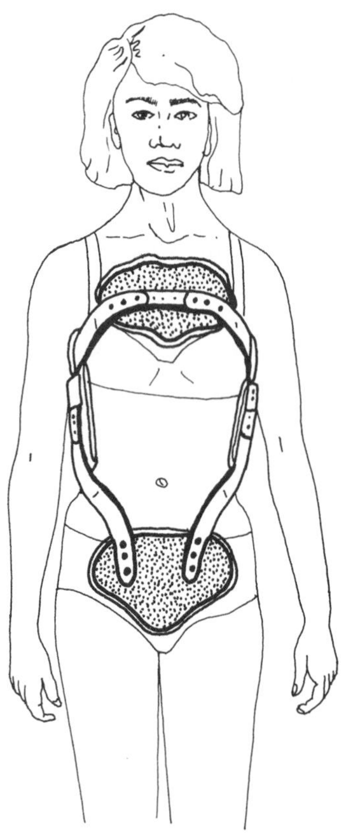

FIGURE 8-4 Jewett brace, a hyperextension brace that immobilizes flexion and extension of the thoracolumbar spine.

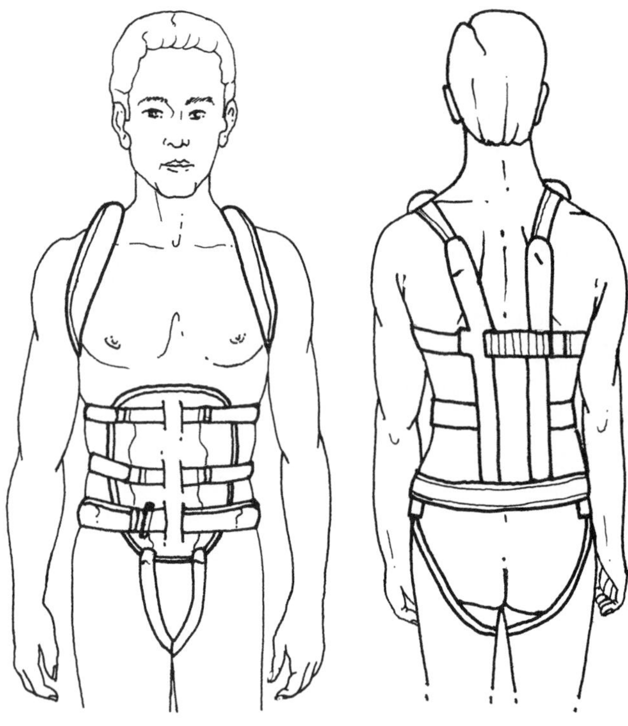

FIGURE 8-5 *(above, left)* Knight-Taylor brace (anterior view) immobilizes the thoracolumbar spine in flexion and extension.

FIGURE 8-6 *(above, right)* Knight-Taylor brace (posterior view). Uprights contain the thoracolumbar spine with fixation to the pelvis.

TABLE 8-1 *Thoracolumbosacral orthoses*

Vertebral Fracture	Brace	Immobilization	Degree of Immobilization
Thoracolumbar Compression Burst Flexion-rotation Postoperative internal fixation	Boston New York	Flexion Extension Rotation	Best
Thoracolumbar Compression	Jewett	Flexion Extension	Fair
Thoracolumbar Compression	Knight-Taylor	Flexion Extension	Fair
Thoracolumbar Compression	Cruciform	Flexion	Fair–poor

Cervical Orthoses

A variety of orthoses are available that provide varying degrees of motion control at the cervical spine. Proper brace use may decrease repetitive stress at the fracture site. Greater fixation is provided in a rigid collar orthosis when containment of the occiput, mandible, or sternum or extension to the thorax is added (examples include the Philadelphia and four-poster collars; Figures 8-7 and 8-8). Fixation is also improved by anchoring a cervical frame into the calvarium with screws, and to the thoracic cage and spine by a vest-type extension. This type of brace, exemplified by a halo vest, is used to provide maximum immobility, particularly for unstable fractures with potential for grave neurologic complications (Figure 8-9). Four-

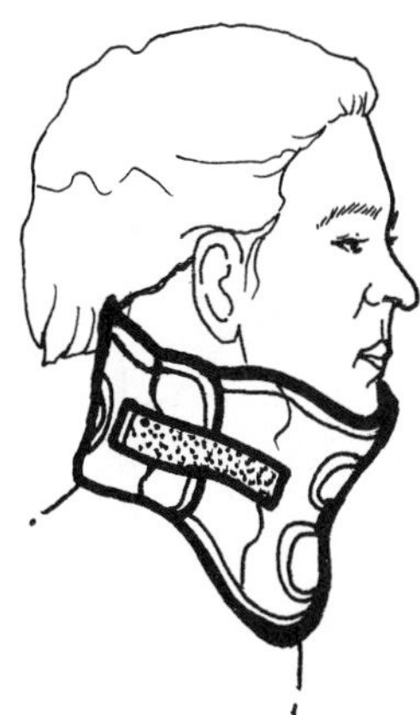

FIGURE 8-7 Philadelphia collar, a rigid cervical collar that contains the cervical spine, occiput, mandible, and a small extension onto the sternum. This helps control flexion, extension, and rotation.

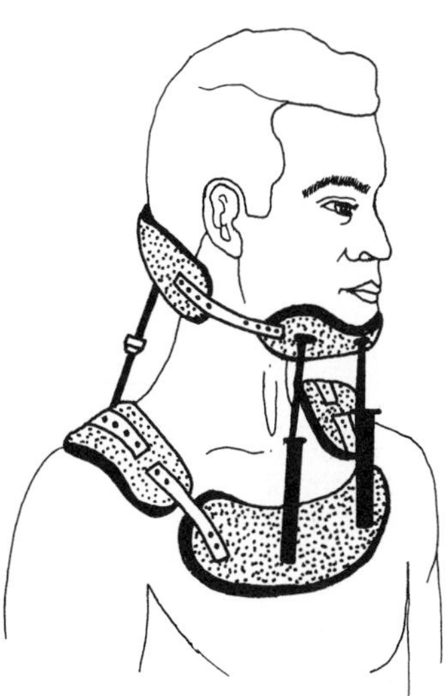

FIGURE 8-8 Four-poster collar. Fixation is provided by immobilizing the occiput and mandible and by extension onto the sternum and posterior aspect of the thorax. Shoulder straps provide additional stability.

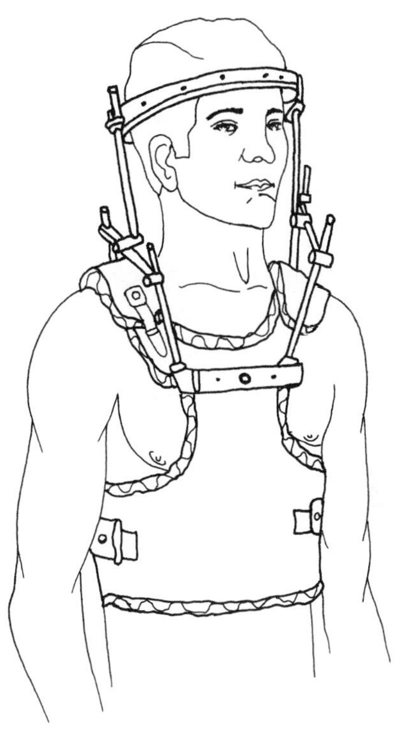

FIGURE 8-9 Halo vest brace. Fixation is provided by anchoring the cervical frame into the calvarium with screws and to the thoracic cage and spine by a vest-type extension. This provides maximum immobilization and is of particular use in unstable fractures with potential for grave neurologic complications.

poster and Philadelphia cervical collars largely immobilize the cervical spine, controlling motion from the occiput to the shoulders. Rigid collars without adequate head or trunk extensions may restrict cervical motion; however, this is often not adequate, particularly for restricting occiput—C1-2 segmental motion (Figure 8-10). In general, the use of soft cervical braces (collars) is not recommended because they provide limited support to the fractured cervical spine and minimal restriction of cervical motion (Figure 8-11).

Most cervical immobilization is done in a neutral position, as close as possible to the patient's position of comfort (Table 8-2).

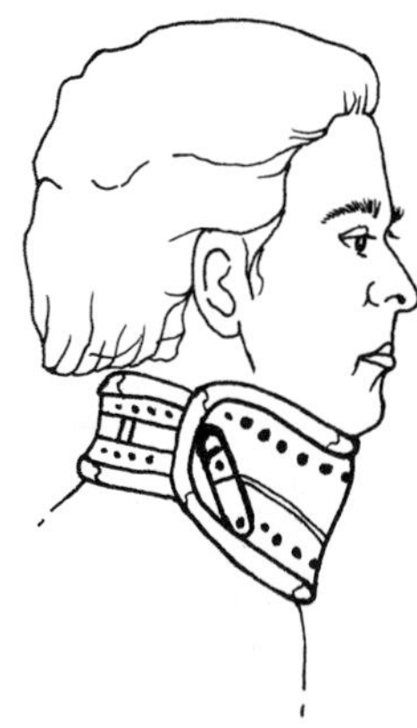

FIGURE 8-10 Firm collar (standard cervical collar) does not provide adequate head or trunk support and thus is not adequate for restricting occiput C1-2 segmental motion.

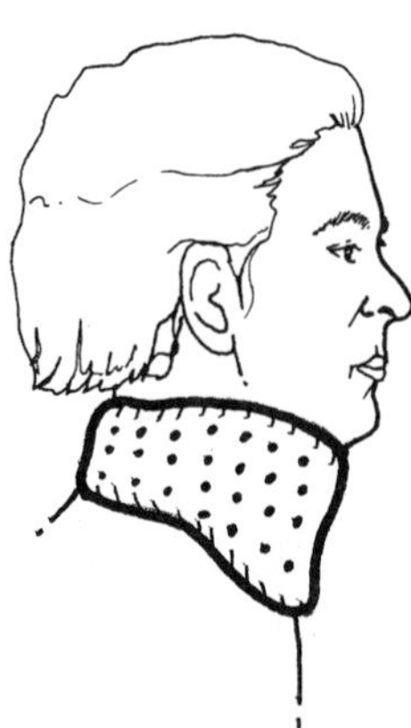

FIGURE 8-11 Soft cervical collar provides minimum or limited support to the fractured cervical spine and minimum restriction of motion. It is rarely used. It may be used in the late stages of cervical spine healing to provide nighttime support.

TABLE 8-2 *Cervical Orthoses*

Vertebral Fracture	Brace	Immobilization	Degree of Immobilization
C1–2 Odontoid Jefferson Hangman's	Halo vest	Flexion Extension Rotation	Best
C3–7	SOMI (sterno-occipital-mandibular immobilizer) Halo vest	Flexion Extension Rotation	Best
Burst Compression Facets	Philadelphia and Four poster collars	Flexion Extension Limited rotation	Good
	Rigid collar	Flexion Extension No rotational control	Fair

Soft collars do not provide sufficient immobilization for use with a cervical spine fracture.

SPLINTS AND POSITIONING AIDS

A splint may be applied to achieve the same goal as the orthotics that are commonly used after fracture. Splints provide some stabilization of the fracture site but may be removed for rehabilitation treatment. They serve to restrict or prevent joint movement, shortening, and contracture but must be used with physical therapy to maintain muscle stretch and range of motion and achieve optimal results.

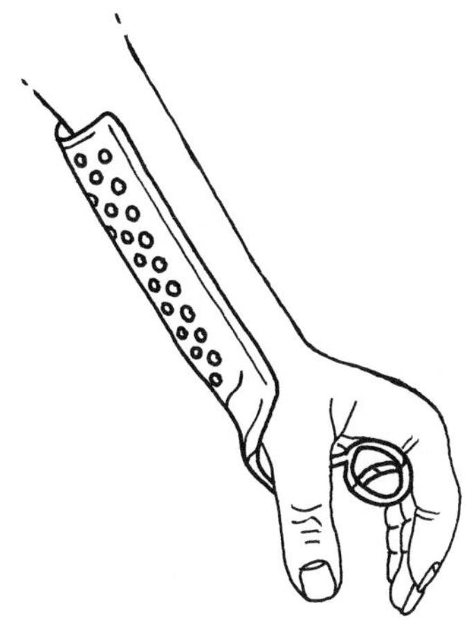

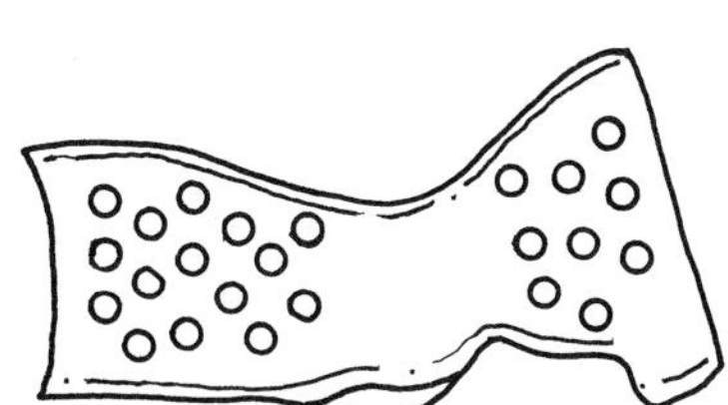

FIGURE 8-12 Prefabricated positioning splint (cock-up splint) positions the wrist and provides some support once some stability is achieved after a Colles' fracture.

A variety of splinting materials provide differing degrees of rigidity and motion control. The posterior shell of a bivalved cast may be used as a splint, or a custom-made splint may be provided. Prefabricated splints may also be adapted to provide joint stability, such as a cock-up splint to position the wrist once some stability is achieved after a Colles' fracture (Figure 8-12).

Splints are frequently used after a cast is first removed during activity or at night to reduce pain and discomfort (Figure 8-13).

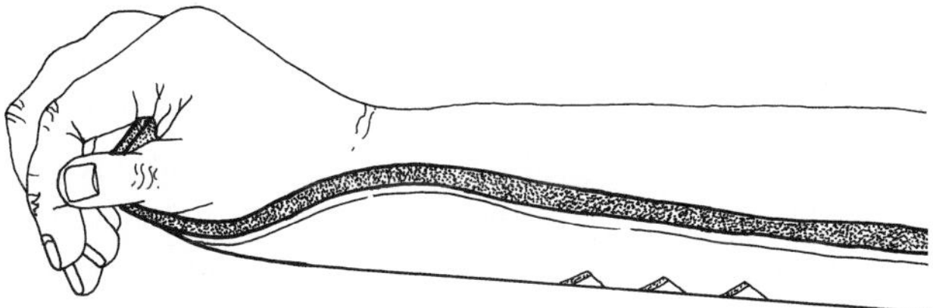

FIGURE 8-13 Forearm splint used after a cast is removed to provide temporary support to the forearm.

Functional splints may be used in select instances to assist the patient in the performance of activities of daily living. An example of this is the use of an outrigger, or lyre, to provide wrist and digit extension after radial nerve palsy related to a humeral fracture. Functional splints are not, however, a component of the rehabilitation prescription after an uncomplicated fracture. Positioning aids are used to prevent muscle shortening and joint contracture. They may also maintain optimal positioning of the fracture site or prevent movement that would jeopardize fracture healing.

These aids are commonly used at the wrist and hand to prevent flexion contracture of the digits due to shortening of the volar forearm muscles, as with a radius or ulnar fracture. They are also used at the ankle and foot to prevent shortening of the triceps surae and a resultant equinus attitude of the foot after a tibial fracture. Positioning aids may be rigid or made of soft materials such as pillows or foam.

BIBLIOGRAPHY

Billig N, Ahmed SW, Kenmore PI. Approaches to senior care no. 1: Hip fracture, depression, and cognitive impairment: a follow-up study. *Orthop Rev*, 17:315–320, 1988.

Borkan JM, Quirk M, Sullivan M. Finding meaning after the fall: injury narratives from elderly hip fracture patients. *Soc Sci Med*, 33:947–957, 1991.

Borquist L, Lindelow G, Thorngren KG. Costs of hip fracture: rehabilitation of 180 patients in primary health care. *Acta Orthop Scand*, 62:39–48, 1991.

Braddom R. *Physical Medicine and Rehabilitation*. Philadelphia: W.B. Saunders, 1996.

Brotzman SB, ed. *Clinical Orthopaedic Rehabilitation*. St. Louis, Mosby, 1996.

Ceder L, Svensson K, Thorngren KG. Statistical predication of rehabilitation in elderly patients with hip fractures. *Clin Orthop*, 152:185–190, 1980.

Goldstein FC, Strasser DC, Woodard JL, Roberts VJ. Functional outcome of cognitively impaired hip fracture patients on a geriatric rehabilitation unit. *J Am Geriatr Soc*, 45:35–42, 1997.

Grundes O, Reiker O. Effect of physical activity on muscle and bone blood flow after fracture: exercise and tenotomy studied in rats. *Acta Orthop Scand*, 62:67–69, 1991.

Hoppenfeld S. *Physical Examination of the Spine and Extremities*. Norwalk, CT: Appleton-Century-Crofts, 1976.

Inman VT, Ralston TR, Todd F. *Human Walking*. Baltimore, Williams & Wilkins, 1981.

Mehta Arun JMB, ed. Rehabilitation of fractures. *State of the Art Reviews in Physical Medicine and Rehabilitation*, Vol. 9, No. 3. Philadelphia: Hanley & Belfus, 1995.

Norkin C, Levangie P. *Joint Structure and Function*, 2nd ed. Philadelphia: F.A. Davis, 1992.

Randell A, Sambrook PN, Nguyen TV, et al. Direct clinical and welfare costs of osteoporotic fractures in elderly men and women. *Osteoporos Int*, 5:427–432, 1995.

Soderberg G. *Kinesiology: Application to Pathological Motion*. Baltimore: Williams & Wilkins, 1986.

Perry J. *Gait Analysis: Normal and Pathological Function*. Thorofare, NJ: Slack, 1992.

CHAPTER *Nine*

Management and Classification of Compound Fractures

ROBERT TAFFET, MD

CONTRIBUTIONS BY BABAK SHEIKH, MD

INTRODUCTION

Patients who sustain compound, or open, fractures present several unique management problems. Compound fractures are often caused by high-energy accidents and accompanied by multiple injuries, both orthopaedic and nonorthopaedic. The stabilization of the fracture, which is discussed in more detail later, is dictated largely by the integrity of the soft-tissue envelope and therefore may be a less-than-ideal biomechanical construct. In addition, the patient may require multiple débridements and ultimately soft-tissue coverage procedures that delay rehabilitation. The amount of energy imparted to the bone and soft tissues at the time of injury is probably the most important variable in determining the treatment and outcome of an open fracture.

The ultimate goal is to restore these patients to their pretrauma status, or as close to that as possible, in as little time as possible. With this in mind, it is important for the orthopaedic trauma surgeon to consider when primary amputation would be beneficial for a severely mangled extremity rather than putting a patient through 2 years of multiple reconstructive procedures and prolonged rehabilitation, when the ultimate outcome would be a limb that will never function well enough to allow the patient to return to work. Primary amputation and early prosthetic fitting may be the treatment of choice for many severely mangled extremities.

The prognostic classification system of Gustillo and Anderson is a qualitative assessment of the soft-tissue and bony injuries as they relate to the risk for infection. An open fracture may occur from either a low-energy or a high-energy mechanism. For example, an elderly patient stepping off a curb may sustain a twisting or bending injury that could, because of poor bone and soft-tissue quality, produce significant enough displacement to create a wound of compounding. The resulting soft-tissue injury would be minor, provided there is no complicating infection, and the patient should do quite well. At the opposite end of the spectrum, a young, healthy motorcyclist who collides at high speed with another vehicle or a stationary object would typically sustain severe abrasions and lacerations as well as crushing injuries to the limbs. The wounds would likely be contaminated secondary to the lack of protection, and the fractures tend to be severely displaced or comminuted. This patient presents a completely different set of problems from the elderly patient and is likely to have a much more protracted course, both in terms of management of the multiple injuries and in requiring multiple débridements for establishing a healthy soft-tissue envelope.

GUSTILLO AND ANDERSON CLASSIFICATION SYSTEM

The Gustillo and Anderson classification system was developed many years ago and remains the standard classification system for open fractures. It initially was designed to describe open fractures of the tibia, which are fairly distinct from open fractures in general, partly because of the sparse soft-tissue coverage over the tibia and the vascularity of that bone.

The Gustillo and Anderson system is based on the findings after surgical débridement and not on a crude assessment in the emergency department. The size of the wound of compounding does not necessarily indicate the degree of soft-tissue injury. This is a potential pitfall when attempting to classify fractures based only on the size of the wound of compounding. The true nature of the soft-tissue injury must be determined at the time of initial débridement. To reveal fully the severity of the soft-tissue injury, débridements must be fairly extensive.

A type I compound fracture results from a relatively low-energy injury, with a small, clean wound of compounding and very little soft-tissue damage. This is a spiral-type fracture with no comminution; the wound of compounding is less than 1 cm in size, with no contusion of the skin or surrounding muscle. In general, the prognosis for a patient with such a low-grade injury is excellent because the surrounding soft tissues have not been damaged enough to become necrotic and require significant débridement or to provide a nidus for bacterial colonization.

A type II injury is a higher-energy injury with more extensive soft-tissue damage. The wound of compounding is from 1 to 10 cm in size and the muscle contusion is moderate, with minimal periosteal stripping from the fracture fragments (Table 9-1 and Figure 9-1).

TABLE 9-1 ***The Gustillo-Anderson Classification of Soft-Tissue Injury in Open Fractures***

	Type I	Type II	Type III[a]
Wound size	<1 cm	1–10 cm	>10 cm
Injury	Low velocity/energy	High velocity/energy	High velocity/energy
Soft tissue	Minimal soft-tissue damage	No extensive soft-tissue damage, flap, or avulsion	Extensive soft-tissue damage, including muscle, skin, and (often) neurovascular structures
Crush	No signs of crush	Slight to moderate crush	Extensive crush
Fracture	Usually simple, transverse, or short oblique with little comminution	Moderate fracture comminution	Great degree of fracture comminution and instability
Contamination	Little contamination	Moderate contamination	High degree of contamination

[a]See Table 9-2.

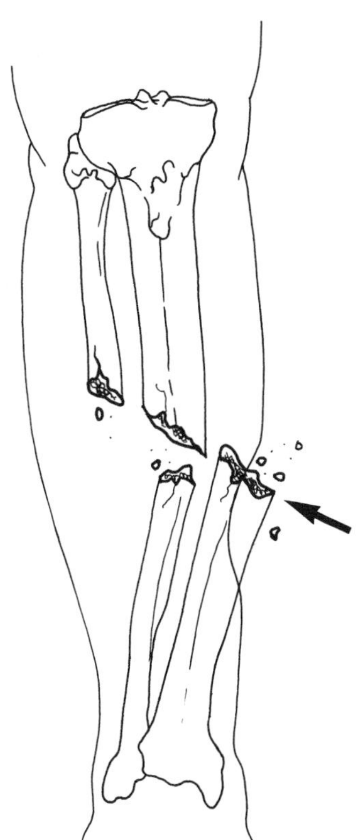

FIGURE 9-1 Type II open tibia and fibular fracture, moderate comminuted, with 2 to 10 cm of skin opening and without neurovascular injury.

TABLE 9-2 ***Type III Soft-Tissue Injury in Open Fractures***

	Type III-A	Type III-B	Type III-C
Wound size	>10 cm	>10 cm	>10 cm
Injury	High velocity/energy	High velocity/energy	High velocity/energy
Soft tissue	Extensive soft-tissue laceration, adequate bone coverage after débridement. Free flaps are not necessary to cover bone. Segmental fractures, such as gunshot injuries.	Extensive sot tissue injury with periosteal stripping and exposed bone after débridement. Requires local or free flap to cover bone.	Same as type IIIB
Vascular injury	Not significant	Not significant	Vascular injury requiring repair for limb salvage
Contamination	High degree	Massive	Massive

A type III-A open fracture has a wound of compounding greater than 10 cm in length, with severe soft-tissue damage and crushing of skin and muscle, possibly requiring débridement of skin and muscle. After surgical débridement, there is adequate soft tissue in the wound locally to provide coverage of the bone without either local rotational myoplasty or free tissue transfer (Table 9-2).

A type III-B fracture is a high-energy injury with severe crushing of muscle and extensive periosteal stripping. There may be severe bone comminution and wound contamination. These patients are at great risk for problems with their fractures, including infection and difficulty obtaining fracture union, and often require multiple débridements before soft-tissue coverage of the bone can be established. In a type III-B fracture, at the conclusion of débridement there is inadequate soft-tissue coverage of bone, and either local muscle flap coverage or free tissue transfer is necessary. Often there are also devitalized bone fragments, which are removed at the time of débridement and require later bony reconstruction (*see* Table 9-2).

The most severe fracture in this classification system is the type III-C fracture, which is a compound fracture with a limb-threatening vascular injury. A single-vessel injury to the tibia below the trifurcation of the popliteal artery that does not require revascularization for limb survival should not be considered a type III-C fracture. Such a patient requires stabilization of the fracture and vascular repair or reconstruction and, depending on the time to reperfusion, may or may not require fasciotomy to prevent compartment syndrome. Typically, a fasciotomy should be performed (*see* Table 9-2).

A patient with a severe open fracture involving soft-tissue injury and bony comminution represents a distinct challenge in terms of (a) reestablishing a healthy soft-tissue envelope surrounding the fracture; (b) obtaining fracture union and bony reconstruction; and (c) rehabilitating the limb. The management of compound fractures thus can be divided into the acute phase, the reconstructive phase, and the rehabilitative phase. Often rehabilitation and reconstruction occur concurrently, and in general these two phases should not be regarded as distinct.

ACUTE PHASE

The goals during the acute phase of compound fracture management are obtaining stability at the fracture site and stabilizing the soft-tissue envelope. The latter cannot occur in the presence of an unstable fracture, and therefore some form of skeletal stabilization must be instituted. The choice of treatment for any fracture is based on multiple factors, including the patient's age and nutritional status, the nature of the fracture (intraarticular vs. extraarticular), the displacement and stability of the fracture, the degree of comminution, and the severity of the associated soft-tissue injury. Multiple treatment options exist for every fracture type. Simply stated, a fracture may be managed by closed or open treatment. Closed treatment can consist of closed reduction and application of a cast, closed reduction and application of an external fixator, application of skeletal traction, or, for stable fractures of many types, merely splinting.

When a fracture is associated with a wound of compounding, the choice of skeletal stabilization is largely determined by the degree of soft-tissue injury and contamination. When a patient is admitted through the emergency department with a compound fracture, initial management should consist of preliminary assessment of the wound, the patient's neurovascular status, and the bony injury. A sterile povidone-iodine–soaked gauze should be applied to the wound of compounding and the limb splinted provisionally. The patient should be taken to the operating room for emergency irrigation and débridement of the wound of compounding and stabilization of the fracture within 6 hours. Delays in treatment beyond this period have been associated with higher rates of infection.

Débridement of the open fracture usually requires extending the wound of compounding, and skin flaps should be fasciocutaneous. Ideally, the extensions of the wound of compounding are not extended directly over bone, as for example over the subcutaneous surface of the tibia. After the wound is thoroughly assessed, a form of stabilization of the fracture needs to be selected. For a very severe soft-tissue injury with significant contamination, external fixation provides the safest form of skeletal stabilization. Lesser degrees of soft-tissue injury and contamination allow the more liberal use of orthopaedic implants, including plates or intramedullary devices. The wound of compounding is packed open, and no tension should be exerted on the skin when attempting to close its extensions. Fasciotomies for compartment syndrome or impending compartment syndrome should be liberally used. A patient with a compound fracture treated in this manner should be returned to the operating room within 24 to 48 hours for a second-look irrigation and débridement. Plan for delayed primary closure or, if this is not possible, soft-tissue coverage with fasciocutaneous flaps, rotational myoplasty, or free tissue transfer no later than 10 days after injury. Delays of greater than 10 days in obtaining soft-tissue coverage have been associated with significantly higher rates of infection. Some surgeons perform primary free tissue transfer if they believe this will ultimately be required; however, most trauma surgeons prefer to allow the wound to declare itself within the initial 24 to 48 hours to see how the soft-tissue injury progresses.

As mentioned, stabilization of the fracture provides the optimal environment for wound healing and allows the wound to settle down, thereby shortening the inflammatory phase of healing. The method of stabilization will have an important bearing on the rehabilitation of the extremity.

Intramedullary Fixation

Intramedullary fixation, in general, is the ideal way to stabilize fractures of the major weight-bearing long bones—the femur and the tibia. Multiple studies have shown that it is safe to use a reamed intramedullary nail to stabilize a compound-fractured femur with a type III-A soft-tissue injury. With compound fractures of the tibia, fractures up to type III-A and occasionally III-B injuries are stabilized with intramedullary nails. However, in this situation, except for type I and II fractures, it is preferable to perform nonreamed intramedullary nailing to avoid further damage to the endosteal circulation, which is already damaged by the fracture. Reaming is thought to be more destructive to the bone's blood supply than inserting smaller-diameter, nonreamed nails.

In intramedullary fixation, the fixation device is placed centrally in the mechanical axis of the bone rather than placed eccentrically. Therefore, it is less subject to bending loads than a plate, which is applied on the tension side of the bone. Ideally, the intramedullary device acts as a load-sharing device in which both the bone and the implant receive the load. The bone must not be completely shielded from weight bearing because weight bearing is a major stimulus for fracture healing. This is particularly important in the weight-bearing bones of the lower extremity. When a fractured long bone is not severely comminuted and can be treated with an intramedullary device so that the major bone fragments are in contact and have inherent axial stability, the rods may be interlocked to provide a dynamic mode of fracture fixation. This allows more loading of the fracture and thus facilitates fracture union. When the fracture is severely comminuted and there is no contact between the proximal and distal fragments, there is no inherent axial stability to the fracture, and the rod initially absorbs all the load crossing the fracture until there is sufficient healing for the bone to absorb some load. In this situation, static interlocking is required and the rod is partially load sparing (stress shielding). Nonreamed nails usually are small in diameter and not necessarily as strong as larger, reamed nails, and may not provide as tight a fit in the intramedullary canal. If there is evidence that fracture union is not progressing well, an unreamed nail is often replaced with a larger-diameter, reamed nail after the soft-tissue envelope has been reestablished.

External Fixation

External fixation for compound fractures of the lower extremity tends to be reserved for those that have very severe soft-tissue injuries with severe contamination or vascular injury and require rapid stabilization of the bone and restoration of circulation to the limb. In addition, the external fixator is particularly useful for rapid stabilization of compound or even closed lower extremity fractures in a patient with multiple injuries who is critically ill and cannot be subjected to prolonged operative time or significant bleeding. The external fixator is a partial load-sparing device that can be used for provisional or definitive stabilization of fractures. In the tibia, where the external fixator is most commonly used for open fractures, this device has fallen into some disfavor because of problems related to delayed fracture union, typically seen with severe compound fractures and subsequent malunion, or problems with pin tract infections. Although the external fixator is initially applied as a load-sparing (stress-shielding) device, when used for definitive stabilization it can be dynamized and converted into a load-sharing (stress-sharing) device. External fixation for compound fractures of the femur is used only under the most extreme circumstances.

In the upper extremity, external fixation is rarely used, except in fractures about the wrist, because internal fixation with plates, screws, or intramedullary devices is biomechanically superior and tolerated better because of the improved vascularity of the upper extremity. In fractures of the distal radius, either open or closed external fixation is commonly used. With fractures of the radius and ulnar shafts in which restoration of anatomy is crucial for maintaining forearm motion, the use of plates is preferred, even in fairly severe compound fractures.

Internal Fixation with Plate and Screws

Internal fixation of fractures of the weight-bearing long bones (except in the periarticular or articular regions) is best accomplished with intramedullary devices. Plate fixation of open tibial fractures has been associated with much higher rates of infection than either external fixation or intramedullary stabilization. The application of a plate requires periosteal stripping, which further compromises the vascularity of the bone and potentially prolongs fracture healing and increases the risk of infection. The plate is a completely load-sparing (stress-shielding) device that tends to protect the underlying bone from stress. The plate is applied eccentric to the weight-bearing axis of the bone and is subject to bending loads. This prohibits early weight bearing to prevent plate fracture or disruption of the fracture site.

Femoral shaft fractures in adults are rarely treated with plates in the United States because the same mechanical problems exist for the femur and the tibia, both major weight-bearing bones. In some cases, however, application of a plate is required, and because of the improved vascularity in the thigh, plate fixation of the femoral shaft appears to be better tolerated in terms of infection. In the upper extremity, anatomic reduction of radius and ulnar fractures in adults may be obtained using plate fixation. For fractures of the humerus, the severity of the soft-tissue injury, the contamination, and the fracture pattern dictate which device is used. Caution must be exercised with external and internal fixation of the humerus because of the risk of neurovascular injury in light of the proximity of the radial nerve to the bone. The placement of proximal pins requires careful attention to the location of the axillary nerve.

Cast Treatment

Cast treatment is reserved only for the lowest-grade compound fractures because a cast interferes with repeat irrigation and débridements and wound care. The use of a cast for open fractures, therefore, tends to be reserved for type I injuries and is more common in the treatment of children than adults.

Soft Tissue Coverage

A limb that requires soft-tissue coverage has a very–high-grade compound fracture, often with muscle and skin loss. This limb cannot be expected to return to its normal function. The rehabilitative phase of treatment for such an injury is initiated relatively late. Typically, no rehabilitation starts before the soft-tissue coverage procedure; after either a local or free tissue flap for soft-tissue coverage, the limb is kept elevated and no range of motion is initiated until the flap has set. This may take several weeks. Particularly with lower extremity flaps, the amount of time that the limb can be kept dependent is limited initially, and in several weeks before the limb can be kept dependent for even as long as 30 minutes. A rotational flap performed on a lower extremity may have a significant effect on the strength of that limb and possibly the range of motion of either the knee or the ankle, as well as some alteration of gait. The same strength and range-of-motion concerns apply to the upper extremity. Nevertheless, the outcome of a successful limb salvage procedure in which bone and soft-tissue reconstruction has been performed and infection avoided is preferable to chronic osteomyelitis and soft-tissue loss.

Early and successful soft-tissue coverage is crucial not only in avoiding infection but for reconstructive procedures. Often there is bone loss that requires bone grafting; revision of the fixation may be necessary. As mentioned earlier, with respect to the tibia, where nonreamed intramedullary nails are frequently placed, it is not unusual to perform a delayed exchange intramedullary nailing with a reamed intramedullary nail; this cannot safely be accomplished until the soft-tissue envelope is healed.

RECONSTRUCTIVE AND REHABILITATIVE PHASES

The care of patients with open or closed fractures with severe soft-tissue injuries is complicated by the fact that many of these patients have multiple injuries. The reconstructive and rehabilitative phases of management for these injuries overlap. In general, these phases begin approximately 2 weeks after the injury and continue for at least 1 year.

Procedures

During this time, the patient may require multiple surgical procedures to facilitate bony union, which may involve autogenous iliac crest bone grafting. In addition, it is not uncommon for fixation devices to be exchanged (either small, reamed nails for larger nails or external fixation for internal fixation devices). Osteotomies may be required to correct deformities. Soft-tissue releases and tendon-lengthening procedures may also be required to restore joint motion. Severely traumatized joints that develop rapid posttraumatic arthrosis will certainly adversely affect rehabilitation and may ultimately require arthrodesis or arthroplasty. In some instances, especially in injuries about the elbow or hip or in patients with neurologic injuries, there may be significant heterotopic bone formation despite prophylactic treatment with antiinflammatory medication (e.g., indomethacin). Heterotopic bone may require excision, which cannot be performed before this bone has a mature trabecular pattern as seen on radiographs. This may take more than 1 year from the time of injury and clearly will adversely affect joint motion and the rehabilitation of the limb.

Compound fractures in general, and particularly in the tibia, have problems with union related to soft-tissue stripping and devascularization of the fracture site secondary to disruption of both the endosteal and periosteal circulations. Once a healthy soft-tissue envelope has been reestablished, rehabilitation of the limb can begin and range-of-motion and strengthening exercises can be initiated. Depending on comminution, bone loss, or the stability of the fixation, secondary procedures may be needed. Early and close follow-up is required to observe these patients' soft-tissue status.

Weight Bearing

The weight-bearing status of the limb is determined by the amount of comminution and bone loss, the type of fixation, and the progress of healing. Weight bearing may be allowed based on the inherent stability of the fracture and the type of implant considered as a biomechanical construct. For example, a short, oblique-type tibial fracture stabilized with an intramedullary device that has been locked either dynamically or statically permits early weight bearing. A patient with this type of fracture is usually allowed partial weight bearing for 6 to 8 weeks until some evidence of callus formation is visible radiographically; weight-bearing status is then progressed.

At the other end of the spectrum is a severe open fracture, perhaps a type III-B injury with either severe comminution or bone loss requiring free tissue transfer and stabilized initially with an external fixation device. The patient will have had several trips to the operating room during the first 96 hours for irrigation and débridement and usually has soft-tissue coverage within 7 to 10 days of the injury. In this situation, it is 6 weeks before the limb is allowed to be in a dependent position for more than very brief periods. During that time, the patient is non-weight bearing on that extremity. If the soft-tissue envelope is stabilized completely by 6 to 8 weeks, early bone grafting is preferred. The patient's weight-bearing status usually progresses to toe-touch weight bearing after the acute recovery from the bone graft procedure, and monthly radiographs are obtained to observe the progression of fracture healing. Once adequate consolidation of the bone graft is noticed on radiographs, the patient progresses to partial weight bearing, and perhaps the external fixator is removed and a cast applied. (The external fixator could also be used for definitive stabilization of the fracture and the fixator dynamized.) In general, it is hoped that bony union will have occurred by 6 to 8 months. It is not unusual, however, for such a fracture to take 1 year to heal. This would be the best-case scenario for an injury of this severity; in the worst case, the patient contracts an infection that might require multiple débridements and bone excision with either massive bone grafting or bone transport using ring fixators, or subsequent amputation.

Rehabilitation Outcome

The rehabilitation outcome of compound fractures usually is delayed compared with uncomplicated fractures. The patient frequently does not regain muscle strength and joint range of motion to his or her pretrauma level. With loss of muscle bulk and muscle damage, there is loss of strength; muscle shortening and scarring may also occur. Contractures lead to shortening of the tendons and ligaments, leading in turn to decreased range of motion. Joint capsule tightness also leads to decreased range of motion. Prolonged immobilization secondary to myoplastic and bone procedures and external fixation devices crossing joints usually causes joint stiffness, disuse atrophy of the muscle, and weakness. Secondary to neural compromise or nerve damage, the patient may permanently need to use a brace or orthosis for ambulation (e.g., a leaf brace in cases of foot drop).

Loss of bone may lead to shortening of the limb, which in turn causes limping. The origin and insertion points of the muscle may come closer together, resulting in muscle weakness and inefficiency in muscle contraction. To normalize the gait pattern, shoe lifts should be considered for limb-length discrepancy.

CONCLUSION

The management of patients with severe compound fractures is a challenging, labor-intensive, time-consuming process that involves careful planning from the management of the acute injury through the reconstructive and rehabilitative phases. These patients often have multiple injuries that adversely affect the rehabilitation of any one injury—and the patient in general. At the time of injury, it is important for the orthopaedist to plan carefully for a management strategy that will not burn any bridges but will also, ideally, provide definitive treatment at the time of injury. It is not always possible to provide definite skeletal fixation with the initial stabilization procedure, and there should be a clear plan for the stages of reconstruction of the limb. It is essential to communicate effectively with patients and their families about the gravity of their injuries and the significant risk of infection and perhaps the loss of the limb. Patients often get depressed and discouraged because of the multiple procedures required, and psychiatric intervention is frequently necessary.

BIBLIOGRAPHY

Bach AW, Hansen ST Jr. Plate versus external fixation in severe open tibial shaft fractures: a randomized trial. *Clin Orthop*, 241:89–94, 1989.

Chapman MW. Role of bone stability in open fractures. *Instr Course Lect*, 3:75–87, 1982.

Gustilo RB, Anderson JT. Prevention of infection in the treatment of one thousand and twenty-five open fractures of long bones. *J Bone Joint Surg Am*, 58:453–458, 1976.

Hansen ST Jr. The type IIIC tibial fracture: salvage or amputation [Editorial]. *J Bone Joint Surg Am*, 69:799–800, 1988.

Llowe DW, Hansen ST Jr. Immediate nailing of open fractures of the femoral shaft. *J Bone Joint Surg Am*, 70:812–819, 1988.

Moed BR, Kellam JF, Foster RJ, et al. Immediate internal fixation of open fractures of the diaphysis of the forearm. *J Bone Joint Surg Am*, 68:1008–1017, 1986.

CHAPTER *Ten*

Clavicle Fractures

RICARDO F. GAUDINEZ, MD

STANLEY HOPPENFELD, MD

CONTRIBUTIONS BY MARK A. THOMAS, MD

INTRODUCTION

Definition

There is more than one accepted classification for clavicle fractures. The following is Craig's classification:

Group I—fracture of the middle one third (most clavicular fractures are group I fractures; Figures 10-1 and 10-2)

Group II—fracture of the lateral or distal one third (Figure 10-3)

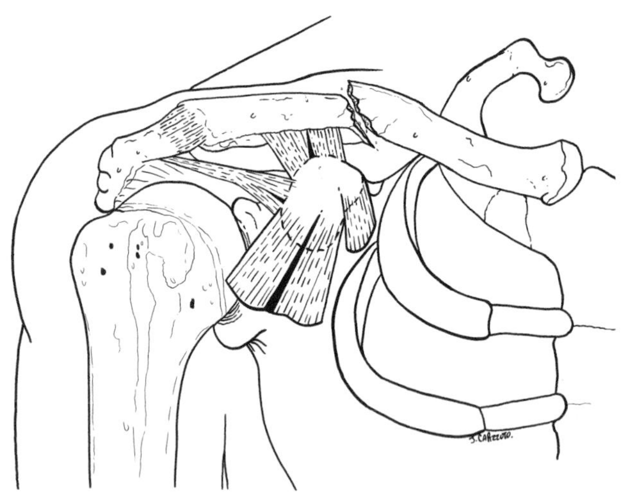

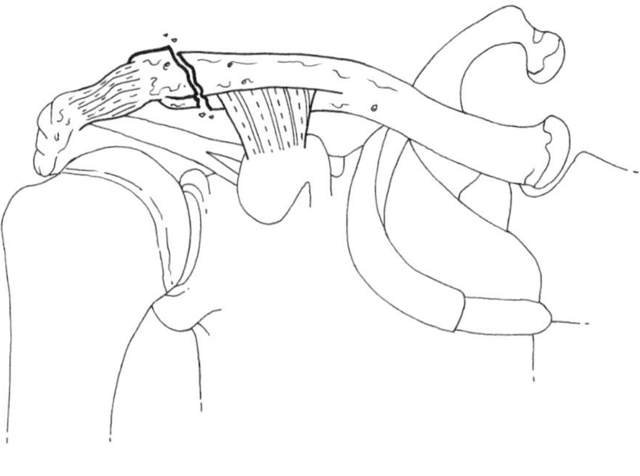

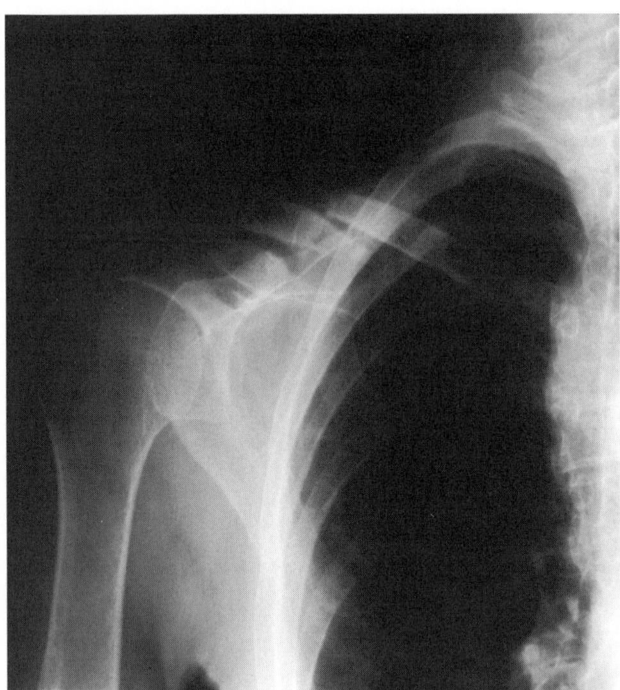

FIGURE 10-1 *(above left)* Fracture of the middle one third of the right clavicle with minimum displacement. This is the most common clavicular fracture.

FIGURE 10-2 *(left)* Radiograph of fracture of the middle one third of the clavicle. Note the displacement. This is best treated with a sling. The neurovascular bundle running immediately beneath the fracture is rarely involved.

FIGURE 10-3 *(above right)* Fracture of the distal one third of the clavicle. There is minimum displacement. The coraco-clavicular ligament is intact, which prevents displacement.

Type I—minimally displaced

Type II—displaced secondary to a fracture medial to the coracoclavicular ligament complex

Type III—fracture of the articular surface

Type IV—ligaments intact to the periosteum, with displacement of the proximal fragment

Type V—comminuted

Group III—fracture of the medial one third

Type I—minimally displaced

Type II—displaced

Type III—intraarticular

Type IV—epiphyseal separation

Type V—comminuted

Fractures of the distal clavicle (lateral one third) are further subclassified into three types by Neer:

Type I—lateral to the coracoclavicular ligament complex, and thus stable.

Type II—medial to the coracoclavicular ligaments, leaving the distal clavicle and the acromioclavicular joint intact but separate from the underlying coracoclavicular ligament complex. These are associated with increased risk of nonunion.

Type III—involving the articular surface of the distal portion of the clavicle. These are usually associated with major ligamentous disruption (Figure 10-4).

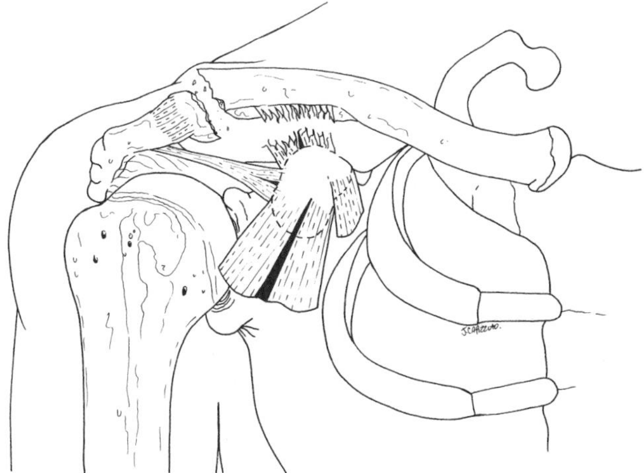

FIGURE 10-4 Fracture of the lateral or distal one third of the clavicle with disruption of the coracoclavicular ligament. This allows the medial end of the fracture to displace, which causes tenting of the skin.

Mechanism of Injury

Most clavicle fractures are caused by a fall or other direct trauma to the shoulder, usually with the clavicle bending and breaking over the fulcrum of the first rib. Falls on an outstretched hand, although commonly cited, account for a smaller percentage of clavicle fractures.

Treatment Goals

Orthopaedic Objectives

Alignment

Achieve anteroposterior and lateral alignment of the fracture because the clavicle is a curvilinear bone.

Stability

Stability is achieved by means of external immobilization for most fractures or, less commonly, by open reduction and internal fixation for more difficult fractures.

Rehabilitation Objectives

Range of Motion

Restore and improve the range of motion of the shoulder (Table 10-1).

TABLE 10-1 *Shoulder Range of Motion*[a]

Motion	Normal	Functional[b]
Abduction	180°	120°
Adduction	45°	30°
Flexion (forward elevation)[c]	180°	120°
Extension (posterior elevation)[d]	60°	40°
Internal rotation with arm at side	70°	30°
External rotation with arm at side	80°	45°
Internal rotation with arm in abduction	65–70°	50°
External rotation with arm in abduction	10°	50°

[a]The clavicle has very little motion. Most of it occurs in rotation as the arm is abducted and externally rotated above the level of the shoulder. The clavicle acts as a strut to keep the shoulder girdle from rolling in.

[b]One third to one half of the full range of motion is considered functional.

[c]To reach maximal flexion or forward elevation, slight abduction and external rotation are required.

[d]To reach maximal extension or posterior elevation, slight internal rotation is required.

Muscle Strength

Improve the strength of the following muscles:

Sternocleidomastoid (neck rotation)
Pectoralis major (arm adduction)
Deltoid (arm abduction)

Functional Goals

Improve and restore the function of the shoulder for activities of daily living and vocational and sports activities.

Expected Time of Bone Healing

Six to 12 weeks. A longer period of healing is required if there is significant comminution or if bone grafting is required.

Expected Duration of Rehabilitation

Ten to 12 weeks.

Methods of Treatment

Sling or Supportive Immobilization

Biomechanics: Stress-sharing device.

Mode of Bone Healing: Secondary, with callus formation.

Indications: This is the method of choice for most clavicle fractures. Many comparisons of plain sling treatment to figure-of-eight bracing in adults have shown no difference. However, figure-of-eight bracing can lead to skin breakdown as well as neurovascular compromise in the axillary region (Figure 10-5).

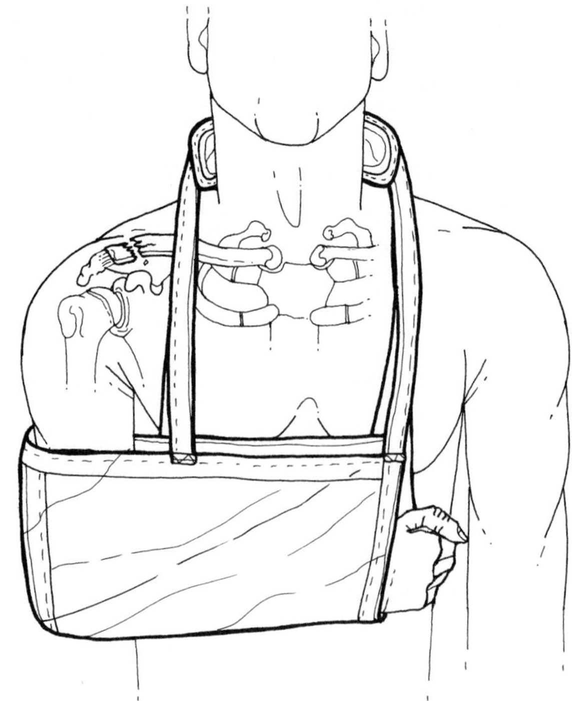

FIGURE 10-5 Sling immobilization. This is the method of choice for most clavicular fractures.

Open Reduction and Internal Fixation

Biomechanics: Stress-shielding with plate and screw fixation; stress-sharing with pin fixation.

Mode of Bone Healing: Primary, unless rigid fixation is not achieved with plate fixation; secondary with pin fixation.

Indications: Open reduction and internal fixation is the method of choice for open fractures, cases of multitrauma, fractures associated with neurovascular compromise requiring immediate exploration, fractures that tent the skin (especially in patients with head injuries or neurologic disorders), and completely displaced fractures of the middle one third in selected patients. In addition, Neer type II distal clavicle fractures are best treated open, either with Kirschner wire or suture loop fixation. This type of fixation is otherwise rarely used (Figure 10-6).

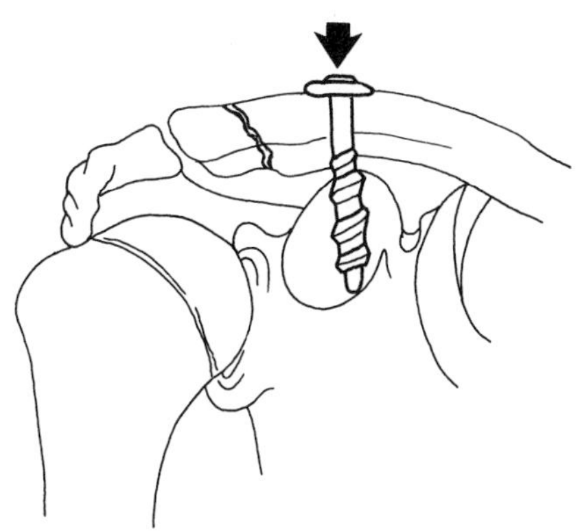

FIGURE 10-6 Fracture of the lateral one third of the clavicle with disruption of the coracoclavicular ligament, treated with a Bosworth screw.

Special Considerations of the Fracture

Age

Elderly patients are at greater risk for development of joint stiffness secondary to the fracture and its treatment.

Articular Involvement

Neer type III lateral distal clavicle fractures are associated with posttraumatic degenerative changes, few of which benefit from a distal clavicle resection.

Delayed Union and Nonunion

Although delayed union and nonunion are uncommon, the risk increases with high-energy injuries, high degrees of displacement, open fractures, and soft-tissue (trapezius) interposition at the fracture site. The middle third of the clavicle, a region almost devoid of cancellous bone and muscle coverage and subject to the most pronounced bending and rotational stress, is at highest risk. Delayed union also occurs with Neer type II lateral third fractures or with open reduction and internal fixation secondary to periosteal stripping.

Cosmetic Deformity and Malunion

Angulation, displacement, or shortening are common after closed management of clavicle fractures. Cosmetic deformity alone is not an indication for corrective osteotomy. Scars from open reductions are often noticeable and frequently noncosmetic.

Pin Migration

Clavicle fractures treated with intramedullary devices are at risk for pin migration, particularly if smooth pins are used. If the patient starts mobilization too early, these devices can break. Most surgeons prefer plate fixation for this reason.

Associated Injury

1. Bony injuries associated with these fractures include scapular fractures, especially after high-energy injuries, and rib fractures.
2. The acromioclavicular and sternoclavicular joints should be evaluated. Pneumothorax, although rare, can be secondary to a puncture from a clavicle fracture or concurrent rib fractures.

Neurovascular Injuries

The subclavian artery and vein are at risk with clavicle fractures. Abnormal vascular findings or an ipsilateral asymmetric bruit warrants further vascular investigation, usually arteriography. Brachial plexus injuries can be secondary to direct trauma or stretch, leading to neuropraxia (stretch) or neurotmesis (lacerations). The middle cord of the brachial plexus is especially at risk because of its proximity to the overlying clavicle and the underlying first rib. Both of these injuries are uncommon.

Weight Bearing

Weight bearing is not permitted.

Gait

Arm swing is reduced.

TREATMENT

Treatment: Early to Immediate (Day of Injury to One Week)

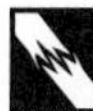

BONE HEALING

Stability at fracture site: None.

Stage of bone healing: Inflammatory phase. The fracture hematoma is colonized by inflammatory cells, and débridement of the fracture begins.

X-ray: No callus.

Orthopaedic and Rehabilitation Considerations

Physical Examination

Check for capillary refill, sensation, and the active and passive range of motion of the affected extremity, including the elbow, wrist, and digits. Instruct the patient to elevate the extremity if there is swelling. Evaluate any incision site for drainage, erythema, fluctuance, or other signs of infection. Evaluate the patient's neurovascular status with a thorough brachial plexus assessment. Check the sling for proper fit and padding at the axillary area and back of the neck. The arm should be in internal rotation and the elbow should be in approximately 90 degrees of flexion, with free movement of the digits and wrist to prevent stiffness.

Dangers

Check for excessive swelling. Dependent edema and skin discoloration are common, with resultant sausage-shaped digits. Check for excessive skin tenting and possible skin breakdown over the fracture site, although this is uncommon.

Radiography

Anteroposterior, 45-degree cephalic, and 45-degree caudal tilt radiographic views are recommended to evaluate the degree of displacement and angulation.

For fractures of the distal one third of the clavicle, also recommended is an anteroposterior view of both shoulders with 10 pounds of weight suspended from each wrist to assess for concomitant ligamentous injury.

Shortening of the clavicle greater than 17 mm is associated with abduction weakness.

Articular fractures of the clavicle may require tomography or computed tomography scanning.

Check for displacement and angulation. Compare later radiographs with immediate postreduction or postoperative radiographs. In open reduction and internal fixation, check for loss of correction, angulation, displacement, or pin migration.

Weight Bearing

No weight bearing on the affected extremity.

Range of Motion

The shoulder is held in adduction and internal rotation. Range of motion of the shoulder is avoided. The elbow is maintained at 90 degrees of flexion if a sling is used. Full, active range of motion is encouraged to the wrist, hand, and digits.

Muscle Strength

Because exercise is too painful, no strengthening exercises are given to the shoulder.

Begin gentle isometric exercises to the elbow and wrist 3 to 4 days after the fracture, once the pain subsides. Active flexion and extension of the elbow is encouraged to maintain the strength of the biceps and triceps.

Functional Activities

Dressing: The patient needs assistance in upper extremity dressing because of shoulder immobilization. The patient can don a shirt or blouse on the unaffected extremity and drape it over the affected extremity.

Personal hygiene: Self-care activities are performed with the uninvolved extremity.

Bed mobility: The patient is instructed to roll over to the unaffected side to come to a sitting position in bed. The patient may initially feel more comfortable sleeping in a reclining chair.

Methods of Treatment: Specific Aspects

Sling

Check for the proper fit of the sling or figure-of-eight brace.

Open Reduction and Internal Fixation

Check the wound for erythema, discharge, or purulence. Begin gentle shoulder pendulum exercises 3 to 5 days after stable fixation.

Prescription

DAY ONE TO ONE WEEK

Precautions Shoulder is held in adduction and internal rotation. Elbow is maintained at 90 degrees of flexion.

Range of Motion No range of motion to the shoulder.

Muscle Strength No strengthening exercises to the shoulder.

Functional Activities The uninvolved extremity is used in self-care and personal hygiene.

Weight bearing None.

Treatment: Two Weeks

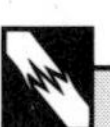

BONE HEALING

Stability at fracture site: None to minimal.

Stage of bone healing: Beginning of reparative phase. Osteoprogenitor cells differentiate into osteoblasts, which lay down woven bone.

X-ray: None to early callus; fracture line is visible.

Orthopaedic and Rehabilitation Considerations

Physical Examination

Check the range of motion of the shoulder and elbow. Check the brachial plexus distribution for any neurologic deficits. Check the sling for comfort and check for skin abrasions. Pad the sling appropriately, especially around the neck. The elbow should be at 90 degrees of flexion, and the shoulder in internal rotation. There should be full range of motion of the wrist and digits.

Radiography

Check radiographs for angulation and displacement; compare them with previous radiographs. Check for possible pin migration in open reduction and internal fixation cases.

Weight Bearing

No weight bearing on the affected extremity.

Range of Motion

Continue range of motion of the elbow, as well as the wrist, hand, and digits. Start gentle pendulum exercises to the shoulder as tolerated. Active range of motion is allowed at the wrist and digits.

Muscle Strength

Continue isometric exercises of the elbow and wrist and begin isotonic exercises to the digits. Begin isometric deltoid strengthening.

Functional Activities

The uninvolved extremity is used for hygiene and self-care. The patient needs assistance in dressing and still needs to drape the affected extremity.

Methods of Treatment: Specific Aspects

Sling

Check for the proper fit of the sling or figure-of-eight brace and adjust as necessary. Check that skin is not tented over the fracture site.

Open Reduction and Internal Fixation

Remove any staples or sutures. Check the wound for evidence of erythema, drainage, or induration.

Prescription

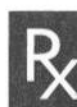

TWO WEEKS

Precautions Shoulder is held in adduction and internal rotation. Elbow is held at 90 degrees of flexion.

Range of Motion Gentle pendulum exercises to the shoulder in the sling as pain permits.

Muscle Strength No strengthening exercises to the shoulder. Start gentle isometric exercises to the deltoid.

Functional Activities The uninvolved extremity is used in self-care and personal hygiene.

Weight bearing None.

Treatment: Four to Six Weeks

BONE HEALING

Stability at fracture site: With bridging callus, the fracture is usually stable; confirm with physical examination.

Stage of bone healing: Reparative phase. There is further organization of the callus, and formation of lamellar bone begins. However, the strength of the callus, especially with torsional load, is significantly lower than that of normal bone. Further protection of bone (if not further immobilization) is required to avoid refracture.

X-ray: Bridging callus is visible. Fracture line is less distinct.

Orthopaedic and Rehabilitation Considerations

Physical Examination

Assess for paresthesias due to pressure from a hypertrophic malunion on the subclavian vessels or on the brachial plexus (secondary to the callus).

Check the fracture site for tenderness and stability.

Continue the sling if the fracture site is tender or if there is motion on palpation. If the fracture site is nontender, without motion, and with abundant callus, discontinue the sling.

Contact sports should be avoided for approximately 2 more months.

Dangers

Assess for paresthesias due to pressure from hypertrophic malunion or nonunion on the brachial plexus or subclavian vessels.

Check for reflex sympathetic dystrophy (RSD), characterized by trophic changes, vasomotor disturbances, hyperesthesia, pain, and tenderness out of proportion to the stage of fracture healing. RSD requires aggressive therapy. It is a rare occurrence with clavicular fractures.

Radiography

Check radiographs for additional callus and the disappearance of the fracture line.

Weight Bearing

No weight bearing on the affected extremity. Patients who use a walker for ambulation may benefit from a hemiwalker or a quad cane, using the unaffected extremity.

Range of Motion

At the end of 6 weeks, once there is good callus formation and the fracture site is stable, the sling is removed. Gentle active range of motion to the shoulder is allowed. Care is taken to limit abduction to 80 degrees and external rotation to avoid stress on the fracture site. Elbow flexion and extension are allowed to full range. Initially, there may be limitations in elbow extension secondary to immobilization. Continue with wrist and digit range of motion.

Muscle Strength

At the end of 6 weeks, start rotator cuff strengthening exercises and continue isometric exercises to the elbow flexors and extensors. Pendulum exercises are prescribed to the shoulder with gravity eliminated.

Maintain wrist flexor and extensor strength. Silly Putty exercises are given to maintain the patient's grip and grasp.

Functional Activities

The patient can don a shirt with the affected extremity first and doff it from the unaffected extremity first.

Methods of Treatment: Specific Aspects

Sling

No significant changes.

Open Reduction and Internal Fixation

Look for infection at the suture line.

Prescription

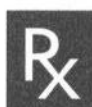

FOUR TO SIX WEEKS

Precautions Limit abduction.

Range of Motion At the end of 6 weeks, gentle active range of motion to the shoulder is allowed. Abduction is limited to 80 degrees.

Muscle Strength Pendulum exercises are prescribed to the shoulder with gravity elimination. Start isometric exercises to the rotator cuff and deltoids.

Functional Activities The patient uses the affected extremity for some self-care and personal hygiene.

Weight bearing None.

Treatment: Six to Eight Weeks

BONE HEALING

Stability at fracture site: With bridging callus, the fracture is usually stable; confirm with physical examination.

Stage of bone healing: Reparative phase. There is further organization of callus, and formation of lamellar bone continues.

X-ray: Bridging callus is more apparent. Fracture line is less distinct.

Orthopaedic and Rehabilitation Considerations

Physical Examination

Ensure that the patient is regaining adequate range of motion without crepitus at the fracture site. If brachial plexus palsy is still present, consider an electromyographic evaluation.

Dangers

Check for possible RSD.

Radiography

If the fracture is clinically and radiographically healed at 4 to 6 weeks, no new radiographs are needed. If it is not, repeat radiographs to check for further bony union and consider open reduction and internal fixation and bone grafting if the patient's pain persists.

Weight Bearing

If the fracture is clinically and radiographically healed, the patient may begin gradual weight bearing when pushing off from a chair or bed or using axillary crutches or a cane.

Range of Motion

Continue range of motion to the shoulder in all planes until satisfactory range is achieved.

Strength

Begin resistive strengthening of the shoulder girdle. The patient can use the unaffected extremity to offer resistance while flexing and extending the affected extremity at the shoulder joint.

Functional Activities

The patient may use the involved extremity for hygiene and self-care as well as for light activities.

Methods of Treatment: Specific Aspects

Sling

No change. The sling may be discontinued, if this has not already been done.

Open Reduction and Internal Fixation

No change.

Prescription

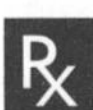

SIX TO EIGHT WEEKS

Precautions None. Avoid contact sports.

Range of Motion Active to active-assistive range of motion in all planes.

Muscle Strength Resistive exercises to the shoulder girdle muscles.

Functional Activities The patient uses the involved extremity for personal hygiene, self-care, stabilization, and light activities.

Weight bearing Gradual weight bearing is allowed.

Treatment: Eight to Twelve Weeks

BONE HEALING

Stability at fracture site: Stable.

Stage of bone healing: Remodeling phase. There is further organization of the callus, and formation of lamellar bone continues.

X-ray: Bridging callus is very visible. The fracture line becomes even less distinct.

Orthopaedic and Rehabilitation Considerations

Physical Examination

Check for tenderness or motion at the fracture site. Callus is easily palpable because this is a subcutaneous bone. Assess improvements in range of motion and strength. Check for resolution of RSD and the status of any existing ulnar nerve deficits (a branch of the medial cord of the brachial plexus).

Dangers

None.

Radiography

If the fracture was clinically and radiographically united at the last visit, no additional radiographs are needed.

Weight Bearing

Full weight bearing is allowed.

Range of Motion

There may be some limitations in forward shoulder elevation. Gentle stretching may be necessary. Active, active-assistive, and passive range-of-motion exercises are prescribed. Abduction is encouraged.

Muscle Strength

Continue progressive resistive exercises to the shoulder. The resistance is gradually increased. The patient can also use graded weights to improve strength. Continue with isometric and isotonic exercises to the shoulder girdle muscles, pectoralis major, and sternocleidomastoid.

Functional Activities

The patient should use the affected extremity for all activities of self-care, hygiene, feeding, grooming, and dressing.

Methods of Treatment: Specific Aspects

Sling

The sling is removed.

Open Reduction and Internal Fixation

Consider removing pins if they are protruding. All smooth pins must be removed to prevent their migration.

Prescription

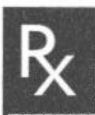

EIGHT TO TWELVE WEEKS

Precautions None.

Range of Motion Active, active-assistive range of motion to the shoulder. Abduction is encouraged.

Muscle Strength Isometric and isotonic exercises are prescribed to the shoulder girdle muscles. Resistive exercises are prescribed.

Functional Activities The involved extremity is used in self-care and functional activities.

Weight bearing Full weight bearing.

LONG-TERM CONSIDERATIONS AND PROBLEMS

The patient should not return to noncontact sports until a painless, full range of motion is present, the fracture is healed, and near-normal strength is restored. This usually requires more than 6 weeks. Contact sports place the clavicle at even greater risk for refracture and should be delayed until the union is solid, at least 4 to 6 months.

Traumatic arthritis at the acromioclavicular joint is a concern, especially if there has been any dislocation at the joint. Resection of the outer portion of the clavicle may be necessary.

Removal of the plate and screws may be necessary if they are causing pain or tenting of the skin.

Nonunion, if it is causing pain, may be treated with bone grafting and internal fixation.

Frequently, it takes years for the large callus to remodel and be less visible cosmetically.

IMMEDIATE TO ONE WEEK

	Nonoperative	*Open Reduction and Internal Fixation*
Stability	None.	Depends on the fixation.
Orthopaedics	Check proper fitting of sling or figure-of-eight brace.	Check wound and proper fitting of sling.
Rehabilitation	Avoid range of motion to the shoulder. Begin active range of motion to elbow, wrist, hand, and digits. Begin isometric exercises to elbow and wrist 3 to 4 days after the fracture, once the pain subsides.	Begin gentle shoulder pendulum exercises and active range of motion of elbow, wrist, hand, and digits. Begin isometric exercises to elbow and wrist as comfort allows.

TWO WEEKS

	Nonoperative	Open Reduction and Internal Fixation
Stability	None to minimal.	Depends on the fixation.
Orthopaedics	Check sling or brace for comfort and pad appropriately. Check that skin is not tented.	Remove sutures. Check sling for comfort and pad appropriately.
Rehabilitation	Start shoulder pendulum exercises, isometric exercises to elbow and wrist, and isotonic exercises to digits. Begin isometric exercises to the deltoid.	Same as for nonoperative.

FOUR TO SIX WEEKS

	Nonoperative	Open Reduction and Internal Fixation
Stability	Partially stable.	Stable.
Orthopaedics	Remove sling or brace.	Remove sling.
	Consider open reduction and internal fixation and bone grafting if not clinically and radiologically healed by 6 weeks.	Consider bone grafting if not radiographically healed by 6 weeks.
Rehabilitation	Start range of motion to shoulder; continue elbow and wrist exercises. Continue deltoid and rotator cuff isometric strengthening.	Same as for nonoperative.

SIX TO EIGHT WEEKS

	Nonoperative	Open Reduction and Internal Fixation
Stability	Stable.	Stable.
Orthopaedics	Discontinue sling. Ensure the patient is gaining adequate range of motion without crepitus at the fracture site.	Same as for nonoperative.
Rehabilitation	Full range of motion to shoulder. Begin resistive strengthening exercises to the shoulder girdle muscles.	Same as for nonoperative.

EIGHT TO TWELVE WEEKS

	Nonoperative	Open Reduction and Internal Fixation
Stability	Stable.	Stable.
Orthopaedics	Consider open reduction and internal fixation and bone grafting if not clinically and radiologically healed.	Consider bone grafting if not radiographically healed.
Rehabilitation	Continue resistive shoulder exercises.	Continue resistive shoulder exercises.

BIBLIOGRAPHY

Abbott LC, Lucas DB. The function of the clavicle: its surgical significance. *Ann Surg*, 140:583–599, 1954.

Allman FL. Fractures and ligamentous injuries of the clavicle and its articulation. *J Bone Joint Surg Am*, 49:774–784, 1967.

Anderson K, Jensen PO, Lauritzen J. Treatment of clavicular fractures: figure-of-eight bandages vs. a simple sling. *Acta Orthop Scand*, 57:71–74, 1987.

Andrews JR, Wilk KE. *The Athlete's Shoulder.* New York: Churchill Livingstone, 1995, pp. 291–303.

Bargar WL, Marcus RE, Ittleman FP. Late thoracic outlet syndrome secondary to pseudoarthrosis of the clavicle. *J Trauma*, 24: 857–859, 1984.

Bowen AD. Plastic bowing of the clavicle in children: a report of two cases. *J Bone Joint Surg Am*, 65:403–405, 1983.

Cohen AW, Otto SR. Obstetric clavicular fractures. *J Reprod Med*, 25:119–122, 1980.

Connolly JF, Dehne R. Nonunion of the clavicle and thoracic outlet syndrome. *J Trauma*, 29:1127–1132, 1989.

Craig EV. Fractures of the clavicle. In: Rockwood CA Jr, Matsen FA III, eds. *The Shoulder*. Philadelphia: W.B. Saunders, 1990, pp. 367–412.

Curtis RJ Jr. Operative treatment of children's fractures of the shoulder region. *Orthop Clin North Am*, 21:315–324, 1990.

Dameron TB Jr, Rockwood CA Jr. Fractures of the shaft of the clavicle. In: Wilkins KE, King RE, eds. *Fractures in Children*. Philadelphia: J.B. Lippincott, 1984, pp. 608–624.

CHAPTER *Eleven*

Proximal Humeral Fractures

RICARDO F. GAUDINEZ, MD

VASANTHA L. MURTHY, MD

STANLEY HOPPENFELD, MD

INTRODUCTION

Definition

Fractures of the proximal end of the humerus involve the humeral head, anatomic neck, and surgical neck of the humerus.

Neer's classification system categorizes these fractures as one-, two-, three-, or four-part fractures based on the displacement and angulation of the parts, which are the head, shaft, greater tuberosity, and lesser tuberosity in the proximal humerus. Displacement of the fracture exceeding 1 cm or angulation of more than 45 degrees constitutes a part or displaced fracture. Fractures that are nondisplaced or angulated less than 45 degrees are considered a one-part fracture. Fractures may have associated dislocations.

A one-part fracture may be an impacted or a nondisplaced fracture. A two-part fracture may be a displaced tuberosity fracture or a displaced/angulated surgical neck fracture. A three-part fracture involves displacement/angulation of the head and shaft with involvement of either the greater or lesser tuberosities. A four-part fracture involves displacement/angulation of all four parts: head, shaft, and greater and lesser tuberosities.

Greater tuberosity fractures with more than 1 cm of displacement are usually associated with rotator cuff tears (Figures 11-1, 11-2, 11-3, 11-4, 11-5, 11-6, and 11-7).

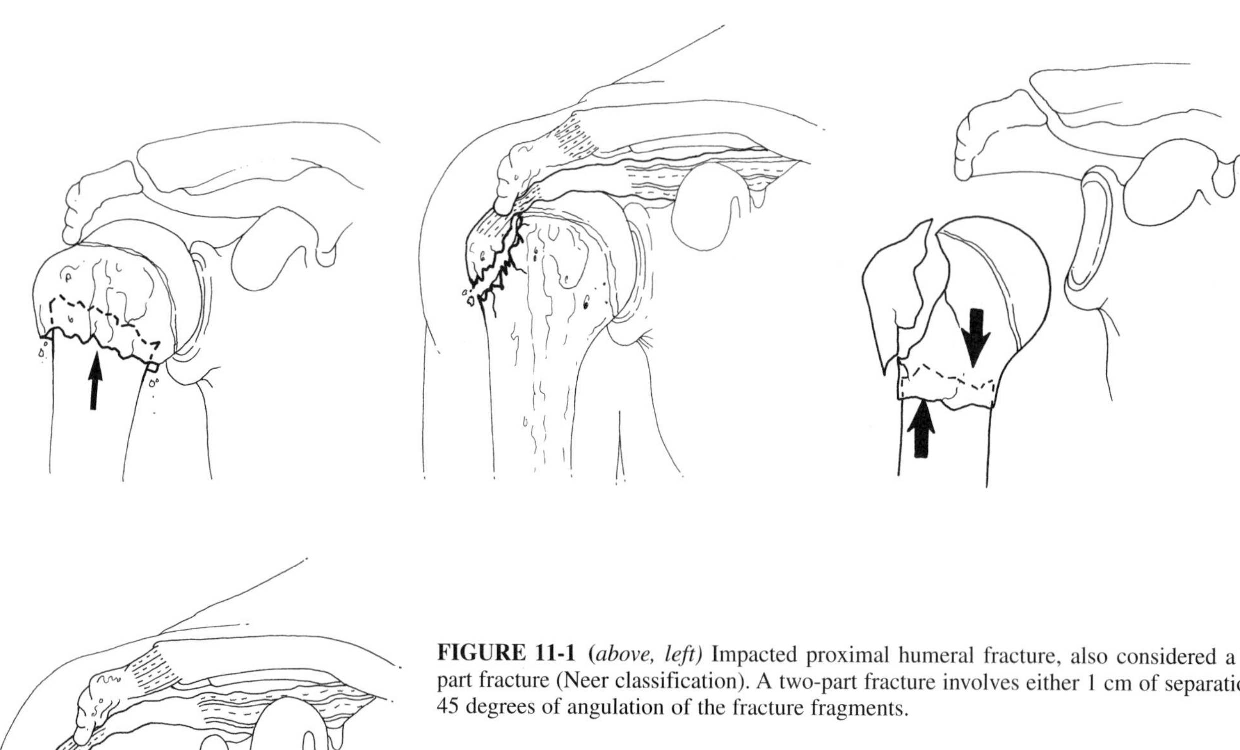

FIGURE 11-1 *(above, left)* Impacted proximal humeral fracture, also considered a one-part fracture (Neer classification). A two-part fracture involves either 1 cm of separation or 45 degrees of angulation of the fracture fragments.

FIGURE 11-2 *(above, middle)* Displaced fracture of the greater tuberosity, also considered a two-part fracture. Rotator cuff injury may occur with this fracture pattern.

FIGURE 11-3 *(above, right)* Three-part fracture of the proximal humerus: one part is the head separated from the shaft at the surgical neck, the second part the shaft, and the third part the greater tuberosity.

FIGURE 11-4 *(left)* Four-part fracture of the proximal humerus. One part is the shaft, the second part the head, the third and fourth parts the greater and lesser tuberosities. The head is left without a blood supply and becomes prone to avascular necrosis.

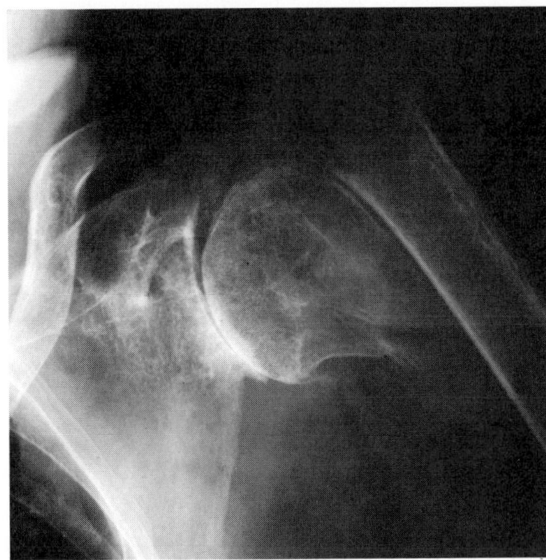

FIGURE 11-5 Two-part fracture of the proximal humerus through the surgical neck with obvious displacement. One part is the head and anatomic neck, the second the displaced shaft of the humerus.

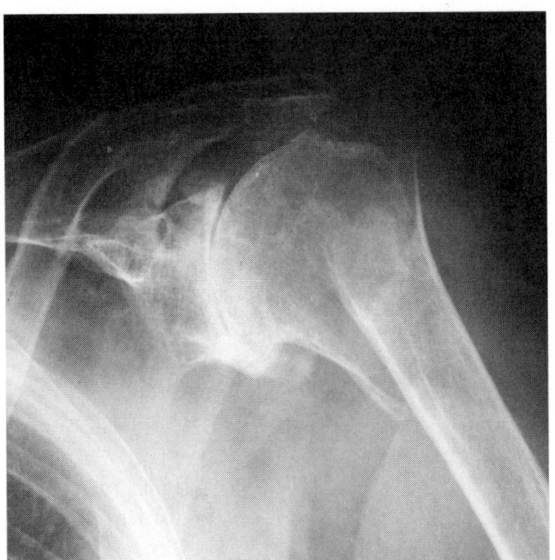

FIGURE 11-6 The same two-part fracture as in Figure 11-5, with partial reduction of the shaft to the surgical neck.

Mechanism of Injury

Proximal humeral fractures can be caused by a fall on an elbow or an outstretched hand, especially in an elderly patient, or by trauma to the lateral aspects of the shoulder. Seizures can occasionally result in fracture/dislocation of the shoulder.

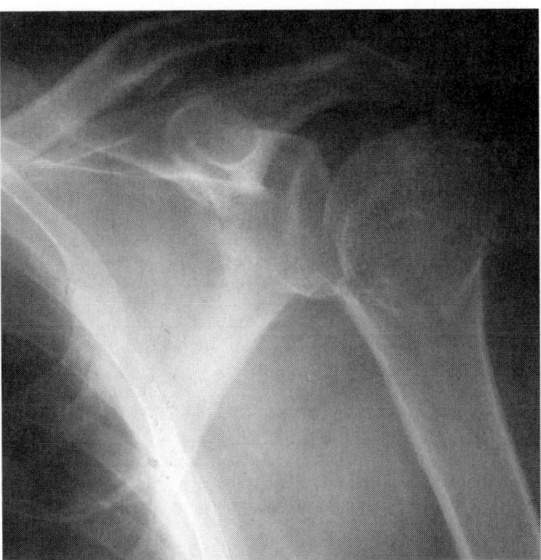

FIGURE 11-7 A three-part fracture of the proximal humerus, with displacement of the head from the shaft and the greater tuberosity from the other two parts.

Treatment Goals

Orthopaedic Objectives

Alignment

Maintain a normal relationship between the humeral head and the glenoid.

Reduce the greater and lesser tuberosities to maintain rotator cuff function.

Obtain a neck shaft angle of 130 to 150 degrees and a retroversion angle of 30 degrees.

Stability

Stability is achieved by means of external immobilization for nondisplaced stable fractures, by internal fixation (open or percutaneous) for displaced two-part or three-part fractures, and by endoprosthesis for four-part fractures.

Rehabilitation Objectives

Range of Motion

Restore the full range of motion of the shoulder in all planes. Frequently, there may be residual loss of range of motion secondary to the fracture (Table 11-1).

TABLE 11-1 *Shoulder Range of Motion*

Motion	Normal	Functional[a]
Abduction	180°	120°
Adduction	45°	30°
Flexion (forward elevation)[b]	180°	120°
Extension (posterior elevation)[c]	60°	40°
Internal rotation with arm at side	100°	80°
External rotation with arm at side	70°	30°
Internal rotation with arm in abduction	80°	45°
External rotation with arm in abduction	90°	45°

[a]One third to one half of the full range of motion is considered functional.

[b]To reach maximal flexion or forward elevation, slight abduction and external rotation are required.

[c]To reach maximal extension or posterior elevation, slight internal rotation is required.

Muscle Strength

Improve the strength of the following muscles and attempt to regain full strength against maximum resistance. Residual loss of strength, especially of the deltoid muscles, 4/5 (5/5 is full strength), may occur frequently (see Chapter 4, Therapeutic Exercise and Range of Motion, Table 4-1) (Table 11-2).

Flexors:

Anterior portion of deltoid (inserts into the deltoid tubercle)

Coracobrachialis (weak flexor of the arm, inserts into the middle of the humerus)

Biceps (originates from the coracoid process, passes through the bicipital groove)

Pectoralis major (clavicular head, inserts into the lateral lip of the bicipital groove)

Shoulder abductors:

Middle portion of the deltoid (inserts into the deltoid tubercle)

Supraspinatus (inserts into the greater tuberosity of the humerus—one of the rotator cuff muscles)

Shoulder adductors:

Pectoralis major (inserts into the lateral lip of the bicipital groove)

Latissimus dorsi (inserts into the floor of the bicipital groove)

Teres major

Shoulder external rotators:

Infraspinatus (inserts into the greater tuberosity of the humerus)

Teres minor (inserts into the greater tuberosity of the humerus)

Posterior portion of the deltoid (inserts into the deltoid tubercle)

Shoulder internal rotators:

Subscapularis (inserts into the lesser tuberosity of the humerus)

Pectoralis major

Latissimus dorsi

Teres major

Shoulder extensors:

Posterior portion of the deltoid

Latissimus dorsi

Rotator cuff:

Supraspinatus

Infraspinatus

Teres minor

Subscapularis

TABLE 11-2 *Shoulder Motion—Prime Movers*

Motion	Prime Movers
Flexion	Anterior deltoid Coracobrachialis
Abduction	Deltoid Supraspinatus
Adduction	Pectoralis major Latissimus dorsi
Extension	Latissimus dorsi Teres major Posterior deltoid
Internal rotation	Subscapularis Pectoralis major Teres major Latissimus dorsi
External rotation	Infraspinatus Teres minor

Functional Goals

Improve and restore the function of the shoulder in self-care, dressing, and grooming. In addition, shoulder movement and strength are vital in almost all sports activities.

Expected Time of Bone Healing

Six to 8 weeks.

Expected Duration of Rehabilitation

Twelve weeks to 1 year.

Methods of Treatment

Sling

Biomechanics: Stress-sharing device.

Mode of Bone Healing: Secondary.

Indications: Nondisplaced, impacted, or minimally displaced proximal humeral fractures usually are immobilized for 2 to 3 weeks until the patient's pain subsides. Eighty-five percent of proximal humeral fractures are minimally displaced.

Open Reduction and Internal Fixation

Biomechanics: Stress shielding with plate fixation; stress sharing for pin or tension band fixation.

Mode of Bone Healing: Primary when rigid fixation is achieved and no callus forms; secondary when rigid fixation is not achieved and callus forms.

Indications: Open reduction and internal fixation is indicated for two- and three-part fractures and those that may also require repair of the rotator cuff (Figures 11-8 and 11-9).

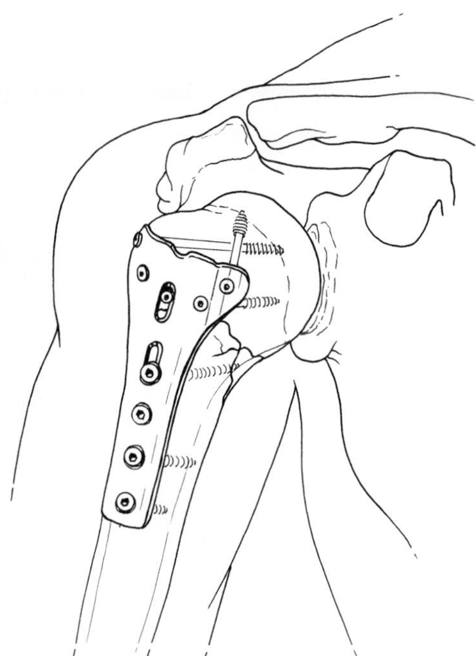

FIGURE 11-8 Plate and screw fixation of a three-part fracture of the proximal humerus. Rigid fixation is achieved and no callus forms.

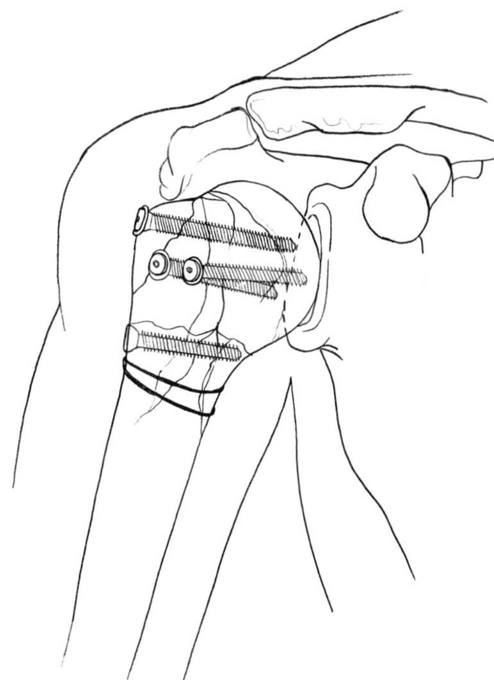

FIGURE 11-9 Screw and wire fixation of a four-part fracture of the proximal humerus. Rigid fixation is not achieved and callus forms.

Closed Reduction and Percutaneous Fixation/Cannulated Screw Tension Banding

Biomechanics: Stress-sharing device.

Mode of Bone Healing: Secondary, with callus formation.

Indications: This method is used for two-part fractures with no significant rotator cuff tears. It is the method of choice for displaced surgical neck fractures (Figure 11-10).

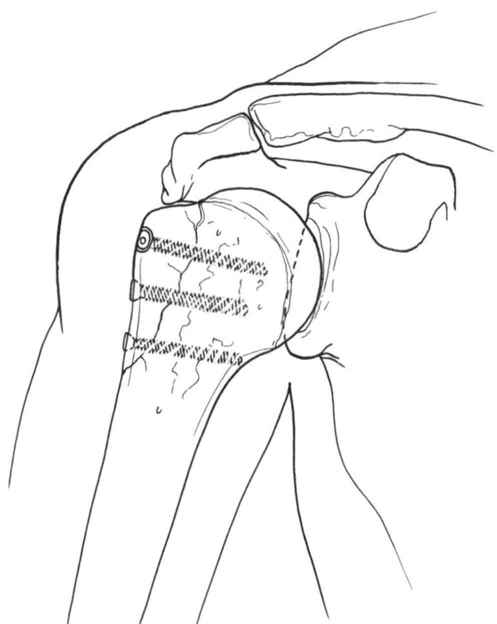

FIGURE 11-10 Screw fixation of a greater tuberosity fracture of the proximal humerus.

Prosthetic Arthroplasty

Biomechanics: Stress-sharing device.

Mode of Bone Healing: Tuberosities heal secondarily, with callus formation.

Indications: This method is indicated for fractures with significant risk of avascular necrosis (four-part fractures, three-part fractures in osteoporotic elderly patients, head-splitting fractures, or head impression fractures greater than 40%). It has the advantage of allowing physical therapy to begin once soft-tissue healing has occurred (Figures 11-11, 11-12, and 11-13).

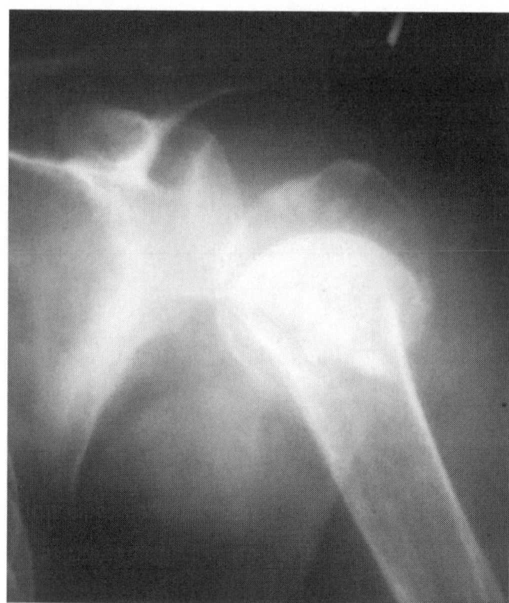

FIGURE 11-11 A four-part fracture of the proximal humerus. Note the rotation and displacement of the four parts.

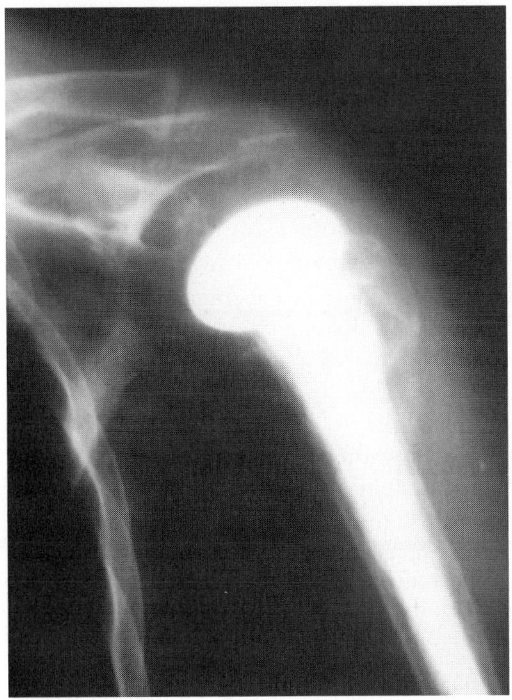

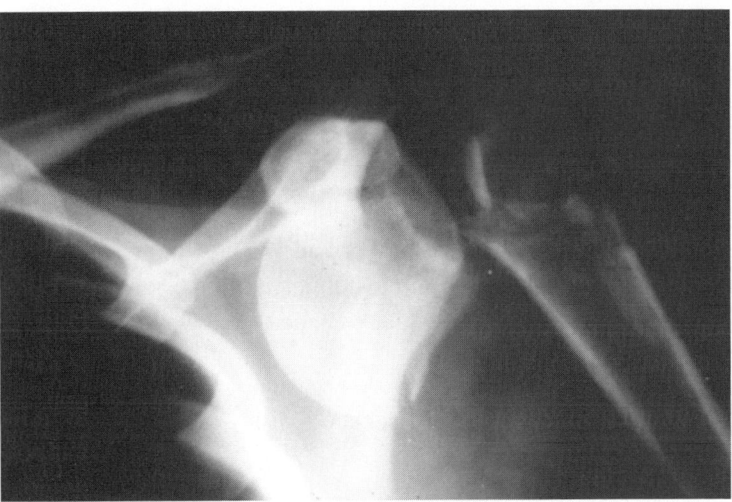

FIGURE 11-12 *(left)* A hemiarthroplasty of the proximal humerus as performed on a four-part fracture of the proximal humerus. (Courtesy of Dr. Louis Bigliani.)

FIGURE 11-13 *(above)* A four-part fracture/dislocation of the proximal humerus with anteroinferior dislocation of the remaining humeral head. The patient required prosthetic replacement and a hemiarthroplasty of the proximal humerus. (Courtesy of Dr. Louis Bigliani.)

Closed Reduction and Immobilization

Biomechanics: Stress-sharing device.
Mode of Bone Healing: Secondary.
Indications: This method of treatment may be used if satisfactory reduction is achieved. However, this rarely occurs, and so this method of treatment is not discussed further.

External Fixator

Biomechanics: Stress-sharing device.
Mode of Bone Healing: Secondary, with callus formation.
Indications: External fixation is used for open and severely comminuted fractures. More rarely, it is indicated for two- or three-part fractures with open wounds and occasionally for two- or three-part fractures extending into the shaft when Kirschner wires cannot be used. This method is not discussed further because it is used infrequently.

Special Considerations of the Fracture

Age

Elderly patients are at greater risk for development of joint stiffness than younger patients.

Articular Involvement

Fractures that split the head of the humerus with greater than 50% involvement of the articular surface may require hemiarthroplasty. Articular indentation of the glenoid fossa predisposes the patient to degenerative changes (*see* Figures 11-4 and 11-11).

Avascular Necrosis

Avascular necrosis can occur after four-part fractures and is seen in anatomic neck fractures as well as fractures with extensive soft-tissue and periosteal stripping.

Malunion/Nonunion

Malunions are well tolerated in these fractures; however, they can develop subacromial impingement. Nonunion is uncommon. It may occur because of soft-tissue interposition or inadequate immobilization.

Associated Injury

Rotator Cuff Tears

Rotator cuff tears are associated with displacement of either tuberosity and require repair (*see* Figure 11-2).

Neurovascular Injuries

Neurovascular injuries are associated with anterior or inferior dislocations. These may involve the axillary nerve or posterior cord of the brachial plexus. Electromyography (EMG) should be considered approximately 3 weeks after the injury because denervation potentials are seen then. Axillary nerve paresthesias are the most common symptoms of nerve injury.

Four-Part Fractures

Four-part fractures may be associated with axillary artery injuries.

Posterior Dislocation

Posterior dislocation may occur with isolated tuberosity fractures.

Weight Bearing

The involved extremity should be non-weight bearing. The patient should avoid supporting the body's weight when using a walker, axillary crutches, or a cane or during push-off from a bed or chair until the fracture is clinically and radiographically united.

Gait

Arm swing is initially absent and may be reduced on a long-term basis.

TREATMENT

Treatment: Early (Day of Injury to One Week)

BONE HEALING

Stability at fracture site: None.

Stage of bone healing: Inflammatory phase. The fracture hematoma is colonized by inflammatory cells, and débridement of the fracture begins.

X-ray: No callus. The fracture line is visible.

Orthopaedic and Rehabilitation Considerations

Physical Examination

Pay special attention to complaints of pain, paresthesia, pin discomfort, drainage, and malodor, all signs of infection. Assess capillary refill, sensation, and active and passive range of motion. Decreased range of motion could be due to swelling. Check all wounds for erythema, discharge, or purulence. Because neurovascular injuries occur in 5% to 30% of complex proximal humerus fractures, reassess sensation, especially along the axillary nerve distribution as well as along the forearm and hand. Check for excessive swelling, skin blisters, and dependent edema of the fingers.

Dangers

Increasing swelling at the shoulder and proximal arm, pallor, and paresthesias may indicate a vascular injury, and angiography should be performed without delay. Carefully examine the neurologic status, both motor and sensory, of the

1. Axillary nerve
2. Musculocutaneous nerve
3. Radial nerve
4. Median nerve
5. Ulnar nerve

Because the axillary nerve is the most susceptible to injury, and an intact sensory examination of the skin overlying the lateral deltoid is not always indicative of an intact axillary nerve, all three slips of the deltoid muscle must be palpated for active contraction. However, immediately after the fracture, the muscle may not be able to contract because of reflex inhibition from pain and direct trauma.

Radiography

Check radiographs (anteroposterior, Y-scapula, and axillary views) for loss of correction and compare them with immediate postreduction or postoperative radiographs. If there is significant displacement, consider performing closed reduction or operative intervention. Expect inferior migration of the humeral head because of deltoid atony.

Weight Bearing

No weight bearing on the affected extremity.

Range of Motion

The shoulder is immobilized in a shoulder immobilizer or sling and no motion is allowed. For stable, nondisplaced fractures, simple pendulum exercises may be started. The elbow is also immobilized by the sling. The patient should be encouraged actively to flex and extend the wrist in the sling and to deviate the wrist radially and ulnarly. Full active range of motion to the digits is prescribed.

Muscle Strength

Sometimes the muscle strength of the deltoid is lost secondary to reflex inhibition even though the axillary nerve is intact. Because the fracture site is unstable, no active contraction of the muscle is allowed. Because of muscle soreness, no strengthening exercises to the shoulder and elbow are prescribed during the immediate phase. At the end of the first week, isometric and isotonic exercises are prescribed to the wrist flexors, extensors, and intrinsic muscles of the hand to maintain strength.

Functional Activities

Patients may use the uninvolved upper extremity for self-care, hygiene, feeding, grooming, and dressing and need assistance initially.

Patients who require a walker for ambulation cannot bear weight on the affected extremity and should be shown how to use a quad cane or hemiwalker.

When dressing, the patient dons clothes on the involved extremity first and doffs them from the uninvolved extremity first. Initially, the patient may don a shirt or blouse with the uninvolved arm first and drape it over the arm in the sling.

Patients should sleep with a few pillows under their back or prop up the head of the bed 30 to 45 degrees. This helps maintain the fracture alignment in patients treated with a sling and makes them more comfortable.

Methods of Treatment: Specific Aspects

Sling

Check the sling to ensure that the elbow is at approximately 90 degrees of flexion with free motion of the wrist and the digits. Ensure that adequate padding is present, especially around the axilla and the posterior aspect of the neck, to prevent skin chafing. Immobilize the shoulder joint in neutral flexion and adduction with 90 degrees of internal rotation. Immobilize two-part lesser tuberosity fractures in internal rotation across the chest to increase adduction to relax the pull of the subscapularis muscle and assist in reduction of the lesser tuberosity. To provide support and comfort, place the patient in a sling for the first 2 weeks regardless of the type of fixation.

Open Reduction and Internal Fixation

Check the wound. Avoid stress to the rotator cuff and tuberosity repairs. A patient with a repair of the rotator cuff is *not* allowed active flexion (forward elevation), active external rotation, or assistive internal rotation until 6 weeks after surgery.

Closed Reduction, Percutaneous Fixation, and Cannulated Screws

Check the wound and pin sites for skin tenting, erythema, drainage, or induration. Clean pin sites with hydrogen peroxide-soaked swabs, release any skin tenting, and treat the patient if a wound or pin site infection is suspected.

Hemiarthroplasty

Patients who undergo prosthetic replacement participate in an early rehabilitation program. Motion is immediately begun to prevent the formation of function-threatening adhesions. Pendulum exercises with gravity elimination are started. Rehabilitation is aimed at maintaining joint stability and obtaining range of motion with reasonable muscle control.

Prescription

DAY ONE TO ONE WEEK

Precautions Avoid shoulder motion.

Range of Motion None at the shoulder and elbow. Gentle pendulum exercises with elimination of gravity are allowed for nondisplaced fractures and hemiarthroplasty.

Muscle Strength No strengthening exercises to the elbow or shoulder are permitted.

Functional Activities One-handed activities with the uninvolved extremity. The patient needs assistance in dressing, grooming, and preparing meals.

Weight Bearing None on affected extremity.

Treatment: Two to Four Weeks

BONE HEALING

Stability at fracture site: None to minimal.

Stage of bone healing: Beginning of reparative phase. Osteoprogenitor cells differentiate into osteoblasts, which lay down woven bone.

X-ray: No callus; fracture line is still visible.

Orthopaedic and Rehabilitation Considerations

Physical Examination

Pay special attention to complaints of pain, paresthesia, pin discomfort, drainage, or malodor. Assess the patient's neurovascular status and examine for concurrent neurovascular injuries, including axillary artery and vein as well as brachial plexus injuries.

Check all wounds for erythema, discharge, or purulence. Remove any sutures.

Assess the active and passive range of motion in the affected extremity, including the elbow, wrist, and digits. Encourage wrist and hand motion to reduce dependent edema.

Dangers

The fracture is still unstable and may lose reduction and alignment.

Check for reflex sympathetic dystrophy (RSD), characterized by trophic changes, vasomotor disturbances, hyperesthesia, pain, and tenderness out of proportion to the stage of fracture healing. RSD may require stellate ganglion blocks.

Radiography

Check radiographs for any loss of correction, the position of the hardware, and possible early callus formation; compare them with previous radiographs. Correct any deformity operatively or by closed reduction.

Weight Bearing

No weight bearing on the affected extremity.

Range of Motion

The sling is removed at the end of 3 weeks. Patients who had conservative treatment with a sling only can start gentle, active range-of-motion exercises to the shoulder in flexion, extension, adduction, and abduction because these fractures are nondisplaced or minimally displaced to start with. Gravity-eliminated or dependent-pendulum exercises are also taught; these usually do not go through the full arc initially. Internal and external rotation should be avoided because they displace the fracture. Continue with active range-of-motion exercises to the elbow, wrist and digits. Applying moist heat before and ice after exercises minimizes swelling.

Muscle Strength

Start isometric exercises to the shoulder girdle muscles only if the fracture was treated conservatively with a sling. Patients may complain of soreness.

Continue with wrist extension and flexion exercises. The patient should do ball-squeezing exercises to maintain the strength of the intrinsic muscles of the hand.

Functional Activities

The patient should continue with one-handed activities and still needs assistance in dressing, grooming, and preparing meals.

Methods of Treatment: Specific Aspects

Sling

A sling should keep the elbow at 90 degrees of flexion with free motion at the wrist and digits. The shoulder joint should be immobilized to neutral flexion and adduction with approximately 90 degrees of internal rotation. In two-part lesser tuberosity fractures, immobilize the extremity in internal rotation across the chest, which increases adduction, to maintain the reduction of the lesser tuberosity. Pad and adjust the sling appropriately, particularly around the axilla and the posterior aspect of the neck.

At the end of 2 weeks, the sling is removed and the patient can perform gentle, active range-of-motion exercises, avoiding internal and external rotation of the shoulder. Lying supine, the patient can try to flex the shoulder up to 180 degrees using the other arm.

The sling is replaced at night for support or during the day when the patient feels a need for it. The patient should continue with pendulum exercises.

Open Reduction and Internal Fixation/Closed Reduction and Immobilization/Closed Reduction and Percutaneous Fixation

Remove sutures or staples from the operative site at 2 weeks and check for evidence of superficial infection (erythema, drainage) or deep infection (fluctuance, induration, pitting edema).

Any pin sites should be clean, without evidence of purulent drainage. If a superficial pin tract infection is suspected, consider a 7- to 10-day course of oral antibiotics.

Patients with a tenuous repair of the rotator cuff are not permitted active flexion (forward elevation), active external rotation, or assisted internal rotation until 6 weeks after surgery.

No active range of motion to the shoulder is allowed because the patient may try to pull or contract the shoulder girdle muscles, which can disturb the fracture. The fracture is not rigid unless plate fixation was done, and this is uncommon.

Gentle passive-assistive range-of-motion exercises in the supine position can be given to tolerance to decrease or prevent shoulder tightness and contracture.

Hemiarthroplasty

The fixation is stable and early range of motion is continued with passive-assistive range of motion. Remove any sutures or staples.

Prescription

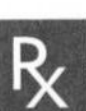

Two to Four Weeks

Precautions Avoid internal/external rotation of the shoulder.

Range of Motion Patients treated *conservatively* with a sling can continue with pendulum exercises. Active to gentle passive-assistive exercises to the shoulder. Patients treated *surgically* should start passive-assistive range of motion in supine position. No active range of motion to the shoulder.

Muscle Strength Isometric shoulder exercises in patients treated with sling only. No strengthening exercises for patients treated with surgical intervention.

Functional Activities Patient continues with one-handed activities and needs assistance in dressing, grooming, and preparing meals.

Weight Bearing None on affected extremity.

Treatment: Four to Six Weeks

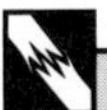

Bone Healing

Stability at fracture site: With bridging callus, the fracture is usually stable; confirm with physical examination.

Stage of bone healing: Reparative phase. Further organization of the callus and formation of lamellar bone begins. Once callus is observed bridging the fracture site, the fracture is usually stable. However, the strength of this callus, especially with torsional load, is significantly lower than that of normal bone. Further protection (if not further immobilization) is required to avoid refracture.

X-ray: Bridging callus is visible. With increased rigidity of the fixation, less bridging callus is noted, and healing with endosteal callus predominates. Expect less callus in end-of-bone fractures than in midshaft fractures.

Orthopaedic and Rehabilitation Considerations

Physical Examination

Check for capillary refill, sensation, and the active and passive range of motion of the digits. Assess for signs of infection.

Although the patient continues in a sling, perform the examination out of the sling. Assess the stability, tenderness, and range of motion of the shoulder joint. Ensure that the fracture fragments are moving as a unit and no crepitus is palpable during range of motion. Replace the sling if there is still tenderness, motion at the fracture site, or inadequate radiographic healing (no visible callus).

Remove percutaneous pins if they were used.

Dangers

Check for early evidence of adhesive capsulitis (frozen shoulder), especially if the patient is not compliant with the rehabilitation program.

If injury to the axillary nerve is suspected by clinical findings, an EMG should be obtained and can be used as a baseline for further comparisons of recovery of function.

Radiography

Check radiographic alignment. If the pins are removed, compare radiographs from before and after the removal of the pins. This is to ensure maintenance of the reduction. Check for callus formation.

Weight Bearing

None on the affected extremity.

Range of Motion

Continue with active and passive-assistive range of motion to the shoulder for patients who were treated conservatively.

If the patient is nontender and has no crepitus or motion at the fracture site and abundant callus on radiography, advance the pendulum exercises. The patient can start these exercises against gravity, as well as internal and external rotation, because there is sufficient callus formation at this stage. The patient is instructed in wall-climbing exercises (fingers against the wall and reaching up) to improve flexion of the shoulder. Wheel exercises are prescribed to allow range of motion in all planes.

Continue with active range-of-motion exercises to the elbow, wrist, and digits.

Muscle Strength

Continue with ball-squeezing and isometric exercises to the shoulder girdle muscles for patients treated conservatively.

Functional Activities

Patients treated with a sling only can start using the affected extremity for dressing and self-care. They can begin to bear weight on the extremity at the end of 6 weeks. Patients treated surgically still need assistance and cannot bear weight.

Gait

Arm swing is reduced.

Methods of Treatment: Specific Aspects

Patients treated surgically (open reduction and internal fixation; closed reduction–percutaneous pinning) should remain non-weight bearing. They can continue gentle passive-assistive range-of-motion exercises to the shoulder and continue with active range-of-motion exercises to the elbow and wrist. No isometric exercises are prescribed to the deltoid because this muscle is incised during surgery.

Hemiarthroplasty

Continue active and active-assistive range-of-motion exercises.

Prescription

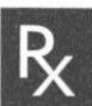

FOUR TO SIX WEEKS

Precautions Do not apply force in attempting to regain the full range of motion.

Range of Motion

Shoulder—limited range

Flexion/abduction up to 100 to 110 degrees

Internal/external rotation—limited

Pendulum exercises against gravity

Elbow—full range of motion in flexion, extension, supination, and pronation

Surgically treated patients may continue with passive-assistive range-of-motion exercises

Muscle Strength

Shoulder—avoid exercises to the deltoid if it is incised during surgery

Elbow—isometric and isotonic exercises

Functional Activities Involved extremity used for dressing and grooming as tolerated. Patient still needs assistance in house cleaning and preparing meals.

Weight Bearing None on affected extremity.

Treatment: Six to Eight Weeks

BONE HEALING

Stability at fracture site: With bridging callus, the fracture is usually stable; confirm with physical examination.

Stage of bone healing: Reparative phase. There is further organization of the callus and formation of lamellar bone. Once callus is observed bridging the fracture site, the fracture is usually stable. Further protection of bone (if not further immobilization) may be required to avoid refracture. However, the strength of this callus, especially with torsional load, is significantly lower than that of normal lamellar bone.

X-ray: Bridging callus is visible. With increased rigidity, less bridging callus is noted, and healing with endosteal callus predominates. The fracture line is less distinct.

Orthopaedic and Rehabilitation Considerations

The fracture is usually healed and the pins removed. Immobilization is discontinued. The patient should have achieved a functional range of motion.

Physical Examination

Ensure that the patient is regaining adequate range of motion without crepitus. Check for resolution of RSD if it was present.

Dangers

Check for RSD. The patient may have adhesive capsulitis secondary to the immobilization and trauma to the shoulder.

Radiography

Check for further callus formation. Check for bony union of tuberosities to the shaft. Evaluate for malunion, especially of the greater tuberosity, and subsequent bony acromion impingement. Evaluate for delayed union.

Weight Bearing

Begin weight bearing as tolerated.

Range of Motion

Gentle active range of motion is given in all planes at this point because there is enough callus formation to reduce the threat of fracture displacement. If signs of adhesive capsulitis are present, aggressive therapy is instituted in the form of gentle passive range of motion.

Active-assistive and passive-assistive exercises are prescribed to the shoulder for all shoulder fractures. Pulley exercises, wheel exercises, and wall-climbing exercises can be prescribed. Some of the suggested exercises are

Begin supine active flexion (forward elevation). Eliminating gravity makes flexion (forward elevation) easier.

Progress flexion in an erect position using a broomstick in the unaffected hand to assist the involved arm in forward elevation.

Perform stretching for flexion (forward elevation) by grabbing the top of a door or wall and leaning to or through door jamb.

Raise the arm over the head with the arms clasped.

Perform external rotation and abduction of the arms by placing the hands behind the head.

Help with internal rotation by using the uninvolved arm to pull the involved arm into internal rotation.

Passive assistance with the elimination of gravity or the opposite arm is important so as not to overstress the healing fracture and the rotator cuff.

Continue full active range-of-motion exercises to the elbow, wrist, and fingers.

Muscle Strength

Continue with isometric exercises to the shoulder. Start active-resistive exercises using weights, beginning with 2 pounds for patients treated conservatively with a sling. If the patient experiences pain, weight should be decreased.

The patient can start resistive exercises to the elbow and wrist using weights.

Functional Activities

The patient is encouraged to use the affected extremity in all activities of self-care, although reduced abduction and internal rotation may limit such actions as unhooking a bra or washing the back. A long-handled sponge to scrub the back may be helpful, and long-handled devices may be used for reaching objects overhead. The patient can bear weight on the involved extremity and can lift light objects.

Gait

Arm swing is beginning to improve, although it is still reduced.

Methods of Treatment: Specific Aspects

Sling

Discontinue immobilization. Prescribe gradual progressive resistive exercises with weights, starting at two pounds and gradually increasing the weight to the patient's tolerance. The patient should have at least 180 degrees of abduction and forward flexion by now.

Patients Treated with Internal Fixation

Discontinue all immobilization if union is demonstrated clinically and radiographically. Start active range-of-motion exercises to the shoulder because the fracture site is stable with adequate callus formation.

Fracture dislocation is now less likely. Initially, range of motion of the shoulder, especially in flexion, abduction, and internal rotation, may be limited because of the previous position of immobilization. Active-assistive exercises should be continued to minimize the limitations of range of motion.

The patient may also have significant loss of strength in the deltoid, biceps, and triceps secondary to disuse and injury.

Strengthening exercises should be started. The patient can offer resistance using his or her other extremity.

Prescription

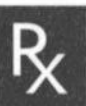

Six to Eight Weeks

Precautions Avoid forced range of motion.

Range of Motion Active, active-assistive, and passive range of motion to the shoulder and elbow in all planes, to tolerance.

Muscle Strength

Continue isometric exercises to the shoulder.

Continue with isometric and isotonic exercises to the elbow.

Start progressive resistive exercises for patients treated with a sling.

Functional Activities The involved extremity is used for self-care and feeding. The patient may still need to use the uninvolved extremity for some self-care activities.

Weight Bearing Weight bearing as tolerated.

Treatment: Eight to Twelve Weeks

Bone Healing

Stability at fracture site: Stable.

Stage of bone healing: Remodeling phase. Woven bone is replaced with lamellar bone. The process of remodeling takes months to years for completion.

X-ray: Abundant callus; fracture line begins to disappear. With time, there will be reconstitution of the medullary canal.

Orthopaedic and Rehabilitation Considerations

Physical Examination

Discontinue the sling, if this has not already been done. Examine the extremity for tenderness, crepitus, and motion at the fracture site. Ensure that the range of motion is adequate and improving in all planes and that shoulder strength is improving.

Dangers

Ensure that clinical and radiographic union is satisfactory before advancing the patient's rehabilitation program. Look for signs of avascular necrosis, which occurs in 3% to 25% of three-part fractures and as many as 90% of four-part fractures.

Radiography

Confirm radiographic union of the fracture. Look for resorption or collapse of the articular segment, indicating avascular necrosis. Evaluate for malunion and delayed union.

Weight Bearing

The patient may bear weight as tolerated.

Range of Motion

Active, active-assistive, and passive range of motion to the shoulder are prescribed in all planes. The patient should have full functional range of motion by this time (e.g., shoulder abduction and flexion up to 130 degrees) and should continue with wall-climbing and wheel exercises.

Active and passive range-of-motion exercises are continued to the elbow. The patient should not have any restriction in elbow flexion or extension.

Muscle Strength

Progressive resistive exercises are prescribed to the deltoids, biceps, triceps, and rotator cuff muscles. Resistance is provided in the form of weights, increased gradually from 2 to 10 pounds. Isokinetic exercises using appropriate equipment are encouraged to build up strength and endurance. If the patient complains of pain when using weights and equipment, consider decreasing the weight or resistance.

Functional Activities

By the end of 12 weeks, the patient should be able to use the involved extremity for all activities of daily living without any significant limitations.

Swimming is allowed by 12 weeks. Contact sports like basketball and football are usually allowed after 6 months, depending on the patient's pain tolerance and healing of the fracture. Tennis and golf can be resumed after 3 months.

Gait

The patient should attempt a normal arm swing.

Methods of Treatment: Specific Aspects

The fracture is healed. Hardware is removed as appropriate. Therapy is directed to obtaining full range of motion and strength and achieving functional goals.

Prescription

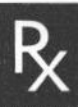

EIGHT TO TWELVE WEEKS

Precautions None.

Range of Motion Active and passive range of motion to the shoulder and elbow in all planes.

Muscle Strength Resistive exercises to the shoulder with gradual increases in weights. Isokinetic exercises using appropriate equipment to improve strength and endurance.

Functional Activities Patient should be able to use the affected extremity without significant limitations in activities of daily living and self-care.

Weight Bearing Full weight bearing.

LONG-TERM CONSIDERATIONS

Reflex sympathetic dystrophy may lead to a decrease in range of motion and strength and to severe pain. Residual loss of motion may be permanent, especially in internal and external rotation. Deltoid strength may be permanently decreased.

Avascular necrosis of the proximal fragment may be present, especially in four-part fractures. This may have to be treated by hemiarthroplasty to provide functional improvement.

Malunion can cause significant functional limitations. When the greater tuberosity heals in a superior or medial position, the space beneath the subacromial arch is limited, and impingement occurs when the arm is abducted or externally rotated.

Nonunion is not uncommon, particularly in two-part displaced shaft fractures and three-part fractures, because of interposition of soft tissue, excessive soft-tissue dissection (in surgically treated patients), inadequate immobilization, poor patient compliance, and overaggressive physical therapy. If nonunion occurs, the patient will require open reduction and internal fixation, bone grafting, and possibly spica cast immobilization.

IMMEDIATE TO ONE WEEK

	Nonoperative Fixation	*Operative Fixation*	*Endoprosthesis, Intact Rotator Cuff*	*Endoprosthesis, Tissue-Deficient*
Stability	None.	Depends on bone quality and fixation.	Depends on cuff repair.	Depends on cuff repair.
Orthopaedics	Check fitting of shoulder immobilizer or orthosis.	Check wound for infection and stability of fixation.	Check for wound infection.	Check for wound infection.
Rehabilitation	Pendulum exercises to shoulder.	No range of motion to the shoulder.	Pendulum exercises to shoulder.	Pendulum exercises to shoulder.

TWO TO FOUR WEEKS

	Nonoperative Fixation	*Operative Fixation*	*Endoprosthesis, Intact Rotator Cuff*	*Endoprosthesis, Tissue-Deficient*
Stability	None to minimal.	Depends on bone quality and fixation.	Depends on cuff repair.	Depends on cuff repair.
Orthopaedics	Elevate involved extremity to decrease swelling.	Remove sutures and elevate involved extremity to decrease swelling.	Remove sutures.	Remove sutures.
Rehabilitation	Gentle active range of motion to the shoulder in flexion, extension, abduction, and adduction. Gravity-eliminated pendulum exercises to the shoulder. Avoid internal external rotation.	No active range of motion to the shoulder. Gentle passive-assistive range-of-motion exercises to the shoulder in supine position.	Begin passive-assistive shoulder range of motion (avoiding internal and external rotation).	Begin passive-assistive shoulder range of motion with limited elevation and external rotation.

FOUR TO SIX WEEKS

	Nonoperative Fixation	*Operative Fixation*	*Endoprosthesis, Intact Rotator Cuff*	*Endoprosthesis, Tissue-Deficient*
Stability	Partially stable.	Partially stable.	Partially stable.	Partially stable.
Orthopaedics	Discontinue shoulder immobilizer.	Remove external fixator or percutaneous pins, if applicable.		
Rehabilitation	Advance isometric exercises.	Continue with passive-assistive range of motion.	Continue with passive-assistive range of motion.	Continue passive shoulder range of motion with limited elevation and external rotation.

SIX TO EIGHT WEEKS

	Nonoperative Fixation	*Operative Fixation*	*Endoprosthesis, Intact Rotator Cuff*	*Endoprosthesis, Tissue-Deficient*
Stability	Stable.	Stable.	Stable.	Stable.
Orthopaedics	Consider open reduction and internal fixation (ORIF) and bone grafting if clinically and radiographically not healing.	Consider ORIF and bone grafting if clinically and radiographically not healing.	Discontinue immobilization.	Discontinue immobilization.
Rehabilitation	Begin active range of motion with terminal stretching, emphasizing elevation and external rotation.	Begin active range of motion with terminal stretching, emphasizing elevation and external rotation.	Begin active shoulder range of motion, emphasizing elevation and external rotation. Advance isometric shoulder exercises in all planes.	Begin active shoulder range of motion, including elevation and external rotation. Advance isometric shoulder exercises in all planes.

EIGHT TO TWELVE WEEKS

	Nonoperative Fixation	*Operative Fixation*	*Endoprosthesis, Intact Rotator Cuff*	*Endoprosthesis, Tissue-Deficient*
Stability	Stable.	Stable.	Stable.	Stable.
Orthopaedics	Consider ORIF and bone grafting if clinically and radiographically not healing.	Consider ORIF and bone grafting if clinically and radiographically not healing.	Ensure that patient is not developing function-threatening adhesions.	Ensure that shoulder joint is stable and that the patient has reasonable muscle control.
Rehabilitation	Begin resistive shoulder exercises and continue terminal capsular stretching.	Begin resistive shoulder exercises and continue terminal capsular stretching.	Begin resistive shoulder exercises and continue terminal capsular stretching.	Begin resistive shoulder exercises and continue terminal capsular stretching. *Note: Some patients will never enter this phase.*

TWELVE + WEEKS

	Nonoperative Fixation	*Operative Fixation*	*Endoprosthesis, Intact Rotator Cuff*	*Endoprosthesis, Tissue-Deficient*
Stability	Stable.	Stable.	Stable.	Stable.
Orthopaedics	Consider ORIF and bone grafting if clinically and radiographically not healing.	Consider ORIF and bone grafting if clinically and radiographically not healing.	Ensure that patient is not developing function-threatening adhesions.	Ensure that shoulder joint is stable and that the patient has reasonable muscle control.
Rehabilitation	Continue resistive exercises with increasing resistance. Continue capsular stretching.	Continue resistive exercises with increasing resistance. Continue termainal capsular stretching.	Continue resistive shoulder exercises and continue terminal capsular stretching.	Continue resistive shoulder exercises and continue terminal capsular stretching. *Note: Some patients will never enter this phase.*

BIBLIOGRAPHY

Bengner U, Johnell O, Redlund-Johnell I. Changes in the incidence of fractures of the upper end of the humerus during a 3-year period: a study of 2125 fractures. *Clin Orthop*, 231:179–182, 1988.

Callahan DJ. Anatomic considerations: closed reduction of proximal humeral fractures. *Orthop Rev*, 13:79–85, 1984.

Cofield RH. Comminuted fractures of the proximal humerus. *Clin Orthop*, 230:49–57, 1988.

Des Marchais JE, Morais G. Treatment of complex fractures of the proximal humerus by Neer hemiarthroplasty. In: Bateman JE, Welsh RP, eds. *Surgery of the Shoulder*. Philadelphia: B.C. Decker, 1984, pp. 60.

Dingley A, Denham R. Fracture-dislocation of the humeral head: a method of reduction. *J Bone Joint Surg Am*, 55:1299–1300, 1973.

Heppenstall RB. Fractures of the proximal humerus. *Orthop Clin North Am*, 6:467–475, 1975.

Jakob RP, Kristiansen T. Classification and aspects of treatment of fractures of the proximal humerus. In: Bateman JE, Welsh RP, eds. *Surgery of the Shoulder*. Philadelphia: B.C. Decker, 1984, pp. 330–343.

Krakovi M, et al. Indications and results of operation in proximal humeral fractures. *Montsschr Unfallheilkd*, 78:326–332, 1975.

Neer CS. Four-segment classification of displaced proximal humeral fractures. *Instr Course Lect*, 24:160–168, 1975.

Neer CS, Rockwood CA Jr. Fractures and dislocations of the shoulder. In: Rockwood CA Jr, Green DP, eds. *Fractures*, 2nd ed. Philadelphia: J.B. Lippincott, 1984, pp. 675–707.

CHAPTER Twelve

Humeral Diaphysis or Midshaft Fractures

JONATHAN D. LEWIN, MD

VASANTHA L. MURTHY, MD

INTRODUCTION

Definition

Fractures of the humeral shaft are those that involve the diaphysis or midshaft and do not involve the articular or metaphyseal regions proximally or distally (Figures 12-1 and 12-2).

It is useful to classify these fractures by anatomic location because the effect of muscle forces causes different displacement patterns depending on the level of the fracture.

Fractures above the pectoralis major insertion lead to abduction and external rotation of the proximal

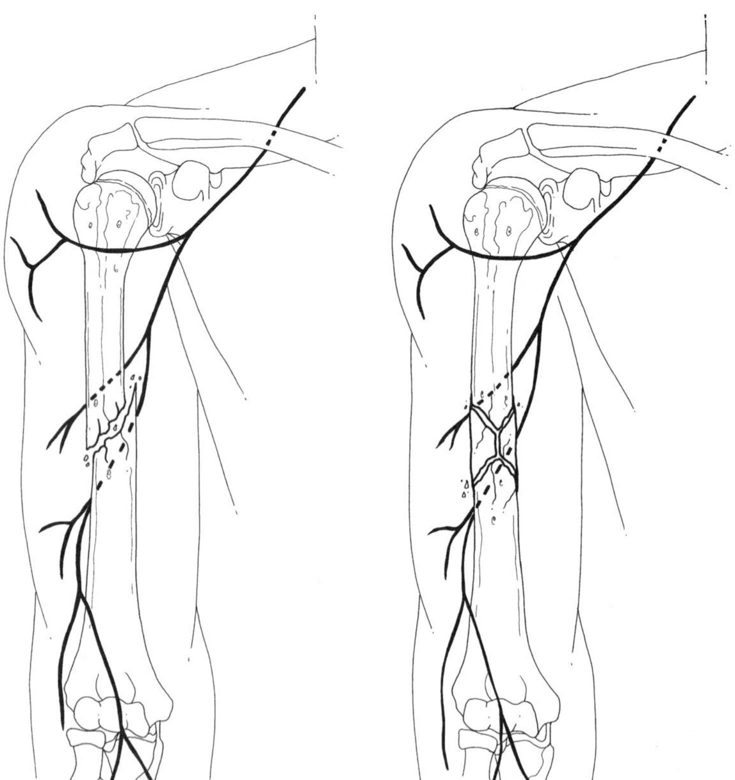

FIGURE 12-1 *(far left)* Oblique fracture of the humeral shaft. Note the proximity of the vessels and nerves running at the posterior aspect of the fracture site.

FIGURE 12-2 *(left)* Comminuted fracture of the humeral shaft. Note the proximity of the radial nerve at the posterior aspect of the fracture site. Nerve injury causes a wrist drop.

humerus secondary to the pull of the rotator cuff muscles.

Fractures below the pectoralis major insertion and above the deltoid lead to adduction of the proximal fragment (under the influence of the pectoralis major) and proximal and lateral displacement of the distal fragment (under the influence of the deltoid).

Fractures below the deltoid insertion lead to abduction of the upper fragment (under the strong influence of the deltoid).

Humeral fractures are further classified as closed or open, transverse, oblique, spiral, segmental, or comminuted. Additional classifications address nerve or arterial injury and whether the fracture is through pathologic bone.

Mechanism of Injury

Humeral fractures are caused by a direct blow, twisting force, fall onto the arm, or penetrating trauma and are frequently associated with motor vehicle accidents.

Treatment Goals

Orthopaedic Objectives

Alignment

The alignment of the fracture when healed should not place the elbow and arm in excessive varus or valgus. Cosmetically and functionally, varus is a greater problem than valgus.

Stability

When healed, the metaphysis of the humerus should be stable in weight bearing (e.g., while doing push-ups). There should be shoulder and elbow range of motion without motion at the fracture site. If there is nonunion (motion at the fracture site), no weight bearing is allowed until the fracture is fixed.

Rehabilitation Objectives

Range of Motion

Restore the full shoulder range of motion in all planes (Table 12-1).

Restore the full elbow range of motion (Table 12-2).

TABLE 12-1 *Shoulder Range of Motion*

Motion	Normal	Functional[a]
Abduction	180°	120°
Adduction	45°	30°
Flexion (forward elevation)[b]	180°	120°
Extension (posterior elevation)[c]	60°	40°
Internal rotation with arm at side	100°	80°
External rotation with arm at side	70°	30°
Internal rotation with arm in abduction	80°	45°
External rotation with arm in abduction	90°	45°

[a] Range of motion that is one half to two thirds of full range of motion is considered functional.

[b] To reach maximal flexion or forward elevation, slight abduction and external rotation are required.

[c] To reach maximal extension or posterior elevation, slight internal rotation is required.

TABLE 12-2 *Elbow Range of Motion*

Motion	Normal	Functional
Flexion	135°	0–90°
Extension	0–5°	−20–30°
Supination	90°	50°
Pronation	90°	50°

Muscle Strength

Improve the strength of the following muscles that are injured secondary to the fracture; attempt to regain strength 5/5.

Pectoralis major: shoulder adductor
Deltoid: shoulder flexor, extensor, and abductor
Biceps: elbow flexor and shoulder flexor
Triceps: elbow extensor

The rotator cuff muscles, supraspinatus, infraspinatus, and teres minor do not usually require aggressive rehabilitation.

Functional Goals

Improve and restore the function of the involved extremity in self-care and personal hygiene. Shoulder movement and strength are vital in almost all sports activities.

Expected Time of Bone Healing

Eight to 12 weeks in uncomplicated cases.

Expected Duration of Rehabilitation

Twelve to 16 weeks.

Methods of Treatment

Coaptation Splint

Biomechanics: Stress-sharing device, using tissue forces and soft tissue integrity around the fracture, to stabilize the fracture.

Mode of Bone Healing: Secondary, with callus formation.

Indications: This method usually is used for initial management of fractures before functional bracing (Figures 12-3, 12-4, 12-5, 12-6, 12-7, 12-8, 12-9, 12-10).

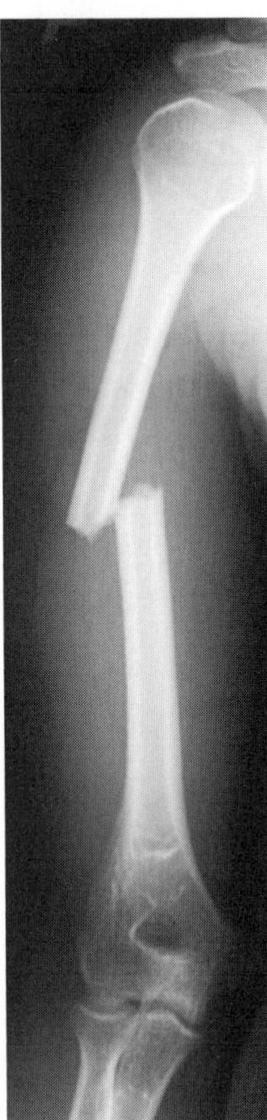

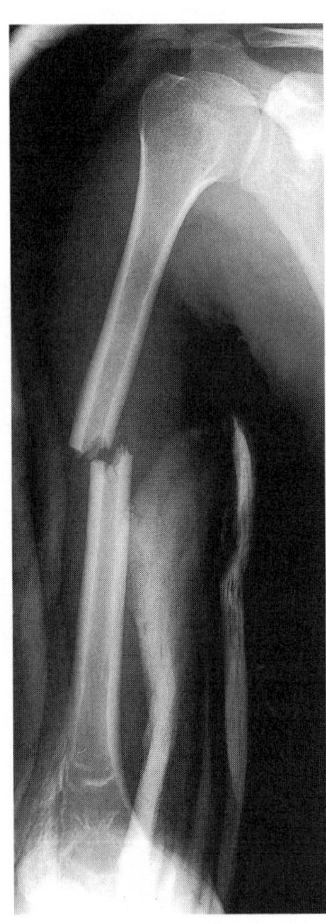

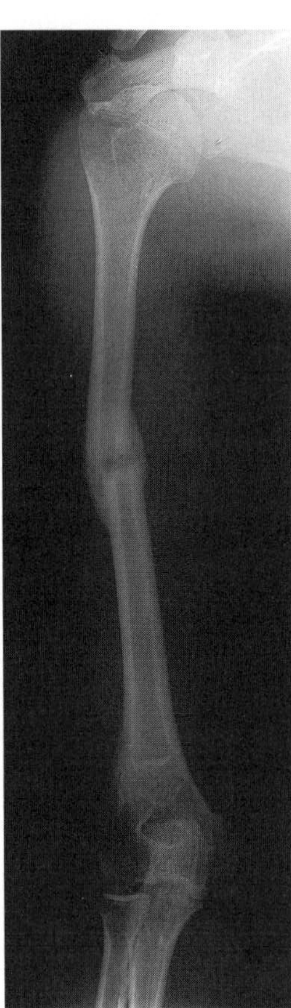

FIGURE 12-3 *(far left)* Transverse fracture of the humeral midshaft with displacement of the two parts.

FIGURE 12-4 *(middle left)* Transverse fracture of the humeral shaft treated in a coaptation splint. Note the reduction of the fracture fragments.

FIGURE 12-5 *(left)* Healing of a transverse fracture of the humeral shaft with abundant callus formation.

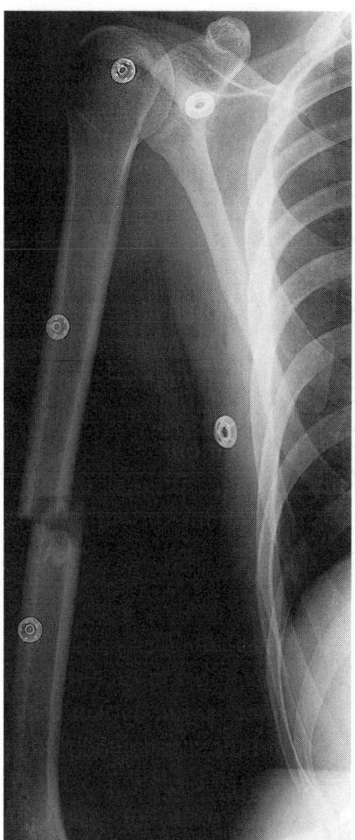

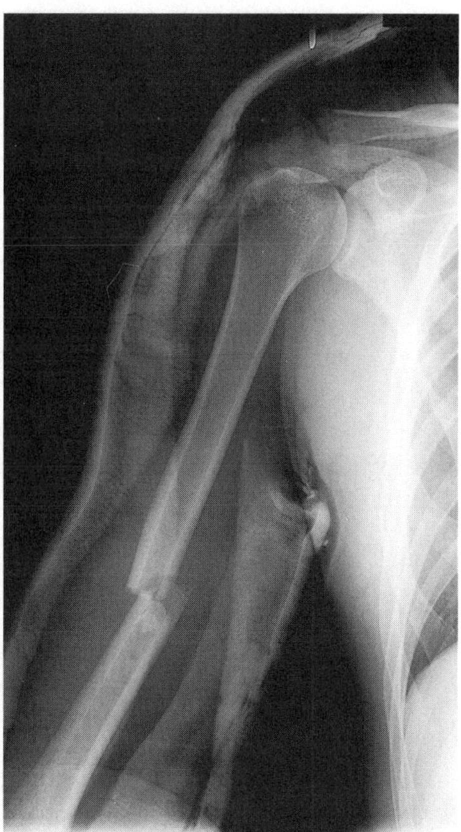

FIGURE 12-6 *(far left)* Transverse fracture of the humeral midshaft with minimal comminution.

FIGURE 12-7 *(left)* Transverse fracture of the humeral shaft treated in a coaptation splint.

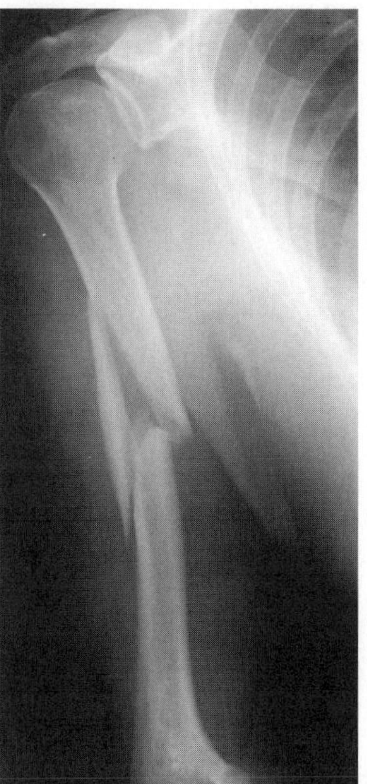

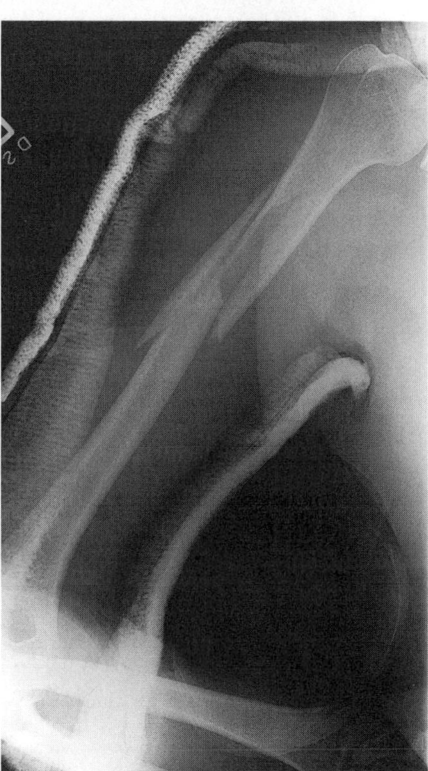

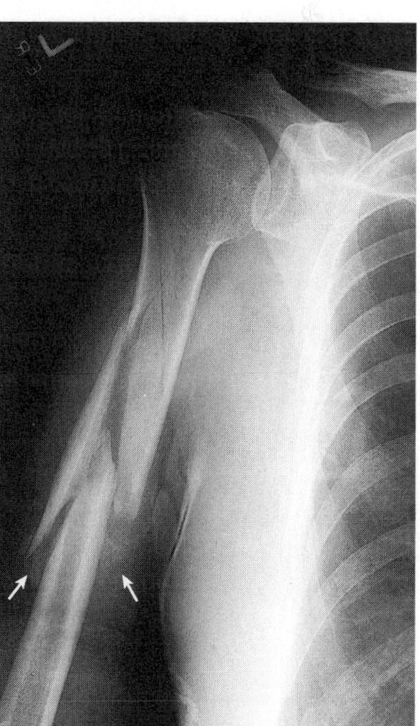

FIGURE 12-8 *(above, left)* Displaced spiral fracture of the humeral shaft with a butterfly fragment.

FIGURE 12-9 *(above, middle)* Treatment of a spiral fracture of the humeral midshaft in a coaptation splint. Note the anatomic alignment of the proximal and distal shaft.

FIGURE 12-10 *(above, right)* Further treatment of a spiral fracture of the humeral shaft in a hanging cast. Note the hard callus formation around the fracture site indicating healing.

Functional Bracing

Biomechanics: Stress-sharing device, using hydraulic tissue forces to maintain fracture alignment.

Mode of Bone Healing: Secondary, with callus formation.

Indications: This is the treatment of choice for most closed fractures of the humeral diaphysis.

Velpeau Dressing

Biomechanics: Stress-sharing device, relies on inherent soft tissue integrity to maintain stability.

Mode of Bone Healing: Secondary, with callus formation.

Indications: A Velpeau dressing is used for nondisplaced or minimally displaced fractures, especially in the young or elderly. This mode of treatment is not commonly used and is not discussed further in this chapter.

Intramedullary Nail/Rod

Biomechanics: Stress-shielding device when the rod is statically locked; stress-sharing device when it is not locked and acts as an internal splint while bone heals (e.g., Kirschner rod).

Mode of Bone Healing: When the nail is stress shielding, bone healing is primary (no callus), unless the nail is not well fixed, in which case it is secondary (Figure 12-11).

When the nail is stress sharing, bone healing is secondary (with callus; Figures 12-12, 12-13, 12-14, and 12-15).

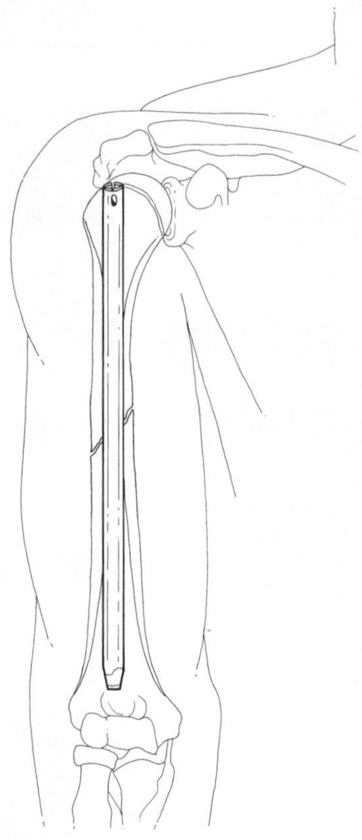

FIGURE 12-11 Unlocked intramedullary rod used to treat an oblique diaphyseal fracture of the humerus.

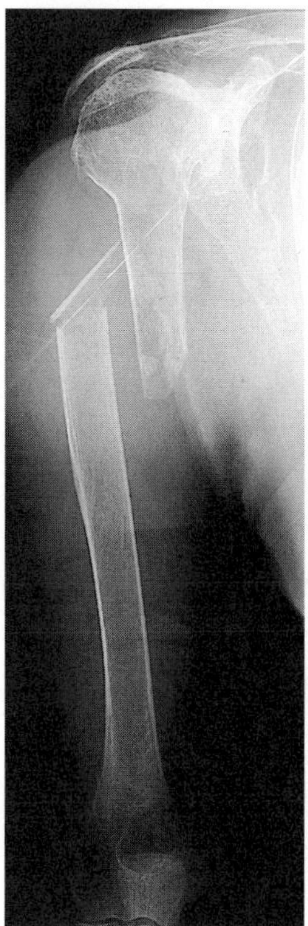

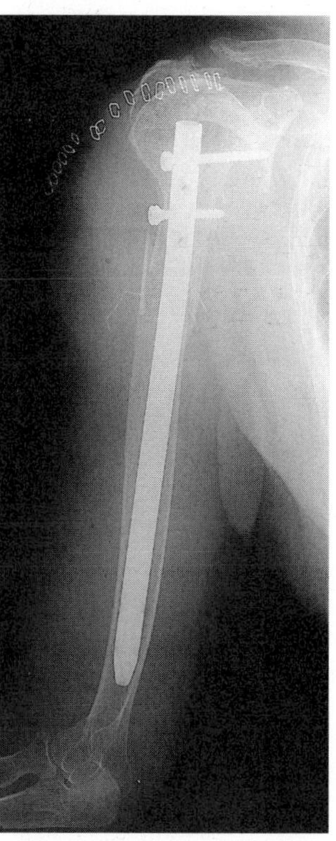

FIGURE 12-12 *(far left)* Displaced proximal diaphyseal fracture of the humerus with comminution.

FIGURE 12-13 *(left)* Proximally locked intramedullary nail used to treat a comminuted proximal diaphyseal fracture of the humerus. Locking of the nail prevents rotation of the fragments.

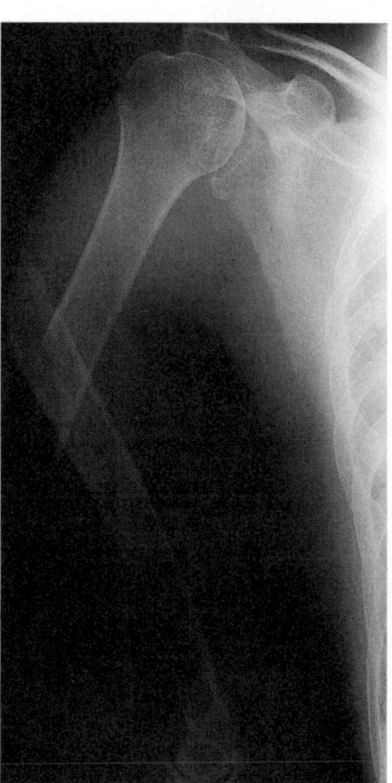

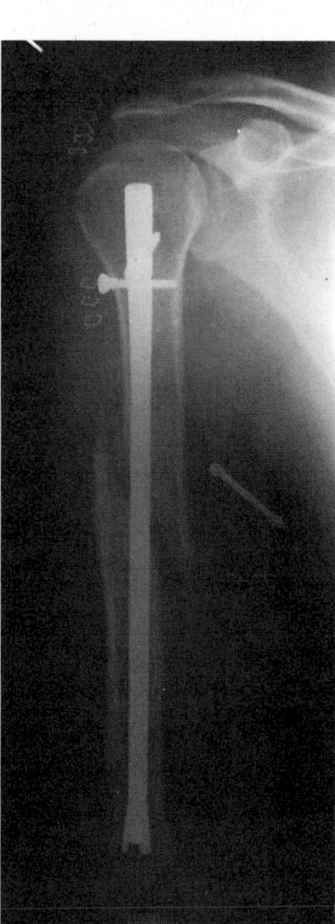

FIGURE 12-14 *(far left)* Spiral fracture in the diaphyseal region of the humerus. Note the angulation and shortening of the fracture.

FIGURE 12-15 *(left)* Statically locked intramedullary nail used to treat a spiral midshaft humeral fracture. The nail is locked at its proximal end with interlocking screws and at its distal end using a flaring device. Locking prevents rotation of the proximal and distal fragments.

Indications: Intramedullary nailing is used for fractures that cannot maintain closed reduction, low-grade open injuries, pathologic fractures, segmental fractures, and multitrauma patients with multiple fractures. The rod is commonly interlocked, making it stress shielding.

Plate Fixation

Biomechanics: Stress-shielding device. Broad plates are used to achieve compression of the fracture and allow lag screw fixation of the fragments.

Mode of Bone Healing: Primary, endosteal bone healing without callus.

Indications: This method is used for open humerus fractures where there is bone loss, interarticular injuries not amenable to intramedullary rodding, or failure to maintain closed reduction (Figures 12-16, 12-17, and 12-18).

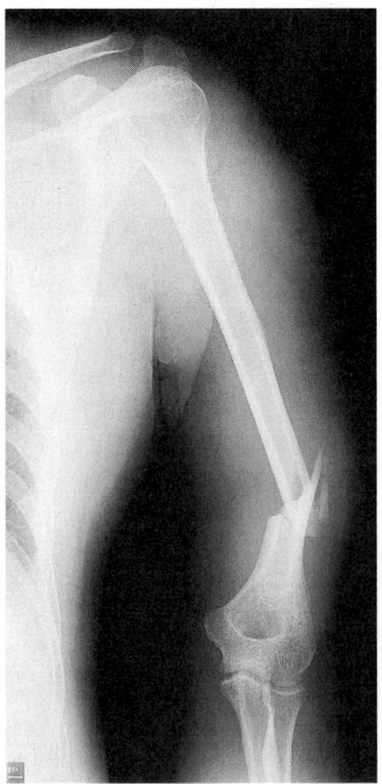

FIGURE 12-16 Oblique fracture of the humerus with varus angulation and a small butterfly fragment.

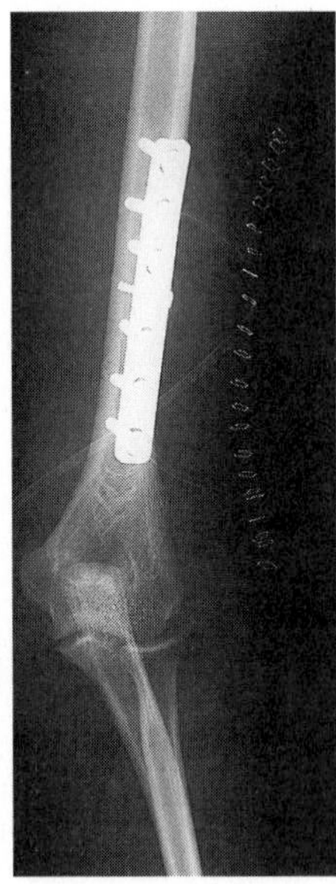

FIGURE 12-17 Fracture of the humeral shaft treated with compression plate fixation (anteroposterior view). Range of motion of the elbow joint should eventually be normal.

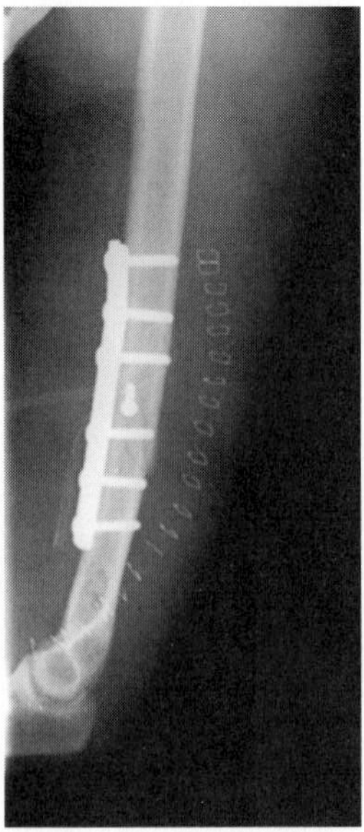

FIGURE 12-18 Fracture of the humeral shaft treated with plate fixation (lateral view). Note the lag screw in the center fixing the two oblique fragments.

External Fixation

Biomechanics: Stress-sharing device. Fixation relies on the rigidity of the pins and frame to maintain fragment alignment.

Mode of Bone Healing: Secondary, with callus.

Indications: External fixation is used for open humeral shaft fractures or closed shaft fractures with severe soft tissue trauma or thermal injury, for fractures with extensive comminution, for floating elbow fractures, or for segmental humerus fractures (Figure 12-19).

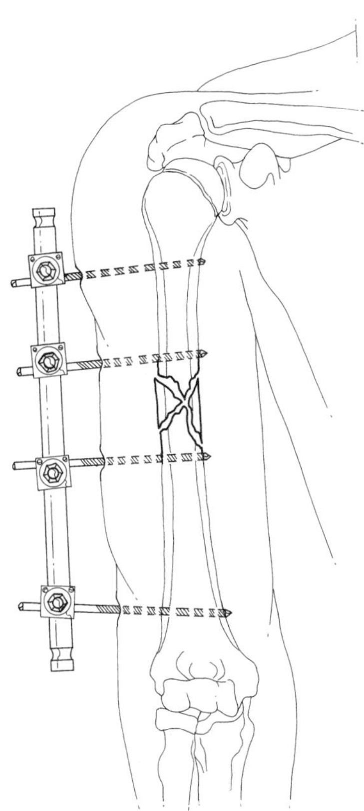

FIGURE 12-19 An external fixator used as a treatment for a comminuted diaphyseal humeral fracture. Care must be taken not to injure the radial nerve when inserting the fixator pins.

Special Considerations of the Fracture

Open Fractures

The more severe the soft tissue injury, the more appropriate is treatment with external fixation. Small-grade open injuries can be managed with plate or rodding techniques.

Pathologic Fractures

Fractures of pathologic bone (e.g., from osteoporosis, Paget's disease, metatastic disease) are best managed using reamed intramedullary rodding because plates rely on strong bone for purchase.

Multiple Trauma Patients

Seriously consider operative stabilization of all multitrauma patients. This enables quicker mobilization and decreased complications from multiple long bone fractures. If the patient must use crutches, intramedullary rodding is most appropriate because it allows early weight bearing on the extremity, whereas plate fixation precludes weight bearing for 4 to 6 weeks.

Age

Elderly patients may be more difficult to immobilize because they are less able to tolerate treatment (e.g., they are more vulnerable to axillary irritation from a coaptation splint).

Joint Stiffness

Elderly patients in particular need early, aggressive rehabilitation to avoid loss of joint motion. The shoulder and elbow are particularly susceptible when closed treatment is undertaken because of immobilization by the coaptation splint. Functional bracing as well as surgical intervention address this problem.

Associated Injuries

Nerves

Radial nerve palsy occurs in approximately 20% of closed fractures, with greater than 90% of these resolving spontaneously in 4 to 5 months' time. Most of these injuries are neuropraxic. The importance of the initial neurologic examination cannot be overemphasized because a new loss of nerve function after manipulation necessitates operative exploration. If nerve function shows *no signs* of recovery, consider electromyography (EMG) after 3 weeks because denervation potentials are seen at this time. If radial nerve palsy is seen at the time of presentation in the emergency room, follow the patient. This may be a neuropraxia due to nerve stretch. If radial nerve palsy occurs *on reduction*, the nerve has been pinched by bone and needs to be explored. In a high percentage of cases, the nerve actually becomes entrapped in the fragments (*see* Figures 12-1 and 12-2).

Vessels

The brachial artery can be injured with humeral fractures. Immediate repair is mandatory and fasciotomy is recommended. Note that ligation of the artery above the profunda brachii results in limb loss (amputation) in 50% of cases, whereas ligation distal to the profunda brachii incurs a 25% risk of limb loss.

Muscles

The mechanism of injury determines the extent of muscle damage. Industrial accidents, motor vehicle accidents, and open injuries will likely cause more soft tissue and muscle damage than a discrete blow or a single penetrating injury.

Weight Bearing

No weight bearing is allowed until an adequate callus has formed or, with plates, until primary healing has taken place. Early weight bearing is allowed with intramedullary rodding.

Gait

Arm swing is initially absent. This improves as the fracture heals.

TREATMENT

Treatment: Early to Immediate (Day of Injury to One Week)

BONE HEALING

Stability at fracture site: None.

Stage of bone healing: Inflammatory phase. The fracture hematoma is colonized by inflammatory cells, and débridement of the fracture begins.

X-ray: No callus.

Orthopaedic and Rehabilitation Considerations

Physical Examination

Inspection of open fracture wounds is of paramount importance. In addition, assess complaints of pain, swelling, and paresthesia. Be alert for developing compartment syndrome. Check capillary refill and sensation, as well as the active and passive range of motion of the wrist and digits. Pay special attention to radial nerve function; if it is not intact at the time of injury, a cock-up wrist splint should be added to avoid permanent wrist drop. If the radial nerve dysfunction occurred after initial treatment, consider nerve exploration. Swelling and discoloration of the arm and wrist are common. Inspect the axilla for irritation.

Dangers

Compartment syndrome of the arm is rare but possible. Resolve any questions with compartment pressure measurement.

Radiography

Examine anteroposterior and lateral radiographs of the humerus at 1 week to assess the position of the fracture fragments.

Weight Bearing

Early weight bearing is impossible unless the fracture was treated with an intramedullary rod. Weight bearing in a functional brace is limited by pain.

Range of Motion

No range of motion is allowed to the shoulder and elbow because they are in a splint or brace. Active range of motion is allowed to the wrist and digits to reduce dependent edema and stiffness.

Muscle Strength

No strengthening exercises are prescribed to the shoulder or elbow.

Functional Activities

The patient should use the uninvolved extremity for self-care and personal hygiene.

Gait/Ambulation

Usually there is no arm swing at this stage, because of pain.

Methods of Treatment: Specific Aspects

Coaptation Splint and Functional Bracing

The coaptation splint is used at this time. For fractures amenable to functional bracing, a brace may be ordered so that it will be available at the next visit.

Check splint integrity, padding, and sling position. Pay special attention to the axilla for evidence of chafing.

The patient should be instructed to use only the unaffected extremity for activities of daily living. Stress the importance of maintaining an upright or semiupright body position to aid in fracture alignment. No range of motion is allowed to the elbow or shoulder.

Open Reduction/Intramedullary Nail/Rod

Check the wound. Examine radiographs for integrity of fixation.

Depending on the stability of the fixation, the patient should be encouraged to use the affected extremity for light activities such as writing and eating. If complete stabilization has not been achieved, activity should be limited accordingly.

If the fixation is rigid and stable, active-assistive range of motion and active range of motion are allowed to the shoulder. Gentle gravity-assisted pendulum exercises are instituted to the shoulder toward the end of first week. The patient is allowed to use the stabilized extremity for light activities like eating and writing. No lifting is allowed.

Plate Fixation

See Intramedullary Nail/Rod.

External Fixation

Check the wound and pin site. Note any drainage, erythema, or skin tenting. Make sure that pins are not tethering tendon or muscle. Review pin care with the patient. Check radiographs for fracture alignment.

The patient is allowed to use the involved extremity for light activities of self-care. Gentle pendulum exercises are allowed to the shoulder. Active and active-assistive range of motion to the elbow are instituted.

Prescription

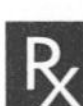

Day One to One Week

Precautions No lifting with the affected extremity.

Range of Motion *If in brace or splint*: no range of motion to shoulder and elbow allowed. *Open reduction and internal fixation (ORIF) and external fixator*: gentle active and active-assistive range of motion to shoulder and elbow allowed if fixation is stable. Pendulum exercises with gravity eliminated to shoulder.

Muscle Strength No strengthening exercises to the elbow or shoulder.

Functional Activities Uninvolved extremity may be used for self-care and activities of daily living.

Weight Bearing No weight bearing on affected extremity.

Treatment: Two Weeks

Bone Healing

Stability at fracture site: None to minimal.

Stage of bone healing: Beginning of reparative phase. Osteoprogenitor cells differentiate into osteoblasts, which lay down woven bone.

X-ray: None to very early callus.

Orthopaedic and Rehabilitation Considerations

Physical Examination

Assess complaints of pain, swelling, and paresthesia. Check capillary refill and sensation, as well as the active and passive range of motion of the wrist and digits. Evaluate the patient's ability to perform pendulum exercises, if these have been previously started. If a neurologic injury has occurred, maintain an appropriate splint for the wrist and hand and encourage the passive range of motion of the wrist and fingers if active motion is not possible. Evaluate the axilla. Swelling and discoloration of the arm are common.

Dangers

Radial nerve injury is still a concern. Reflex sympathetic dystrophy is always a concern in injuries of the upper extremity. Ensure adequate motion of the wrist and fingers.

Radiography

Evaluate anteroposterior and lateral radiographs of the humeral shaft.

Weight Bearing

No weight bearing is permitted with external fixation, a plate, or a functional brace. Limited weight bearing is permitted for other types of treatment (e.g., rod).

Range of Motion

Active and active-assistive range of motion is prescribed to the shoulder, elbow, and wrist.

Muscle Strength

No strengthening exercises are prescribed to the shoulder or elbow. Prescribe isotonic exercises to the forearm muscles with wrist flexion and extension and ball-squeezing exercises.

Functional Activities

The patient should use the uninvolved extremity for self-care and personal hygiene.

Gait/Ambulation

Arm swing during gait is minimal secondary to pain and discomfort.

Methods of Treatment: Specific Aspects

Coaptation Splint and Functional Bracing

If arm swelling has decreased, the coaptation splint may be changed to a functional brace.

Check radiographs for loss of reduction. Correct for angulation by adjusting the sling, adding medial bolsters, or reapplying a splint. If a functional brace has been applied, check the fracture position in the brace.

Gentle pendulum exercises may be started. The shoulder should not be abducted greater than 60 degrees. If a functional brace is applied, elbow range-of-motion exercises can be started.

Open Reduction/Intramedullary Nail/Rod

Check the wound and remove stitches. Check radiographs for integrity of fixation. Full active and active-assistive range of motion is allowed to the shoulder and elbow. The involved extremity is used for feeding, light grooming, and writing activities. No heavy lifting is allowed. Limited weight bearing is allowed.

Plate Fixation

See Intramedullary Nail/Rod. No weight bearing is allowed.

External Fixation

Check the wound and pin site. Review pin care with the patient. Any skin tethering may be released with a scalpel.

Check radiographs for fracture alignment and for lucency about the pins, which may signify infection.

Full active and active-assistive range of motion is allowed to the shoulder and elbow. The involved extremity is used for feeding, light grooming, and writing activities. No heavy lifting is allowed.

Prescription

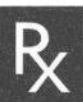

TWO WEEKS

Precautions No lifting with the affected extremity.

Range of Motion Active and active-assistive range of motion to the elbow and shoulder. With a *splint or brace*, no abduction of the shoulder beyond 60 degrees.

Muscle Strength Gentle pendulum exercises to the shoulder. No strengthening exercises to the elbow or shoulder.

Functional Activities Uninvolved extremity may be used for activities of daily living. In *ORIF and external fixation*, involved extremity used for feeding, light grooming, writing.

Weight bearing No weight bearing on affected extremity. Limited weight bearing with rodding.

Treatment: Four to Six Weeks

BONE HEALING

Stability at fracture site: Bridging callus and moderate stability.

Stage of bone healing: Reparative phase. Organization of callus continues and lamellar bone deposition begins. Bridging callus is still weaker than normal bone.

X-ray: Bridging callus is visible.

Orthopaedic and Rehabilitation Considerations

Physical Examination

Assess complaints of pain, swelling, and paresthesia. Check capillary refill and sensation. Check the active and passive motion of the shoulder, elbow, wrist, and fingers. Evaluate the patient's ability to perform pendulum exercises. Maintain appropriate splinting and encourage the passive range of motion of the wrist and fingers if active motion is not possible.

Dangers

Monitor the radial nerve. Assess the arm for signs of reflex sympathetic dystrophy.

Radiography

Examine anteroposterior and lateral radiographs of the humerus.

Weight Bearing

In a functional brace, the patient may begin to feel comfortable bearing some weight on the arm. With an intramedullary rod, weight bearing should be relatively pain free and encouraged. With plate fixation, light weight bearing is allowed.

Range of Motion

Active and active-assistive range of motion is instituted to the shoulder and elbow, wrist, and digits. Continue pendulum exercises. Continue supination and pronation of the forearm.

Muscle Strength

Continue strengthening exercises to the wrist and digits with isotonic exercises to the forearm muscles against resistance. At the end of 6 weeks, gentle isometric exercises may be instituted to the biceps and triceps if good callus formation is present.

Functional Activities

The patient may use the involved extremity for basic self-care and personal hygiene. No heavy lifting is allowed.

Gait/Ambulation

Arm swing should be returning at this point. Intramedullary rodding treatment allows the earliest return.

Methods of Treatment: Specific Aspects

Coaptation Splint and Functional Bracing

If the functional brace was not previously applied, it should now be used. Check for stability at the fracture site.

Check radiographs for the presence of bridging callus and alignment at the fracture site. Check the position of the fracture in a functional brace if it was just applied. In some patients, correction of angulation is still possible and may be accomplished by the adjustment of a sling or the addition of medial bolsters.

The patient should work on active and active-assistive abduction up to 90 degrees. Continue with pendulum exercises.

Open Reduction/Intramedullary Nail/Rod

Check radiographs for integrity of fixation and note the presence of bridging callus.

The patient may continue to use the extremity for basic activities of daily living, other than lifting heavy objects. Continue full range of motion to the shoulder and elbow.

Plate Fixation

See Intramedullary Nail/Rod. Light weight bearing is allowed.

External Fixation

Check the wound and pin site. Strong consideration should be given to removing the external fixator and applying a functional brace if the skin condition allows. Check the stability of the fracture site if the external fixator has been removed.

Check radiographs for fracture alignment and for lucency about the pins, which may signify infection. Check for the presence of bridging callus.

The patient may continue to use the extremity for basic activities of daily living, other than lifting.

Prescription

Four to Six Weeks

Precautions No heavy lifting with the affected extremity.

Range of Motion Active and active-assistive range of motion to the shoulder and elbow.

Muscle Strength Isometric and isotonic exercises to the forearm muscles. After 6 weeks, isometric exercises to the biceps and triceps.

Functional Activities Involved extremity may be used for basic self-care and personal hygiene.

Weight bearing Early weight bearing is allowed with internal fixation.

Treatment: Eight to Twelve Weeks

Bone Healing

Stability at fracture site: Stable callus.

Stage of bone healing: Remodeling phase. Woven bone is replaced by lamellar bone. Remodeling occurs over months to years.

X-ray: Abundant callus, fracture line begins to disappear, reconstitution of medullary canal. Nonunion is clearly evident.

Orthopaedic and Rehabilitation Considerations

Physical Examination

Check for tenderness at the fracture site and evaluate the stability of the humerus. Check the active and passive motion of the shoulder, elbow, wrist, and fingers. If neurologic injury has occurred, check for resolution. If the patient has persistent wrist drop, EMG and nerve conduction studies should be scheduled. The radial nerve may need to be formally explored and repaired if there is no return of function.

Dangers

Evaluate for reflex sympathetic dystrophy. Radial nerve injury is still a concern.

Radiography

Examine anteroposterior and lateral radiographs of the humerus.

Weight Bearing

For fractures treated with an intramedullary rod, weight bearing should be painless. If healing has progressed, the patient can continue progressive weight bearing on a fracture treated with a plate or by external fixation.

Range of Motion

Full range of motion in all planes is instituted to the shoulder and elbow. Once there is good callus formation, passive range of motion is encouraged if full range is not present at these joints.

Muscle Strength

Continue isometric exercises to the shoulder and elbow. Progressive resistive exercises can be instituted with a gradual increase in weights to the shoulder and elbow.

Functional Activities

The involved extremity may now be used in self-care and personal hygiene. Light lifting is allowed. No heavy contact sports are allowed.

Gait/Ambulation

Arm swing should now be fully integrated into the gait.

Methods of Treatment: Specific Aspects

Functional Bracing

Check radiographs for angulation and the presence of callus. If the fracture site is stable and nontender and the radiograph demonstrates ample callus, the functional brace may be discontinued. If the fracture is not united, operative intervention should be considered.

The patient may begin light lifting. Stress the importance of compliance and the possibility of refracture. The patient should understand that this risk decreases over time. No sports are allowed.

Open Reduction/Intramedullary Nail/Rod

Check radiographs for the integrity of fixation and note the presence of callus.

The patient may begin light lifting. Stress the importance of the possibility of refracture from overlifting. The patient should understand that this risk decreases over time. No sports are allowed.

Plate Fixation

See Open Reduction/Intramedullary Nail/Rod. Increase weight bearing. Plate removal is usually not necessary.

External Fixation

Remove the apparatus, if this has not already been done. Functional bracing may be used if the fracture is not well healed.

Check radiographs for maintenance of alignment and fracture healing after the apparatus is removed.

Prescription

EIGHT TO TWELVE WEEKS

Precautions No contact sports.

Range of Motion Active, active-assistive, and passive range of motion to the elbow and shoulder.

Muscle Strength Progressive resistive exercises to the shoulder and elbow.

Functional Activities Involved extremity may be used in activities of daily living. Light lifting is allowed with the affected extremity.

Weight bearing Full weight bearing is allowed.

LONG-TERM CONSIDERATIONS AND PROBLEMS

Uneventful healing is the rule in uncomplicated closed fractures. Transverse fractures and open fractures have a higher incidence of nonunion. If limited healing or nonhealing is evident, consider the possibility of delayed union or impending nonunion. Bone grafting or, less commonly, electrical stimulation may be necessary. Reflex sympathetic dystrophy is a concern after treatment has been discontinued. Radial nerve exploration may be reconsidered if there is no return of function after four months.

Plate removal is usually not necessary. If removed, the fracture site must be protected to prevent refracture in the weakened bone cortex under the plate.

IMMEDIATE TO ONE WEEK

	Cast/Brace	*Rod*	*Plate*
Stability	None.	Stability depends on fit of rod and comminution of fracture. If well fitting, arm is stable.	Stability depends on accuracy of reduction and stability of fixation. If minimal comminution is present, the arm is usually stable.
Orthopaedics	Examine radial nerve function. Inspect axilla for irritation. Ensure wrist and finger motion and check arm swelling. Examine radiographs for displacement.	Check surgical wounds. Check radiographs.	Check surgical wounds and radiographs.
Rehabilitation	Move digits to diminish hand swelling. No strengthening or ranging to elbow or shoulder.	If stable fixation, the patient may begin moving the shoulder and elbow as pain allows.	If stable fixation, the patient may range the shoulder and elbow as pain allows. If unstable, no range of motion.

TWO WEEKS

	Cast/Brace	*Rod*	*Plate*
Stability	None to minimal.	Variable.	Variable.
Orthopaedics	Examine axilla. Examine radial nerve. Check radiographs for loss of reduction.	Check surgical wounds; remove stitches. Check for early reflex sympathetic dystrophy (RSD).	Check surgical wounds; remove stitches. Check radiographs.
Rehabilitation	Begin gentle range of motion to elbow and shoulder. No strengthening.	Progress with range of motion to shoulder and elbow. Pendulum exercises to the shoulder. Limited weight bearing is allowed.	Progress with range of motion to shoulder and elbow. Pendulum exercises to the shoulder. No weight bearing.

FOUR TO SIX WEEKS

	Cast/Brace	*Rod*	*Plate*
Stability	Partially stable.	Increasingly stable.	Increasingly stable (especially if bone graft was used in surgery).
Orthopaedics	All casts should be converted to . braces by week 4. Check radial nerve. Check for RSD. Check radiographs for evidence of callus and maintenance of reduction	Check radiographs for callus and fracture position. Check healed wounds. Check for return of radial nerve if originally lost.	Check radial nerve. Check healed wounds. Check radiographs for cortical continuity or hardware failure.
Rehabilitation	Aggressive range of motion to shoulder and elbow. Strengthening with isometric and isotonic exercises.	If callus is evident, weight bearing is to be progressed.	Light weight bearing allowed. Aggressive ranging and light strengthening to shoulder and elbow.
	Light weight bearing to extremity. Use extremity for activities of daily living.	Isotonic and isometric strengthening, and ranging to elbow and shoulder.	

EIGHT TO TWELVE WEEKS

	Cast/Brace	*Rod*	*Plate*
Stability	Stable.	Stable.	Stable.
Orthopaedics	Abundant callus usually present on radiographs. No motion or tenderness at fracture sites. Reexamine radial nerve. Electromyography if needed.	Abundant callus on radiographs. No tenderness. Healed wounds.	Full cortical continuity on radiographs. No fracture line evident. All wounds well healed.
Rehabilitation	Full weight bearing, ranging, and progressive resistive exercises for strengthening.	Full activities.	Full activities.

BIBLIOGRAPHY

Balfour GW, Mooney V, Ashby M. Diaphyseal fractures of the humerus treated with a ready made fracture brace. *J Bone Joint Surg Am*, 64:11–13, 1982.

Bone L. Fractures of the shaft of the humerus. In: Chapman MW, ed. *Operative Orthopedics*, Vol 1. Philadelphia: J.B. Lippincott, 1988, pp. 221–234.

Connolly JF, Mendes M, Browner B. Principles of closed management of common fractures. In: Browner DB, et al., eds. *Skeletal Trauma*. Philadelphia: W.B. Saunders, 1992, pp. 211–230.

Epps CH Jr, Grant RE. Fractures of the shaft of the humerus. In: Rockwood C, ed. *Rockwood and Green's Fractures in Adults*, Vol 1, 3rd ed. Philadelphia: J.B. Lippincott, 1991, pp. 843–870.

Ward EF, Savoie FH, Hughes JL. Fractures of the diaphyseal humerus. In: Browner DB, et al., eds. *Skeletal Trauma*. Philadelphia: W.B. Saunders, 1992, pp. 1177–1200.

CHAPTER *Thirteen*

Distal Humeral Fractures

SAMUEL A. HOISINGTON, MD

MARK A. THOMAS, MD

INTRODUCTION

Definition

Fractures of the distal humerus involve the metaphysis. They may or may not extend into the intraarticular surface.

Intraarticular fractures include medial and lateral condylar fractures (single column) as well as T and Y intercondylar (two-column) fractures. The articular surface has been disrupted in each, but with unicondylar fractures, one fragment is still connected to the shaft. In bicondylar fractures, both columns are fractured and the articular fragments are separate from the humeral shaft. Intraarticular distal humeral fractures pose a great challenge for the treating physician (Figures 13-1, 13-2, 13-3, 13-4, 13-5).

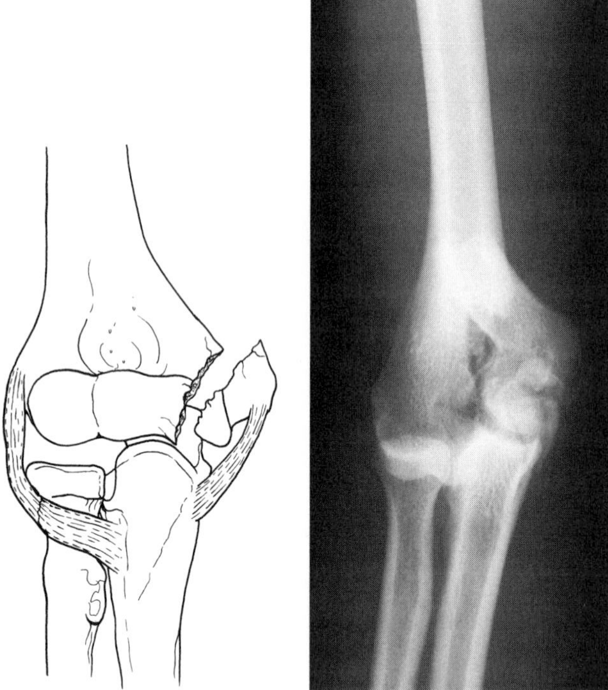

FIGURE 13-1 *(above, left)* Intraarticular single-column fracture involving the medial condyle (trochlea) of the distal humerus.

FIGURE 13-2 *(above, right)* Radiograph illustrating an intraarticular fracture involving a single column, the medial condyle of the distal humerus. Note the associated fracture of the olecranon.

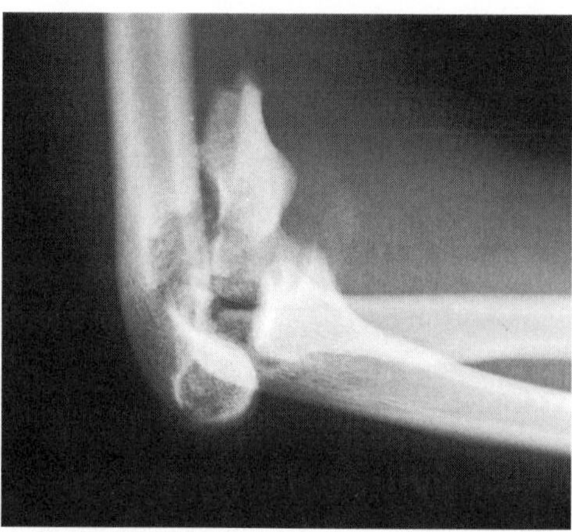

FIGURE 13-3 Lateral radiograph of an intraarticular single-column fracture involving the medial condyle of the distal humerus. Note the associated anterior radial head dislocation and olecranon fracture.

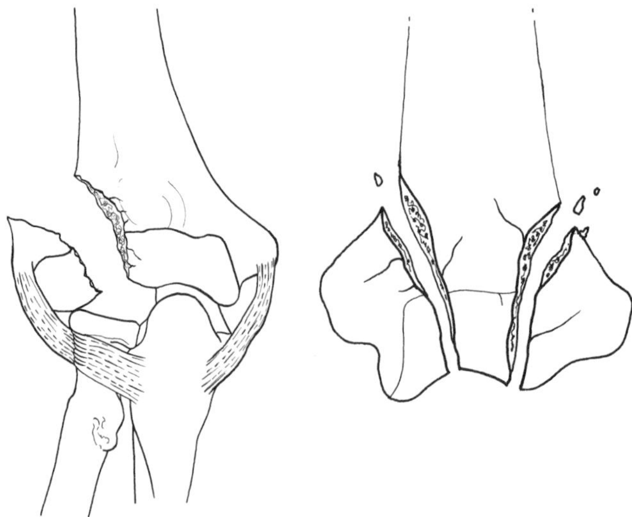

FIGURE 13-4 *(above, left)* Lateral condyle fracture of the distal humerus. This is an intraarticular single-column fracture of the distal humeral capitellum.

FIGURE 13-5 *(above, right)* Y intracondylar fracture of the distal humerus. This is a two-column intraarticular fracture.

Extraarticular fractures include supracondylar (extracapsular), transcondylar (intracapsular), and medial and lateral epicondylar fractures (extracapsular). Supracondylar and transcondylar fractures may be further subdivided into extension or flexion type, depending on the mechanism of injury and the location of the distal fragments. With an extension-type fracture there is posterior displacement of the distal end of the humerus, whereas the flexion-type injury leads to anterior displacement of the distal fragment and elbow joint (Table 13-1 and Figures 13-6, 13-7, 13-8, 13-9, 13-10, 13-11, and 13-12).

TABLE 13-1 *Distal Humeral Fractures*

Intraarticular fractures		Extraarticular fractures	
Single Column	**Two Column**	**Extracapsular**	**Intracapsular**
Medial condyle	T Intercondylar	Supracondylar	Transcondylar
Lateral condyle	Y Intercondylar	Medial and lateral epicondylar	

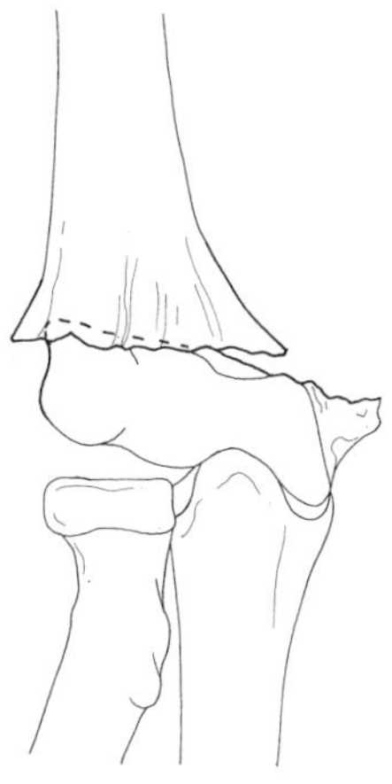

FIGURE 13-6 Displaced transcondylar fracture. This is an intracapsular extraarticular fracture.

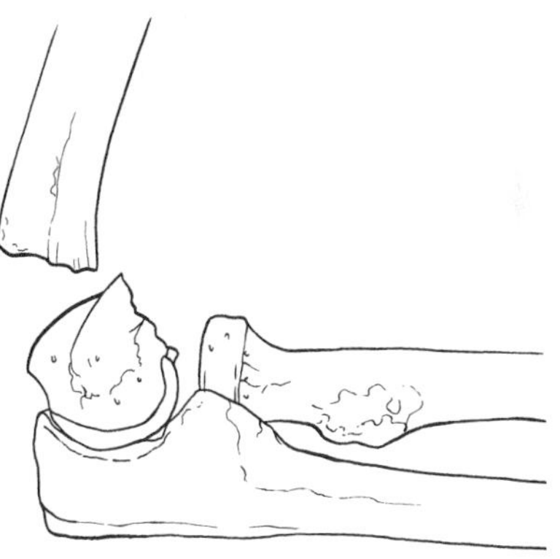

FIGURE 13-7 Lateral illustration of a transcondylar fracture bordering on a supracondylar fracture. This fracture is extraarticular.

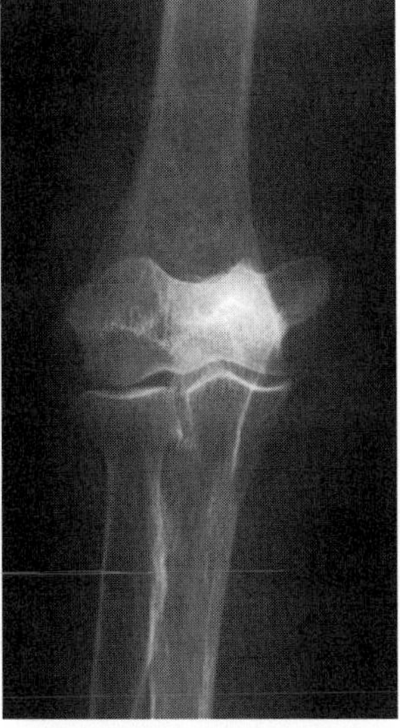

FIGURE 13-8 Displaced transcondylar fracture. This fracture is extraarticular and intracapsular.

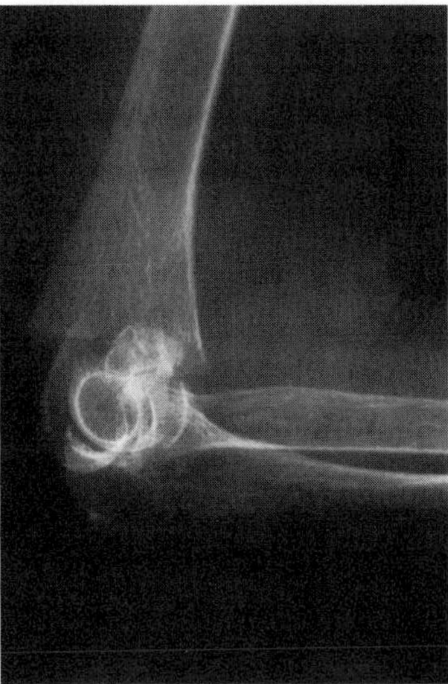

FIGURE 13-9 Lateral radiograph of a transcondylar fracture.

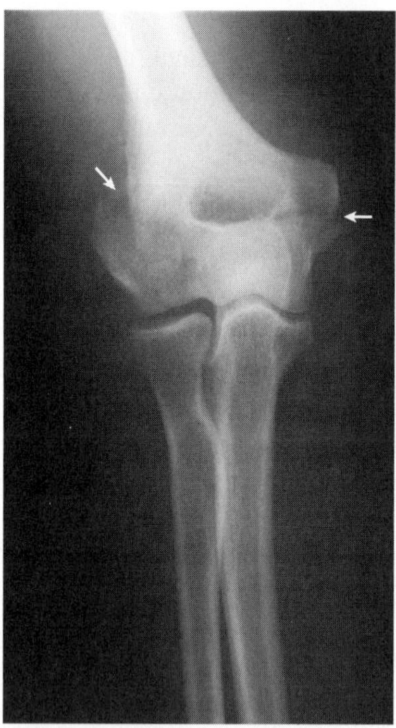

FIGURE 13-10 Anteroposterior radiograph of a transcondylar fracture with possible intraarticular extension into the lateral condyle (capitellum).

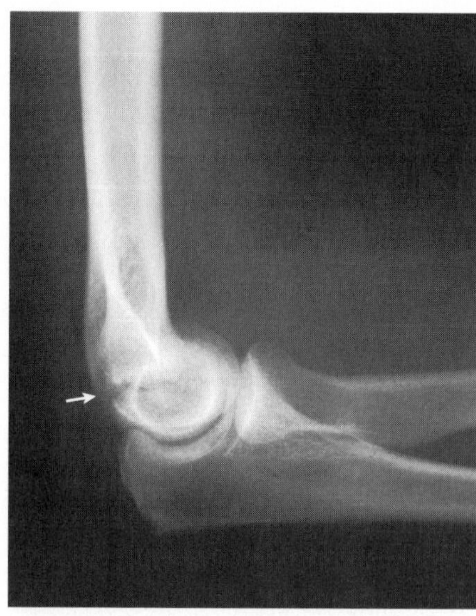

FIGURE 13-11 Lateral radiograph of a transcondylar fracture.

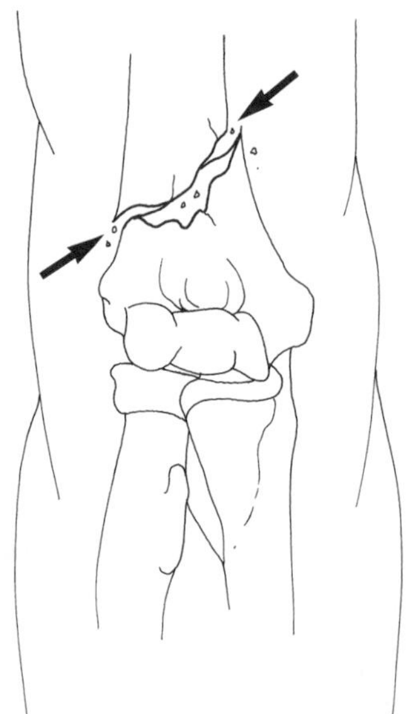

FIGURE 13-12 Oblique supracondylar fracture in the metaphyseal region of the distal humerus. This fracture is extraarticular and extracapsular.

Mechanism of Injury

Intraarticular fractures result from compression forces across the elbow. The points of application and direction of the force in combination with a varus or valgus stress concentrate the force to either the medial or lateral column of the distal humerus, whereas a direct impaction of the ulna into the trochlear groove may cause a condylar split. Extension-type supracondylar or transcondylar fractures generally result from a fall on an outstretched hand or a direct blow to the elbow, whereas flexion-type fractures result from a direct force against the posterior aspect of the elbow. Extension-type supracondylar humeral fractures are the most common extraarticular injury.

Treatment Goals

Orthopedic Objectives

Alignment

Accurate alignment of the distal humerus avoids the disability and cosmetic deformity associated with an abnormal carrying angle, whereas accurate reduction of the intraarticular surface is necessary to reduce the risk of posttraumatic arthritis.

Stability

Displaced distal humeral fractures are unstable injuries. Surgical stabilization allows early rehabilitation and return to function. When healed, the distal humerus should be stable on weight bearing.

Rehabilitation Objectives

Range of Motion

Restore and maintain the full range of motion of the elbow, protect the normal carrying angle of the elbow, and reestablish the full range of shoulder motion (Table 13-2).

TABLE 13-2 *Elbow Range of Motion*

Motion	Normal	Functional
Flexion	135°	0–90°
Extension	0–5°	–20–30°
Supination	90°	50°
Pronation	90°	50°

Muscle Strength

Improve the strength of the following muscles:

Elbow extensor: triceps

Elbow flexor: biceps

Secondary muscles:

Forearm supinators and pronators

Wrist extensors:

Extensor carpi radialis longus and brevis

Extensor carpi ulnaris

Wrist flexors:

Flexor carpi radialis long

Flexor carpi ulnaris

Deltoid

Functional Goals

Restore activities that require flexion/extension and supination/pronation, such as feeding, personal hygiene, dressing, and grooming.

Expected Time of Bone Healing

Eight to 12 weeks.

With open fractures or fractures that require periosteal stripping for fixation, expect a delay in bone healing.

Expected Duration of Rehabilitation

Twelve to 24 weeks.

Methods of Treatment

Cast or Posterior Splint

Biomechanics: Stress-sharing device.

Mode of Bone Healing: Secondary.

Indications: A long arm cast or posterior long arm splint is indicated for nondisplaced fractures of the distal humerus and for displaced fractures amenable to closed reduction. For most injuries, the elbow is placed at 90 degrees. Greater flexion may be needed to maintain reduction in extension-type injuries, but the ability to achieve this flexion may be limited by swelling. Controversy exists as to the best position of forearm immobilization, but placing the forearm in neutral is usually preferred for adult patients. Care should be taken to protect the normal carrying angle of the elbow (5° to 15° valgus) as well as the normal 30° anterior angulation of the distal humerus. In nondisplaced injuries, the extremity is immobilized for 2 to 3 weeks, followed by supervised active range of motion for another 4 to 6 weeks. For fractures following closed reduction, immobilization is usually required for 4 to 6 weeks and rehabilitation of the elbow is started only when radiographic evidence of healing and clinical stability is present. The use of a hinged cast or functional brace should be considered when mobilization begins. Close clinical and radiographic follow-up is necessary with closed treatment of these types of fractures. Any fracture in which closed reduction has led to neurologic compromise requires exploration.

Percutaneous Pinning with Cast or Splint

Biomechanics: Stress-sharing device.

Mode of Bone Healing: Secondary.

Indications: Closed reduction and percutaneous pin fixation, although commonly used in children, is used less often in adults and is best reserved for extraarticular distal humeral fractures. The pins are left in place for 4 to 6 weeks, with the arm in a splint or cast, the elbow at a right angle, and the forearm in neutral. Following pin removal, gentle protected active elbow range of motion is begun if clinical stability and the progression of radiographic union allows (Figures 13-13, 13-14, 13-15, 13-16).

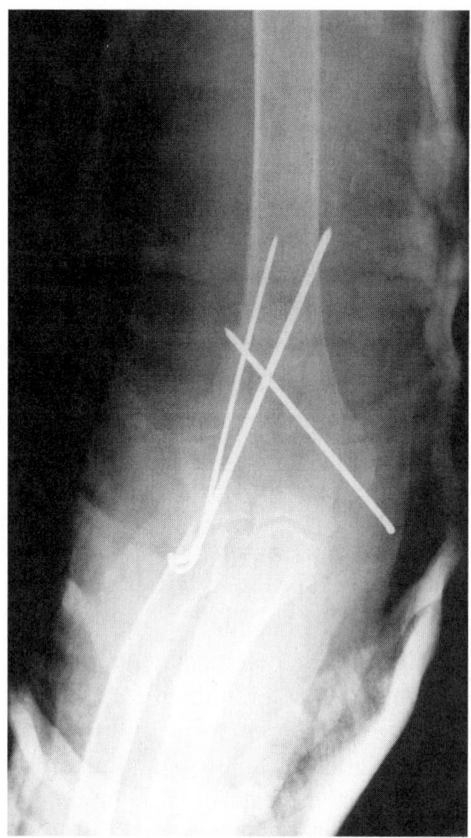

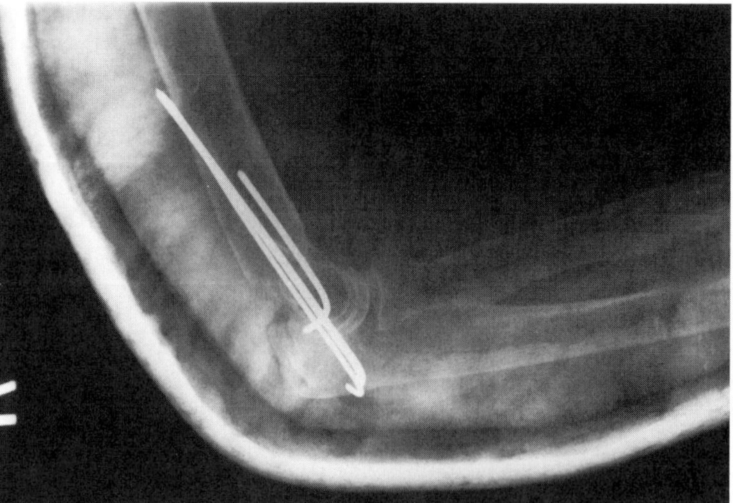

FIGURE 13-13 *(above, left)* Pin fixation of a transcondylar fracture with the limb placed in a posterior splint.

FIGURE 13-14 *(above)* Lateral radiograph of a transcondylar fracture treated with pin fixation and the extremity placed in a posterior splint.

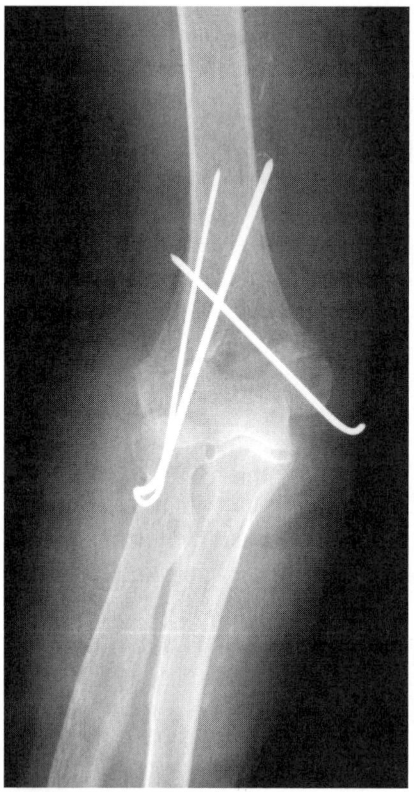

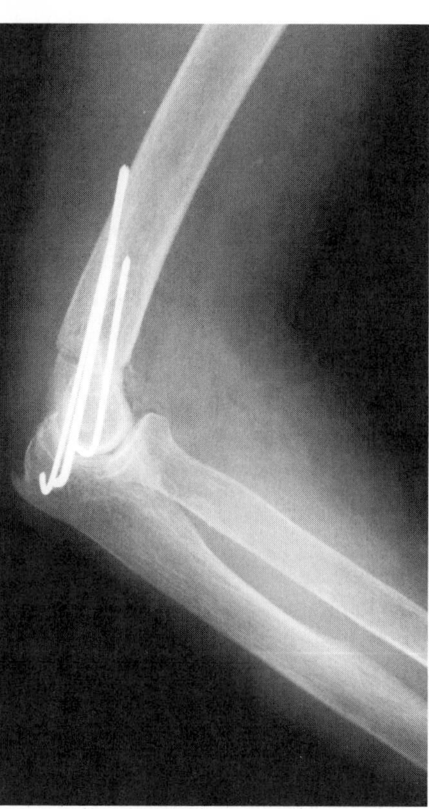

FIGURE 13-15 *(far left)* Transcondylar fracture treated with pin fixation.

FIGURE 13-16 *(left)* Lateral radiograph of a transcondylar fracture treated with pin fixation. The pins are generally left in place for 4 to 6 weeks.

Open Reduction and Internal Fixation

Biomechanics: Stress-shielding device. Stress sharing may occur if there is inadequate internal fixation.

Mode of Bone Healing: Secondary healing occurs if solid fixation is not achieved.

Indications: Fixation with lag screws or medial and lateral reconstruction plates is used for intraarticular injuries with persistent step-off and for extraarticular injures that do not reduce with closed manipulation. Careful preoperative planning is necessary. Plates placed at right angles to each other yield the greatest stability in all planes. Plate placement ultimately depends on the fracture configuration, but usually the lateral plate may be placed along the posterior surface of the lateral column and the medial plate along the medial aspect of the medial column. Ulnar nerve subcutaneous transposition may be required if the hardware impinges on the cubital tunnel. Open reduction and internal fixation is also indicated for open fractures that require irrigation and débridement, fractures with associated neurovascular injury that require exploration, and floating elbows (Figures 13-17, 13-18, 13-19, 13-20, 13-21, 13-22, 13-23, 13-24.)

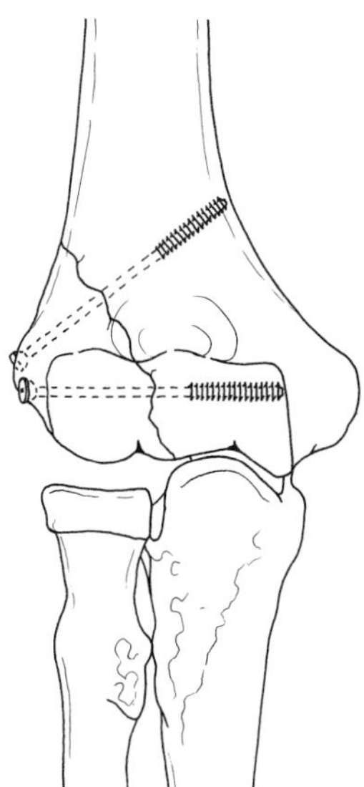

FIGURE 13-17 Lateral condylar fracture treated with screw fixation. This is an intraarticular fracture that requires anatomic reduction of the articular surface.

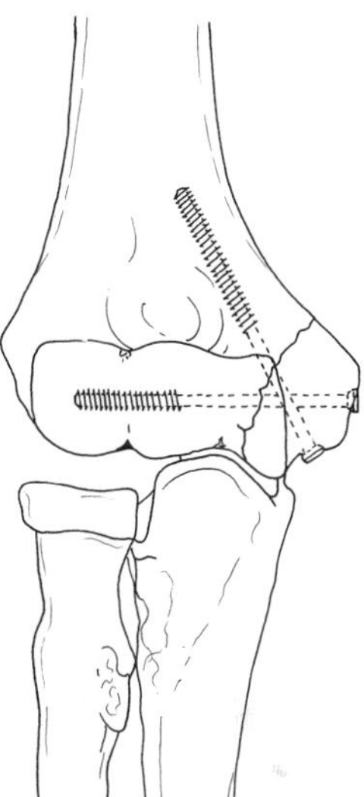

FIGURE 13-18 A medial condylar fracture of the distal humerus treated with screw fixation. This is an intraarticular single-column fracture that requires anatomic reduction of the articular surface.

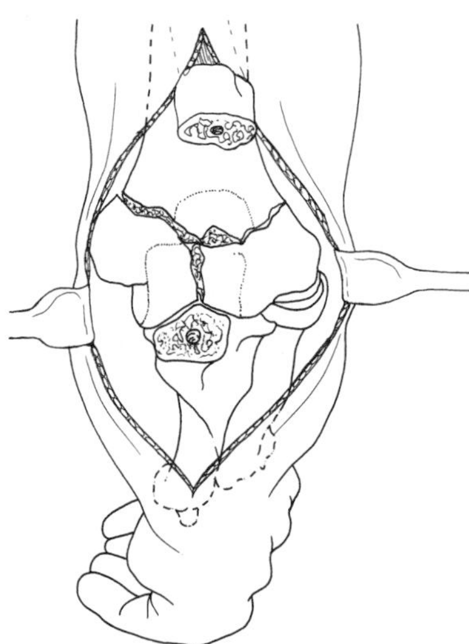

FIGURE 13-19 Illustration of a posterior surgical approach to the elbow using an olecranon osteotomy for visualization of the posterior articular surface of the elbow. This approach is used for intraarticular fractures; in this case, a T intercondylar fracture of the distal humerus is noted.

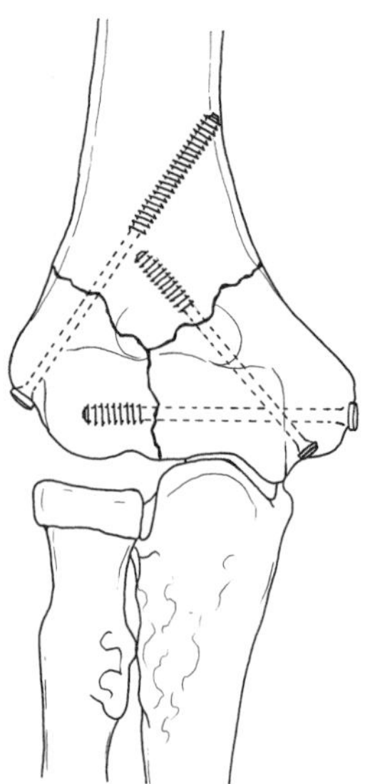

FIGURE 13-20 T intercondylar fracture of the distal humerus, treated with screw fixation.

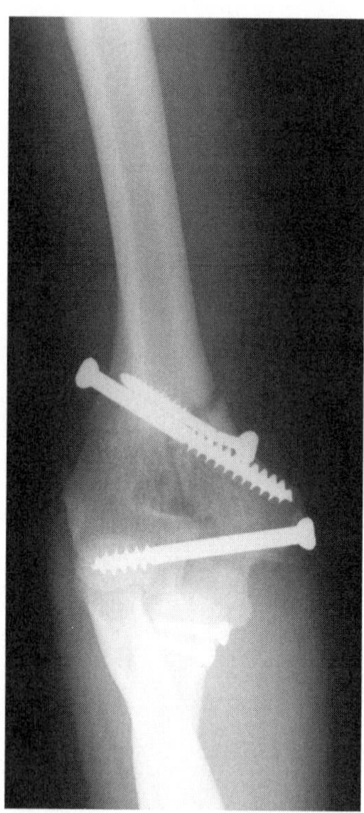

FIGURE 13-21 T intercondylar fracture of the distal humerus, treated with screw fixation. Note the screw fixation of the olecranon fracture. This is an intraarticular two-column fracture.

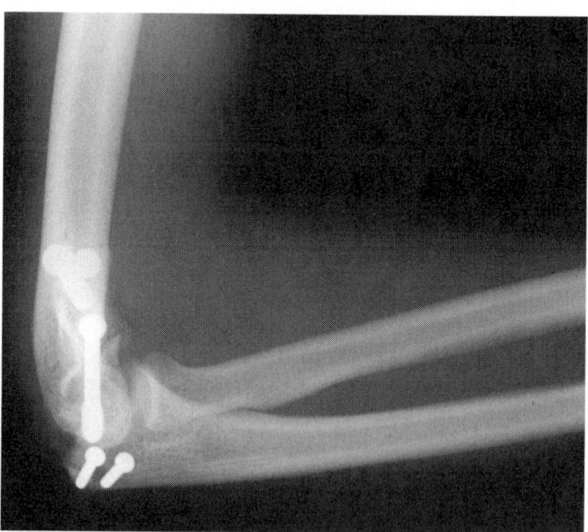

FIGURE 13-22 Lateral radiograph showing an intraarticular two-column fracture of the distal humerus, treated with screw fixation. Note the screw fixation of the olecranon fracture.

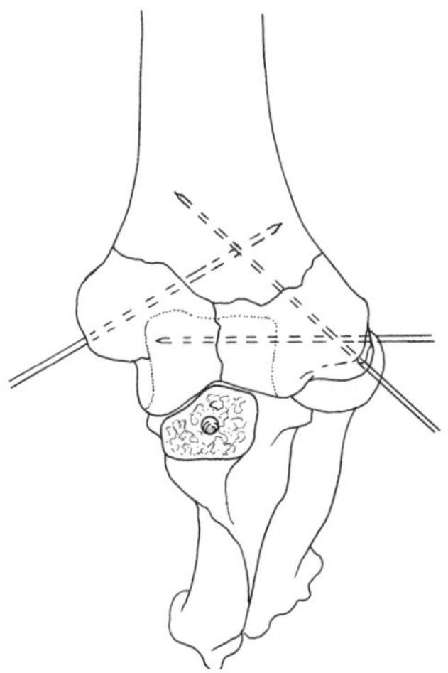

FIGURE 13-23 T intercondylar fracture of the distal humerus, treated with pin fixation. This intraarticular two-column fracture requires anatomic reduction of the articular surface through an extensile posterior approach to the elbow and an olecranon osteotomy. See Figure 13-19.

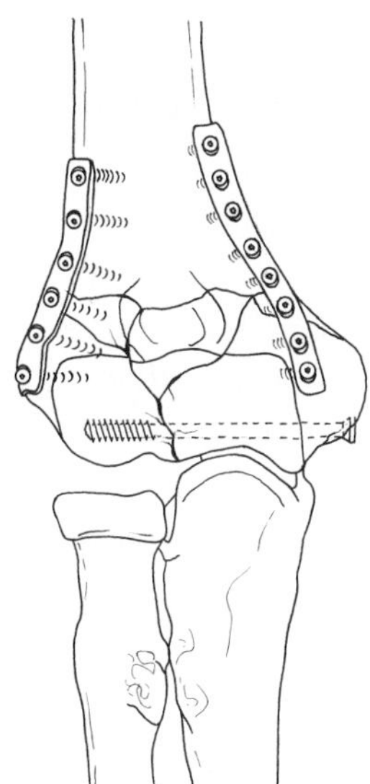

FIGURE 13-24 Comminuted intraarticular fracture of the distal humerus with plate and screw fixation. This intraarticular fracture requires anatomic reduction of the articular surface through an extensile posterior approach to the elbow and an olecranon osteotomy. See Figure 13-19.

External Fixation

Biomechanics: Stress-sharing device.

Mode of Bone Healing: Secondary.

Indications: External fixation is used only for grossly contaminated open injuries.

Skeletal Traction

Biomechanics: Stress-sharing device.

Mode of Bone Healing: Secondary.

Indications: Olecranon pin traction is not commonly used with adults. It is useful only for fractures that do not achieve reduction by standard techniques, for achieving proper length and alignment before surgical management, and for reduction of edema in the grossly swollen elbow. Overhead traction is preferable to lateral skeletal traction because it maintains the elbow in an elevated position. Skeletal traction is rarely a definitive treatment and is later converted to splint or cast immobilization when possible.

Special Considerations of the Fracture

Loss of Motion

The most common complication of fractures around the elbow is loss of motion. This may result from poor treatment of the fracture, scarring after operative management, malunion, the development of myositis ossificans, or the production of excess callus. Full extension of the elbow is the hardest to achieve. Most functions of the elbow require motion from 30° to 130°; consequently, a 30° extension lag has little functional significance. Early physical therapy with active range-of-motion exercises is crucial. Myositis ossificans is especially common after elbow dislocations and radial head fractures. It is also associated with passive range-of-motion exercises, which should be avoided.

Age

In elderly patients, joint stiffness is more likely to develop and they are also more likely to have comminuted intraarticular fractures as a result of the osteoporotic nature of their bone. Osteoporosis makes open reduction and internal fixation more difficult and reduces the strength of the fixation.

Articular Involvement

Intraarticular fractures may result in posttraumatic degenerative changes of the elbow joint unless anatomic reduction is achieved. (*See* Figures 13-19, 13-20, 13-21, 13-22, 13-23, and 13-24.)

Elbow Dislocation or Ligamentous Injury

Concurrent elbow dislocation may be present at the time of the initial evaluation. The relationship of a condylar fracture to the lateral trochlear ridge is important to the stability of the elbow. When the lateral trochlear ridge is included in a condyle fracture, it is considered a fracture/dislocation. Condylar fractures are often associated with ligamentous and capsular injuries.

Open Fractures

Open fractures involving the distal end of the humerus may be associated with significant periosteal stripping. A delay in bone and soft tissue healing, as well as the need for a longer period of rehabilitation, are common.

Malunion/Nonunion

Malunion of distal humeral fractures generally results in a cosmetic deformity. Malunion of lateral condylar fractures with a concurrent valgus deformity of the elbow may lead to tardy ulnar nerve palsy. Risk factors for nonunion of distal humeral fractures include significant fracture comminution, inadequate fixation, open fracture, and infection. The management of a distal humerus nonunion is a major challenge.

Delayed Union/Nonunion Following Olecranon Osteotomy

An olecranon osteotomy is done during the posterior approach to the distal humerus. (*See* Figure 13-19.) Careful planning and stable fixation of the olecranon are necessary to avoid this complication. Tension band wiring with parallel pins or a lag screw is preferred, because this allows early mobilization of the elbow. The tension band technique enhances compression across the osteotomy site, which promotes healing. Fixation with compression screws alone should be avoided.

Associated Injury

Nerves

The ulnar nerve lies close to the medial epicondyle and is the most commonly injured nerve in distal humeral fractures, particularly T intercondylar fractures. Malunion of distal humeral fractures can also lead to tardy ulnar nerve palsy. The radial and median nerves may be injured with any distal humeral fracture. Careful evaluation of possible nerve injuries at the time of the fracture and immediately after treatment is of utmost importance. Nerve injuries may occur with closed reduction, percutaneous pin placement, or open surgical treatment. Those that occur as a result of treatment should be explored.

Vessels

Injury to the brachial artery may occur with any humeral fracture, although it is most often associated with supracondylar and T or Y intercondylar fractures. There is generally a concurrent nerve injury, and a compartment syndrome may result. If a brachial artery injury is suspected, an arteriogram must be performed immediately, followed by emergent vascular repair if an injury is present. If the arm or forearm is tense, or if there are any other signs of compartment syndrome, pressures must be measured and appropriate treatment provided. The consequences of a missed compartment syndrome can be devastating, including Volkmann's ischemic contracture or even the loss of the limb.

TREATMENT

Treatment: Early to Immediate (Day of Injury to One Week)

BONE HEALING

Stability at fracture site: No bony stability. Some stability may be afforded by an intact periosteum and ligaments.

Stage of bone healing: Inflammatory phase. The fracture hematoma is colonized by inflammatory cells and debridement of the fracture begins.

X-ray: No callus.

Orthopedic and Rehabilitation Considerations

Physical Examination

Assess complaints of pain, swelling, and paresthesia. Be alert for developing compartment syndrome. Check capillary refill and sensation, as well as the active and passive range of motion of the digits. Swelling and discoloration of the skin are common. Dependent edema should be treated by limb elevation or removal and reapplication of the cast or splint if severe.

Dangers

Compartment syndrome of the arm or forearm may occur. Pay special attention to complaints of pain, paresthesia, and cast or splint discomfort. If compartment syndrome is suspected, compartment pressures should be measured and fasciotomies performed for elevated pressures.

X-rays

Anteroposterior and true lateral radiographs of the elbow should be obtained and checked for loss of reduction and joint congruency. On a true lateral x-ray film of the elbow, the distal humerus is flexed about 30°; however flexion of 10° to 30° is considered acceptable. On the anteroposterior view, the trochlear axis is in 4° to 8° of valgus, which leads to the normal valgus carrying angle of the elbow. Comparison views of the opposite elbow may be obtained.

Weight Bearing

No weight bearing is allowed on the affected extremity.

Range of Motion

Begin active range of motion of the fingers and metacarpophalangeal joints. Instruct the patient in gentle pendulum exercises to allow shoulder range of motion. The patient should be able to perform these exercises once the pain subsides. Avoid internal and external rotation of the shoulder, because this stresses the fracture site.

Muscle Strength

Flexion and extension exercises of the fingers as well as adduction and abduction exercises for intrinsic strengthening are instituted.

Functional Activities

The patient is instructed in using the uninvolved extremity for all functions of daily living. Clothes are donned on the involved extremity first and doffed from the uninvolved extremity first. Clothing may have to be draped around the affected arm for comfort and convenience. Elderly patients are instructed in using a hemi-walker or quad cane instead of a regular walker, because they cannot hold a walker with two hands.

Gait

The arm swing is absent as the extremity is immobilized and usually painful.

Methods of Treatment: Specific Aspects

Cast or Posterior Splint

With casting or splinting, there should be no motion at the elbow. The cast should be trimmed to the proximal palmar crease to allow full range of motion of the metacarpophalangeal joints.

No supination or pronation is allowed if in a splint. Shoulder pendulum exercises may be started, but internal and external rotation movements should be avoided, because they can lead to fracture displacement.

Percutaneous Pinning

The arm is immobilized and there should be no motion at the elbow. The patient follows the same protocol as for a cast or splint.

Open Reduction and Internal Fixation

If there is adequate fixation with a stable construct, immobilization is not required, and gentle active range-of-motion exercises are begun at the wrist, elbow, and shoulder. This may be started within 3 to 5 days as soft tissues, pain, and edema allow. A functional brace or posterior splint may be used for protection. An arm sling alone may also be used. Rotational movements of the shoulder should be avoided because they produce excessive torque at the fracture site. (Pronation and supination of the forearm are allowed if a stable construct has been achieved.) If the bone quality is poor or the fixation inadequate, the arm may be immobilized, but extended postoperative immobilization defeats the purpose of open reduction and internal fixation and may lead to severe stiffness.

Prescription

DAY ONE TO ONE WEEK

Precautions

No internal or external rotation of the shoulder.

No passive range of motion to the elbow.

Range of Motion

Gentle active elbow flexion and extension allowed for stable fractures treated *with open reduction and internal fixation.*

No range of motion to the elbow if treated by other methods.

Strength No strengthening exercises to the elbow.

Functional Activities The uninvolved extremity is used for the activities of daily living and self-care.

Weight Bearing No weight bearing on the affected extremity.

Treatment: Two Weeks

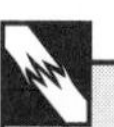

BONE HEALING

Stability at fracture site: None to minimal.

Stage of bone healing: Beginning of reparative phase. Osteoprogenitor cells differentiate into osteoblasts, which lay down woven bone.

X-ray: None to early callus.

Orthopedic and Rehabilitation Considerations

Physical Examination

Carefully assess complaints of pain, swelling, and paresthesia. Check capillary refill and sensation, as well as the active and passive range of motion of the digits. Dependent edema should be treated by limb elevation or removal and reapplication of the cast or splint if severe.

Dangers

Compression neuropathy may occur as a result of swelling and a tight cast.

X-rays

Anteroposterior and true lateral x-ray films of the elbow should be obtained and checked for loss of reduction and joint congruency.

Weight Bearing

No weight bearing is allowed on the affected extremity.

Range of Motion

Continue active range of motion of the digits. If the fingers are swollen, instruct the patient in retrograde massage from the tips of the fingers toward the palm. Continue pendulum exercises at the shoulder to prevent adhesive capsulitis. Internal and external rotation of the shoulder should be avoided, because this stresses the fracture site.

Muscle Strength

The patient may squeeze a sponge, ball, or putty to strengthen the fingers.

Functional Activities

Continue one-handed activities, using the uninvolved extremity for all self-care.

Gait

Arm swing is still reduced.

Methods of Treatment: Specific Aspects

Cast or Posterior Splint

Check the margins of the cast or splint and make sure that it is well padded; if it is loose, it should be reapplied. The patient should avoid rotatory movements of the shoulder. Because the pain usually subsides by this time, the patient can perform isometric exercises of the wrist flexors and extensors as well as ulnar and radial deviators within the cast. This is done by applying a gentle pressure against the confines of the cast. For nondisplaced fractures that are stable and did not require reduction, gentle supervised active range-of-motion exercises may be started at 2 or 3 weeks. For those that required closed reduction, supervised active-assistive flexion from 90° with posterior splint protection may be started at 2 to 3 weeks as tolerated by the patient. Immobilization should continue for extension-type supracondylar humeral fractures that required reduction. Between sessions, the patient must remain in a splint.

Percutaneous Pinning

Check the wound. The pins should remain in place with continued immobilization of the arm. The rehabilitation protocol is the same as for cast or splint treatment.

Open Reduction and Internal Fixation

The patient should continue active range-of-motion exercises at the wrist, elbow, and shoulder. Postoperative elbow stiffness is a major problem and active flexion and extension exercises of the elbow help prevent this problem. No passive range-of-motion exercises should be performed at the elbow because the risk of myositis ossificans is increased with passive motion. The patient uses a functional brace, posterior splint, or simply an arm sling for support and protection between therapy sessions.

Prescription

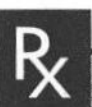

Two Weeks

Precautions
No internal or external rotation of the shoulder.
No passive range of motion to the elbow.

Range of Motion
Gentle active flexion and extension exercises to the elbow for fractures only when treated with open reduction and internal fixation.
Gentle assistive supervised active flexion and extension for nondisplaced stable fractures.

Strength No strengthening exercises to the elbow.

Functional Activities The uninvolved extremity is used for the activities of daily living and self-care.

Weight Bearing No weight bearing on the affected extremity.

Treatment: Four to Six Weeks

Bone Healing

Stability at fracture site: Once callus is observed bridging the fracture site, the fracture is usually stable. This should be confirmed by physical examination. The strength of this callus is significantly lower than that of normal bone, especially with torsional load.

Stage of bone healing: Reparative phase. Organization of callus continues, and lamellar bone deposition begins.

X-ray: Bridging callus is visible. With increased rigidity, less bridging callus is noted, and healing with endosteal callus predominates.

Orthopedic and Rehabilitation Considerations

Physical Examination

Check stability and tenderness at the fracture site and the range of motion of the elbow joint.

X-ray

Anteroposterior and true lateral x-ray films of the elbow should be obtained with the extremity out of the cast or splint.

Weight Bearing

No weight bearing is allowed on the affected extremity.

Range of Motion

Continue range of motion of the fingers and pendulum exercises of the shoulder.

Muscle Strength

Continue grip strengthening and isometric exercises of the forearm musculature.

Functional Activities

The uninvolved extremity is still used as the dominant extremity for self-care and personal hygiene. If rigid internal fixation was preformed, the patient may use the involved extremity for eating and similar light activities.

Methods of Treatment: Specific Aspects

Cast or Posterior Splint

For nondisplaced fractures that are stable and did not require reduction, gentle supervised active range-of-motion exercises that were started at 2 to 3 weeks should be continued and a home program added. Patients with extension-type supracondylar humeral fractures should continue supervised flexion exercises from 90° with posterior splint protection. Pending clinical stability and radiographic evidence of early union, a full program of gentle active elbow range of motion may be started for these and other distal humeral fractures. At first, this should be in a supervised setting, but a home program can be added by 6 weeks. Between sessions, the patient must remain in a splint. If there is motion at the fracture site or significant tenderness without radiographic evidence of healing, cast or splint immobilization should be continued.

Percutaneous Pinning

Once there is radiographic evidence of healing, the pins are removed and active elbow range of motion is started. Initially, the elbow can be quite stiff. This can be eased with hydrotherapy or by applying a hot pack before exercising. Supervised elbow active-assistive range of motion is performed at first, with a home program implemented early. Wrist range of motion is also performed. Between sessions, the patient should remain in an orthoplast or equivalent splint or in a functional brace.

Open Reduction and Internal Fixation

The patient should continue active and active-assistive range-of-motion exercises at the wrist, elbow, and shoulder. The patient uses a functional brace, posterior splint, or an arm sling for support and protection between therapy sessions. The patient should be performing exercises at home.

Prescription

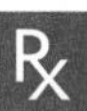

TREATMENT: FOUR TO SIX WEEKS

Precautions Avoid rotational stresses across the elbow.

Range of Motion Active flexion and extension to the elbow. Active-assistive range of motion to the elbow.

Strength No strengthening exercises to the elbow.

Functional Activities The uninvolved extremity is used for the activities of daily living and self-care.

Weight Bearing No weight bearing on the affected extremity.

Treatment: Eight to Twelve Weeks

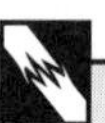

BONE HEALING

Stability at fracture site: Stable.

Stage of bone healing: Remodeling phase. Woven bone is replaced with lamellar bone. The process of remodeling takes months to years for completion.

X-ray: Callus is present but less than in midshaft. The fracture line begins to disappear. Reconstitution of the medullary canal occurs with time.

Orthopedic and Rehabilitation Considerations

Physical Examination

Check for stability and tenderness at the fracture site and the range of motion of the wrist, elbow, and shoulder joints. Pay special attention to limitations in elbow flexion and extension.

X-rays

Anteroposterior and true lateral radiographs of the elbow should be obtained and checked for malunion, delayed union, and nonunion.

Weight Bearing

The affected extremity may be used for support. After 3 months, full weight bearing should be possible if radiographic union is present.

Range of Motion

If the fracture is united, passive range-of-motion exercises should be combined with the active program that has already been instituted. At this point, the risk of myositis ossificans related to passive motion of the elbow has decreased significantly. Emphasis should be placed on achieving full flexion, extension, supination, and pronation. Considerable stiffness may yet be present at the elbow joint and dynamic splinting may also be attempted. Range-of-motion exercises of the fingers, wrist, and shoulder should continue.

Muscle Strength

Gentle resistive exercises may begin with elbow flexion/extension. Weights (starting with 1 to 2 pounds and gradually increasing) are lifted against gravity. Kinetic activities are taught, such as range-of-motion wheel exercises or holding a rod with two hands, raising it above the head, and moving it from side to side. These exercises, when repeated many times, improve the range of motion of the elbow and shoulder in all planes. Grip strengthening should also continue.

Functional Activities

The involved extremity should not be used for any functional activity, including personal hygiene.

Methods of Treatment: Specific Aspects

For all treatment modalities, the protective splint or functional brace may be discontinued when the fracture is united radiographically. This is expected by 10 to 12 weeks but may be apparent as early as 8 weeks. Many patients who had open reduction and internal fixation with a rigid construct have already had their bracing or splinting removed.

Prescription

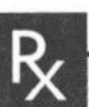

Eight to Twelve Weeks

Precautions Avoid heavy lifting or pushing.

Range of Motion Active and passive range of motion to the elbow.

Strength Progressive resistive exercises to the elbow musculature.

Functional Activities The involved extremity used for self-care and personal hygiene.

Weight Bearing Full weight bearing by 12 weeks.

LONG-TERM CONSIDERATIONS AND PROBLEMS

Range of Motion

The most common long-term consequence of distal humeral fractures, whether intraarticular or extraarticular, is loss of elbow range of motion. This may be caused by capsular contractures or myositis ossificans. Most activities require elbow motion between 30° and 130°, with loss of extension being less significant than loss of flexion. Supination and pronation may also suffer, but they have less effect on the activities of daily living. The treatment for severe capsular contractures or myositis ossificans is surgical release or resection, respectively. Myositis ossificans should only be resected when mature, usually by 1 year, to reduce the chance of recurrence. Treatment of an elbow with severely limited range of motion is difficult and the results are often poor. The best approach is prevention with adequate postinjury rehabilitation.

Post-traumatic Arthritis

An incongruent articular surface will lead to post-traumatic arthritis, causing significant disability and pain. Operative treatment of severe elbow arthritis includes total elbow arthroplasty or elbow fusion. Neither gives a good result in a young, active patient and conservative treatment may be the best option in this situation. If intraarticular displacement is not allowed at the time of the initial treatment, the incidence of post-traumatic arthritis is significantly reduced.

IMMEDIATE TO ONE WEEK

	Cast/Splint	*Percutaneous Pinning*	*Open Reduction and Internal Fixation*
Stability	None.	Stability afforded by pin fixation only.	Stability afforded by fixation only.
Orthopedics	Long arm cast or posterior splint.	Long arm cast or posterior splint.	Functional brace, posterior splint, or arm sling.
	Trim cast or splint to distal palmar crease volarly and metacarpophalangeal prominences dorsally to allow free finger and metacarpophalangeal motion.	Trim cast or splint to distal palmar crease volarly and metacarpophalangeal prominences dorsally to allow free finger and metacarpophalangeal motion.	
	Dependent edema treated with elevation or cast/splint removal and reapplication if severe.	Dependent edema treated with elevation or cast/splint removal and reapplication if severe.	Dependent edema treated with elevation.
Rehabilitation	Active range-of-motion exercises to the digits.	Active and passive range-of-motion exercises to the digits.	Assuming a stable construct, begin gentle active range of motion exercises to the entire extremity, including elbow, fingers, wrist, and shoulder within 3 to 5 days as soft tissues allow.
	Active and active-assistive range-of-motion exercises to the shoulder.	Active and active-assistive range-of-motion exercises to the shoulder. Isometric exercises to biceps, triceps, and deltoid.	
	Avoid elbow motion.		
	No shoulder internal/external rotation exercises.	Avoid elbow motion.	
		No shoulder internal/external rotation exercises.	Avoid passive range of motion exercises to the elbow to reduce the risk of myositis ossificans.

TWO WEEKS

	Cast	Percutaneous Pinning	Open Reduction and Internal Fixation
Stability	None to minimal.	Stability mainly afforded by pin fixation, with minimal contribution from organization at the fracture site.	Stability mainly afforded by fixation, with minimal contribution from organization at the fracture site.
Orthopedics	Long arm cast or posterior splint.	Long arm cast or posterior splint.	Functional brace, posterior splint, or arm sling alone for protection.
Rehabilitation	Active range-of-motion exercises to the digits.	Active range-of-motion exercises to the digits.	Continue gentle active range-of-motion exercises to the entire extremity including elbow, fingers, wrist, and shoulder.
	Active and active-assistive range-of-motion exercises to the shoulder. Isometric exercises to biceps, triceps, and deltoid; add isometric exercises for forearm musculature.	Active and active-assistive range of motion exercises to the shoulder. Isometric exercises to biceps, triceps, and deltoid; add isometric exercises for forearm musculature.	
	Begin grip-strengthening exercises with ball or putty.	Begin grip-strengthening exercises with ball or putty.	Begin grip-strengthening exercises with ball or putty.
	No pronation/supination or shoulder internal/external rotation exercises.	No pronation/supination or shoulder internal/external rotation exercises.	Avoid passive range-of-motion exercises to the elbow to reduce the risk of myositis ossificans.
	For extension type supracondylar humerus fractures, may add supervised elbow flexion from 90° up with posterior splint immobilization between sessions.		

FOUR TO SIX WEEKS

	Cast/Splint	*Percutaneous Pinning*	*Open Reduction and Internal Fixation*
Stability	Bridging callus provides stability.	Stability afforded by pin fixation and bridging callus.	Stability afforded by fixation and bridging callus.
Orthopedics	Functional brace or posterior splint.	Remove pins once there is radiographic evidence of healing. Functional brace or posterior splint used for protection.	Consider discontinuing functional brace or posterior splint at 6 to 8 weeks if bridging callus is present and fixation is stable. Continue with sling for protection.
Rehabilitation	Once clinical stability and radiographic healing are present, begin supervised active elbow range of motion. Usually, a home program may be added by 6 weeks. Between sessions the patient should be protected.	Once clinical stability and radiographic healing are present, begin supervised active elbow range of motion. Usually, a home program may be added by 6 weeks. Between sessions the patient should be protected.	Continue active and active-assistive range-of-motion exercises to the entire extremity including elbow, fingers, wrist, and shoulder.
	Continue grip-strengthening exercises with ball or putty.	Continue grip-strengthening exercises with ball or putty.	Continue grip-strengthening exercises with ball or putty.
	Avoid passive range-of-motion exercises to the elbow to reduce the risk of myositis ossificans.	Avoid passive range-of-motion exercises to the elbow to reduce the risk of myositis ossificans.	Avoid passive range-of-motion exercises to the elbow to reduce the risk of myositis ossificans.

EIGHT TO TWELVE WEEKS			
	Cast	*Percutaneous Pinning*	*Open Reduction and Internal Fixation*
Stability	Stable.	Stable.	Stable.
Orthopedics	Discontinue bracing, splinting, and sling with radiographic evidence of union. This is usually present by 10 to 12 weeks, although sometimes as early as 8 weeks.	Discontinue bracing, splinting, and sling with radiographic evidence of union. This is usually present by 10 to 12 weeks, although sometimes as early as 8 weeks.	Discontinue bracing, splinting, and sling with radiographic evidence of union.
Rehabilitation	Continue active and add passive range-of-motion exercises to all joints of the extremity while focusing on flexion/extension of the elbow and pronation/supination of the forearm.	Continue active and add passive range-of-motion exercises to all joints of the extremity while focusing on flexion/extension of the elbow and pronation/supination of the forearm.	Continue active and add passive range-of-motion exercises to all joints of the extremity while focusing on flexion/extension of the elbow and pronation/supination of the forearm.
	Continue grip-strengthening exercises with ball or putty. Introduce resistive exercises using weights in gradation, starting with 1 to 2 pounds.	Continue grip-strengthening exercises with ball or putty. Introduce resistive exercises using weights in gradation, starting with 1 to 2 pounds.	Continue grip-strengthening exercises with ball or putty. Introduce resistive exercises using weights in gradation, starting with 1 to 2 pounds.
	The risk of myositis ossificans related to passive range of motion of the elbow has significantly decreased.	The risk of myositis ossificans related to passive range of motion of the elbow has significantly decreased.	The risk of myositis ossificans related to passive range of motion of the elbow has significantly decreased.

BIBLIOGRAPHY

Asprinio D, Helfet DL. Fractures of the distal humerus. In: *Trauma: Orthopaedic Knowledge Update.* Rosemont, IL: American Academy of Orthopaedic Surgeons, 1996, pp. 35–45.

Crenshaw AH. Fractures of shoulder girdle, arm, and forearm. In: Crenshaw AH, ed. *Campbell's Operative Orthopaedics,* Vol. 2, 8th ed. St. Louis: Mosby, 1992, pp. 1016–1025.

Helfet DL, Hotchkiss RN. Internal fixation of the distal humerus: a biomechanical comparison of methods. *J Orthop Trauma,* 4: 260–264, 1990.

Helfet DL, Schmeling GJ. Bicondylar intraarticular fractures of the distal humerus in adults. *Clin Orthop,* 292:26–36, 1993.

Henley MB, Bone LB, Parker B. Operative management of displaced intraarticular fractures of the distal humerus. *J Orthop Trauma.* 1:24–35, 1987.

Hotchkiss RN, Green DP. Fractures and dislocations of the elbow. In: Rockwood CA, ed. *Fractures in Adults,* Vol. 1, 3rd ed. Philadelphia: J.B. Lippincott, 1991, pp. 739–841.

Jupiter JB. Complex fractures of the distal part of the humerus and associated complications. *J Bone Joint Surg,* 76A:1252–1264, 1994.

Jupiter JB. The surgical management of intraarticular fractures of the distal humerus. In: Morrey BF, ed. *Master Techniques in Orthopaedic Surgery, The Elbow.* New York: Raven Press, 1994, pp. 53–70.

Jupiter JB, Mehne DK. Trauma to the adult elbow and fractures of the distal humerus. In: Browner BD, ed. *Skeletal Trauma,* Vol. 2, 1st ed. Philadelphia: W.B. Saunders, 1992, pp. 1125–1176.

Schatzker J. Fractures of the distal end of the humerus. In: Schatzker J, Tile M, eds. *The Rationale of Operative Fracture Care.* Berlin: Springer-Verlag, 1987, pp. 71–87.

CHAPTER *Fourteen*

Olecranon Fractures

RICARDO F. GAUDINEZ, MD

VASANTHA L. MURTHY, MD

STANLEY HOPPENFELD, MD

INTRODUCTION

Definition

An olecranon fracture involves the proximal end of the ulna. It may be extraarticular or intraarticular, displaced or nondisplaced. These fractures can be further classified as transverse, oblique, comminuted, stable, or unstable. Displaced fractures are generally defined as those with a separation of greater than 2 mm between fracture fragments (Figure 14-1; *see* Figures 14-5 and 14-6). The fracture is considered stable if it does not separate or if the degree of separation does not increase with flexion of the elbow to 90 degrees.

Olecranon fractures may cause disruption of the extensor mechanism. To test this, the patient should be asked to attempt extension of the elbow against gravity. If the patient is unable to do this, the extensor mechanism is interrupted and will require operative repair.

Olecranon fractures may be associated with coronoid fractures as well as elbow fracture/dislocations.

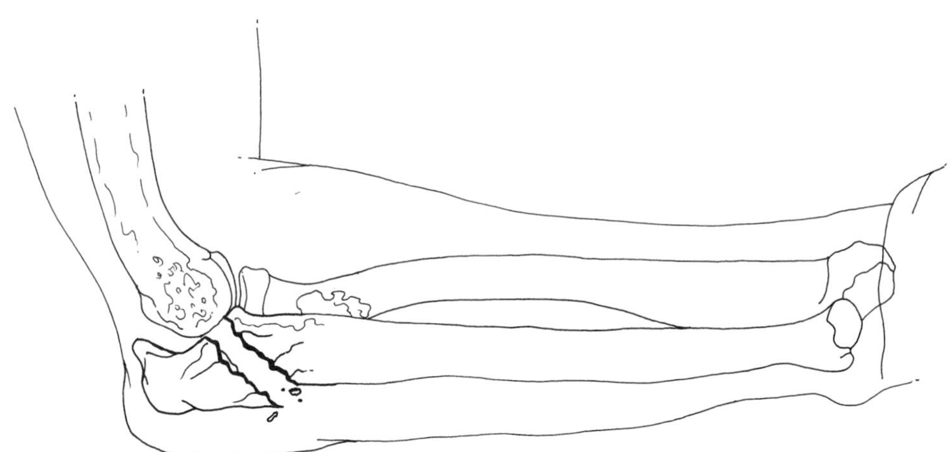

FIGURE 14-1 Oblique olecranon fracture with displacement of greater than 2 millimeters. The coronoid process is not involved. This is an intraarticular fracture.

The stability of the elbow should be tested, including the medial collateral ligament (MCL), following operative fixation by subjecting the elbow joint to varus and valgus stress in both full extension and moderate flexion.

Intraarticular fractures account for the majority of olecranon fractures and are generally associated with joint effusions and hematomas. Extraarticular fractures include avulsion fractures and are most commonly seen in the elderly.

Mechanism of Injury

Because the olecranon is a subcutaneous structure, it is especially vulnerable to direct trauma. Direct blows are the most common injuries to the olecranon, followed by falls on an outstretched hand with the elbow in flexion, leading to contraction of the triceps. High-energy trauma, such as a car accident, may also cause an associated radial head fracture or elbow dislocation.

Treatment Goals

Orthopaedic Objectives

Alignment

Articular restoration.

Stability

The olecranon forms the greater sigmoid notch, which articulates with the trochlea of the distal humerus, and its architecture adds to the intrinsic stability of the elbow.

Rehabilitation Objectives

Range of Motion

Restore and improve elbow range of motion and maintain the range of motion of the shoulder and wrist (Table 14-1).

TABLE 14-1 *Forearm and Elbow Range of Motion*

Motion	Normal	Functional
Flexion	150°	90°
Extension	−5°–0°	Lacking 20°–30°
Pronation	90°	50°
Supination	90°	50°

Muscle Strength

Improve the strength of the following muscles:

Triceps: extensor of the elbow

Biceps: flexor of the elbow

Supinators of the forearm and wrist

Pronators of the forearm and wrist

Wrist extensor group:

- Extensor carpi radialis longus and brevis
- Extensor carpi ulnaris
- Extensor digitorum longus

Wrist flexor group:

- Flexor carpi radialis
- Flexor carpi ulnaris
- Flexor digitorum longus and sublimis

Functional Goals

Restore and normalize activities of daily living such as grooming, feeding, dressing and self-care.

Even though there may be some permanent loss of extension, the patient should eventually be able to perform self-care and activities of daily living independently.

Expected Time of Bone Healing

Ten to 12 weeks.

Expected Duration of Rehabilitation

Ten to 12 weeks.

Methods of Treatment

Closed Reduction and Splint or Cast

Biomechanics: Stress-sharing device.

Mode of Bone Healing: Secondary, with callus formation.

Indications: This method is used for nondisplaced, stable fractures. The elbow should be held in 90-degree flexion for 4 weeks. If less than 45-degree flexion is required to maintain the reduction, open reduction and internal fixation (ORIF) is recommended. Closed treatment requires close observation with routine follow-up, including radiographs to ensure that no displacement of the fracture fragments has occurred.

Open Reduction and Internal Fixation

Biomechanics: Stress-sharing device for both tension band and plate and screw fixation (Figure 14-2).

Mode of Bone Healing: Secondary, with callus formation. Because rigid fixation cannot be obtained in most olecranon fractures, primary bone healing with no visible callus is rare.

Indications: ORIF is the method of choice for displaced and comminuted fractures. Use of the Kirschner wire (K-wire) loop remains the most common method of fixation, using the principles of tension banding. This method allows for early active elbow range of motion. In severely comminuted fractures in which tension band wiring will not be effective, plate fixation is necessary, which acts as a neutralization device (Figures 14-3, 14-4, 14-5, 14-6, 14-7, and 14-8).

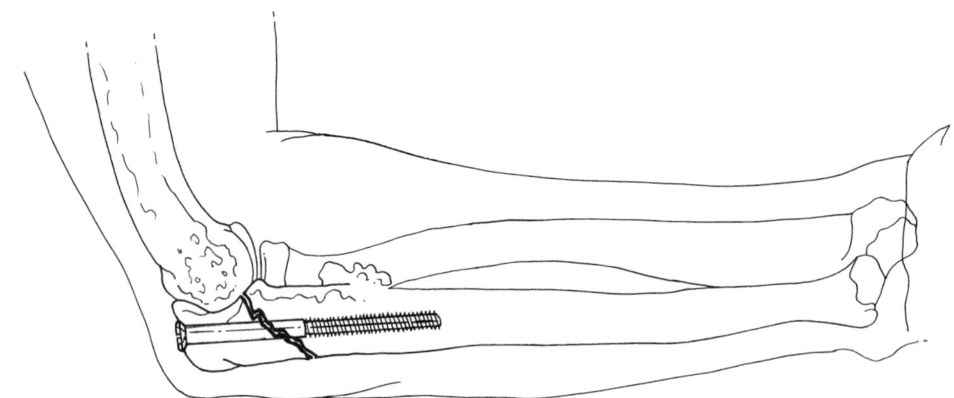

FIGURE 14-2 Screw fixation of an intraarticular displaced olecranon fracture. Note the lag effect of the screw compressing the fracture fragments. Early range of motion may be started.

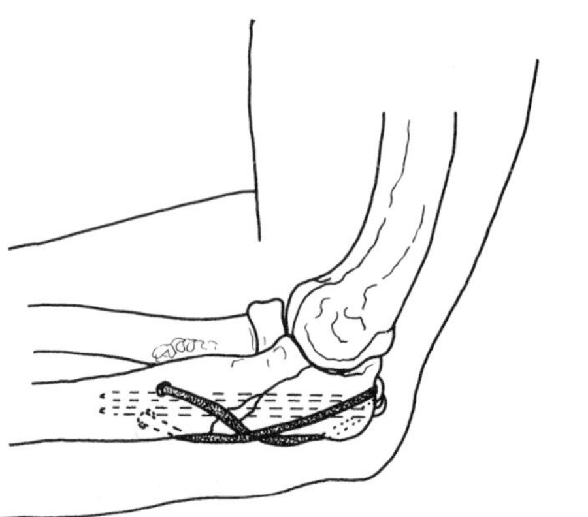

FIGURE 14-3 Tension band fixation of an oblique olecranon fracture (lateral view).

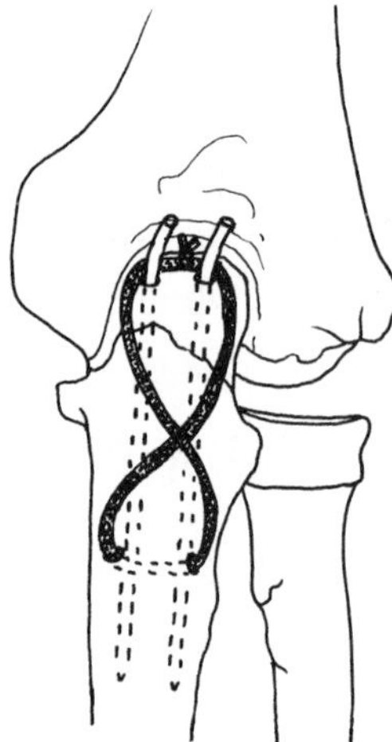

FIGURE 14-4 Tension band fixation of an olecranon fracture (posterior view). This is the most common method of treatment. As the elbow flexes, the looped wire tightens, creating compression at the fracture site as the fracture fragments are forced to slide together along the direction of the K-wires (the tension band effect).

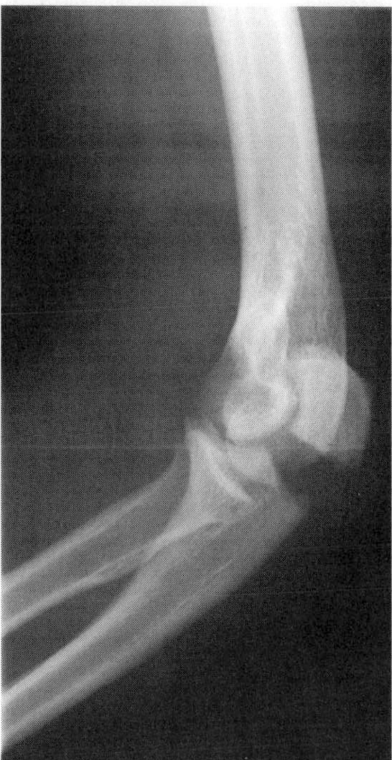

FIGURE 14-5 Transverse olecranon fracture with marked displacement. The pull of the triceps displaces the proximal fragment.

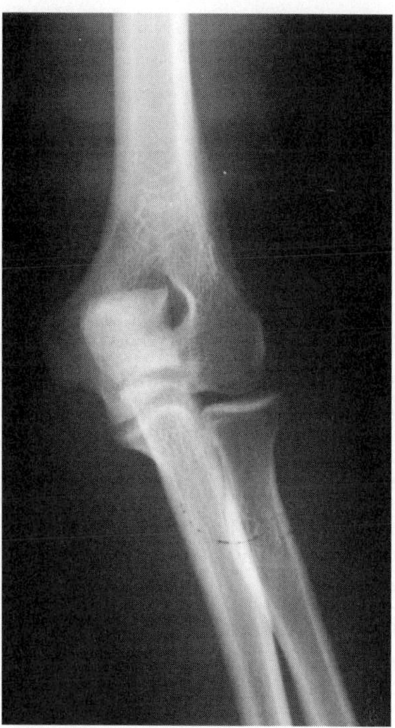

FIGURE 14-6 Transverse olecranon fracture (anteroposterior view).

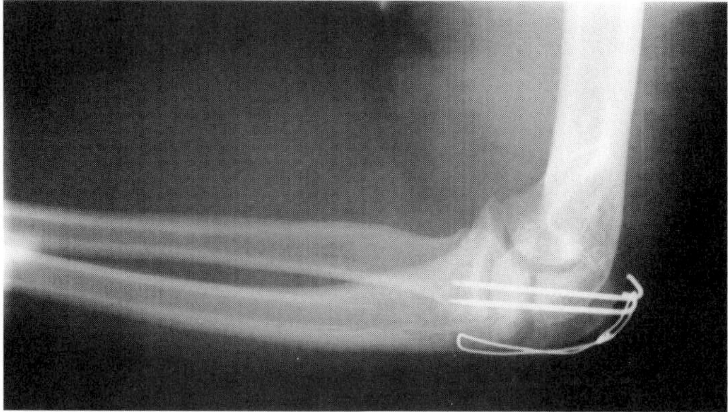

FIGURE 14-7 Treatment of a transverse olecranon fracture with tension band wiring. Note the restoration of the articular surface. As the elbow flexes, the wire tightens, causing compression at the fracture site.

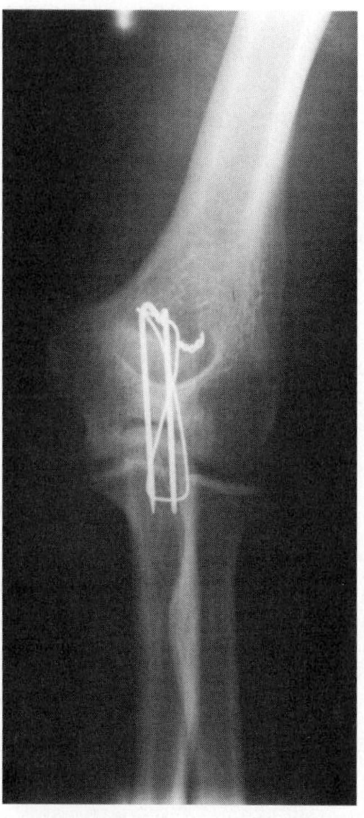

FIGURE 14-8 Anteroposterior view of transverse olecranon fracture treated with tension band wiring. The patient is usually placed in a sling postoperatively. Early range of motion is encouraged.

Excision and Triceps Advancement and Reattachment

Biomechanics: Stress-sharing device.

Mode of Bone Healing: Soft tissue–to–bone healing.

Indications: In elderly patients with osteoporotic bone or for significantly comminuted fractures, excision of the olecranon should be considered. As long as the coronoid process and the anterior portion of the ulnar collateral ligament are intact, as much as two thirds of the olecranon can be excised without the risk of elbow instability. This technique has the added advantage of avoiding posttraumatic arthritis secondary to joint incongruity and nonunion or malunion. Excision of the olecranon fragments does not lead to pain, decreased motion or instability in contrast to internal fixation. Debate exists whether excision and triceps reattachment is functionally as effective as internal fixation.

Special Considerations of the Fracture

Age

Elderly patients are more at risk for development of joint stiffness secondary to the fracture and its treatment. They also have more osteoporotic bone, which determines the choice of fixation for displaced fractures. Stable fixation with K-wires or cancellous screws may be difficult. Excision and triceps reattachment may be more appropriate.

Articular Involvement

More severe injuries, including intraarticular and open fractures, require more time for bony healing and rehabilitation. With intraarticular fractures, posttraumatic degenerative changes can be problematic, causing pain and limitation of motion, but they are not common. Every effort should be made to restore the articular congruity at the time of fracture management. Up to 2 mm of step-off is considered acceptable. Loss of elbow motion, including an extensor lag and flexion contractures, is not uncommon with these injuries, especially when associated with fracture/dislocations of the elbow.

Associated Injury

Ulnar nerve neuropraxia or injury has been reported in approximately 2% to 10% of olecranon fractures. Careful examination at the time of initial evaluation should identify any ulnar nerve deficits. If there is no recovery of the ulnar nerve with time, an ulnar nerve decompression with transposition should be undertaken. During surgical treatment of displaced fractures, care must be taken to protect the ulnar nerve.

The elbow joint can be unstable if there is a concomitant fracture of the coronoid process or an injury to the MCL. The MCL should be evaluated before and during any operative management. With injury to the coronoid process or MCL, care should be taken in excision of olecranon fragments because this can lead to further instability, a difficult problem to manage.

Weight Bearing

No weight bearing on the affected extremity.

Gait

Arm swing is reduced.

TREATMENT

Treatment: Early to Immediate (Day One to One Week)

BONE HEALING

Stability at fracture site: None.

Stage of bone healing: Inflammatory phase. The fracture hematoma is colonized by inflammatory cells, and débridement of the fracture begins.

X-ray: No callus.

Orthopaedic and Rehabilitation Considerations

Physical Examination

Check for capillary refill, sensation, and active and passive range of motion of the digits. Pay special attention to ulnar nerve function, because an ulnar nerve injury may accompany an olecranon fracture.

Dangers

Check for excessive swelling. Dependent edema and skin discoloration are common, with resultant sausage-shaped digits. If a splint or cast is applied, care must be taken to avoid pressure on the antecubital fossa from the cast or Ace bandage supporting the splint, because this may lead to a compartment syndrome.

Evaluate by passively extending all the digits; pain out of proportion to what is expected when moving the digits may be an early sign of compartment syndrome.

Radiography

Check for loss of reduction and displacement of the fracture fragments. Compare with immediate postreduction or postoperative radiographs.

Weight Bearing

No weight bearing on the affected extremity.

Range of Motion

Begin active range of motion of the shoulder and wrist (if the cast or splint permits), the hand and the digits. The digits and hand may be edematous as a result of the fracture. Retrograde massage helps reduce the edema.

Muscle Strength

No strengthening exercises are prescribed for the elbow. Gentle isometric exercises to the wrist may begin 3 to 4 days after the fracture, once the patient's pain subsides. The patient flexes and extends the wrist and deviates the wrist within the cast or splint. Active flexion and extension of the digits is encouraged to maintain the strength of the long extensors and flexors.

Functional Activities

The patient should use the uninvolved upper extremity for self-care, hygiene, feeding, grooming, and dressing. The patient is instructed in donning clothes on the involved extremity first and doffing them from the uninvolved extremity first. If the patient is in a cast, he or she may drape a blouse or shirt over the affected extremity first.

Methods of Treatment: Specific Aspects

Closed Reduction and Splint or Cast

Check the adequacy of the cast padding and look for skin breakdown at the edges of the cast or splint. Trim the cast to the distal palmar crease volarly and to the metacarpophalangeal joints dorsally to allow for full motion at the interphalangeal and metacarpophalangeal joints.

Open Reduction and Internal Fixation

Check the wound for erythema, discharge, or purulence. Gentle active elbow flexion is begun 3 to 5 days following stable tension band fixation.

Excision and Triceps Advancement and Reattachment

Check the wound for erythema, drainage, or induration. The elbow is kept in a bulky dressing for the first 10 days with a posterior splint. The sutures are then removed and a long arm cast is applied. No range of motion is allowed.

Prescription

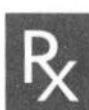

DAY ONE TO ONE WEEK

Precautions Avoid premature elbow motion.

Range of Motion

No range of motion to the elbow or wrist in a cast or splint.

Gentle active elbow flexion and active range of motion to the wrist if treated surgically.

Strength

No strengthening exercises to the elbow.

Three to 4 days after fracture, isometric exercises to the wrist within the cast.

Functional Activities One-handed activities. The patient uses the uninvolved extremity for personal hygiene and self-care.

Weight Bearing None.

Treatment: Two Weeks

BONE HEALING

Stability at fracture site: None to minimal.

Stage of bone healing: Beginning of reparative phase. Osteoprogenitor cells differentiate into osteoblasts, which lay down woven bone.

X-ray: None to early callus. Fracture line is visible.

Orthopaedic and Rehabilitation Considerations

Physical Examination

Check active and passive range of motion of all digits, sensation, and capillary refill, and for excessive swelling. If immobilization is still required (for a nondisplaced fracture, severe osteoporosis, or a tenuous repair), ensure that the cast or splint has not loosened. If it has, a better-fitting cast or splint may be necessary.

Dangers

Ensure that there is no pressure from the cast in the antecubital fossa, which may lead to compartment syndrome.

Radiography

Check radiographs for any loss of reduction and compare them with previous radiographs. If loss of reduction is noted, consider ORIF.

Weight Bearing

No weight bearing on the affected extremity. Patients who rely on a walker for ambulation may benefit from using a platform walker because no weight is borne through the fracture when such a walker is used.

Range of Motion

Continue active range of motion of the shoulder as well as the wrist (if the cast or splint permits), hand, and digits in the cast or splint.

Muscle Strength

Begin gentle isometric exercises of the biceps. Continue isometric exercises to the wrist and isotonic exercises to the digits.

Functional Activities

The patient should use the uninvolved extremity for self-care and hygiene. Elderly patients who use a walker for ambulation are instructed in using a wide-based quad cane or hemiwalker with the unaffected extremity.

Methods of Treatment: Specific Aspects

Closed Reduction and Splint or Cast

Check the cast margins. Trim the cast to allow full range of motion of the metacarpophalangeal joints. The patient is encouraged to flex the elbow within the cast to perform isometric exercises of the elbow flexors. To avoid displacement of the fracture fragments, extension is not allowed.

Open Reduction and Internal Fixation

Remove staples or sutures. Check the wound for erythema, drainage, or induration. Continue elbow flexion if stable tension band fixation was achieved. The patient is instructed in active wrist flexion and extension and ulnar and radial deviation.

Usually after 2 to 3 weeks the splint is removed. It may be used at night for additional support.

Excision and Triceps Advancement and Reattachment

Remove the staples or sutures. Check the wound for erythema, drainage, or induration. The patient should remain in a splint (or, more frequently, in a cast) for the balance of 6 weeks because the suture repair line is still weak. Avoid range of motion.

Prescription

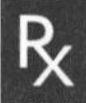

TWO WEEKS

Precautions Cast or splint: no extension to the elbow less than 90 degrees.

Range of Motion

No range of motion to the elbow or wrist in a cast or splint.

Active elbow flexion and active range of motion to the wrist if treated surgically.

Strength

No strengthening exercises to the elbow in extension.

Isometric exercises to the elbow in flexion in a cast.

Isometric exercises to the wrist.

Functional Activities The patient uses the uninvolved extremity for self-care and personal hygiene.

Weight Bearing None.

Treatment: Four to Six Weeks

BONE HEALING

Stability at fracture site: With bridging callus, the fracture is usually stable.

Stage of bone healing: Reparative phase. Further organization of callus and formation of lamellar bone begins. The strength of this callus, especially with torsional load, is significantly lower than that of normal bone, and further protection is recommended.

X-ray: Bridging callus is visible. Fracture line is less distinct. Endosteal callus formation will predominate.

Orthopaedic and Rehabilitation Considerations

Physical Examination

Discontinue the cast or splint, if this has not already been done. Check for fracture site tenderness, crepitus, and motion to assess clinical union. Check the elbow range of motion.

Dangers

Check for reflex sympathetic dystrophy, characterized by trophic changes, vasomotor disturbances, hyperesthesia, pain, and tenderness out of proportion to the stage of fracture healing. Reflex sympathetic dystrophy requires aggressive therapy.

Radiography

Check radiographs for additional callus and disappearance of the fracture line. Check for the formation of heterotopic bone. This may reduce elbow range of motion.

Weight Bearing

No weight bearing. Patients who rely on a walker for ambulation may benefit from use of a platform walker.

Range of Motion

Continue active and active-assistive range of motion to the shoulder, elbow, and wrist. Avoid passive range of motion at the elbow.

Muscle Strength

Advance isometric exercises to the biceps and triceps and isotonic exercises to the long flexors and extensors of the digits.

Functional Activities

The patient should continue one-handed activities. If the splint is removed, the patient can start using the affected extremity for grooming.

Methods of Treatment: Specific Aspects

Closed Reduction and Splint or Cast

The cast is removed when the fracture is nontender, there is no motion at the fracture site, and there is sufficient callus formation. The patient is instructed in gentle active range-of-motion exercises to the elbow in flexion, extension, supination, and pronation, and active and active-assistive range-of-motion exercises to the wrist in all planes. Repetitive active range-of-motion exercises to the wrist help strengthen the muscles. The patient is also taught isotonic exercises to the wrist.

Open Reduction and Internal Fixation

The patient should be able to flex and extend the elbow actively. If the patient is apprehensive, active-assistive exercises may be instructed. The patient can use the unaffected extremity to assist with range-of-motion exercises to the affected extremity.

Excision and Triceps Advancement and Reattachment

Maintain the splint or cast for the full 6 weeks. After 6 weeks, remove the cast and start active and active-assistive range of motion to the elbow. A posterior elbow splint may be used at night for comfort.

Prescription

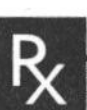

FOUR TO SIX WEEKS

Precautions Active to active-assistive range of motion to the elbow and wrist.

Range of Motion Encourage active range of motion to the elbow in flexion and extension.

Strength Isometric exercises to the elbow and wrist in flexion and extension.

Functional Activities The patient uses the affected extremity for stability and light self-care.

Weight Bearing No weight bearing.

Treatment: Six to Eight Weeks

BONE HEALING

Stability at fracture site: Stable.

Stage of bone healing: Reparative phase. Further organization of callus and formation of lamellar bone continues.

X-ray: Bridging callus is more apparent, especially with less-rigid fixation. Fracture line is less distinct. There is less callus formation if the fracture site is at the end of the ulna than in a midshaft fracture.

Orthopaedic and Rehabilitation Considerations

Physical Examination

Ensure that the patient is regaining adequate range of motion without crepitus. If ulnar nerve palsy is still present, consider an electromyographic evaluation to determine the intactness of the nerve and its recovery.

Radiography

If the fracture is clinically and radiographically healed at 4 to 6 weeks, no repeat radiographs are needed. If it is not, repeat radiographs to check for further bony union and consider bone grafting in the future if nonunion occurs.

Weight Bearing

If the fracture is clinically and radiographically healed, the patient may progressively bear weight when pushing off from a chair or bed, or when using axillary crutches or a cane.

Range of Motion

Continue active and active-assistive range of motion to the elbow and wrist in all planes until satisfactory range is achieved.

Muscle Strength

Begin resistive strengthening of both the biceps and triceps. The patient can use the unaffected extremity to offer resistance while flexing and extending the affected elbow. Continue the previous exercise program.

Functional Activities

The patient may use the involved extremity for hygiene and self-care.

Methods of Treatment: Specific Aspects

Closed Reduction and Splint or Cast

No change.

Open Reduction and Internal Fixation

No change.

Excision and Triceps Advancement and Reattachment

No change.

Prescription

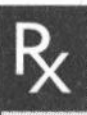

SIX TO EIGHT WEEKS

Precautions None.

Range of Motion Full active to active-assistive range of motion in all planes to the elbow and wrist.

Strength Resistive exercises to the elbow and wrist.

Functional Activities The patient uses the involved extremity for personal hygiene and self-care.

Weight Bearing Gradual weight bearing is allowed.

Treatment: Eight to Twelve Weeks

Bone Healing

Stability at fracture site: Stable.

Stage of bone healing: Remodeling phase. Woven bone is replaced by lamellar bone. The process of remodeling takes months to years for completion.

X-ray: More callus is seen, and fracture line becomes even less distinct.

Orthopaedic and Rehabilitation Considerations

Physical Examination

Check for tenderness or motion at the fracture site. Check for improving range of motion and strength. Check for resolution of reflex sympathetic dystrophy and the status of any existing ulnar nerve deficits.

Radiography

If the fracture was clinically and radiographically united at the last visit, no additional radiographs are needed.

Weight Bearing

Full weight bearing is allowed.

Range of Motion

Remove the cast if this was not previously done. The patient is instructed in active to active-assistive range-of-motion exercises in all planes of the elbow. There may be some limitations in elbow extension. Gentle passive stretching may be necessary. A dynamic splint may be used for passive elbow stretch.

Muscle Strength

Continue progressive resistive exercises to the wrist and elbow, gradually increasing the resistance. The patient can use the unaffected extremity to offer resistance while flexing and extending the affected elbow. The patient can also use graded weights to improve strength.

Functional Activities

The patient should use the affected extremity for all activities of self-care, hygiene, feeding, grooming, and dressing.

Methods of Treatment: Specific Aspects

Closed Reduction and Splint or Cast

No change.

Open Reduction and Internal Fixation

No change.

Excision and Triceps Advancement and Reattachment

Continue active and passive range of motion with no restrictions, because the tendon repair is strong at this point. Heterotopic bone formation is usually not a problem. Splinting is usually not required. Supination and pronation are also encouraged.

Prescription

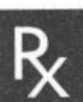

Eight to Twelve Weeks

Precautions None.

Range of Motion Full active and active-assisted range of motion in all planes to the elbow and wrist.

Strength Resistive exercises to the elbow and wrist.

Functional Activities The patient uses the involved extremity for personal hygiene and self-care.

Weight Bearing Full weight bearing is allowed.

LONG-TERM CONSIDERATIONS AND PROBLEMS

Self-care activities rely more on elbow flexion than extension, so lack of terminal extension is usually not problematic. Heterotopic bone formation may significantly reduce elbow range of motion. Additional surgery to excise this bone may be necessary once it is mature.

IMMEDIATE TO ONE WEEK

	Nonoperative	*Open Reduction and Internal Fixation*	*Excision and Triceps Advancement*
Stability	None.	Depends on bone quality.	Depends on bone and soft-tissue quality.
Orthopedics	Elevate the upper extremity to decrease swelling.	Elevate the upper extremity to decrease swelling.	Elevate the upper extremity to decrease swelling.
	Trim cast to metacarpophalangeal (MCP) prominences dorsally and proximal palmar crease volarly.		
Rehabilitation	Range of motion of shoulder and digits.	Range of motion of shoulder and digits, and elbow from 0° to 90° after 3 to 5 days if stable.	Range of motion of shoulder and digits. No range of motion to elbow.

TWO WEEKS

	Nonoperative	*Open Reduction and Internal Fixation*	*Excision and Triceps Advancement*
Stability	None to minimal.	Minimal.	None to minimal.
Orthopedics	Check cast margins to allow full range of motion of MCP joints.	Remove sutures.	Remove sutures.
		Remove splint if not already removed.	Posterior splint or long cast applied.
Rehabilitation	Range of motion of shoulder and digits.	Range of motion of shoulder, wrist, and digits, as well as active elbow flexion.	No range of motion of to the elbow.
	Isometric exercises to wrist as well as elbow flexors within cast.		Range of motion to the shoulder and digits.

FOUR TO SIX WEEKS			
	Nonoperative	*Open Reduction and Internal Fixation*	*Excision and Triceps Advancement*
Stability	Partially stable.	Partially stable.	Partially stable.
Orthopedics	Remove cast if fracture is nontender, there is no motion at fracture site, and there is sufficient callus formation.	Consider bone grafting if not radiographically healed.	Elevate as necessary to decrease swelling. Patient still in a long arm cast.
Rehabilitation	Advance isometric exercises to elbow flexors and extensors, and isotonic exercises to wrist and digits.	Continue active elbow flexion and begin active elbow extension.	No range of motion of the elbow.

EIGHT TO TWELVE WEEKS			
	Nonoperative	*Open Reduction and Internal Fixation*	*Excision and Triceps Advancement*
Stability	Stable.	Stable.	Stable.
Orthopedics	Remove cast. Consider open reduction, internal fixation, and bone grafting if not clinically and radiographically healed.	Consider bone grafting if not radiographically healed.	Elevate as necessary to decrease swelling.
Rehabilitation	Active and active-assisted range of motion to elbow and wrist, and resistive exercises to elbow.	Begin resistive exercises to elbow flexors and extensors.	Begin active to active-assistive range of motion to the elbow. Gentle strengthening exercises to the elbow.

BIBLIOGRAPHY

Adler S, Fay GF. Treatment of olecranon fractures. Indications for excision of the olecranon fragments and repair of the triceps tendon. *J Trauma,* 2:597–602, 1962.

Cabanela ME. Fractures of the proximal ulna and olecranon. In: Morrey BF, eds. *The elbow and its disorders.* Philadelphia: W.B. Saunders, 1985.

Gartsman GM, Sculco TP. Operative treatment of olecranon fractures: excision or ORIF. *J Bone Joint Surg,* 63A:718–721, 1981.

Heim U, Pfeiffer KM. Elbow. In: Heim U, Pfeiffer KM, eds. *ORIF of small fractures,* 3rd ed. Berlin: Springer Verlag 1988, pp. 107–109.

Helm RH, Hornby R, Miller SWM. The complications of surgical treatment of displaced fractures of the olecranon. *Injury,* 12: 48–50, 1987.

Horne JG, Tanzer TL. Olecranon fractures: a review of 100 cases. *J Trauma,* 21:469–472, 1981.

Johnson RP, Roetker A. Olecranon fractures treated with AO screw and tension bands. *Orthopaedics,* 9:66–68, 1986.

Mathewson MH, McCreath SW. Tension band wiring in the treatment of olecranon fractures. *J Bone Joint Surg* 57B:399, 1975.

McKeever FM, Buck RM. Fracture of the olecranon process of the ulna: treatment by excision of fragment and repair of triceps tendon. JAMA 135:1, 1947.

Murphy DF, Green WB. Displaced olecranon fractures in adults. Clinical evaluation. *Clin Orthop* 224:215–223, 1987.

Murphy DF, Greene WB, Gilbert JA, Dameron TB. Displaced olecranon fractures in adults. Biomechanical analysis of fixation methods. *Clin Orthop* 224:210–214, 1987.

CHAPTER *Fifteen*

Radial Head Fractures

LANE SPERO, MD

VASANTHA L. MURTHY, MD

INTRODUCTION

Definition

Fractures of the radial head are classified into four types by Mason:

Type I: Nondisplaced (Figure 15-1A)
Type II: Marginal fractures with displacement, depression, or angulation (*see* Figures 15-1 and 15-9)
Type III: Comminuted fractures of the entire head or completely displaced fractures of the radial head (Figures 15-2, 15-3, and 15-4 and *see* Figure 15-7)

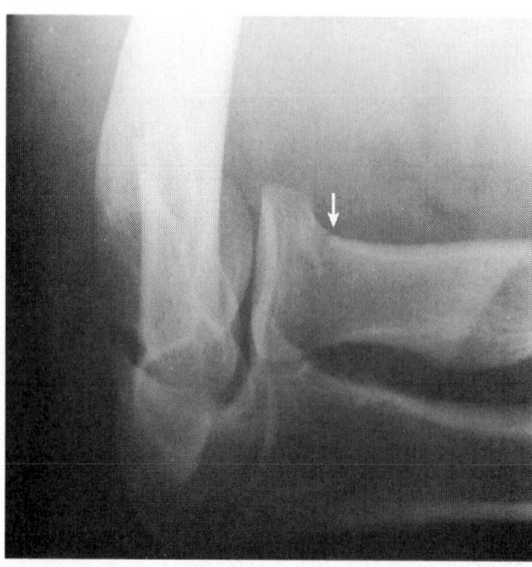

FIGURE 15-1A Fracture of the radial neck type I (Mason classification). It is nondisplaced and there is no angulation.

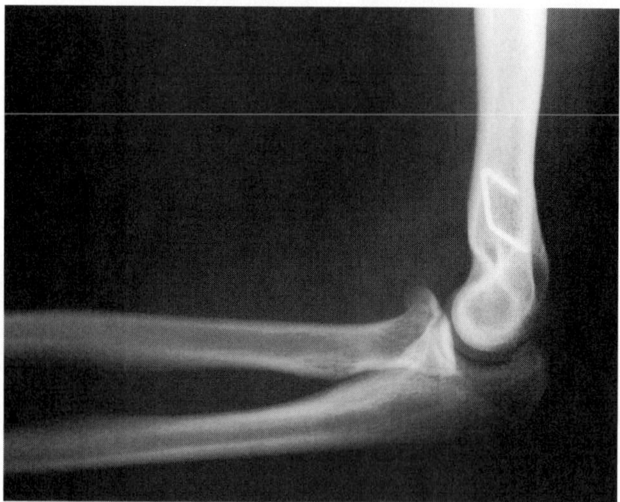

FIGURE 15-1 Lateral radiograph of a marginal fracture of the radial head with angulation. This is a radial head fracture type 2 (Mason classification) involving approximately one third of the radial head.

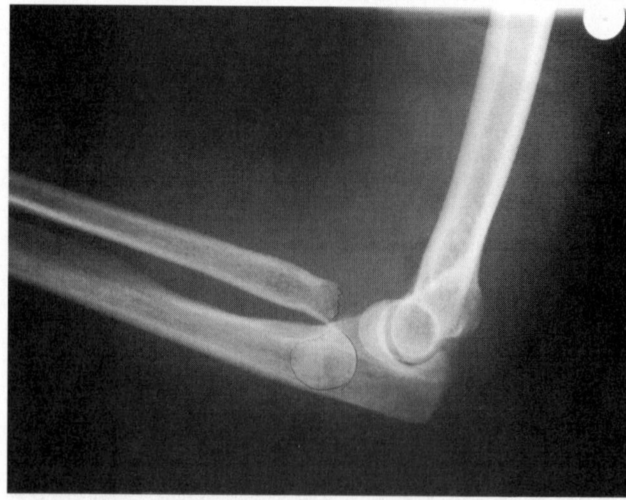

FIGURE 15-2 Completely displaced radial head fracture type 3 (lateral view). The radial head is not comminuted.

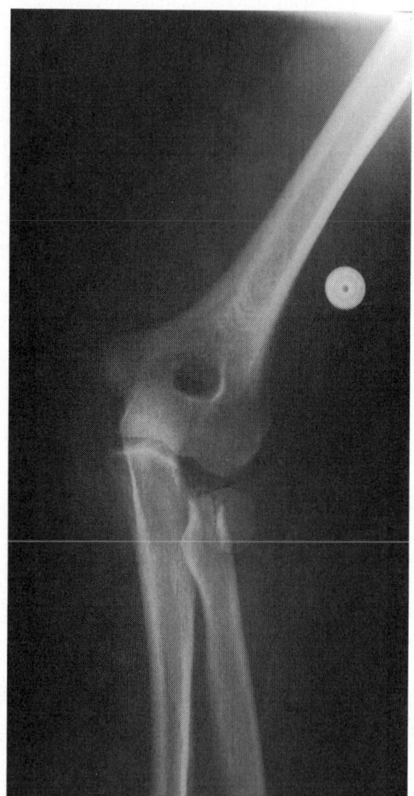

FIGURE 15-3 Completely displaced radial head fracture (anteroposterior view). The radial head is seen in a rotated position lying beside the proximal radius. This is a radial head fracture type 3.

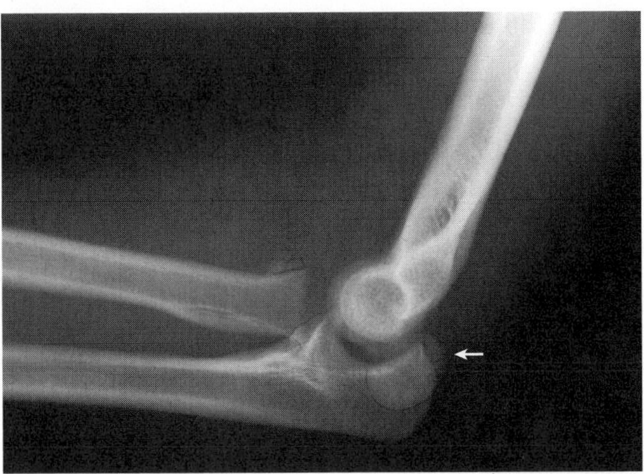

FIGURE 15-4 Completely displaced and comminuted radial head fracture. There is comminution about the proximal radius, and the radial head is seen lying superimposed on the tip of the olecranon. This is a radial head fracture type 3.

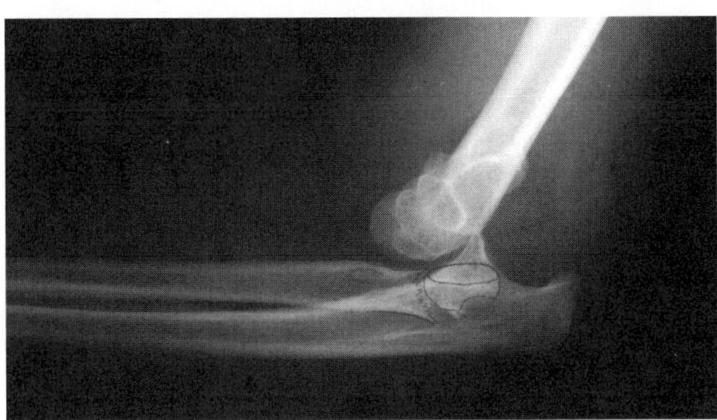

FIGURE 15-5 Completely displaced radial head fracture in association with a posterior elbow dislocation (type 4) (lateral view). Note the radial head lying in a rotated position proximal to the radial shaft.

Type IV: Any of the type I, II, or III patterns with associated elbow dislocation (Figures 15-5 and 15-6)

Radial head fractures can be associated with distal radial ulnar joint injuries or valgus instability of the elbow joint.

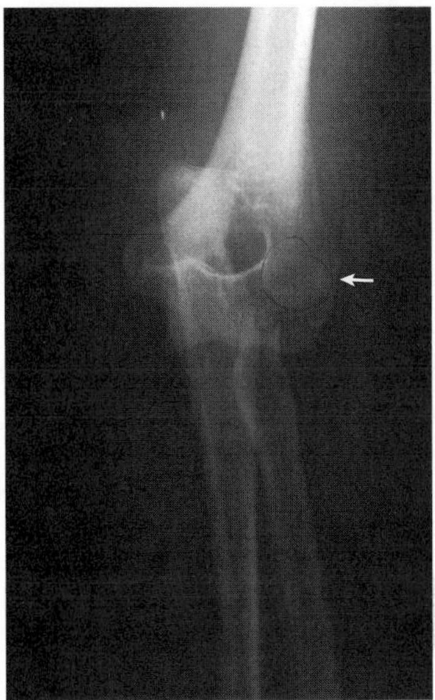

FIGURE 15-6 Completely displaced radial head fracture in association with an elbow dislocation (type 4) (anteroposterior view). Note the radial head lying in a rotated position proximally and laterally to the radial shaft, superimposed on the distal portion of the humerus.

Mechanism of Injury

Radial head fractures are caused by impaction of the capitellum onto the radial head by a valgus force. Injury is usually caused by axial loading on a pronated and partially flexed or outstretched arm.

Treatment Goals

Orthopaedic Objectives

Alignment

Displaced fractures of the radial head may affect the functional and anatomic alignment of the elbow joint. The normal valgus carrying angle is approximately 7 degrees in male patients and 13 degrees in female patients.

Stability

The radial head is the secondary stabilizer of the elbow joint, providing approximately 30% resistance to a valgus force. Fractures of the radial head may cause valgus instability and shortening of the radius, thus increasing the normal carrying angle of the elbow joint and altering its biomechanics.

Rehabilitation Objectives

Range of Motion

1. Restore and maintain the range of motion of the elbow and radioulnar joints in extension, flexion, supination, and pronation (Table 15-1). For most activities of daily living, the arc of elbow flexion is 30 degrees to 130 degrees, and the functional arc of forearm rotation is 50 degrees pronation and 50 degrees supination.
2. Maintain the full range of motion of the wrist, digits, and shoulder.

TABLE 15-1. *Elbow Range of Motion*

Motion	Normal	Functional
Flexion	140° – 160°	130°
Extension	0° – −5°	−30° (lacking)
Supination	80° – 90°	50°
Pronation	70° – 80°	50°

Muscle Strength

Restore and maintain the strength of the following muscles:

Elbow flexors:
- Brachialis
- Biceps
- Brachioradialis

Elbow extensors:
- Triceps
- Anconeus

Elbow supinators:
- Supinator
- Biceps

Elbow pronators:
- Pronator teres
- Pronator quadratus

Wrist flexors:
- Flexor carpi radialis
- Flexor carpi ulnaris

Wrist extensors:
- Extensor carpi radialis longus and brevis
- Extensor carpi ulnaris

Functional Goals

Improve and restore activities of daily living such as grooming, feeding, and dressing, and activities that require supination and pronation such as opening doors and jars or turning keys.

Expected Time of Bone Healing

Six to 8 weeks.

A radial head fracture is an intraarticular fracture, bathed in synovial fluid, and may heal more slowly than an extraarticular fracture.

Expected Duration of Rehabilitation

Six to 12 weeks.

Achieving stability is very important. Once the fracture is stable, range of motion may be initiated. Because a functional range of motion is the goal of rehabilitation, beginning rehabilitation as early as possible reduces the length of rehabilitation.

Methods of Treatment

Aspiration, Early Range of Motion, Sling

Biomechanics: Stress-sharing device (sling or splint).

Mode of Bone Healing: Secondary.

Indications: This method is used for nondisplaced fractures. Aspiration decreases hematoma and capsular distention. This reduces pain and may aid in the diagnosis of occult radial head fractures when a hemarthrosis is detected and no fracture is clearly seen on radiograph.

Joint infiltration of a local anesthetic during aspiration allows painless evaluation of the patient's range of motion and assessment of bony blocks to motion. A sling or splint is then applied for 5 to 7 days, with immediate protected range of motion and a gradual increase in strengthening exercises as tolerated.

Excision of Fracture Fragments or Entire Radial Head

Biomechanics: Stress-sharing sling.

Mode of Bone Healing: Secondary.

Indications: Although this method of treatment has come under question recently, many surgeons opt to excise articular fragments that restrict the range of motion. Recent studies recommend repair of the articular surface to maintain stability. Comminuted fractures that are not amenable to repair require excision. If the elbow is then noted to be unstable secondary to bone loss and ligament damage, a prosthetic spacer is required (Figures 15-7 and 15-8).

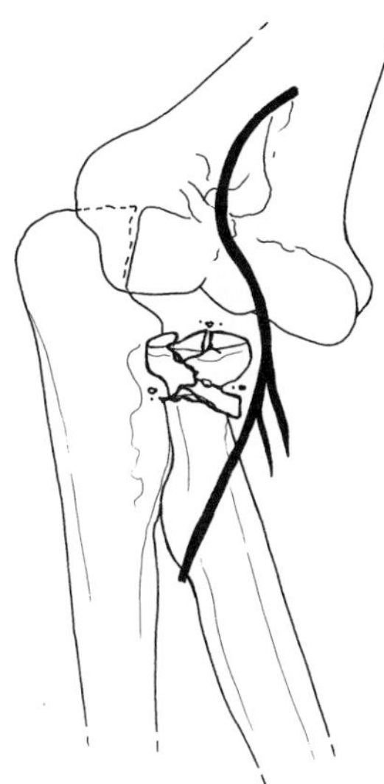

FIGURE 15-7 Comminuted radial head fracture type 3. Because of the extensive comminution, this fracture is best treated by radial head excision or radial head replacement.

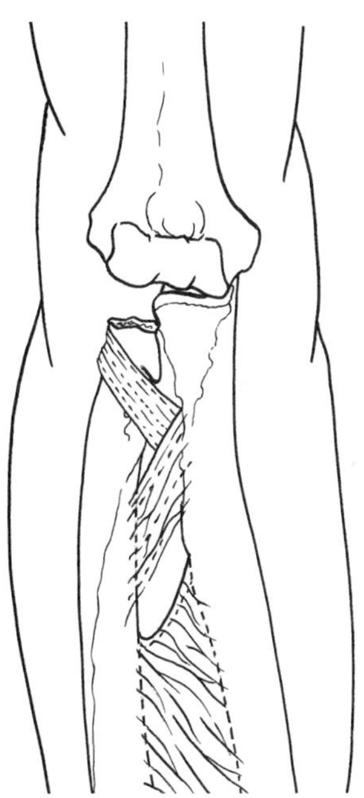

FIGURE 15-8 Proximal radius and elbow after radial head excision. This treatment is for a comminuted radial head fracture with or without an associated elbow dislocation.

Open Reduction and Internal Fixation

Biomechanics: Stress-shielding device.

Mode of Bone Healing: Primary. Secondary if a solid fixation is not achieved.

Indications: This is the treatment of choice for type II radial head fractures that are displaced 2 to 3 mm, with more than 25% to 30% involvement of the articular surface. The radial head is reconstructed with mini fragment screws, Kirschner wires (K-wires), or a mini T-plate, wires, and screws; the screws must be countersunk to avoid impingement on the articular surface of the proximal radioulnar joint. Displaced or angulated fractures should be repaired to preserve the radial head, which is the lateral stabilizer of the elbow. This is especially true with associated elbow dislocation. Open reduction and internal fixation should be performed when possible on displaced fractures to prevent deformity, instability, and compromise of elbow function (Figures 15-9 and 15-10).

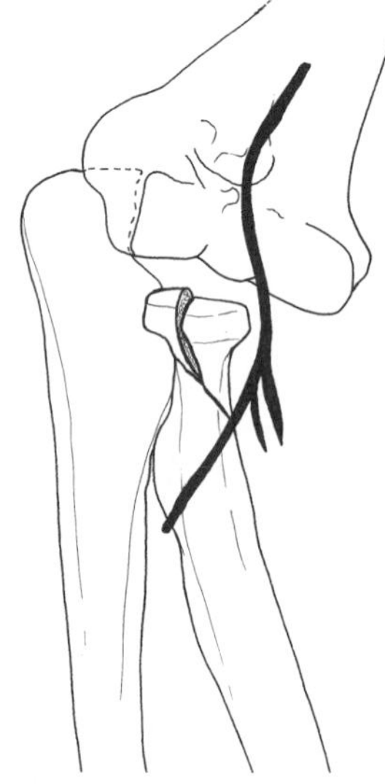

FIGURE 15-9 Displaced split fracture of the radial head type 2 with greater than 2 mm of displacement and involving 50% of the radial head.

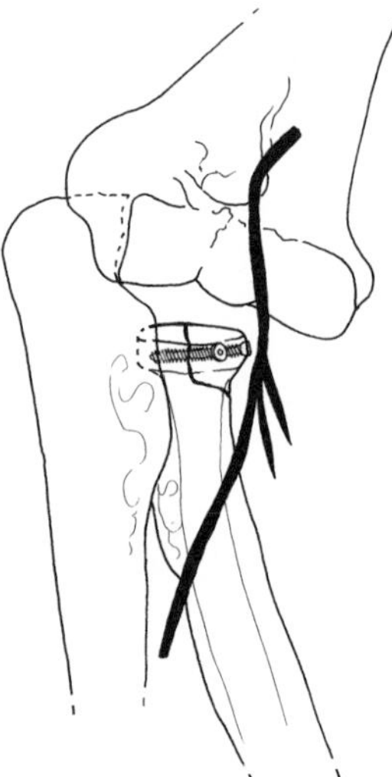

FIGURE 15-10 Split fracture of the radial head after operative treatment with screw fixation. Note the anatomic reduction of the articular surface of the radial head and restoration of radial length. Early range of motion should follow operative fixation.

Special Considerations of the Fracture

Age

In young patients or high-performance athletes, every effort should be made to reconstruct the fracture with open reduction and internal fixation to prevent valgus instability. In elderly patients, if the elbow is stable, early excision of the radial head and immediate range of motion are recommended. Functional range of motion is more difficult to obtain in elderly patients because of joint stiffness.

Comminuted Fractures

These are associated with delayed healing and with the worst posttraumatic complications (greater loss of extension, greater decrease in range of motion, and greater risk of nonunion; *see* Figure 15-7).

Terrible Triad

The combination of a radial head fracture, a coronoid process fracture, and a medial collateral ligament (MCL) injury creates multidirectional instability. In this scenario, the radial head should be preserved or a prosthetic replacement fitted to help stabilize the elbow against valgus stresses.

Type IV Posterior Dislocation

Reduction of the dislocation must be undertaken first. The radial head is then treated according to the type of fracture (*see* Figures 15-5 and 15-6).

The radial head is a major lateral stabilizer of the elbow. This function is of the utmost importance when there is associated coronoid process fracture, MCL injury of the elbow, or destruction of the radioulnar interosseous membrane (other stabilizers of the elbow joint). Excision of the radial head or fracture fragments is indicated when there is a bony block to motion secondary to a fracture fragment or secondary to comminution of the fracture. This procedure is generally associated with decreased grip strength, pain at the wrist, proximal migration of the radius, valgus instability of the elbow joint, heterotopic ossification at the elbow, posttraumatic arthritis, and, if silicon implants are used, synovitis.

Associated Injury

Neurovascular injury to the posterior interosseous nerve or the median nerve may occur. The brachial artery is also at risk because of its close proximity to the radial head. A thorough neurovascular examination must be performed before surgery (*see* Figure 15-10).

Elbow dislocation may occur with a radial head fracture, which may cause disruption of the anterior oblique fibers of the MCL (the primary valgus resister). With this injury, it is very important to either repair or replace the radial head to prevent valgus instability of the elbow joint (*see* Figures 15-5 and 15-6).

Weight Bearing

No weight bearing through the arm (lifting, carrying, pushing up from a chair) is allowed for 4 to 6 weeks in patients treated with internal fixation. After 4 weeks, partial weight bearing is allowed for patients treated conservatively.

Gait

Because the patient is initially in a sling, arm swing is absent.

TREATMENT

Treatment: Early to Immediate (Day of Injury to One Week)

BONE HEALING

Stability at fracture site: None.

Stage of bone healing: Inflammatory phase. The fracture hematoma is colonized by inflammatory cells, and débridement of the fracture begins.

X-ray: No callus.

Orthopaedic and Rehabilitation Considerations

Physical Examination

Assess the patient's capillary refill, sensation, and the active and passive range of motion of the digits. Evaluate the posterior interosseous nerve, which is at risk because of its close proximity to the radial neck. The intactness of the nerve is tested by examining the active extension of the metacarpophalangeal joints. Also evaluate for swelling of the extremity secondary to the dependent position. Assess range of motion of the elbow, including flexion/extension and especially pronation/supination, because it can be limited by bony block. Tenderness over the MCL of the elbow with possible opening (gapping) during valgus stress may indicate an MCL injury and an unstable elbow.

Dangers

Fractures at the elbow create a large amount of soft tissue swelling, and care must be taken to ensure that there is adequate blood flow distal to the elbow. Compartment syndromes of the elbow and forearm do occur.

Whereas active range of motion is acceptable to regain function, passive range of motion should be avoided because of its association with the formation of heterotopic ossification. This is usually associated with a poor functional outcome.

Radiography

Anteroposterior, lateral, and radiocapitellar (angling the x-ray tube 45 degrees from the lateral, directing the beam toward the radial head) views should be obtained. Anteroposterior and lateral x-rays of the wrist should also be obtained to rule out disruption of the distal radioulnar joint. The radiographs at the elbow should be checked for displacement of the fracture fragments or free-floating fragments. Consider excision of comminuted fractures. Fractures involving more than 25% of the articular surface and composed of only a few fragments may be considered for open reduction and internal fixation. Radiographs obtained after internal fixation should be carefully checked for loose, free-floating, or prominent screws.

Weight Bearing

No weight bearing is allowed on the involved extremity.

Range of Motion

Early mobilization of the elbow is crucial to prevent stiffness and contractures, especially if the fracture is intraarticular. Three to 4 days after the fracture and once the pain subsides, gentle active range of motion is provided to the elbow in flexion and pronation. Active range of motion is prescribed to the wrist and shoulder to maintain mobility of these joints. The patient is placed in a sling or an articulating brace after the exercises.

Muscle Strength

No strengthening exercises are prescribed to the elbow yet because they are too painful to perform.

Functional Activities

The uninvolved extremity is used for self-care and the activities of daily living. Because the involved extremity is in a sling, the patient's blouse or shirt is draped over that extremity.

Methods of Treatment: Specific Aspects

Sling/Splint

Check the patient's neck where the strap lies to be sure there is no skin irritation; the strap should be padded for comfort. Check the skin around the elbow to be sure there are no pressure areas from the sling.

The sharp edges of a splint should be trimmed and additional padding placed where appropriate. A splint that is not rigid is acceptable because it allows some flexion and extension.

Open Reduction and Internal Fixation

It is difficult to obtain rigid fixation of radial head fractures, and thus some external immobilization is needed. Usually an articulated brace is used. This must be checked for a comfortable, snug fit without pressure areas. Extra padding may be required over the incision to prevent irritation. Examine the wound for erythema and drainage, which signify infection. Begin the patient on indomethacin at 75 mg per day in divided doses postoperatively to prevent heterotopic bone formation.

Prescription

DAY ONE TO ONE WEEK

Precautions No passive range of motion.

Range of Motion Gentle, active range of motion to the elbow in flexion and pronation.

Strength No strengthening exercises are prescribed to the elbow.

Functional Activities The uninvolved extremity is used for activities of daily living.

Weight Bearing None.

Treatment: Two Weeks

BONE HEALING

Stability at fracture site: None to minimal.

Stage of bone healing: Beginning of reparative phase. Osteoprogenitor cells differentiate into osteoblasts, which lay down woven bone.

X-ray: No callus.

Orthopaedic and Rehabilitation Considerations

Physical Examination

Assess the patient's neurovascular status and the active range of motion of the elbow. Remove the splint and encourage active range of motion. Check wounds for erythema, discharge, or fluctuance. Remove staples or sutures. Avoid passive range of motion because of its high association with heterotopic ossification.

Dangers

Heterotopic ossification, especially after internal fixation, limits or reduces range of motion and function. Radiographs should be examined closely for small foci of heterotopic ossification. Confirm that the patient is taking indomethacin according to the prescribed dosage and frequency. Check for loss of reduction or fixation after internal fixation.

Radiography

Nonoperative Treatment. Radiographs should be checked for further displacement or collapse at the fracture site, which may necessitate operative treatment. Free-floating fragments should be excised to prevent blockage of motion.

Operative Treatment. Poor or prominent screw position may be observed on the anteroposterior radiograph and could cause a problem with motion and loss of reduction. Comparison of the hardware to that in the immediate postoperative radiograph is essential, because small changes may not be otherwise noticed.

Weight Bearing

No weight bearing is allowed on the involved extremity.

Range of Motion

Continue with the active range of motion of the elbow. No passive range of motion is given so as to avoid dislocation or disruption of the callus and hardware. Continue with full range of motion to the shoulder and wrist.

Muscle Strength

No strengthening exercises are given to the elbow. Putty and ball-squeezing exercises are prescribed to the wrist and digits to maintain their strength and decrease dependent edema. Start gentle isometric exercises to the triceps, biceps, and deltoid to prevent disuse atrophy.

Functional Activities

The uninvolved extremity is used for self-care and the activities of daily living.

Methods of Treatment: Specific Aspects

Sling/Splint

Remove the sling to encourage active range of motion. A patient who is apprehensive or experiences pain upon its removal may be weaned from the sling over a few days. It is essential to begin motion.

Remove the splint and encourage active motion. Stiffness of the elbow is not unusual, and a sling may be warranted for a few days until the patient is more comfortable with motion. A hinged orthosis may be useful at night to help control pain.

Open Reduction and Internal Fixation

Proper fit is essential to the comfort and function of an articulated brace. Check the wounds for erythema and discharge and pressure areas for proper padding. The patient should understand that active elbow flexion and extension within the brace are essential, as are active pronation and supination out of the brace. Continue the patient on 75 mg of indomethacin, in divided doses for 3 to 6 weeks.

Prescription

TWO WEEKS

Precautions No passive range of motion to the elbow.

Range of Motion Active range of motion to the elbow.

Strength No strengthening exercises to the elbow. Start isometric exercises to the deltoid, biceps, and triceps.

Functional Activities The uninvolved extremity is used for self-care.

Weight Bearing None.

Treatment: Four to Six Weeks

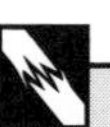

BONE HEALING

Stability at fracture site: With bridging callus, the fracture is usually stable; confirm with physical examination.

Stage of bone healing: Reparative phase. Further organization of the callus and formation of lamellar bone begin. Once callus is observed bridging the fracture site, the fracture is usually stable. However, the strength of this callus, especially with torsional load, is significantly lower than that of normal bone. Further protection of the bone is required to avoid refracture.

X-ray: Bridging callus is visible. With increased rigidity, less bridging callus is noted, and healing with endosteal callus predominates. The amount of callus formation is less at the ends of the long bones, compared to midshaft fractures.

Orthopaedic and Rehabilitation Considerations

Physical Examination

Check the range of motion, the varus and valgus stability of elbow, and the patient's neurovascular status. In particular, assess for reflex sympathetic dystrophy (tropic changes, vasomotor disturbances, hyperesthesia, and pain and tenderness out of proportion to the stage of healing).

Dangers

Reflex sympathetic dystrophy is a potential problem with any fracture. Desensitization modalities should be prescribed early as part of physical therapy. Dislocation is not unusual.

Radiography

Heterotopic ossification is apparent if it is present. Radiocapitellar alignment should be carefully assessed for proper articulation. Callus should be easily seen in nonoperatively treated fractures and less apparent in rigidly or semirigidly repaired fractures.

Weight Bearing

Partial weight bearing is allowed for nonoperatively treated cases. Radiographs should always be obtained shortly after the initiation of weight bearing to assess any changes. Patients with internal fixation should not begin weight bearing yet.

Range of Motion

Continue with full active to active-assistive range of motion to the elbow in all planes. At the end of 6 weeks, if there is some limitation in the range of motion, gentle passive range of motion is allowed. Continue with full range of motion to shoulder, wrist, and digits.

The functional range of motion should be achieved at this point, and more aggressive active-assistive to passive range of motion therapy may be needed for patients with large limitations in motion. Lags in terminal extension and flexion are acceptable, but with more extensive losses heterotopic ossification should be suspected.

Muscle Strength

Continue with isometric exercises to the biceps, triceps, and deltoid. Continue with ball-squeezing exercises to the digits.

Functional Activities

The uninvolved extremity is used for self-care and the activities of daily living. As the splint or sling is removed, the patient may don a shirt or blouse with the involved extremity first and doff it from the uninvolved extremity first.

Methods of Treatment: Specific Aspects

Sling/Splint

These should have been removed by two weeks and active range of motion encouraged.

Open Reduction and Internal Fixation

Healing may be slower than with nonoperative treatment. The patient should continue wearing an articulated brace but should spend more time out of the brace working active and active-assistive pronation and supination. Patients can gradually increase their hours out of brace to be completely out by the end of 6 weeks. Continue with active to passive range of motion to the elbow.

Prescription

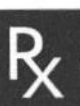

FOUR TO SIX WEEKS

Precautions Avoid valgus stresses to the elbow to avoid stress on the radial head.

Range of Motion Active, active-assistive, and passive range of motion to the elbow for nonoperative cases. Active and active-assistive range of motion for patients with internal fixation.

Strength Isometric exercises to the biceps, triceps, and deltoid.

Functional Activities The uninvolved extremity is used in self-care. The involved extremity is used to assist in gentle activities.

Weight Bearing Partial weight bearing for patients with nonoperative fixation. No weight bearing for patients with internal fixation.

Treatment: Eight to Twelve Weeks

BONE HEALING

Stability at fracture site: Stable.

Stage of bone healing: Remodeling phase. Further organization of callus, which becomes more resistant to torsional forces. The process of remodeling takes years.

X-ray: Visible bridging callus in nonoperative patients. There is less callus with internal fixation.

Orthopaedic and Rehabilitation Considerations

Physical Examination

Assess the patient's active and passive range of motion. Neurovascular status (especially that of the posterior interosseous nerve) should be examined, with particular attention to the patient's ability to extend the metacarpophalangeal joint. With compromised nerve function, electromyographic studies should be obtained at 6 weeks to gain insight as to the location of the lesion.

Dangers

Heterotopic ossification may be the cause of loss of motion, and early excision with soft tissue releases may be considered at 8 to 12 months after injury, when formation is complete.

Radiography

In nonoperative patients, the fracture line should be resolving and forming abundant callus. Pain and tenderness at the fracture site may suggest a nonunion, which is rare.

Patients who have been internally stabilized may have minimal callus. Broken or loosened hardware should raise the question of nonunion.

Weight Bearing

Full weight bearing is allowed for both operatively and nonoperatively treated cases. Operative patients should continue to wear a brace for a total of 3 months to prevent valgus stresses upon the elbow.

Range of Motion

Gain in functional motion is most important at this time. Aggressive passive and active range of motion therapy should continue. There should be at least functional range of motion of the elbow. If, however, there is some diminution in the range, passive stretch motion may begin because the fracture is stable. If necessary, hydrotherapy or fluidotherapy can be administered to facilitate range of motion and decrease the stiffness and pain.

Muscle Strength

Progressive resistive exercises can be started to the elbow flexors, extensors, supinators, and pronators and to the wrist flexors and extensors. Initially the patient can use the uninvolved extremity to offer resistance and thereby monitor his or her own tolerance.

Functional Activities

The involved extremity is used for self-care and light-duty activities. Heavy lifting or pushing with the involved extremity should be avoided. Elderly patients can use the affected extremity for holding a cane as tolerated.

Methods of Treatment: Specific Aspects

All patients undergoing nonoperative treatment or with bony excision should be completely healed. The range of motion should be normal or near normal. Patients with contractures that do not respond to aggressive therapy should be evaluated for soft tissue release.

In patients undergoing surgical intervention, all braces should be discontinued and the patient should continue active and passive range of motion until functional flexion, extension, pronation, and supination are achieved.

Prescription

EIGHT TO TWELVE WEEKS

Precautions No pushing or lifting heavy objects.

Range of Motion Active and passive range of motion to the elbow.

Strength Progressive resistive exercises are given to the elbow flexors, extensors, supinators, and pronators.

Functional Activities The involved extremity is used in self-care.

Weight bearing Weight bearing allowed for self-care and light-duty activities.

LONG-TERM CONSIDERATIONS AND PROBLEMS

Heterotopic Ossification

This is usually a problem after internal fixation has been placed, although approximately 5% of nonoperatively treated fractures also show signs of heterotopic ossification. Severe heterotopic ossification can be the major factor in significant loss of function about the elbow. Surgeons have tried soft tissue releases combined with heterotopic ossification resection, both early and late, with mixed success. The current treatment of choice is prophylactic administration of indomethacin, 75 mg per day, started within 1 week of injury and continued for 3 to 6 weeks.

Loss of Motion

Patients with severe compromise in motion need aggressive surgical treatment by either soft tissue releases, bony excision, or both.

Radial Head Excision

The loss of this stabilizer to valgus stress may be associated with many problems. Proximal migration of the radius and the development of an ulna-positive wrist may cause weakness in grip strength and ulnar-sided impingement of the carpus. These are complicated problems without an easy solution. Silicone synovitis may develop in patients with silicone radial head replacement and the spacer must be removed once the soft tissues are healed (3 to 6 months). Patients lacking both the MCL and the radial head (as in a fracture dislocation) are susceptible to valgus instability and late tardy ulnar nerve palsy.

IMMEDIATE TO ONE WEEK

	Sling/Splint	*Excision*	*Open Reduction and Internal Fixation*
Stability	None	None	None
Orthopedics	Ensure proper fitting of sling and check for pressure sores on neck. Pad as necessary.	Evaluate wound.	Evaluate wound.
	Trim splint to allow free range of motion of metaphalangeal MP joints.	Trim and pad splint as necessary.	Ensure articulated elbow arthrosis is well fitting.
	Add padding to splint as necessary		
Rehabilitation	Active range of motion of elbow after 3 to 4 days of immobilization.	Same.	Same.
	Avoid passive range of motion of the elbow.		
	Active and passive range of motion to shoulder, wrist, and fingers.		

TWO WEEKS

	Sling/Splint	*Excision*	*Open Reduction and Internal Fixation*
Stability	None to minimal	None to minimal	None to minimal
Orthopedics	Should be removed to encourage active range of motion.	Evaluate wound. Remove sutures. Encourage active range of motion.	Evaluate wound. Remove sutures. Encourage active range of motion in articulated orthosis only.
Rehabilitation	Isometric exercises to triceps, biceps, and deltoid.	Same.	Same.
	Active range of motion to the elbow.		
	Active and passive range of motion of shoulder and wrist.		

FOUR TO SIX WEEKS

	Sling/Splint	Excision	Open Reduction and Internal Fixation
Stability	Stable.	Stable.	Partially stable.
Orthopedics	Check active and passive range of motion.	Check active and passive range of motion.	No weight bearing. Active range of motion only. Strengthening exercises.
Rehabilitation	Partial weight bearing. Active and active-assistive range of motion. Strengthening exercises to the biceps, triceps, deltoids, and digits.	Same. Strengthening exercises to the biceps, triceps, deltoids, and digits.	No weight bearing. Active range of motion only.

EIGHT TO TWELVE WEEKS

	Splint/Sling	Excision	Open Reduction and Internal Fixation
Stability	Stable.	Stable.	Stable.
Orthopedics	Full activity.	Full activity.	May remove orthosis at 12 weeks.
Rehabilitation	Active and passive range of motion of the elbow. Resistive exercises to elbow flexors, extensors, supinators, and pronators.	Same.	Same.

BIBLIOGRAPHY

Bakalim G. Fractures of radial head and their treatment. *Acta Orthop Scand,* 41:320–331, 1970.

Broberg MA, Morrey BF. Results of delayed excision of the radial head after fracture. *J Bone Joint Surg,* 68A:669–674, 1986.

Broberg MA, et al. Results of treatment of fracture-dislocations of the elbow. *Clin Orthop,* 216:109–119, 1987.

Edwards GS, Jupiter JB. Radial head fracture with acute distal radio-ulnar dislocation—Essex-Lopresti revisited. *Clin Orthop,* 234:61–69, 1988.

Epner RA, Bowers WH. Ulnar variance—the effect of wrist positioning and roentgen filming technique. *J Hand Surg* 7:298–305, 1982.

Gerald Y, Schernburg F. Anatomical, pathological and therapeutic investigation of fractures of the radial head in adults. *J Bone Joint Surg,* 66B:141, 1984.

Grundy A, Murphy G. The value of the radial head-capitellum view in radial head trauma. *Br J Radiol,* 58:965–967, 1985.

Harrington IL, Tountas AA. Replacement of the radial head in the treatment of unstable elbow fractures. *Injury,* 12:405–412, 1981.

Hotchkiss RN, Weiland AJ. Valgus stability of the elbow. *J Orthop Res* 5:372–377, 1987.

CHAPTER *Sixteen*

Forearm Fractures

SAMUEL A. HOISINGTON, MD

VASANTHA L. MURTHY, MD

INTRODUCTION

Definition

Forearm fractures include fractures of the shaft of the radius, ulna, or both bones. Radial head dislocation in association with fracture of the ulna (Monteggia) and distal radioulnar joint dislocation in association with fracture of the radius (Galeazzi) also occur.

Forearm fractures are further classified according to location (proximal-third, middle-third, or distal-third radius fractures), fracture pattern (transverse, oblique, spiral, comminuted, or segmental), displacement (displaced or nondisplaced), and angulation (volar or dorsal and radial or ulnar) (Figures 16-1, 16-2, 16-3, 16-4, 16-5, and 16-6).

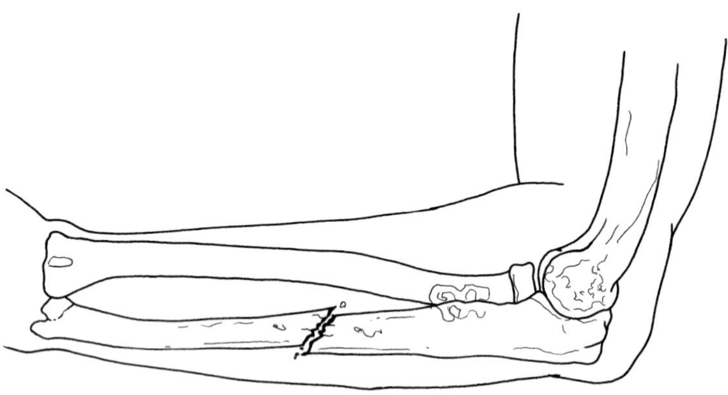

FIGURE 16-1 Minimally displaced oblique fracture of the middle third of the ulna.

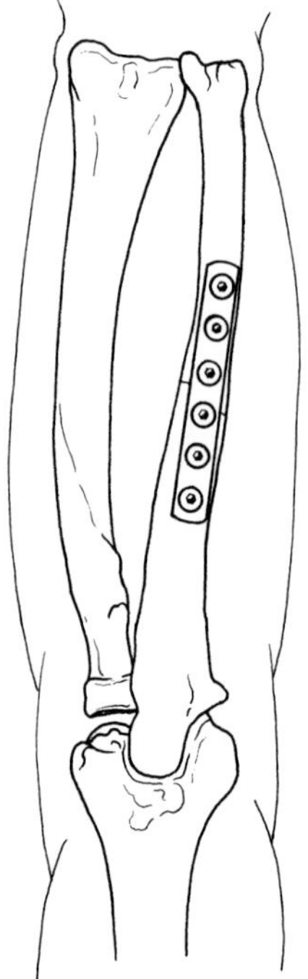

FIGURE 16-2 Midshaft ulnar fracture treated with compression plate fixation. This fixation restores anatomic alignment of the shaft of the ulna and allows early range of motion of the elbow, forearm, and wrist.

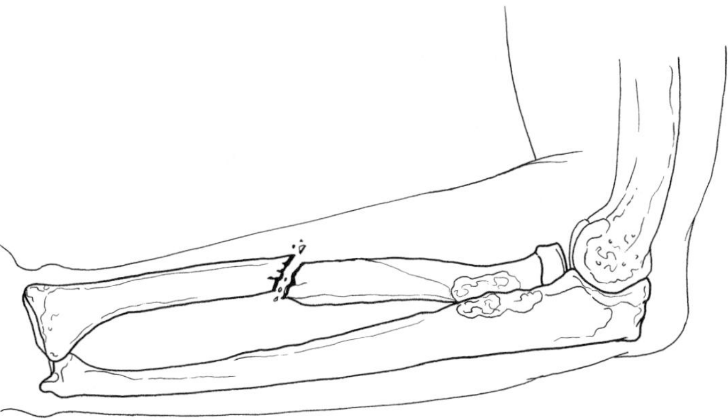

FIGURE 16-3 Displaced oblique fracture of the midshaft of the radius. This fracture generally requires internal fixation to anatomically align the radius and restore radial bow.

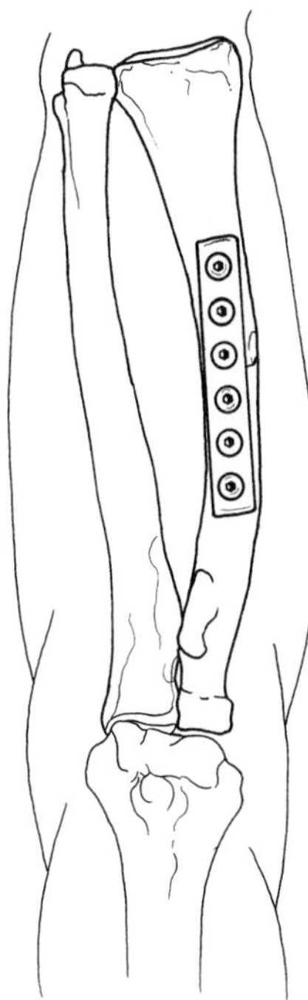

FIGURE 16-4 Midshaft radius fracture treated with compression plate fixation. This fixation restores the anatomic alignment of the radius and the radial bow and allows for early range of motion of the elbow, forearm, and wrist.

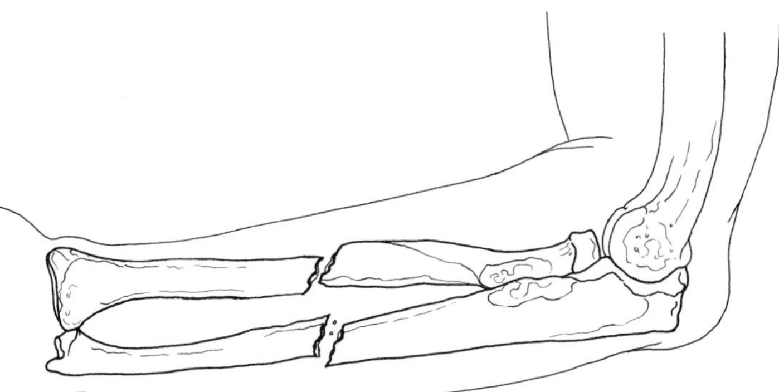

FIGURE 16-5 Oblique displaced midshaft fractures of the radius and ulna (both-bones forearm fracture). These fractures require open reduction and internal fixation with a compression plate in order to restore the anatomic alignment of the radius and ulna and allow early range of motion.

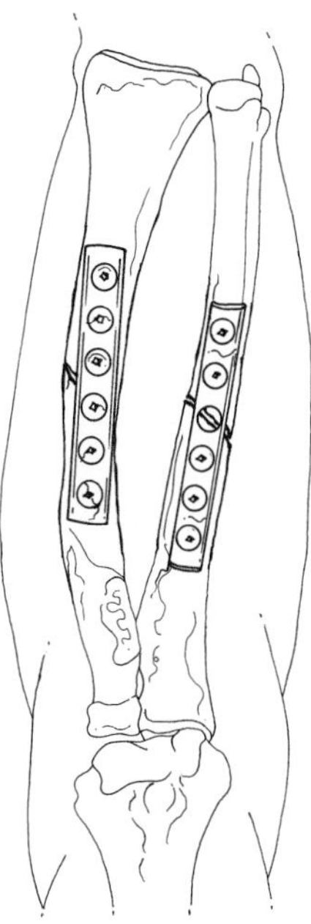

FIGURE 16-6 Both-bones fracture of the forearm treated with compression plate fixation of both the radius and the ulna. This fixation restores the anatomic alignment of the radius and ulna and the radial bow, and allows early range of motion of the elbow, forearm, and wrist.

Types of Forearm Fractures

A *nightstick fracture* is an isolated midshaft (diaphyseal) ulnar fracture resulting from a direct blow. It is usually amenable to closed reduction and cast application (Figures 16-7 and 16-8).

A *Monteggia fracture/dislocation* is a proximal or middle-third ulna fracture with dislocation of the radial head. The radial head may be dislocated anteriorly, posteriorly, or laterally, and in some instances both the radius and ulna are fractured (Figures 16-9 and 16-10, and *see* Figures 16-19 and 16-20).

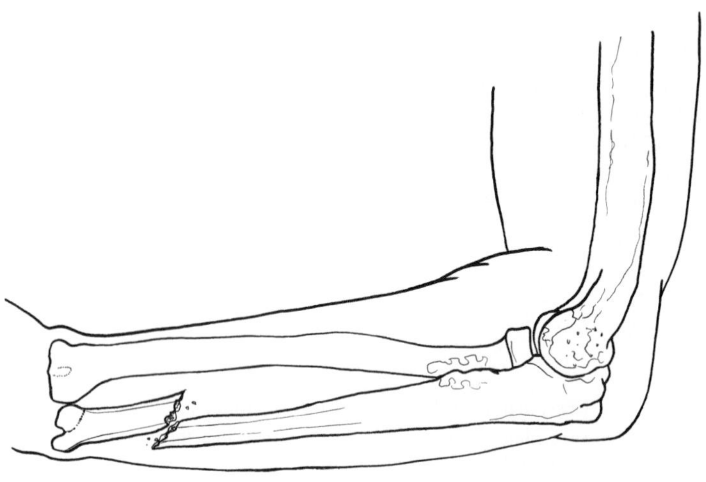

FIGURE 16-7 Displaced oblique fracture of the distal diaphyseal region of the ulna (nightstick fracture). This fracture may be treated with a splint, a cast, or with open reduction and internal fixation.

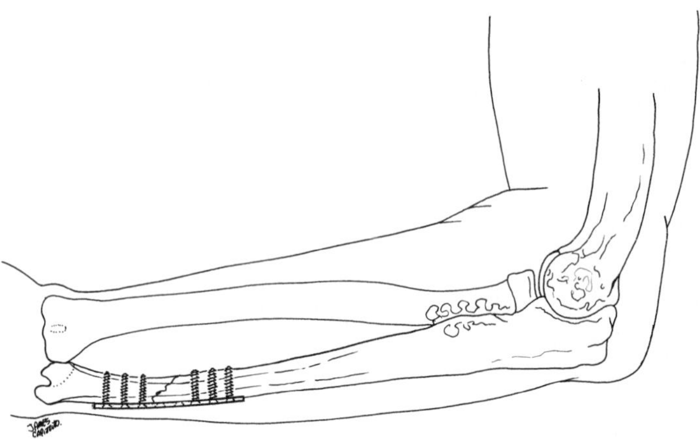

FIGURE 16-8 Distal diaphyseal fracture of the ulna treated with compression plate fixation. This allows early range of motion of the elbow, forearm, and wrist.

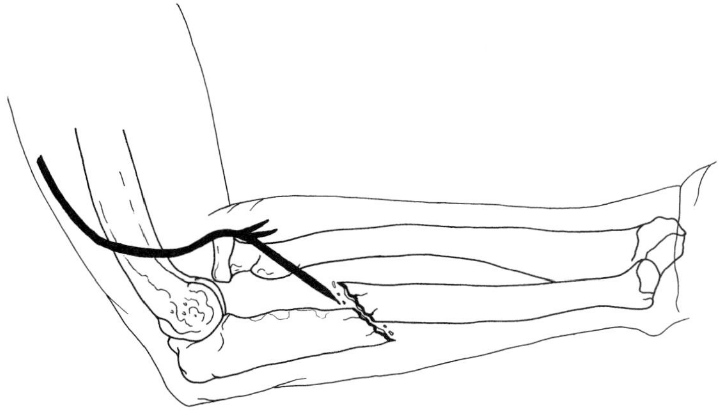

FIGURE 16-9 Fracture of the diaphysis of the ulna with a dislocated radial head. An anterior dislocation of the radial head is a Monteggia fracture type I, as seen here, requiring reduction of the radial head and internal fixation of the ulnar fracture.

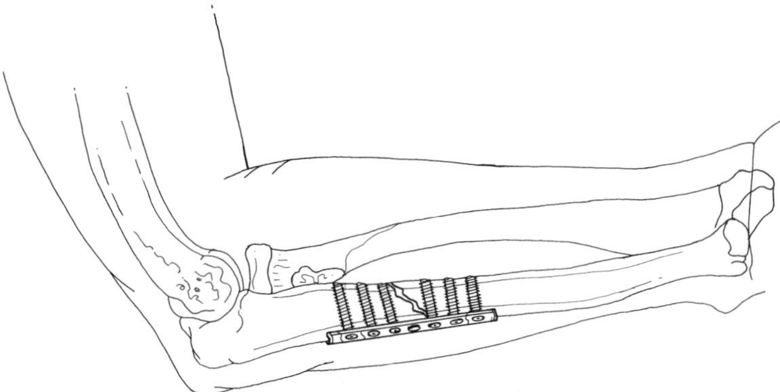

FIGURE 16-10 Reduction of the radial head and internal fixation of the ulnar fracture with compression plating.

A *Galeazzi fracture/dislocation* is a distal-third radius fracture with disruption of the distal radioulnar joint. It is called a fracture of necessity, because, in this injury, it is necessary to provide surgical intervention because of loss of correction and loss of bowing of the radius (Figures 16-11, 16-12, and 16-13, and *see* Figures 16-21 and 16-22).

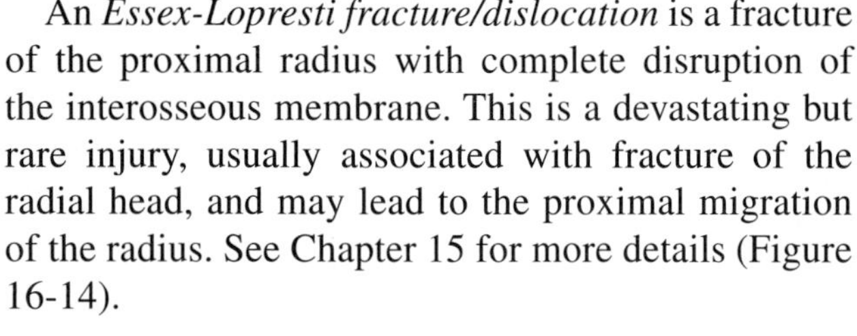

An *Essex-Lopresti fracture/dislocation* is a fracture of the proximal radius with complete disruption of the interosseous membrane. This is a devastating but rare injury, usually associated with fracture of the radial head, and may lead to the proximal migration of the radius. See Chapter 15 for more details (Figure 16-14).

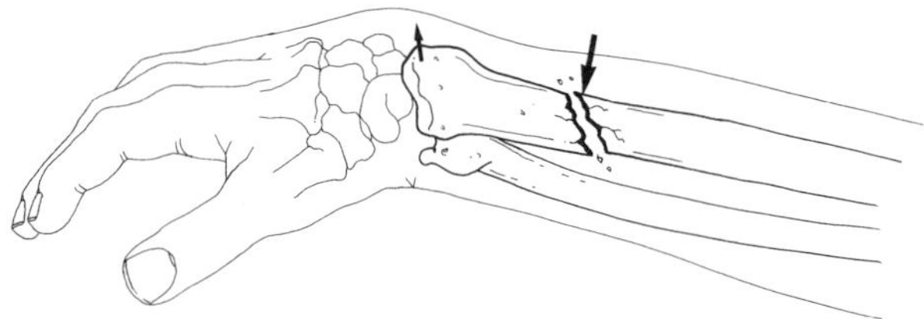

FIGURE 16-11 Fracture of the distal radius with distal radial/ulnar joint disruption (Galeazzi fracture/dislocation).

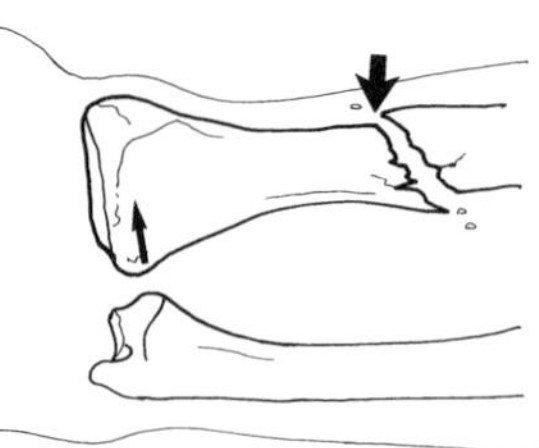

FIGURE 16-12 Galeazzi fracture/dislocation, illustrating a distal radioulnar joint disruption.

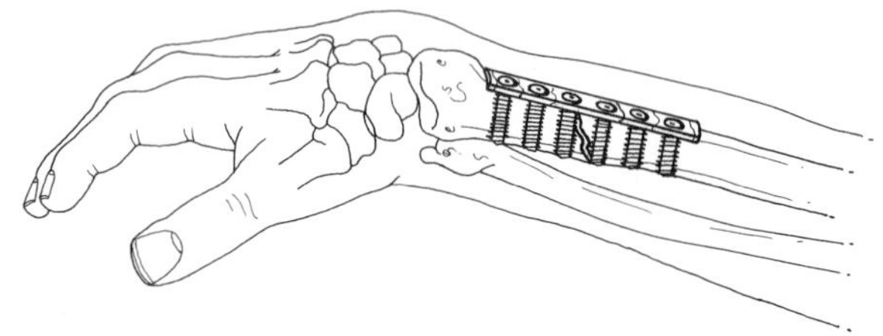

FIGURE 16-13 Reduction of a Galeazzi fracture/dislocation with compression plate fixation of the distal radius and reduction of the distal radioulnar joint.

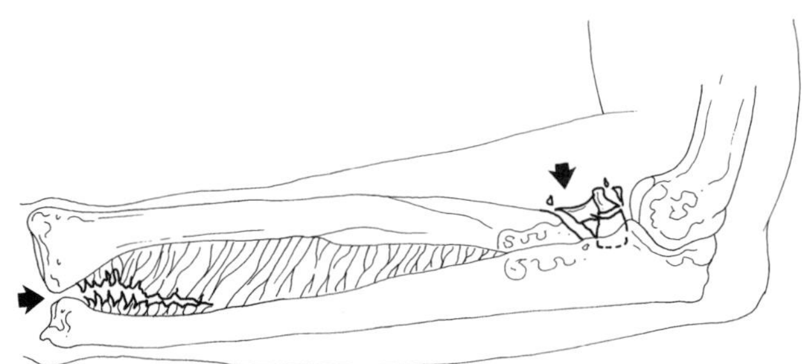

FIGURE 16-14 Fracture of the proximal radius with disruption of the interosseous membrane between the radius and ulna (Essex-Lopresti fracture). This injury is associated with proximal migration of the radius and instability of the distal radioulnar joint.

Mechanism of Injury

Most forearm fractures are the result of either a fall on an outstretched hand or a direct blow sustained in a motor vehicle accident or altercation.

Treatment Goals

Orthopaedic Objectives

Alignment

Accurate reduction of radius and ulna fractures is important. Malunion leads to a loss of pronation, supination, and grip strength. The radial bow and interosseous space should be maintained, as should fragment rotation and length. The exception to this is in isolated ulna fractures in which up to 50% of displacement has not resulted in significant dysfunction.

Stability

Both-bone forearm fractures are unstable injuries. Undisplaced fractures are rare. Fracture stability depends on the amount of energy absorbed during the injury and the forces of the large muscles tending to displace the fragment. Surgical stabilization with a rigid construct allows early mobilization and is preferred.

Rehabilitation Objective

Range of Motion

Restore full supination and pronation of the forearm and maximal wrist and hand motion (Table 16-1).

TABLE 16-1 *Range of Motion of Forearm and Elbow*

Motion	Normal	Functional
Pronation	80°	50°
Supination	80°	50°
Flexion	135°	90°
Extension	0°	20°–30°

Muscle Strength

Improve the strength of the following muscles:

Pronators:

- Pronator quadratus
- Pronator teres

Supinators:

- Supinator
- Brachioradialis

Long flexors:

- Flexor digitorum superficialis (flexes the proximal interphalangeal joints of the digits)
- Flexor digitorum profundus (flexes the proximal and distal interphalangeal joints)
- Flexor pollicis longus (flexes interphalangeal joints of the thumb)
- Flexor carpi radialis (wrist flexor and radial deviator)
- Flexor carpi ulnaris (wrist flexor and ulnar deviator)

Long extensors:

- Extensor digitorum communis (extends the fingers)
- Extensor pollicis longus (extends the thumb)
- Extensor carpi radialis longus and brevis (wrist extensor and radial deviator)
- Extensor carpi ulnaris (wrist extensor and ulnar deviator)
- Extensor indicis propius (extends the index finger)
- Extensor digit minimi propius (extends the small finger)

Functional Goals

Improve and restore activities that require supination and pronation of the forearm (turning a doorknob or key), and improve the flexion and extension of the wrist.

Expected Time of Bone Healing

8 to 12 weeks.

Some fractures require up to 4 months for union to occur. Delayed union is rare.

Expected Duration of Rehabilitation

12 to 24 weeks.

Fractures with associated dislocations, such as Galeazzi and Monteggia fracture/dislocations, require longer rehabilitation.

Methods of Treatment

Cast

Biomechanics: Stress-sharing device.

Mode of bone healing: Secondary.

Indications: Cast immobilization is the treatment of choice for nondisplaced both-bone forearm fractures and isolated ulna fractures. Closed reduction and long arm cast immobilization has been used for displaced forearm fractures but may be unsatisfactory unless the reduction is carefully maintained. The cast should have a good interosseous mold, with an oval rather than a circular cross section, because this helps to maintain the interosseous space. Middle-third fractures are generally treated with a long arm cast with the elbow in 90 degrees of flexion and the forearm in neutral rotation. Reduction of proximal-third radius fractures is assisted by immobilization in supination. This relaxes the deforming pull of the supinator muscle. Distal-third radius fractures should be immobilized in pronation (this relaxes the deforming pull of the pronator quadratus muscle) to achieve the best chance of acceptable alignment. The long arm cast is applied for 4 weeks and then replaced by a short arm cast or functional brace for 2 weeks. The total duration of casting and immobilization is approximately 6 to 8 weeks before union.

Displacement of a both-bones fracture after careful reduction necessitates open reduction and internal plate fixation. In an isolated ulna fracture, up to 10 degrees of angulation and 50% of displacement are permitted. Frequently it is difficult to hold the position following closed reduction, because the forces of the forearm muscles and biceps tend to displace the fracture even in a cast. For the most part, good treatment is anatomic reduction.

Open Reduction and Internal Plate Fixation

Biomechanics: Stress-shielding device.

Mode of bone healing: Primary.

Indications: Most forearm fractures, including isolated radius fractures, both-bone fractures, and fractures involving radial head dislocation or destruction of the distal radioulnar joint require open reduction and internal fixation (Figures 16-15, 16-16, 16-17, and 16-18, and *see* Figures 16-5 and 16-6).

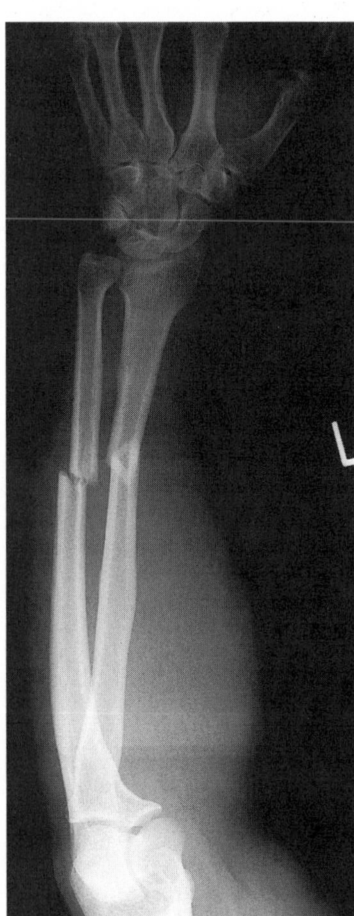

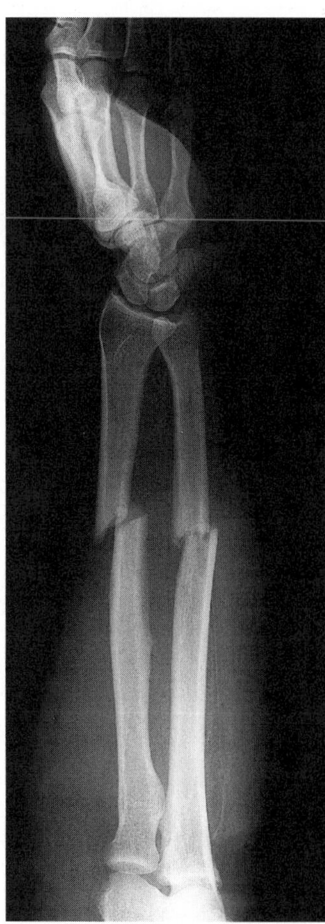

FIGURE 16-15 *(far left)* Both-bones fracture of the forearm. Midshaft diaphyseal fractures of both the radius and the ulna are displaced.

FIGURE 16-16 *(left)* Both-bones fracture of the forearm: middle-third oblique fracture of the radius with minimal comminution and middle-third transverse fracture of the ulna with minimal comminution. Both are displaced.

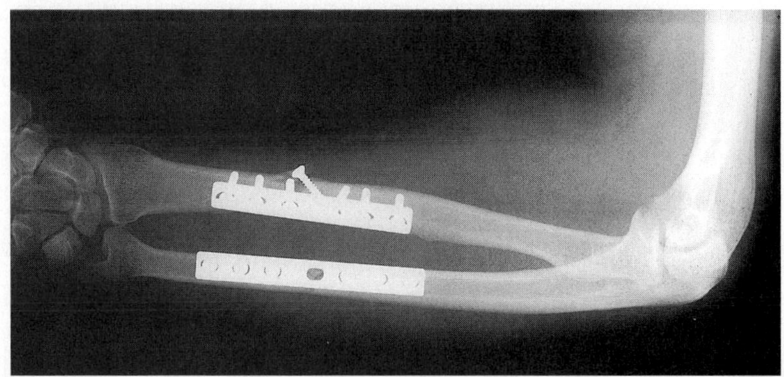

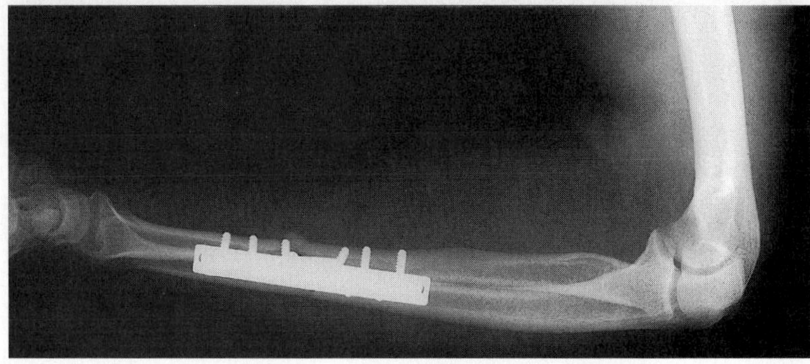

FIGURE 16-17 *(above left)* Both-bones fracture of the forearm treated with open reduction and compression plate fixation along with lag screw fixation. This fixation restores the anatomic axis of the forearm along with the radial bow and allows early range of motion of the elbow, forearm, and wrist.

FIGURE 16-18 *(left)* Both bones fracture of the forearm treated with open reduction and compression plate fixation as seen on a lateral radiograph. This fixation restores the anatomic axis of the radius and ulna.

For Monteggia fractures, closed reduction of the radial head is carried out, followed by the plating of the ulnar fracture. Simultaneous reduction of the radial head occurs as the ulnar shaft fracture is anatomically reduced and fixed. Depending on the stability of the radial head after reduction, postoperative immobilization varies from a long arm cast to a functional brace (Figures 16-19 and 16-20, and *see* Figures 16-9 and 16-10).

For Galeazzi fractures, the radius is anatomically reduced and fixed with a plate. This restores the position of the radioulnar joint. A long arm cast or functional brace holds the forearm in supination for 4 weeks. This is followed by a short arm cast for an additional 2 weeks (Figures 16-21, 16-22, 16-23, and 16-24, and *see* Figures 16-11, 16-12, and 16-13).

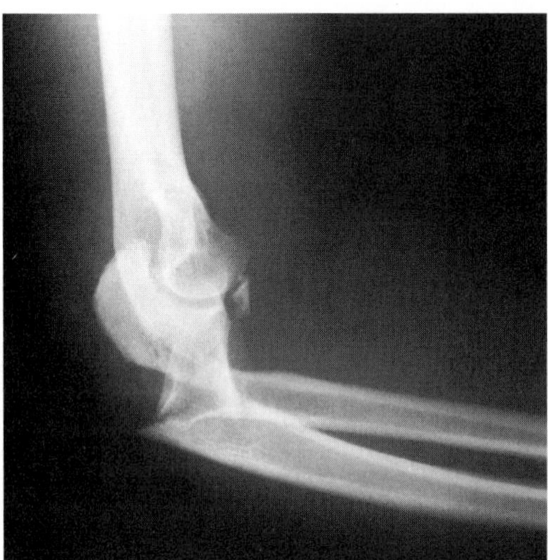

FIGURE 16-19 Displaced oblique fracture of the proximal ulna, posterior dislocation of the radial head, and displaced fracture of the coronoid (Monteggia fracture/dislocation of the proximal forearm). This is a Monteggia type II pattern and requires reduction of the radial head and internal fixation of the proximal ulnar fracture.

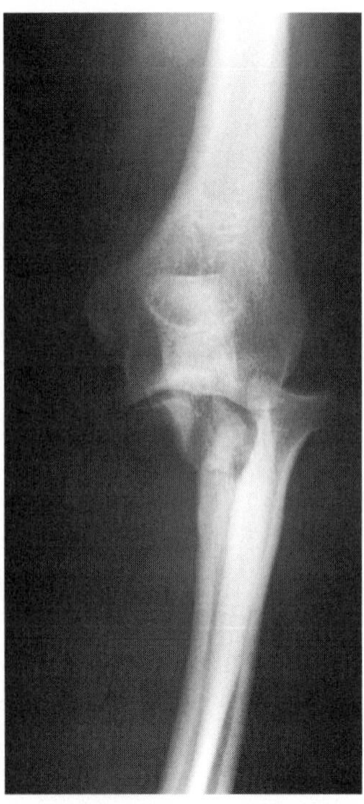

FIGURE 16-20 Comminuted fracture of the proximal ulna with lateral dislocation of the radial head (Monteggia fracture/dislocation of the proximal forearm). This is a Monteggia type III pattern.

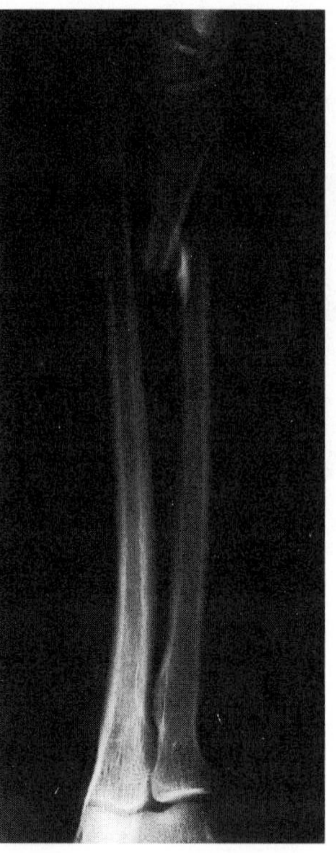

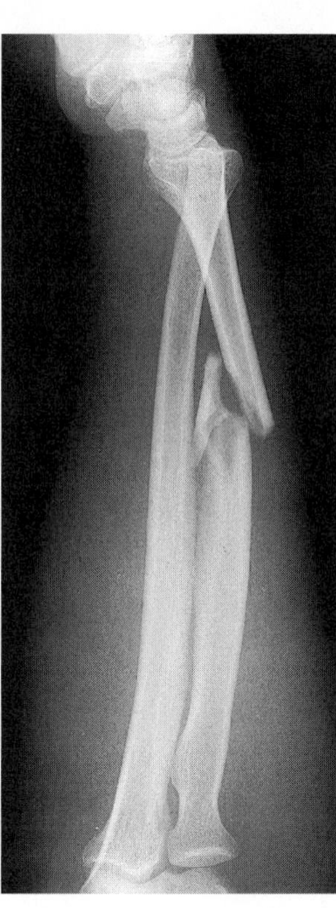

FIGURE 16-21 *(above left)* Comminuted displaced fracture of the distal radius with separation of the distal radioulnar joint (Galeazzi fracture/dislocation of the distal forearm, anteroposterior view).

FIGURE 16-22 *(above right)* Fracture of the middle third of the radius with a butterfly fragment and dorsal dislocation of the distal ulna at the distal radioulnar joint (Galeazzi fracture/dislocation). The distal radioulnar joint generally reduces to a stable position when the radius is restored to its anatomic position and fixed with a compression plate. If the distal radioulnar joint is unstable after fixation of the radius, the forearm may be immobilized in maximal supination to restore the distal radioulnar joint.

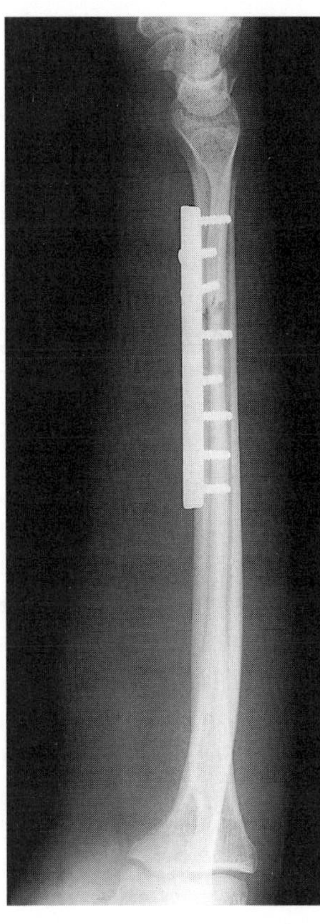

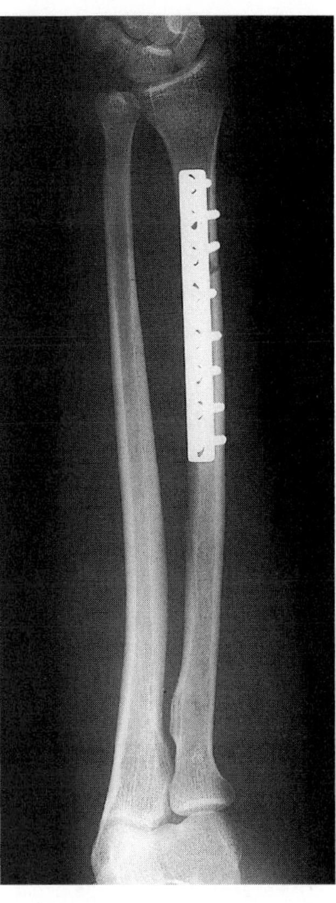

FIGURE 16-23 *(far left)* Galeazzi fracture treated with reduction of the distal radioulnar joint and compression plate fixation of the distal radius. Note that the distal radioulnar joint is restored to its anatomic position.

FIGURE 16-24 *(left)* Galeazzi fracture/dislocation treated with reduction of the distal radioulnar joint and compression plate fixation of the radius. Note the restoration of the radioulnar joint.

External Fixation

Biomechanics: Stress-sharing device.

Mode of bone healing: Secondary.

Indications: This method of treatment is only advocated for severe grade III open forearm fractures and is used in cases of extreme contamination or soft tissue loss. The mainstay of treatment for open injuries is débridement, antibiotics, and stable fixation. Tissue flaps, internal fixation, and bone graft may be used secondarily.

Special Considerations of the Fracture

Age

Elderly patients have a greater risk of development of joint stiffness at the elbow and wrist.

Location

The location of the fracture determines the muscular forces acting on the proximal and distal fragments. A proximal-third radius fracture, between the insertion of the supinator and pronator teres muscles, leads to supination of the proximal fragment by the action of the supinator muscle and pronation of the distal fragment caused by the action of the pronator teres and quadratus muscles. A distal-third radius fracture leads to a proximal fragment held in neutral by the actions of both the supinator and pronator teres muscles, and a distal fragment pronated by the pronator quadratus muscle.

Dislocation of the Radial Head or Distal Ulna

Fractures of the ulna and radius require evaluation of the elbow and wrist, respectively. Satisfactory anteroposterior and lateral radiographs of both joints should be obtained for all forearm fractures. Careful examination of the ulnar styloid and distal radioulnar joint should be performed. Ulnar styloid fractures and widening of the distal radioulnar joint are suggestive of distal radioulnar joint injury and help in diagnosing Galeazzi fractures. Distal radial shortening of greater than 5 mm is also associated with Galeazzi fractures. Prominence of the radial head, pain on radial head palpation, and ulnar shortening without a radius fracture are all associated with radial head subluxation or dislocation and indicate a Monteggia fracture. Galeazzi and Monteggia fractures must be identified, because the joint injury needs to be addressed. There is an increased risk of complications, including loss of motion, malunion, nonunion, and neurovascular compromise (posterior interosseous nerve) associated with these injuries.

Need for Supplementary Bone Graft

The current recommendation is that bone graft should be used when more than one third of the cortex is deficient, although this remains a point of discussion. Sources of bone graft include the iliac crest as well as the distal radius and olecranon.

Delayed Union/Nonunion

These complications are seen with nonrigid fracture fixation, early mobilization of the fracture before stability has been achieved, open reduction and internal fixation with excessive periosteal stripping, and open injuries associated with contamination and periosteal stripping.

Malunion

Angulation of the radius or ulna with narrowing of the interosseous space leads to decreased supination, pronation, and grip strength.

Synostosis

The risk of synostosis is increased when radius and ulna fractures occur at the same level. During operative fixation, approaches to both the radius and ulna through a single incision and the use of bone graft have also been associated with an increased risk of synostosis. Incidence of up to 10% to 15% synostosis has been reported.

Refracture Following Open Reduction and Internal Fixation and Hardware Removal

The patient must be advised that the immediate stability accompanying rigid internal fixation does not imply limitless strength. It should be noted that external callus formation is reduced with anatomic fixation and that the primary bone healing that occurs is initially weaker. Weight-bearing activities must be held until adequate radiographic evidence of bone healing is seen. These issues should be discussed with the patient before operative fixation. See Long-Term Considerations and Problems.

Associated Injury

All forearm nerves are susceptible to injury, although injury to the posterior interosseous is most common. It is especially vulnerable during the radial head dislocation of a Monteggia fracture. Most posterior interosseous nerve injuries are neuropraxias (nerve contusion without disruption) that resolve in 6 to 8 weeks. If no recovery is noted clinically or electrophysiologically after 4 to 6 months, an exploration of the nerve should be performed.

Surgical approaches to the radius and ulna may lead to nerve injury. Nerve injury associated with the application of a plate should be explored immediately. Approach to the ulna may result in injury to the ulnar nerve if subperiosteal elevation of the flexor carpi ulnaris is not performed. The dorsal approach to the radius puts the posterior interosseous nerve at risk, whereas the volar approach is associated with risk to the anterior interosseous nerve, the superficial radial nerve underneath the brachioradialis muscle, and the posterior interosseous nerve with more proximal dissection. Injury to the superficial radial nerve has been known to lead to neuroma formation. Nerve injuries also occur with open fractures, especially with gunshot wounds.

Weight Bearing

The involved extremity should be non-weight bearing until adequate callus formation or primary bone healing has occurred. The patient should avoid supporting the body's weight when using a walker or cane or pushing off from a chair or bed. Platform crutches or a platform walker may be used if necessary.

Gait

The role of arm swing as a balancing and stabilizing force may be temporarily impaired by the presence of a cast or surgery.

TREATMENT

Treatment: Early to Immediate (Day of Injury to One Week)

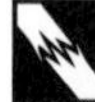

BONE HEALING

Stability at fracture site: None.

Stage of bone healing: Inflammatory phase. The fracture hematoma is colonized by inflammatory cells, and débridement of the fracture begins.

X-ray: No callus.

Orthopaedic and Rehabilitation Considerations

Physical Examination

Assess complaints of pain, swelling, and paresthesia. Pay special attention to the extensor pollicis longus and digit extensors supplied by the posterior interosseous nerve, to the flexor pollicis longus and flexor digitorum longus of the index finger supplied by the anterior interosseous nerve, to finger abduction supplied by the ulnar nerve, and to opposition supplied by the median nerve. Check capillary refill and sensation, as well as the active and passive range of motion of the digits. Be alert for development of compartment syndrome.

Swelling and discoloration of the skin are common. Dependent edema should be treated with elevation or removal and reapplication of the cast if severe.

Dangers

Forearm compartment syndrome does occur, especially with high-energy trauma or open injuries. Pay special attention to complaints of pain, paresthesia, and cast discomfort. Do not refrain from removing a cast for fear of losing an excellent reduction. The sequelae of Volkmann's ischemic contracture are much worse than a lost reduction. If compartment syndrome is suspected, compartment pressures should be measured; if they are elevated, fasciotomies should be performed.

Radiography

Anteroposterior and lateral radiographs of the forearm should be obtained and checked for loss of reduction. Shortening is unacceptable, but up to 10 degrees of angulation is allowed. Gradual loss of reduction should be followed up closely; it may necessitate operative intervention. Wrist or elbow films should also be obtained if the patient has a Galeazzi or Monteggia fracture or if one is suspected.

Weight Bearing

No weight bearing is allowed on the affected extremity.

Range of Motion

For patients in a long arm cast treated conservatively, active range-of-motion exercises are prescribed to the digits, including the interphalangeal and metacarpophalangeal joints, as well as the shoulder. A patient who is in a cast may need assistance in shoulder range of motion. Patients in a short arm cast are also given active elbow exercises. For patients with stable internal fixation who do not require immobilization, gentle active range-of-motion exercises are prescribed for the entire extremity. These are started 3 to 5 days after surgery. The goal is to decrease edema and stiffness of the digits, prevent adhesive capsulitis of the shoulder, and decrease stiffness of the wrist and elbow when stable fixation allows their inclusion in the exercise regimen. Patients with Monteggia or Galeazzi fractures begin active and passive range of motion to the interphalangeal and metacarpophalangeal joints. The patient is usually in too much pain to move the elbow joint. All rotational movement of the forearm must be avoided in Monteggia and Galeazzi fractures.

Muscle Strength

Range of motion should be obtained before strengthening. No strengthening exercises are prescribed initially to the arm and forearm muscles. Patients with rigid fixation are instructed in isometric exercises to biceps, triceps, and deltoid.

Functional Activities

The uninvolved extremity should be used for all functional activities of self-care such as feeding, dressing, and personal hygiene.

Elderly patients using a walker are given a quad cane or hemiwalker for ambulation, because they cannot hold a walker with two hands. The patient should don a shirt with the involved extremity first and doff it from the uninvolved extremity first. Patients with a long arm cast drape the shirt or blouse over the involved extremity.

Gait

Arm swing is reduced secondary to the fracture.

Methods of Treatment: Specific Aspects

Cast

A long arm cast is required for both-bone forearm fractures not treated with open reduction and internal fixation, as well as for Monteggia and Galeazzi fracture/dislocations following fixation. A short arm cast or functional brace may be used for isolated ulna fractures without displacement.

Check the cast margins. Make sure that the cast margin is at the proximal palmar crease to allow full flexion of the metacarpophalangeal joints.

Active range-of-motion exercises are prescribed to the digits when tolerated. This helps in ranging the joints.

Care should be taken not to disrupt the fracture site because flexion and extension of fingers and digits also involve the long flexors and extensors that cross the fracture line. If the digits are edematous, retrograde massage is instituted to decrease pain and improve their range of motion.

Open Reduction and Internal Fixation

If there is adequate fixation with a stable construct, cast immobilization is not required and the patient may begin gentle active range-of-motion exercises to the elbow and wrist in all planes. The shoulder can also be ranged actively. These exercises should be gentle, because no bony stability yet exists. An arm sling should be used when the patient is not performing exercises. If a stable construct does not exist, continue immobilization in a long arm cast and follow the protocol for cast immobilization.

Following fixation, Galeazzi fractures should be maintained in a long arm cast with supination for a full 6 weeks. Monteggia fractures are kept in a long arm cast for 4 to 6 weeks. Following removal of the long arm cast, a short arm cast or functional brace may be used for an additional 4 to 6 weeks.

Prescription

Day One to One Week

Precautions No passive range of motion.

Range of Motion If there is adequate fixation and the forearm is not in a cast, gentle active range-of-motion exercises are prescribed to the elbow and wrist, including supination and pronation exercises.

Strength Isometric exercises to the deltoid, biceps, and triceps if the fracture is rigidly fixed. No strengthening exercises to the forearm if treated with cast only.

Functional Activities The uninvolved extremity is used for self-care.

Weight Bearing No weight bearing on the affected extremity.

Treatment: Two Weeks

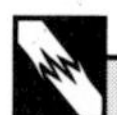

Bone Healing

Stability at fracture site: None to minimal.

Stage of bone healing: Beginning of reparative phase. Osteoprogenitor cells differentiate into osteoblasts, which lay down woven bone.

X-ray: None to early callus.

Orthopaedic and Rehabilitation Considerations

Physical Examination

Carefully assess complaints of pain, swelling, and paresthesia. Check capillary refill and sensation, as well as the active and passive range of motion of the digits. Dependent edema should be treated with elevation or removal and reapplication of the cast if severe.

Dangers

Compression neuropathy may occur with swelling in a tight cast.

Radiography

Anteroposterior and lateral radiographs of the forearm should be obtained and checked for loss of reduction. Gradual loss of reduction should be followed up closely; it may necessitate operative intervention. Wrist or elbow films should also be obtained if the patient has a known or suspected Galeazzi or Monteggia fracture.

Weight Bearing

No weight bearing is allowed on the affected extremity.

Range of Motion

Continue active range of motion of the digits, wrist, elbow, and shoulder for postoperative patients with stable fixation. For patients immobilized in either a short or long arm cast, available joints should be given active range-of-motion exercises. A patient in a cast may require assistance in lifting the arm to perform the range of motion to the shoulder.

Muscle Strength

With patients receiving conservative treatment with a cast, strengthening exercises are not prescribed because the fracture site is unstable. Patients who had rigid fixation can perform isometric strengthening exercises to the biceps and triceps to prevent muscle atrophy. Gentle isotonic exercises with minimal resistance can be instituted to the fingers, such as ball-squeezing and putty exercises. Repetitive flexion and extension of the digits not only improves the range of motion of the joints but also increases the strength of the long flexors and extensors.

Functional Activities

The patient should continue to use the uninvolved extremity for self-care and personal hygiene.

Elderly patients using a walker are given a quad cane or hemiwalker for ambulation, because they cannot hold a walker with two hands.

Gait

If the arm is in a cast, there is no arm swing. Arm swing is reduced for patients undergoing open reduction and internal fixation.

Methods of Treatment: Specific Aspects

Casting

A long arm cast is still required for both-bone forearm fractures not treated with open reduction and internal fixation, as well as for Monteggia and Galeazzi fracture/dislocations following fixation. A short arm cast or functional brace is continued for nondisplaced isolated ulna fractures.

Flexion, extension, abduction, and adduction of the digits should be performed repetitively to maintain the range of motion. Active shoulder motion is important to prevent adhesive capsulitis.

Open Reduction and Internal Fixation

Patients with stable fixation should continue active range-of-motion exercises to the fingers, wrist, elbow, and shoulder. Elbow flexion and extension, forearm supination and pronation, and wrist flexion and extension should be performed regularly to prevent stiffness. Active shoulder motion prevents adhesive capsulitis. No lifting or weight bearing is allowed, although the patient may use the extremity to eat or write. An arm sling should be used when the patient is not performing exercises. Patients without a stable construct or with Galeazzi or Monteggia fracture/dislocations should continue immobilization, continue active range-of-motion exercises to joints not in a cast, and continue isometric strengthening exercises as before. Stitches or staples should be removed.

Prescription

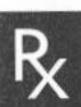

TWO WEEKS

Precautions No passive range of motion.

Range of Motion Gentle active range of motion to the elbow and wrist if there is adequate fixation and the forearm is not in a cast.

Strength No strengthening exercises to the forearm if treated with cast only. Isometric exercises to deltoid, biceps, and triceps with rigid fixation.

Functional Activities The uninvolved extremity is used for self-care.

Weight Bearing No weight bearing on the affected extremity.

Treatment: Four to Six Weeks

BONE HEALING

Stability at fracture site: Once callus is observed bridging the fracture site, the fracture is usually stable. This should be confirmed with physical examination. The strength of this callus is significantly lower than that of normal bone.

Stage of bone healing: Reparative phase. Organization of callus continues, and formation of lamellar bone begins.

X-ray: Bridging callus is visible in patients with a cast. Patients who have had anatomic rigid internal fixation show little or no callus, because primary bone healing predominates. The fracture line becomes less visible.

Orthopaedic and Rehabilitation Considerations

Physical Examination

Examination is performed out of plaster. Check for stability and tenderness about the fracture, and the range of motion of the shoulder, elbow, and wrist. Evaluate flexion and extension as well as supination and pronation. Decreased range of motion may be due to pain, stiffness, or malunion with angulation or loss of the interosseous space.

Radiography

Anteroposterior and lateral radiographs of the forearm should be obtained out of plaster and checked for loss of reduction, evidence of callus formation, and disappearance of the fracture line. Wrist or elbow films should also be obtained if the patient has a known Galeazzi or Monteggia fracture to be sure the proximal or distal radioulnar joint is reduced. Following open reduction and internal fixation, the appearance of significant callus may suggest a lack of rigid fixation with micromotion at the fracture site.

Weight Bearing

No weight bearing is allowed on the affected extremity.

Range of Motion

Continue active range of motion of all joints that are not immobilized. The patient should have no difficulty with shoulder and digit range of motion.

Strength

Whether the patient is immobilized in a cast or maintained in a postoperative sling, flexion and extension of the digits is performed, along with grip-strengthening exercises using a gentle ball-squeezing protocol. Isometric biceps and triceps exercises are used to decrease muscular atrophy.

For rigidly fixed fractures the range of motion of the elbow and wrist joints are usually either full or functional. At 6 weeks, less than 5 lb resistive exercises can be started. At least functional range of motion is needed before offering resistance.

Functional activities

The uninvolved extremity is still used for self-care and personal hygiene.

Methods of Treatment: Specific Aspects

Cast

If tenderness or motion at the fracture site is noted, or if there is little radiographic evidence of healing, replace the long arm cast.

If there is no motion or tenderness at the fracture site and abundant callus is noted on the radiograph, the cast should be removed.

Patients with intermediate findings may be given a short arm cast or functional brace for protection.

After cast removal or conversion to a short arm cast, the patient is instructed in gentle active range-of-motion exercises to the elbow in all planes, including pronation and supination. If casting has been discontinued entirely, the wrist is also actively ranged in all planes. Initially, the patient experiences stiffness, which may be eased with hydrotherapy. Gentle ball-squeezing exercises are prescribed to improve grip strength. If pain develops, the palmar half of the cast may be used as a temporary splint.

Patients who require further long arm cast immobilization should perform active and passive range-of-motion exercises of the shoulder and fingers and continue isometric biceps and triceps exercises.

Open Reduction and Internal Plate Fixation

If the fracture has been treated without a cast from the onset, continue active range-of-motion exercises to the digits, wrist, elbow, and shoulder. At 6 weeks, gentle resistive exercises can be started if callus formation is noted (diaphyseal fracture is slow healing). The patient uses the affected extremity to offer gentle resistance. Isotonic exercises using the pronation/supination board are instituted. Wall-climbing exercises with the affected extremity are prescribed to improve the range of shoulder and elbow motion. These activities will increase muscular strength, along with the range of motion of the affected joints.

For Galeazzi fractures, once the radius is reduced and the forearm held in supination, the distal radioulnar joint is stable and a Kirschner wire (K-wire) is not needed. At 4 weeks after injury, a short arm cast or functional brace may be used and elbow motion started.

With Monteggia fractures, the long arm cast may be replaced with a short arm cast or functional brace at 4 weeks, and gentle active and active-assistive elbow exercises begun.

Prescription

FOUR TO SIX WEEKS

Precautions No passive range of motion to the forearm.

Range of Motion Active to active-assistive range of motion to the elbow and wrist, including supination and pronation if the patient is out of a cast.

Strength If fixation is adequate at end of 6 weeks, start gentle isokinetic exercises to the forearm muscles with less than 5 lb of resistance.

Functional Activities The affected extremity is used for light self-care activities.

Weight Bearing No weight bearing on the affected extremity.

Treatment: Eight to Twelve Weeks

BONE HEALING

Stability at fracture site: Stable.

Stage of bone healing: Woven bone is replaced by lamellar bone. The process of remodeling takes months to years. Patients whose treatment is with rigid fixation have direct bridging osteomes.

X-ray: Abundant callus is present if cast treatment was used. The fracture line begins to disappear, and reconstitution of the medullary canal occurs with time. Patients who have had anatomic rigid internal fixation show little or no callus; rather, the fracture line disappears as primary bone healing progresses. The amount of callus is inversely proportional to the stability.

Orthopaedic and Rehabilitation Considerations

Physical Examination

Remove the cast, if this has not already been done. Examine for tenderness and motion at the fracture site. Evaluate the wrist, elbow, and shoulder range of motion. Pay special attention to the patient's complaints regarding pain and functional disabilities, especially decreased grip strength and decreased forearm pronation and supination, which may result from prolonged casting.

Radiography

Examine anteroposterior and lateral radiographs of the forearm for loss of reduction, evidence of callus formation, and the disappearance of the fracture line. Wrist or elbow films should also be obtained if the patient has a known Galeazzi or Monteggia fracture. Check radiographs for malunion, delayed union, and nonunion.

Weight Bearing

If union has been obtained, weight bearing is progressively allowed past 8 weeks, with full weight bearing as tolerated past 12 weeks.

Range of Motion

Full active and passive range-of-motion exercises are prescribed to all joints of the extremity while focusing on pronation and supination of the forearm. The patient can use the uninvolved extremity in ranging the affected joints, for example, by holding a towel with two hands and raising it above the head and moving it in all planes. Assistive exercises are beneficial if the patient has not been able to achieve the full joint range of motion actively.

Muscle Strength

Putty and ball-squeezing exercises are done to improve grip strength. Progressive resistive exercises using weights are continued. The patient can hold the weights in the hand while flexing and extending the elbow to strengthen the biceps and triceps. Similar exercises are instituted to strengthen the wrist musculature.

Functional Activities

The affected extremity is used for all activities of daily living, including grooming, dressing, feeding, and personal hygiene, if pronation/supination allows. The patient should not use the affected extremity for heavy lifting or sports until full bony union is achieved and should be instructed to lift to tolerance but nothing heavier than a telephone book.

Methods of Treatment: Specific Aspects

If the fracture is united, no immobilization is required and the patient should proceed with range-of-motion and resistive exercises.

Union may take up to 4 months, and if the progression of healing is slow, further immobilization may be used. If no change in fracture union has occurred after 3 to 4 months, a delayed union is present and bone grafting with open reduction and internal fixation should be considered. Delayed union usually occurs only with poor fixation, such as with a K-wire. If surgery has already been performed, bone grafting with or without revision of the fixation may be required. Delayed union and nonunion are unusual with anatomic reduction and rigid fixation, as well as in undisplaced fractures or displaced fractures that have been anatomically reduced with rigid fixation.

Prescription

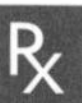

EIGHT TO TWELVE WEEKS

Precautions No heavy lifting or sports activities.

Range of Motion Full active and passive range of motion to the elbow and wrist. Stress supination and pronation of the forearm.

Strength Progressive resistive exercises are prescribed for the forearm muscles. Use free weights of 5 lb and more.

Functional Activities The affected extremity is used for self-care.

Weight Bearing Full weight bearing as tolerated.

LONG-TERM CONSIDERATIONS AND PROBLEMS

Pronation and supination can be limited secondary to the type of the fracture. This hinders functional activities such as personal hygiene and opening doors as well as activities requiring power grip.

Hardware Removal

Plate removal carries a risk of refracture and should be performed only if there is associated pain. Fixation should not be removed for 15 to 24 months, and protection of the forearm for 6 to 12 weeks after removal is prudent. The screw holes will not radiographically fill with callus for 1 to 2 years. The patient should be advised of the risk of refracture following hardware removal. Fracture may occur through one of the screw holes, at the junction of normal bone with the bone that was under the plate (the bone under the plate is thinner than the adjacent bone), or at the original fracture site.

Synostosis

This complication occurs with severe comminution and high-energy injuries, as well as in patients with concomitant head injury. Radius and ulna fractures occurring at the same level, as well as those approached through a single incision, also have an increased risk of synostosis. If the forearm is in a functional position, no treatment may be required. Surgery for a midshaft synostosis can give good results, whereas excision of a distal or proximal synostosis is less successful. This should be taken into account before surgical intervention is undertaken. Resection should be postponed for 1 year until the synostosis has had a chance to mature.

IMMEDIATE TO ONE WEEK

	Cast	*Open Reduction and Internal Fixation of Both-Bone Fractures*	*Open Reduction and Internal Fixation of Galeazzi and Monteggia Fractures*
Stability	None.	Stability afforded by fixation only.	Stability afforded by fixation only.
Orthopedics	Nondisplaced both-bone fractures: long arm cast. Trim cast to distal palmar crease volarly and metacarpophalangeal (MCP) prominences dorsally to allow free finger and MCP motion. Dependent edema treated with elevation or cast removal and reapplication if severe. Isolated ulnar fracture: short arm cast, trimmed proximally if impingement occurs with elbow flexion.	No cast with stable fixation. Dependent edema treated with elevation or cast removal and reapplication if severe.	Long arm cast: trim cast to distal palmar crease volarly and to MCP prominences dorsally to allow for free finger and MCP motion. Dependent edema treated with elevation or cast removal and reapplication if severe.
Rehabilitation	Long arm cast for nondisplaced both-bone fractures: active and passive range-of-motion exercises to the shoulder. Short arm cast for isolated ulnar fracture: active and passive range-of-motion exercises to the digits. Active and active-assistive range-of-motion exercises to the elbow and shoulder.	No cast with stable fixation. Gentle active range-of-motion exercises for the entire extremity, including fingers, wrist, elbow, and shoulder.	Long arm cast: active and passive range-of-motion exercises to the digits. Active and active-assistive range-of-motion exercises to the shoulder. Isometric exercises to the biceps, triceps and deltoid.

2 WEEKS			
	Cast	*Open Reduction and Internal Fixation of Both-Bone Fractures*	*Open Reduction and Internal Fixation of Galeazzi and Monteggia Fractures*
Stability	None to minimal.	Stability mainly afforded by fixation with minimal contribution from organization at fracture site.	Stability mainly afforded by fixation with minimal contribution from organization at fracture site.
Orthopedics	For nondisplaced both-bone fractures: long arm cast. Isolated ulnar fracture: short arm cast.	Long arm cast. No cast with stable fixation.	
Rehabilitation	Long arm cast for nondisplaced both-bone fractures: active and passive range-of-motion exercise to the digits. Active and active-assistive range-of-motion exercises to the shoulder. Short arm cast for isolated ulnar fractures: active and passive range-of-motion exercises to the digits. Active and active-assistive range-of-motion exercises to the elbow and shoulder.	No cast for both-bone fractures after open reduction and stable internal fixation. Gentle active range-of-motion exercises for the entire extremity, including fingers, wrist, elbow, and shoulder.	Long arm cast: active and passive range-of-motion exercises to the digits. Active and active-assistive range-of-motion exercises to the shoulder. Isometric exercises to the biceps, triceps, and deltoid.

FOUR TO SIX WEEKS

	Cast	*Open Reduction and Internal Fixation of Both-Bone Fractures*	*Open Reduction and Internal Fixation of Galeazzi and Monteggia Fractures*
Stability	Bridging callus indicates stability.	Stability afforded by fixation and bridging callus.	Stability afforded by fixation and bridging callus.
Orthopedics	Nondisplaced both-bone fractures: if nontender to palpation, no motion at the fracture site, and abundant callus on x-ray film, the long arm cast may be changed to a short arm cast or functional brace. Isolated ulnar fracture: short arm cast, removed when nontender.	No cast with stable fixation.	Galeazzi fractures: if K-wire is used to reduce distal radioulnar joint, it should be removed at 4 weeks. Long arm cast until 6 weeks in supination, then short arm cast or functional brace. Monteggia fractures: long arm cast replaced with short arm cast or functional brace.
Rehabilitation	When nondisplaced both-bone fractures placed into short arm cast: continue active and passive range-of-motion exercises to the digits. Continue active and active-assistive range-of-motion exercises to the shoulder. Add gentle active range-of-motion exercises to the elbow in all planes, including pronation and supination. Also include ball-squeezing exercises. Isometric exercises to biceps, triceps, and deltoid. When casting of isolated ulnar fracture discontinued: gentle active range-of-motion exercises for the entire extremity, including the fingers, wrist, elbow, and shoulder. Gentle resistive exercises can also be started.	No cast. Gentle active range-of-motion exercises for the entire extremity, including fingers, wrist, elbow, and shoulder. At 6 weeks, gentle resistive exercises can be started. No lifting or weight bearing allowed, although patient may use extremity to eat or write.	When placed in a short arm cast: continue active and passive range-of-motion exercises to the digits. Continue active and active-assistive range-of-motion exercises to the shoulder. Add gentle active range-of-motion exercises to the elbow in all planes including pronation and supination. Include ball-squeezing exercises.

EIGHT TO TWELVE WEEKS

	Cast	*Open Reduction and Internal Fixation of Both-Bone Fractures*	*Open Reduction and Internal Fixation of Galeazzi and Monteggia Fractures*
Stability	Stable.	Stable.	Stable.
Orthopedics	For nondisplaced both-bone fractures: discontinue cast or functional brace upon radiographic evidence of union. Isolated ulnar fractures should be out of cast. In cases of slow healing, immobilization may be extended. If after 3 to 4 months no change in fracture union has taken place, a delayed union has occurred and bone grafting with open reduction/internal fixation should be considered.	Immobilization discontinued when nontender to palpation, no motion at the fracture site, and radiographic evidence of union.	No cast with stable fixation.
Rehabilitation	When immobilization discontinued: full active and passive range-of-motion exercises to all joints of the extremity while focusing on pronation and supination of the forearm. Putty and ball-squeezing exercises improve grip strength. Introduce resistive exercises using weights in gradation.	When immobilization discontinued: full active and passive range-of-motion exercises to all joints of the extremity while focusing on pronation and supination of the forearm. Putty and ball-squeezing exercises improve grip strength. Introduce resistive exercises using weights in gradation.	When immobilization discontinued: full active and passive range-of-motion exercises to all joints of the extremity while focusing on pronation and supination of the forearm. Putty and ball-squeezing exercises improve grip strength. Introduce resistive exercises using weights in gradation.

BIBLIOGRAPHY

Anderson LD, Meyer FN. Fractures of the shafts of the radius and ulna. In: Rockwood CA, ed. *Fractures in Adults,* Vol. 1, 3rd ed. Philadelphia: J.B. Lippincott, 1991, pp. 679–738.

Brostrm LA, Stark A, Svartengren G. Acute compartment syndrome in forearm fractures. *Acta Orthop Scand,* 61:50–53, 1990.

Chapman MW, Gordon JE, Zissimos AG. Compression-plate fixation of acute fractures of the diaphyses of the radius and ulna. *J Bone Joint Surg,* 71A:159–169, 1989.

Crenshaw AH. Fractures of shoulder girdle, arm, and forearm. In: Crenshaw AH, ed. *Campbell's Operative Orthopaedics,* Vol. 2, 8th ed. St. Louis, MO: Mosby, 1992, pp. 1025–1046.

Duncan R, Geissler W, Freeland AE, et al. Immediate internal fixation of open fractures of the diaphysis of the forearm. *J Orthop Trauma,* 6:25–31, 1992.

Grace TG, Eversmann WW Jr. Forearm fractures: treatment by rigid fixation with early motion. *J Bone Joint Surg,* 62A:433–438, 1980.

Kellam JF, Jupiter JB. Diaphyseal fractures of the forearm. In: Browner BD, ed. *Skeletal Trauma,* Vol. 2, 1st ed. Philadelphia: W.B. Saunders, 1992, pp. 1095–1124.

Moed BR. Forearm fractures. In: *Trauma: Orthopaedic Knowledge Update.* Rosemont, IL: American Academy of Orthopaedic Surgeons, 1996, pp. 57–65.

Moore TM, Klein JP, Patzakis MJ, et al. Results of compression-plating of closed Galeazzi fractures. *J Bone Joint Surg,* 67A:1015–1021, 1985.

Rumball K, Finnegan M. Refractures after forearm plate removal. *J Orthop Trauma,* 4:124–129, 1990.

CHAPTER *Seventeen*

Colles' Fracture

BABAK SHEIKH, MD

VASANTHA L. MURTHY, MD

CONTRIBUTIONS BY STANLEY HOPPENFELD, MD

INTRODUCTION

Definition

Colles' fracture is a distal metaphyseal fracture of the radius, usually occurring 3 to 4 cm from the articular surface with volar angulation of the apex of the fracture (silver fork deformity), dorsal displacement of the distal fragment, and a concomitant radial shortening. It may or may not involve an ulnar styloid fracture (Figures 17-1 and 17-2).

An intraarticular variant may involve the distal articular surface of the radius and the distal radiocarpal or radioulnar joints (*see* Figure 17-9A).

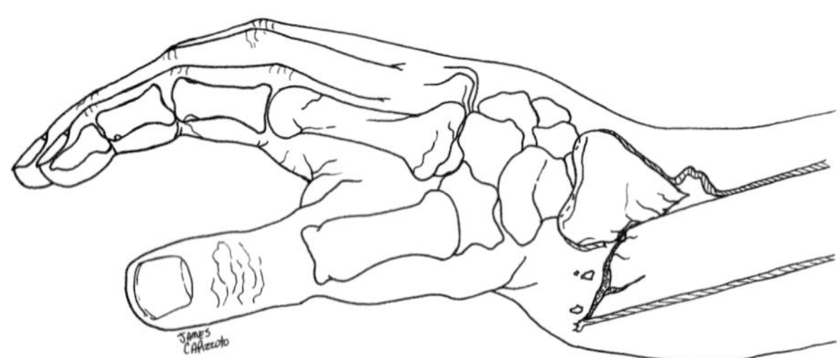

FIGURE 17-1 Classic Colles' fracture involving the distal third of the radius. There is dorsal displacement of the distal fragment causing spoon-shaped deformity.

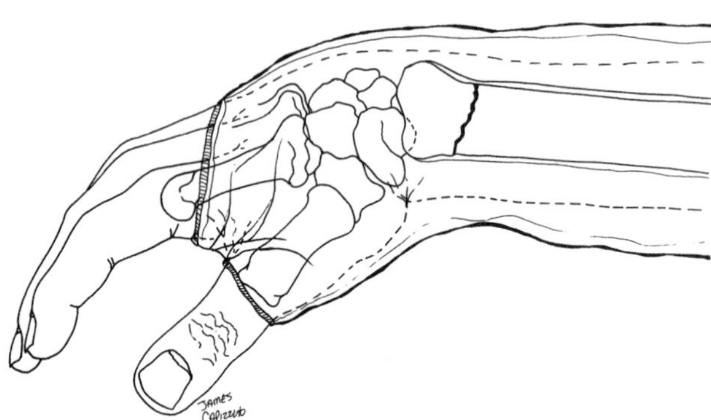

FIGURE 17-2 Reduced Colles' fracture treated with cast immobilization. The anatomic volar tilt of the distal fragment is restored.

Mechanism of Injury

A fall on an outstretched hand leads to fracture and dorsal displacement of the distal radius.

Treatment Goals

Orthopaedic Objectives

Alignment

The objective of alignment is to maintain radial length and a palmar (volar) tilt. To allow for functional wrist mechanics, avoid a change of more than 2 mm in the ulnar variance (the relative lengths of the ulna and the radius at the distal articular surface as determined on a posteroanterior wrist radiograph). Normally, the length of the radius extends slightly distal to that of the ulna, denoting a negative ulnar variance. Positive ulnar variance is seen when the ulna is longer than the radius at the distal articular surface, which may occur after a Colles' fracture if the radius shortens (Figures 17-3A and 17-3B).

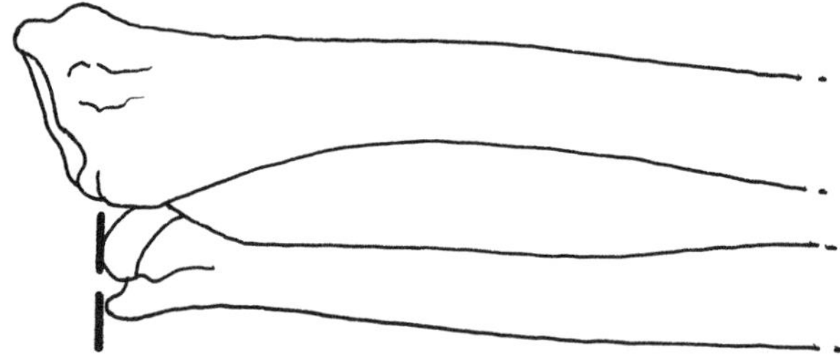

FIGURE 17-3A Negative ulnar variance. The ulna is normally shorter than the radius distally, allowing for ulnar deviation of the wrist.

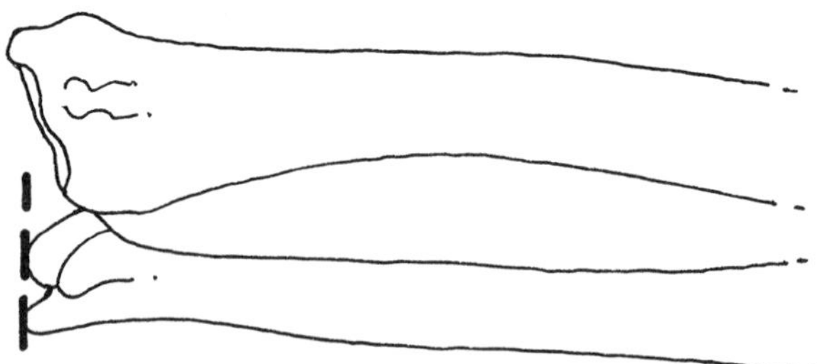

FIGURE 17-3B Positive ulnar variance. This occurs following a comminuted Colles' fracture in which there is shortening of the radius. The relative increase in ulnar length often limits ulnar deviation of the wrist.

Stability

The goal is to provide a stable, pain-free wrist for work and activities of daily living.

Rehabilitation Objectives

Range of Motion

Restore full range of motion to the wrist and digits (Table 17-1).

TABLE 17-1 *Range of Motion*

Wrist	Normal	Functional
Flexion	75°	15°
Extension	70°	30°
Radial deviation	20°	10°
Ulnar deviation	35°	15°

Muscle Strength

1. Improve the strength of the hypothenar and thenar muscles and the lumbricals and interossei.
2. Improve the strength of the muscles that cross the wrist joint to a preinjury level, specifically:

Extensors of the digits:

Extensor digitorum communis

Extensor pollicis longus and brevis

Extensor indicis proprius

Flexors of the digits:

Flexor digitorum superficialis

Flexor digitorum profundus

Flexor pollicis longus

Abductor pollicis longus

Flexor carpi ulnaris

Flexor carpi radialis

Extensor carpi ulnaris

Extensor carpi radialis longus and brevis

Functional Goals

Reestablish power grip, grasp, and pincer grip (Appendix I).

Expected Time of Bone Healing

6 to 8 weeks until the fracture is stable.

Expected Duration of Rehabilitation

12 weeks.

More severe injuries, including intraarticular as well as open fractures, require more time for healing and rehabilitation.

Methods of Treatment

Cast

Biomechanics: Stress-sharing device.

Mode of Bone Healing: Secondary, with callus formation.

Indications: Closed reduction and casting provides fracture management without the need for operative fixation. It is indicated for patients with nondisplaced or minimally displaced fractures without much comminution. Postreduction radiographs should reveal restoration of palmar tilt and radial length (Appendix II). In general, patients older than 60 years of age (physiologically) may undergo treatment with a short arm cast to prevent elbow stiffness. All others receive a long arm cast for the first 3 to 6 weeks, followed by a short arm cast. Long arm casts give better support for unstable comminuted fractures and give rotational control and better pain control. Nondisplaced fractures may be treated with a short arm cast (Figures 17-4A, 17-4B, 17-5A, and 17-5B, and *see* Figure 17-2).

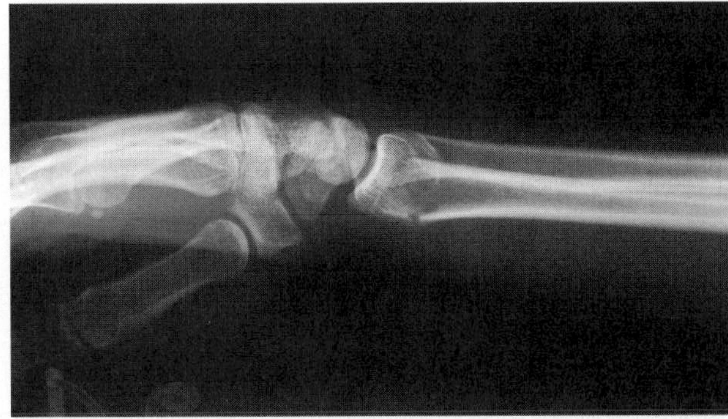

FIGURE 17-4A Lateral radiograph of the wrist showing a Colles' fracture. Note the loss of the normal 10-degree volar angular tilt of the distal radius.

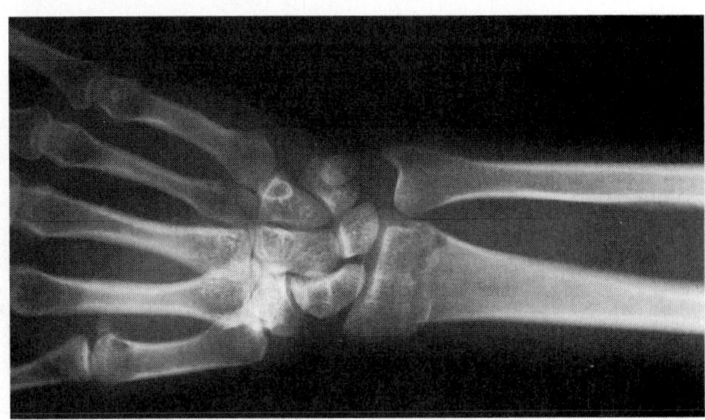

FIGURE 17-4B Classic extraarticular Colles' fracture (anteroposterior view). There is no shortening of the radius. The patient should have no difficulty in regaining ulnar deviation.

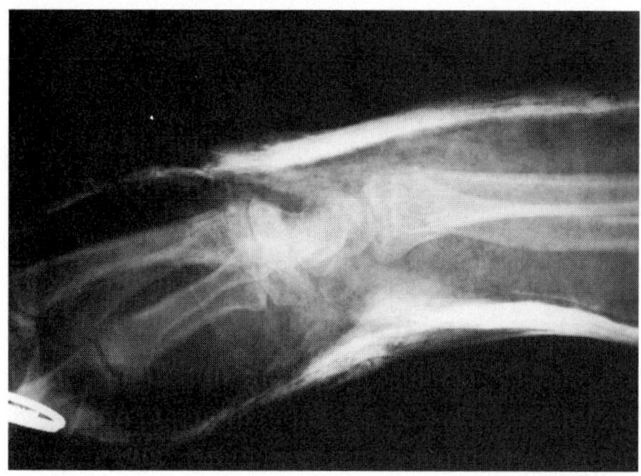

FIGURE 17-5A Colles' fracture after reduction and cast immobilization (lateral view). Note the restoration of volar tilt of the distal radius.

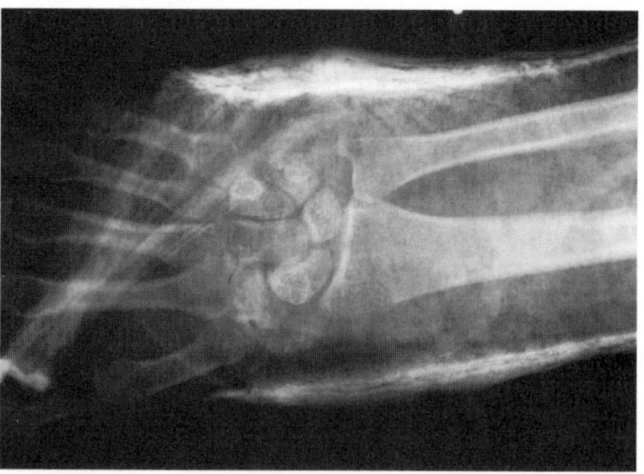

FIGURE 17-5B Colles' fracture after reduction and cast immobilization (anteroposterior view). Cast must be trimmed proximal to the metacarpophalangeal joints to allow full flexion of the joints and the fingers.

External Fixator

Biomechanics: Stress-sharing device (more rigid and therefore more shielding than a cast).

Mode of Bone Healing: Secondary, with callus formation.

Indications: An external fixator is useful for comminuted, displaced, or open fractures not amenable to closed reduction or internal fixation. Occasionally, percutaneous pinning or internal fixation may be used as adjuncts to external fixation (Figures 17-6, 17-7A, 17-7B, 17-7C, and 17-8).

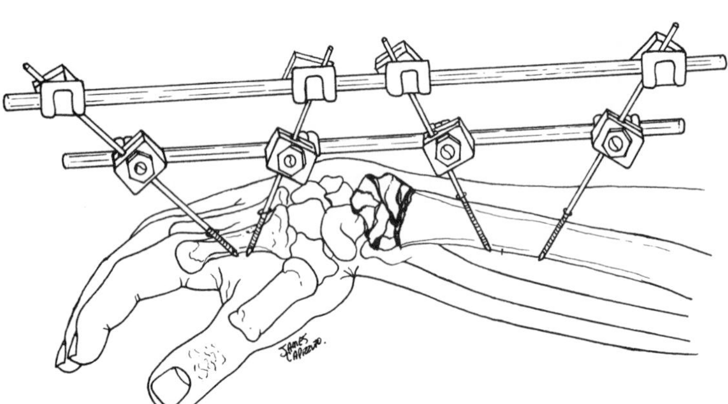

FIGURE 17-6 External-fixator immobilization of a comminuted intraarticular Colles' fracture. This helps restore the length of the distal radius.

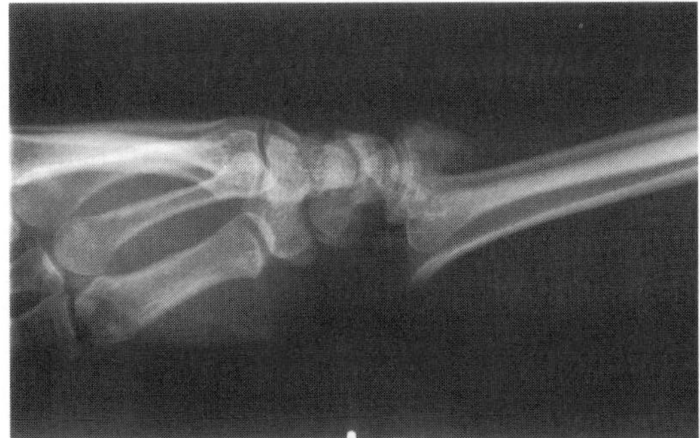

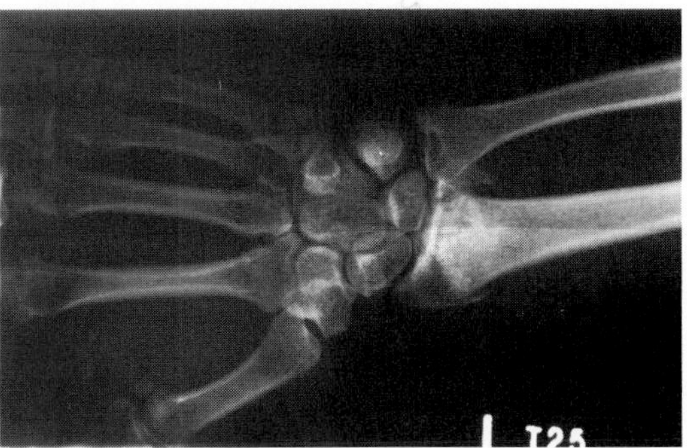

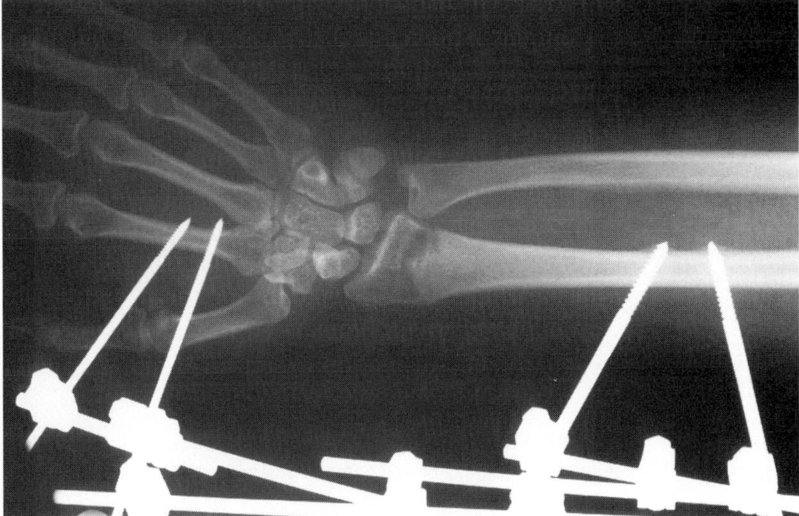

FIGURE 17-7A *(above, left)* Colles' fracture with marked dorsal displacement of the intraarticular fracture (lateral view).

FIGURE 17-7B *(above)* Anteroposterior radiograph of the wrist. Note the intraarticular comminution and shortening of the radius-ulnar positive variance.

FIGURE 17-7C *(left)* Reduction and immobilization of the Colles' fracture with an external fixator. Note the restoration of the length of the radius, causing a normal ulnar negative variance as well as anatomic reduction of the articular surface of the distal radius.

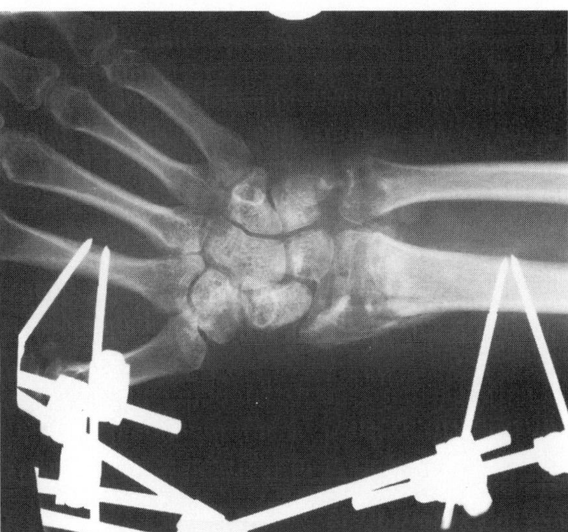

FIGURE 17-8 Intraarticular Colles' fracture immobilized with an external fixator. Note the evidence of healing, the intraarticular nature of the fracture, and the ulnar styloid fracture. There is callus formation bridging the fracture and a decrease in the visibility of the fracture lines.

Open Reduction and Internal Fixation (Plates or Percutaneous Pins)

Biomechanics: Stress-shielding device for plate fixation and stress-sharing device for pin fixation.

Mode of Bone Healing: Primary, when solid fixation is achieved with a plate, allowing no callus to form. Secondary, when solid fixation is not achieved, or with percutaneous pins.

Indications: This method is primarily indicated for displaced articular fractures. Postoperative casting is generally recommended for 2 to 6 weeks, depending on stability of fixation (Figures 17-9A and 17-9B).

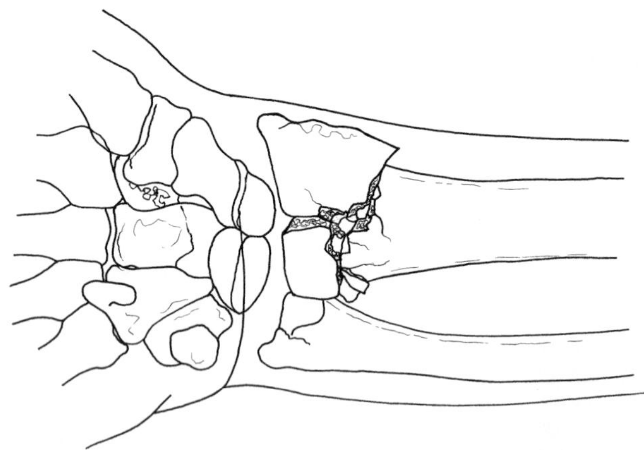

FIGURE 17-9A Comminuted intraarticular Colles' fracture with shortening of the radius. These fractures tend to cause stiffness at the radiocarpal joint and may need more extensive therapy.

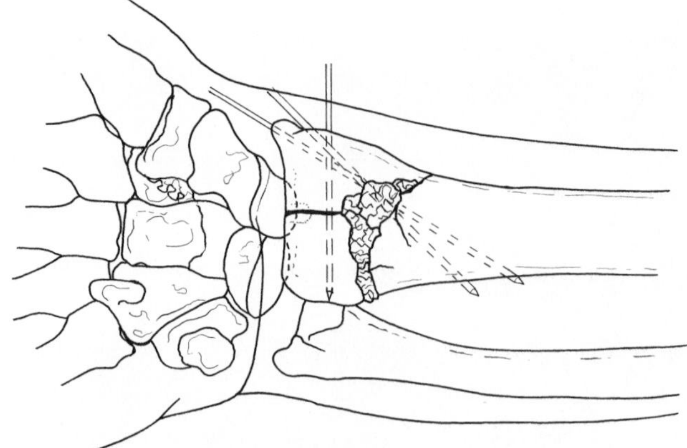

FIGURE 17-9B Intraarticular Colles' fracture treated with percutaneous pinning to obtain anatomic restoration of the distal articular surface of the radius.

Special Considerations of the Fracture

Age

Elderly patients are more at risk of development of joint stiffness secondary to the fracture and its treatment. Osteoporosis in elderly patients coupled with a fall on the outstretched hand makes them more susceptible to this type of fracture.

Articular Involvement

Patients with involvement of the distal radioulnar joints and radial shortening usually end up with weaker grip strength, poorer range of supination, and difficulty writing secondary to decreased ulnar deviation.

Associated Injury

Tendons

Rupture of extensor pollicis longus and peritendinous adhesions of both the flexor and extensor compartments may occur. It is speculated that tendon ischemia, from swelling within the tight confines of the extensor retinaculum, results in rupture of the extensor pollicis longus.

Nerves

Nerve injuries include median nerve contusion, resulting in the development of acute carpal tunnel syndrome (Figure 17-10). Late carpal tunnel may be seen secondary to residual deformity. Nerve damage could be due to forced hyperextension at the time of injury, direct trauma from fracture fragments, edema, or compartment syndrome, or it may be iatrogenic. Ulnar nerve entrapment at Guyon's canal may result, but this is uncommon.

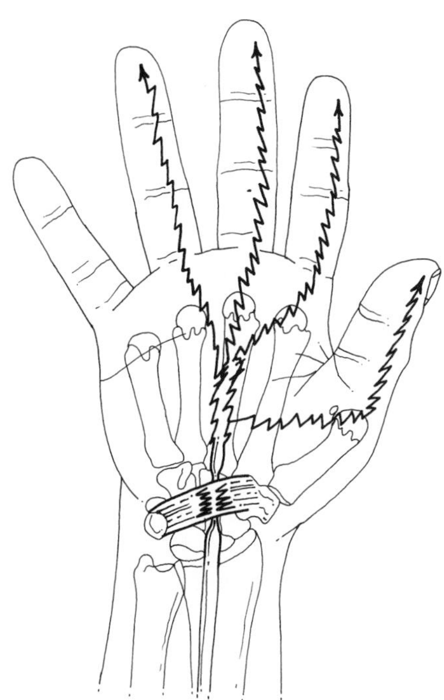

FIGURE 17-10 Median nerve compression or contusion resulting in the development of acute carpal tunnel syndrome. Late carpal tunnel syndrome may be seen secondary to residual deformity. Decompression of the median nerve by transecting the transverse carpal ligament may be necessary to relieve the neurologic symptoms.

Open Injuries

Lacerations of tendons as well as the neurovascular bundle may result. This is uncommon.

Bone

The ulnar styloid process may also be fractured, causing pain over the process.

Weight Bearing

The involved extremity is non-weight bearing. The patient should avoid supporting the body's weight when using a walker or cane or during push-off from a bed or chair.

Gait

The role of arm-swing as a balancing and stabilizing force may be affected by the affected arm not being able to swing in tandem with the opposite extremity.

TREATMENT

Treatment: Early to Immediate (Day of Injury to One Week)

BONE HEALING

Stability at fracture site: None.

Stage of bone healing: Inflammatory phase. The fracture hematoma is colonized by inflammatory cells and débridement of the fracture begins.

X-ray: No callus; fracture line is visible.

Orthopaedic and Rehabilitation Considerations

Physical Examination

Pay special attention to complaints of pain, paresthesia, and cast discomfort as an indicator of compartment syndrome. Consider the tightness or looseness of the cast and check for swelling. Dependent edema as well as discoloration of skin are common, with resultant sausage-shaped digits. This causes decreased range of motion of the fingers. If swelling is noted, explain retrograde massage: the patient should elevate the extremity and milk the swelling from the fingertips toward the palm.

Check for function of all tendons, especially extensor pollicis longus, the most commonly injured tendon. Although rare, tendon entrapment may develop at the fracture site.

Check the digits for capillary refill, sensation, and active and passive range of motion.

Dangers

Look for carpal tunnel syndrome (acute compression neuropathy). It is less common with an external fixator than with casting, because no external soft tissue compression is present with a fixator. Look for compartment syndrome as discussed previously.

Radiography

Check radiographs for loss of correction, but compare them with immediate postreduction films (*see* Appendix II).

Weight Bearing

The patient should not use the affected extremity to push off from a chair or bed, because the fracture is non-weight bearing.

Range of Motion

Active range of motion (flexion, extension, and opposition) is encouraged to the digits and thumb to prevent stiffness and swelling. However, this motion is usually painful for the patient. Elbow flexion and extension is allowed actively, except in a long arm cast. Active range of motion to the shoulder is instructed to prevent adhesive capsulitis (frozen shoulder). In a short arm cast, avoid supination and pronation because this is usually painful and may result in loss of reduction.

Muscle Strength

Once the swelling and pain subside, the patient can perform isometric exercises to abductor digiti minimi and opponens of the thumb, as well as abduction and adduction of the digits to maintain strength of the intrinsic muscles, by applying resistance to the digits using the other hand, as tolerated.

Functional Activities

Patients may use the uninvolved extremity for self-care, hygiene, feeding, grooming, and dressing. The patient is instructed in donning clothes with the involved arm first and doffing clothes with the uninvolved arm first. Elderly patients who rely on a walker for ambulation should be shown how to use a wide-based quad cane or a hemiwalker, because they cannot bear weight on the affected wrist.

Methods of Treatment: Specific Aspects

Cast

Trim the cast to the proximal palmar crease volarly and to the metacarpophalangeal prominences dorsally to allow for free finger and metacarpophalangeal joint motion. This permits free finger flexion up to 90 degrees at the metacarpophalangeal joints. Pay special attention to full range of motion of the index metacarpophalangeal joint, located at the proximal palmar crease and often ignored in casts of the hand. To allow for opposition, the cast loop must be trimmed so that the thumb can oppose the fifth digit. Check for adequate padding at the edges of the cast; look for skin breakdown at cast edges. Also check for cast softening and repair appropriately. Perform retrograde massage to control finger edema. Proceed with active range of motion of the shoulder. If a short arm cast is applied, elbow flexion/extension exercises are instituted. Avoid rotatory movement of the elbow to prevent displacement of the fracture. Encourage active and active-assisted range of motion of the digits.

External Fixator

Check the wound and pin sites for erythema, discharge, or skin tenting. Treat any problems encountered: clean pin sites with peroxide-soaked swabs to foam away debris; release any skin tenting; admit the patient if pin sites are infected. Instruct the patient on pin care. Pay special attention to complaints of pain, pin discomfort, drainage, or malodor. These could indicate an impending infection. Beware of intraoperative skewing of tendons and nerves, especially the superficial radial nerve. This can be manifested by paresthesia or inability to extend the digits.

The patient can perform supination and pronation exercises of the forearm because the pins do not go through both the ulna and the radius and the fracture site is stabilized. However, supination and pronation range of motion is usually limited secondary to the injury and pain. A posterior splint may be used as a support to the fracture.

Open Reduction and Internal Fixation

After surgery, a cast is applied. Cast care as well as rehabilitation protocols are similar to those discussed in the cast section. Casting is to allow for soft tissue healing and pain control and is not intended for protection of the fracture.

Prescription

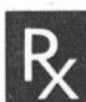

EARLY TO IMMEDIATE (DAY ONE TO ONE WEEK)

Precautions

No supination and pronation.

No range of motion to wrist.

Range of Motion

Full active range of motion of digits of metacarpal phalangeal joint.

Full opposition of thumb.

Strength Attempt isometric exercises to the intrinsic muscles of the hand.

Functional Activities Use the uninvolved extremity for self-care and activities of daily living.

Weight Bearing No weight bearing on the involved extremity.

Treatment: Two Weeks

BONE HEALING

Stability at fracture site: None to minimal.

Stage of bone healing: Beginning of reparative phase of fracture healing. Osteoprogenitor cells differentiate into osteoblasts, which lay down woven bone.

X-ray: None to early callus; fracture line is visible.

Orthopaedic and Rehabilitation Considerations

Physical Examination

Check for swelling and function of all tendons, especially the extensor pollicis longus.

Dangers

Look for carpal tunnel syndrome (acute compression neuropathy).

Radiography

Check anteroposterior and lateral radiographs for loss of correction and compare with previous films for maintenance of reduction. Most correction is lost within the first 2 weeks. Re-reduction may be necessary.

Weight Bearing

No weight bearing on affected extremity.

Range of Motion

Continue with active range-of-motion exercises to the digits and the thumb. As swelling decreases, the range of motion improves at the metacarpophalangeal and interphalangeal joints. Maintain elbow flexion and extension as well as shoulder range of motion, as permitted by the cast.

Muscle Strength

Continue with isometric exercises to the intrinsics of the hand. The patient may begin isometric exercises to the wrist flexors and extensors; this does not cause fracture displacement.

Functional Activities

The patient still uses the uninvolved extremity for self-care, hygiene, feeding, grooming, and dressing. In two-handed activities, the patient may start using the involved extremity for stabilization purposes.

Methods of Treatment: Specific Aspects

Cast

Check the integrity of the cast. If the cast is loose, it should be replaced. If the cast has slipped distally toward the fingers but is not very loose, it may be necessary to trim the leading edge to the proximal palmar crease. If the fracture was reduced in extreme flexion and ulnar deviation, the extremity may be recasted in less flexion and ulnar deviation.

External Fixator

Evaluate the pin sites for any signs of infection. Hydrotherapy may be instituted for mechanical débridement of wounds and pin sites. Continue with active range of motion of the digits. Encourage active supination and pronation.

Open Reduction and Internal Fixation

Discontinue the cast. Check the wound for erythema, discharge, or fluctuance. Remove sutures and replace the cast. If the fracture is rigidly fixed, there is no need for further casting. However, a temporary volar splint may provide additional support, especially at night. If the internal fixation at the time of surgery was not rigid, for example in the case of poor bone stock, then maintain the patient in the cast. If the cast has been removed, begin active range of motion of the wrist.

Prescription

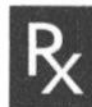

TWO WEEKS

Precautions

No supination and pronation if treated with cast and open reduction and internal fixation

No passive range of motion.

Range of Motion

Full range of motion of metacarpophalangeal and interphalangeal joints.

Attempt gentle active range of motion of wrist if treated by open reduction and internal fixation and fixation is rigid.

Strength Isometric exercises given to intrinsic muscles of the hand and wrist flexor and extensor.

Functional Activities Uninvolved extremity is used for self-care and activities of daily living.

Weight Bearing No weight bearing on the affected extremity.

Treatment: Four to Six Weeks

BONE HEALING

Stability at fracture site: With bridging callus, the fracture is usually stable; confirm with physical examination.

Stage of bone healing: Reparative phase. Further organization of the callus and formation of lamellar bone begins. Once callus is observed bridging the fracture site, the fracture is usually stable. However, the strength of this callus, especially with torsional load, is significantly lower than normal lamellar bone.

X-ray: Bridging callus is visible. With increased rigidity, less bridging callus is noted, and healing with endosteal callus predominates. The fracture line is less distinct (Figure 17-11).

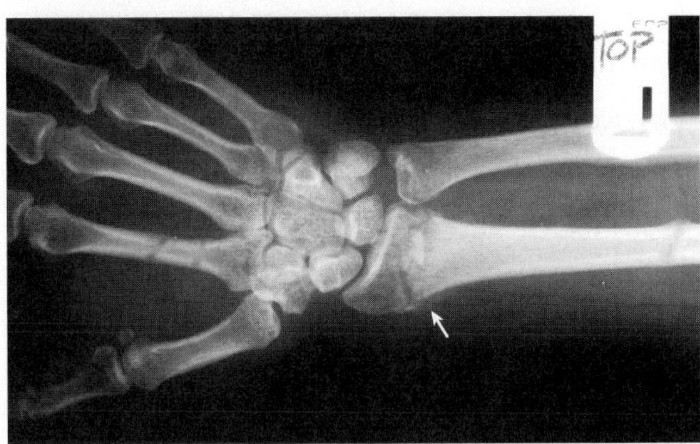

FIGURE 17-11 Healing Colles' fracture. Note the callus formation bridging the fracture. The external fixator has been removed.

Orthopaedic and Rehabilitation Considerations

Physical Examination

Finger swelling is generally resolved and discoloration of the digits is improved.

Dangers

Check for reflex sympathetic dystrophy, characterized by trophic changes, vasomotor disturbances, hyperesthesia, pain, and tenderness out of proportion to the stage of fracture healing. Associated skin changes can vary depending on the stage. If discovered, this syndrome requires aggressive therapy.

Radiography

Check radiographs for callus formation and disappearance of the fracture line. Loss of correction usually does not occur at this time (*see* Figures 17-8 and 17-11).

Weight Bearing

Non-weight bearing.

Range of Motion

Fluidotherapy and hydrotherapy can be used to minimize patient discomfort, thereby allowing for greater range-of-motion activities. Continue with shoulder, elbow, and digit range-of-motion exercises as discussed previously. Kinetic exercises in which range of motion is achieved through activity are instituted to enhance ulnar-radial deviation, pronation, and supination motions. These exercises may include scooping beans and dumping them in a box, as well as using a pronation/supination board. Supination is usually limited more than pronation after the fracture has been immobilized. Achieving at least 50 degrees of supination is very important for functional activities, such as eating, self-care, and hygiene. If supination at the radioulnar joint is limited, functional activities may require the patient to externally rotate the glenohumeral joint. Ulnar deviation exercises should also be emphasized to improve power grip and writing skills.

Muscle Strength

Gentle resistive exercises such as ball squeezing and putty exercises are prescribed. Repetition increases strength.

Functional Activities

It is of utmost importance to start retraining the affected hand to restore its previous function. The patient is instructed in the use of the affected extremity for functional activities. Bimanual activities are not only encouraged but stressed. However, the fracture requires further protection in a cast or splint to avoid refracture.

Methods of Treatment: Specific Aspects

Cast

Discontinue the cast. X-ray and examination are performed out of plaster. Check for stability, tenderness, and range of motion. If tenderness or motion is present at the fracture site, or if poor radiographic healing or inadequate callus is visualized, replace the cast, because the fracture remains potentially unstable. At this time, the fracture should be sticky enough to allow replacement with a short arm cast. If there is no tenderness or motion at the fracture site and a callus appears on radiograph, discontinue the cast, because the fracture site is stable. As the cast is removed, full active range of motion of the wrist is instituted. Initially, the range of wrist joint motion may be limited secondary to immobilization. For patient comfort, a bivalve cast or a cock-up splint may be used for support at night.

External Fixation

Keep the pins clean and encourage range of motion of the digits. Pins are maintained for at least 6 to 8 weeks. If the pins sites are infected, remove the external fixator and replace it with a cast.

Open Reduction and Internal Fixation

Discontinue the cast. Radiographs are obtained and examination is performed out of plaster. Check for stability, tenderness, and range of motion. Because the fracture site is stable, gentle resistive exercises to the wrist are prescribed. The patient may use the good hand to offer resistance to the involved extremity. Because this exercise is patient controlled, it can be performed to the patient's tolerance.

Prescription

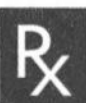

FOUR TO SIX WEEKS

Precautions No passive range of motion.

Range of Motion

Full active range of motion of wrist, and metacarpophalangeal and interphalangeal joints.

Supination and pronation encouraged. Active ulnar deviation and radial deviation.

Strength Gentle resistive exercises given to the digits of the hand.

Improve power grip Isometric exercises to wrist flexors, extensors, and radial and ulnar deviators. Gentle resistive exercises given to the wrist if treated by open reduction and internal fixation.

Functional Activities The involved extremity may be used as a stabilizer in two-handed activities. The patient may attempt self-care with involved extremity.

Weight Bearing Avoid weight bearing until the end of 6 weeks.

Treatment: Six to Eight Weeks

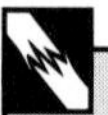

BONE HEALING

Stability at fracture site: With bridging callus, the fracture is usually stable; confirm with physical examination.

Stage of bone healing: Reparative phase. Further organization of the callus and formation of lamellar bone begins. Once callus is observed bridging the fracture site, the fracture is usually stable. However, the strength of this callus, especially with torsional load, is still less than that of normal lamellar bone.

X-ray: Bridging callus is visible. With increased rigidity, less bridging callus is noted and healing with endosteal callus predominates. The fracture line is less distinct.

Orthopaedic and Rehabilitation Considerations

Physical Examination

Pay special attention to the patient's comments on his or her activity level or any functional disabilities, especially decreased grip strength and inability to ulnar deviate.

Check for resolution of reflex sympathetic dystrophy and for carpal tunnel syndrome development.

Radiography

Check radiographs for callus formation and disappearance of the fracture line. Evaluate for malunion (especially radial shortening), delayed union, and nonunion.

Weight Bearing

The patient may begin a progressive increase in weight-bearing using the involved extremity.

Range of Motion

Active range-of-motion exercises to the wrist joint are continued. If the joint is stiff, active-assistive as well as gentle passive range-of-motion exercises are instituted and the patient is instructed on using the unaffected hand to perform the needed movements. Hydrotherapy or fluidotherapy reduces the patient's discomfort and allows increased range of motion.

Muscle Strength

Continue with gentle resistive exercises to the digits and wrist. The patient uses the uninvolved extremity to offer resistance.

Functional Activities

The patient may use the affected extremity for any activity. Activities such as writing, turning doorknobs to open doors, and wiping oneself for personal hygiene are all performed with the affected extremity.

Methods of Treatment: Specific Aspects

Cast

Discontinue the cast, if this has not already been done. Examine for tenderness and motion at the fracture site.

External Fixator

Discontinue the fixator. Minimally, 6 to 8 weeks of fixator is required to decrease the chance of loss of reduction. If the fracture is unstable with motion present at the fracture site, tenderness or poor radiographic healing (i.e., minimal or no callus), replace the fixator with a short arm cast. Leave the cast on for an additional 4 weeks. If the fracture is stable and nontender with a good callus, and no motion is present at the fracture site, casting may not be required if the patient is reliable.

Check fracture alignment on radiograph without the fixator and look especially for radial shortening or collapse at the fracture site. Evaluate the first dorsal interosseous space for scarring, especially if the external fixator pins have penetrated this space. Once the fixator is removed and the fracture is stable, begin full range of motion of the wrist. A splint may be used at night for patient comfort.

Open Reduction and Internal Fixation

Discontinue the cast if this has not already been done. Examine for tenderness or motion at the fracture site. If stable, continue with resistive exercises and passive range of motion to the wrist.

Prescription

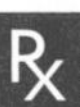

SIX TO EIGHT WEEKS

Precautions None, unless pseudarthrosis or nonunion is suspected.

Range of Motion

Full range of motion of all joints of upper extremity. Stress supination and ulnar deviation.

Active assistive to passive range of motion attempted or initiated.

Strength

Gentle resistive exercises to digits and wrist.

Improve power grip.

Functional Activities Involved extremity used for self-care and activities of daily living.

Weight Bearing Weight bearing as tolerated, because the fracture is stable.

Treatment: Eight to Twelve Weeks

BONE HEALING

Stability at fracture site: Stable.

Stage of bone healing: Remodeling phase. Woven bone is replaced with lamellar bone. The process of remodeling takes months to years for completion.

X-ray: Callus is seen. The fracture line begins to disappear; with time, the contour of the bone is being restored. Metaphyseal areas do not produce as much callus as diaphyseal regions.

Orthopaedic and Rehabilitation Considerations

Physical Examination

Check for resolution of reflex sympathetic dystrophy.

Radiography

Check radiographs for malunion, delayed union, and nonunion.

Weight Bearing

Full weight bearing.

Range of Motion

By this time, the patient should have full range of motion of the digits, thumb, and wrist in all planes. Continue with ulnar-radial deviation, supination, and pronation exercises. Stress supination and ulnar deviation exercises, because these are important for daily functional activities.

Muscle Strength

The affected muscles are all strengthened with progressive resistive exercises using weights in graduation to improve strength.

Functional Activities

The patient is allowed to bear weight at the wrist region. Elderly patients may use the affected wrist to support themselves while using a walker or to raise themselves from a chair or bed. Encourage the patient to work on power grip, pincer grip, writing, and turning doorknobs with the affected wrist. Forceful activities such as hammering or chopping wood are not done for approximately 16 weeks, when sufficient callus formation will prevent the patient from experiencing pain.

Methods of Treatment: Specific Aspects

No change.

Prescription

EIGHT TO TWELVE WEEKS

Precautions None.

Range of Motion Full range of motion, active and passive in all planes to the wrist and digits. Stress supination and ulnar deviation.

Strength Progressive resistive exercises to the wrist and digits and to all groups of muscles.

Functional Activities The patient may use the involved extremity in self-care and activities of daily living.

Weight Bearing Full weight bearing as tolerated on the involved extremity.

LONG-TERM CONSIDERATIONS AND PROBLEMS

Patients need to be warned about the possibility of future degenerative osteoarthritis, a risk that is significantly increased in cases of intraarticular fracture. Other possible hazards may include decreased range of motion, residual deformity (especially radial shortening), and prolonged swelling secondary to injury. Some loss of ulnar deviation may be present, which may lead to decreased power grip. In the event of an ulnar positive variance with marked limitation of ulnar deviation, resection of the distal ulna is considered (Darrach procedure) (Figure 17-12).

If supination is limited, the patients need to adapt themselves for personal hygiene and feeding by substituted motions. The patient may require assistive devices to turn keys in a hole or to turn doorknobs, or open doors.

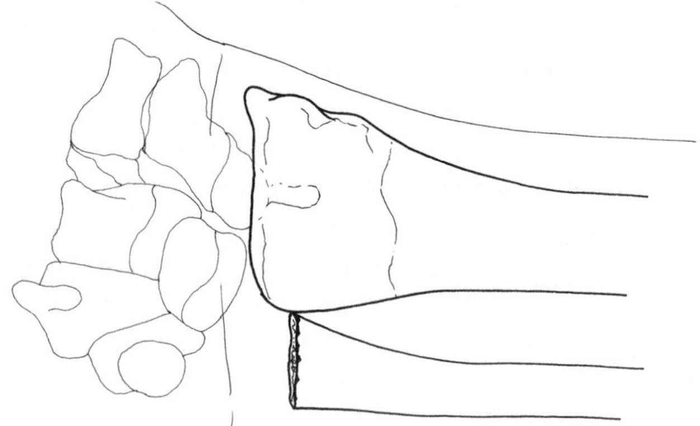

FIGURE 17-12 Darrach procedure. Resection of the distal ulna is performed in the event of a positive ulnar variance with marked limitation of ulnar deviation.

If an external fixator was used, considerable stiffness may be present, because a fixator is generally used for intraarticular fractures that have the most propensity for degenerative joint disease and stiffness.

APPENDIX I

A good level of function following treatment:

1. ≥45 degrees of wrist dorsiflexion and ≥30 degrees of palmar flexion
2. ≥15 degrees of radial deviation/≥15 degrees ulnar deviation
3. 50 degrees of pronation/50 degrees of supination
4. Minimal discomfort and cosmetic deformity with no disability

These values serve only as a guide. Each patient's fracture pattern and clinical situation must always be considered. These levels of achievement may not be attainable in every patient.

APPENDIX II

Minimal Acceptable Values

1. Radial inclination ≥12 degrees
2. Loss of radial length ≤ 5 mm
3. Palmar tilt of 0 degree
4. Change in ulnar variance ≤ 2 mm—must compare with radiographs of opposite wrist
5. Articular incongruity < 2 mm

These values serve only as a guide. Each patient's fracture pattern and clinical situation must always be considered.

IMMEDIATE TO ONE WEEK

	Cast	*External Fixator*	*Open Reduction and Internal Fixation*
Stability	None.	None.	None.
Orthopedics	Trim cast to metacarpophalangeal (MCP) prominences dorsally and to proximal palmar crease volarly.	Evaluate pin sites and tendon functions.	Trim cast to MCP prominences dorsally and to proximal palmar crease volarly.
Rehabilitation	Range of motion of shoulder and digits.	Range of motion of shoulder, elbow, and digits.	Range of motion of shoulder, elbow, and digits.

TWO WEEKS

	Cast	*External Fixator*	*Open Reduction and Internal Fixation*
Stability	None to minimal.	None to minimal.	None to minimal.
Orthopedics	Trim cast to MCP prominences dorsally and to proximal palmar crease volarly.	Evaluate pin sites and tendon functions.	Remove sutures and cast. Replace cast if fixation is not rigid.
Rehabilitation	Range of motion of shoulder and digits.	Range of motion of the shoulder, elbow, and digits.	Range of motion of the shoulder, elbow, and digits. Active range of motion to the wrist if fixation is rigid.

FOUR TO SIX WEEKS

	Cast	*External Fixator*	*Open Reduction and Internal Fixation*
Stability	Stable.	Stable.	Stable.
Orthopedics	Shorten or remove cast. May still need a night splint.	Remove fixator at 6 to 8 weeks. Replace with cast if unstable.	Remove cast.
Rehabilitation	Begin active range of motion of wrist if cast removed.	Begin active range of motion of wrist if cast removed.	Begin active range of motion of wrist if cast removed.

SIX TO EIGHT WEEKS			
	Cast	*External Fixator*	*Open Reduction and Internal Fixation*
Stability	Stable.	Stable.	Stable.
Orthopedics	Remove cast if not already done.	Remove fixator. Night splint for comfort. Cast applied if fracture not healed.	Remove cast if not already done.
Rehabilitation	Active and passive range of motion to wrists. Gentle resistive exercises to the wrist.	Active and passive range of motion to the wrist as tolerated. Gentle resistive exercises to the wrist.	Active and passive range of motion to the wrists. Gentle resistive exercises to the wrist.

EIGHT TO TWELVE WEEKS			
	Cast	*External Fixator*	*Open Reduction and Internal Fixation*
Stability	Stable.	Stable.	Stable.
Orthopedics	Remove cast if not already done.	Remove fixator if not already done. Remove cast.	
Rehabilitation	Active and passive range of motion and progressive resistive exercises.	Active and passive range of motion and progressive resistive exercises.	Active and passive range of motion and progressive resistive exercises.

BIBLIOGRAPHY

Cohen MS, McMurtry R, Jupiter J. Fractures of the distal radius. In: Browner DB, et al., eds. *Skeletal Trauma,* Vol. 2. Philadelphia: W.B. Saunders, 1998, pp. 1063–1095.

Cooney PW, Linscheid LR, Dobyns HJ. Chapter 8. In: Rockwood AC, Green PD, and Bucholz WR, eds. *Fractures and Dislocations of the Wrist,* Vol. 1. Philadelphia: J.B. Lippincott, 1996, pp. 563–601.

Geissier WB, Fernandez DL, Lamey DM. Distal radioulnar joint injuries associated with fractures of the distal radius. *Clin Orthop*, 327:135–146, 1996.

Glowacki KA, Weiss AP, Akelman E. Distal radius fractures: concepts and complications. *Orthopedics,* 19:601–608, 1996.

Gustilo BR, Kyle FR, Templeman D, eds. Fractures and dislocations of the carpus including the distal radius. *Fractures and Dislocations,* Vol. 1. pp. 553–585, 1993.

Hutchinson F. Decision making in distal radius fractures. *J South Orthop Assoc,* 4:290–306, 1995.

Kihara H, et al. The effect of dorsally angulated distal radius fractures on distal radioulnar joint congruency and forearm rotation. *J Hand Surg [Am]*, 21:40–47, 1996.

Kreder HJ, et al. X-ray film measurements for healed distal radius fractures. *J Hand Surg [Am]*, 21:31–39, 1996.

Levine MA, ed. Fractures of the distal radius. *Orthopedic Knowledge Update, Trauma,* Rosemont, IL: American Academy of Orthopaedic Surgeons, 1996, pp. 67–82.

Lipton AH, Wollstein R. Operative treatment of intraarticular distal radius fractures. *Clin Orthop Rel Res,* 327:110–124, 1996.

Melone PC Jr, ed. Distal radius fractures: changing concepts of management. *Orthopedic Clinics of North America.* pp. 205–382, 1993.

Putnam MD, Gustilo BR, Kyle FR, Templeman D, eds. Fractures and dislocations of the carpus including the distal radius. *Fractures and Dislocations,* Vol. 1. St. Louis, MO: Mosby, 1993, pp. 553–585.

Rikli DA, Regazzone P. Fractures of the distal end of the radius treated by internal fixation and early function. A preliminary report of 20 cases. *J Bone Joint Surg [Br]*, 78:588–592, 1996.

Szabo R. Fractures of the distal radius. In: Chapman WM, et al., eds. *Operative Orthopaedics.* Vol. 2. Philadelphia: J.B. Lippincott, 1993, pp. 1351–1361.

CHAPTER Eighteen

Scaphoid (Navicular) Fractures

SAMUEL A. HOISINGTON, MD

VASANTHA L. MURTHY, MD

INTRODUCTION

Definition

Fractures of the scaphoid may occur at any point in the bone, including the distal pole, waist, proximal pole, or tubercle (Figure 18-1). They are characterized as stable or unstable. Unstable fractures are displaced more than 1 mm or have greater than 60-degree scapholunate angulation or greater than 15-degree radiolunate angulation. Eighty percent of the surface of the scaphoid is covered by articular cartilage. Fractures with continuity of the cartilage envelope have greater stability.

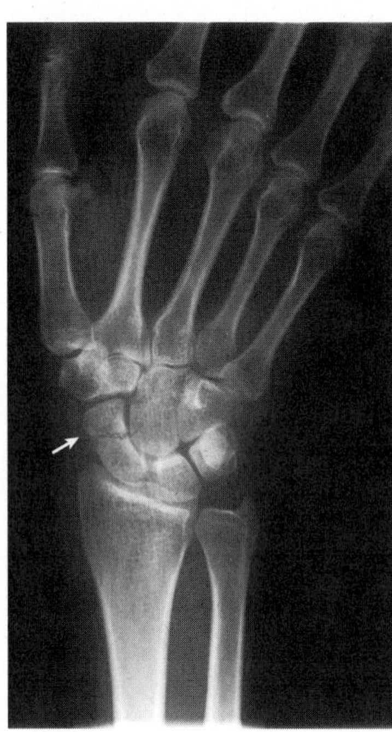

FIGURE 18-1 Fracture of the scaphoid involving the waist of the bone (anteroposterior view).

Mechanism of Injury

A scaphoid fracture occurs during a fall on an outstretched hand with the wrist dorsiflexed and radially deviated. In 95 to 100 degrees of wrist extension, the proximal pole of the scaphoid remains fixed while the distal pole moves dorsally, leading to a waist fracture.

Treatment Goals

Orthopaedic Objectives

Alignment

Anatomic reduction of the scaphoid is necessary. The distal pole of the scaphoid tends to flex in unstable fractures, leading to the humpback deformity and malalignment. Malunion in this position must be avoided because it leads to carpal instability, loss of wrist extension, weakness of grip, and ultimately carpal collapse.

Stability

Normally aligned (anatomic) scaphoid union usually leads to carpal stability, depending on the severity of the initial injury. Any associated ligamentous injury, such as that resulting in a perilunate or lunate dislocation, must be recognized and treated. In the case of scaphoid nonunion, the distal scaphoid may flex when the proximal scaphoid and lunate extend. This leads to malalignment and carpus instability similar to that associated with scapholunate dissociation (ligamentous injury). The scaphoid articulates with five bones: radius, lunate, capitate, trapezium, and trapezoid.

Rehabilitation Objectives

Range of Motion

Restore and improve the range of motion at the thumb and wrist.

Muscle Strength

Restore and improve the strength of the following muscles:

Abductor pollicis longus and brevis: abducts the thumb.
Extensor pollicis brevis: extends the metacarpophalangeal joint of the thumb; the abductor pollicis longus and extensor pollicis brevis form the palmar border of the anatomic snuff box.
Extensor pollicis longus: extends the interphalangeal joint of the thumb, forming the dorsal border of the anatomic snuff box: the scaphoid or navicular bone forms the floor of the anatomic snuff box.
Flexor carpi radialis: flexes and deviates the wrist radially.
Flexor carpi ulnaris: flexes and deviates the wrist in an ulnar direction.
Flexor pollicis longus and brevis: flexes the metacarpophalangeal and interphalangeal joints of the thumb.

Functional Goals

Improve and restore hand and wrist function with attention to power grip, pincer grasp, activities associated with thumb abduction, flexion, and opposition, and activities of daily living such as grooming, self-care, writing, and opening doors.

Expected Time of Bone Healing

Four weeks to 12 months depending on the fracture location.

Four to 6 weeks for fractures of the tuberosity.

Ten to 12 weeks for waist fractures.

Sixteen to 20 weeks for proximal pole fractures.

Failure to heal by 4 to 6 months indicates a delayed union; beyond this, a nonunion.

Expected Duration of Rehabilitation

Three to 6 months.

Methods of Treatment

Cast

Biomechanics: Stress-sharing device.

Mode of Bone Healing: Mostly primary.

Indications: Thumb spica cast immobilization is the treatment of choice for nondisplaced or minimally displaced scaphoid fractures. The inclusion of the thumb reduces motion at the scaphoid waist. The wrist should be maintained in neutral flexion/extension and neutral to radial deviation (Figure 18-2).

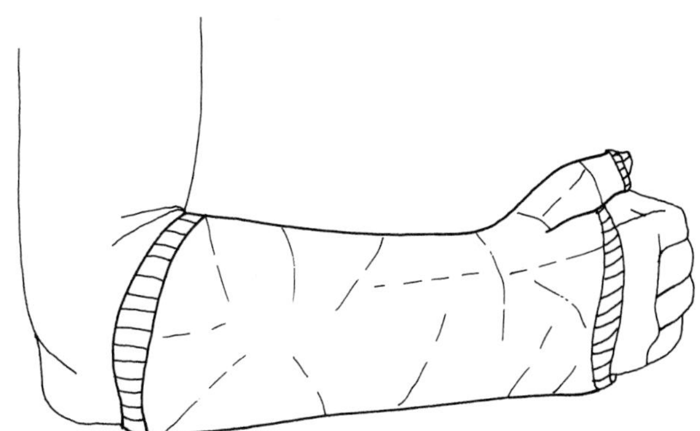

FIGURE 18-2 Thumb spica cast for immobilization is the treatment of choice for nondisplaced or minimally displaced scaphoid fractures.

A short arm thumb spica may be used for tuberosity fractures. Tuberosity fractures are associated with the lowest risk of delayed union.

A long arm thumb spica should be used for all other fractures. Higher rates of union have been noted with long arm thumb spica cast immobilization for 6 weeks followed by 6 weeks of short arm thumb spica casting. An above-elbow cast prevents forearm pronation and supination, which is thought to jeopardize fracture healing by allowing motion at the fracture site.

Casting may be combined with pulsed electromagnetic field electrical stimulation. This method is still experimental but is sometimes suggested to treat scaphoid nonunion following bone grafting. (Further studies are required to evaluate efficacy.)

Open Reduction and Internal Fixation

Biomechanics: Stress-shielding device.

Mode of Bone Healing: Primary. If a solid fixation is not achieved, secondary healing will also occur.

Indications: Operative treatment is used for new displaced fractures as well as delayed unions or nonunions. Fresh fractures may be treated with a Herbert compression screw or Kirschner wires (K-wires), whereas delayed unions or nonunions require bone grafting. Cast immobilization is required postoperatively. Herbert screw fixation provides compression at the fracture site, which may shorten the postoperative period of cast immobilization (Figures 18-3, 18-4, 18-5, 18-6, and 18-7).

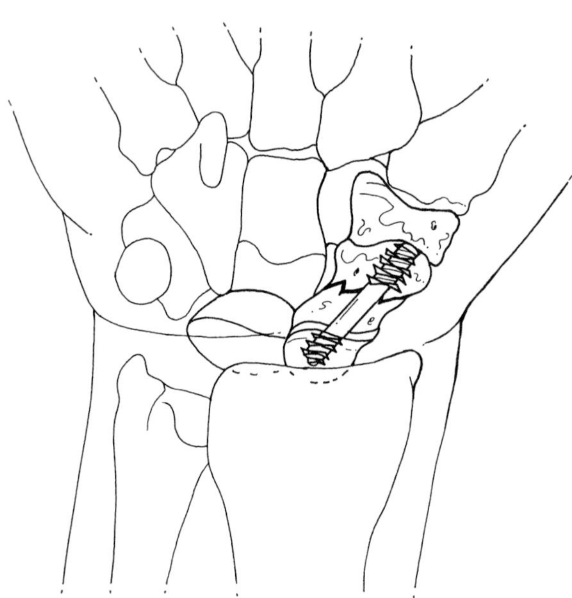

FIGURE 18-3 Herbert screw fixation of navicular fractures provides compression at the fracture site.

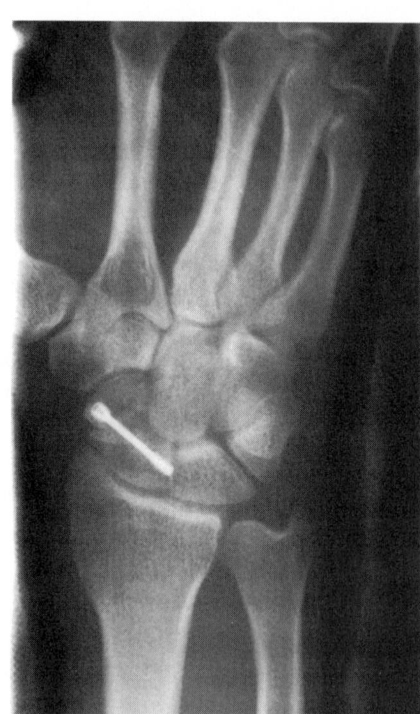

FIGURE 18-4 Herbert screw fixation of navicular fracture (anteroposterior view). This may shorten the postoperative period of cast immobilization.

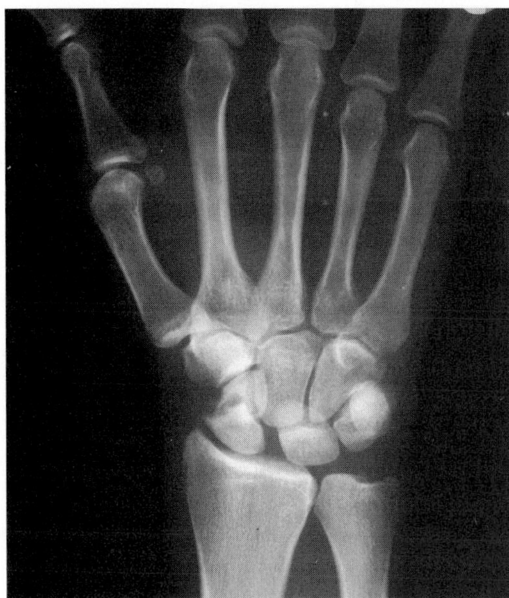

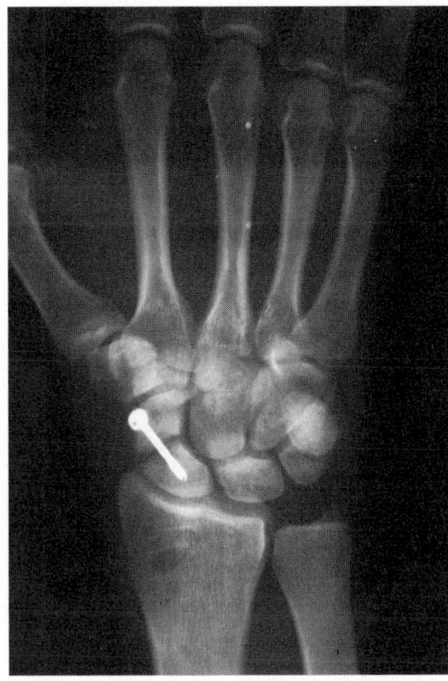

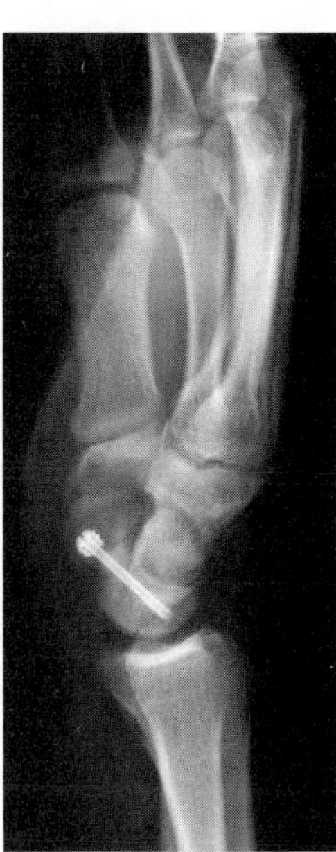

FIGURE 18-5 *(above, left)* Displaced fracture of the waist of the scaphoid (navicular). The blood supply to the proximal pole may be in jeopardy because of the retrograde blood flow from the distal to the proximal pole in the scaphoid.

FIGURE 18-6 *(above, center)* Transverse fracture at the waist of the scaphoid fixed with an AO compression screw. Note that the gap at the fracture site is due to bone grafting.

FIGURE 18-7 *(above, right)* Lateral view of a fracture of the waist of the scaphoid treated with an AO compression screw.

Special Considerations of the Fracture

Fracture Location and Blood Supply

The precarious blood supply to the scaphoid accounts for the variability in healing time. Approximately 80% of the blood supply to the scaphoid is via branches of the radial artery. These enter distally and dorsally, so the blood supply is retrograde, that is, from distal to proximal (Figure 18-8). Fractures through the waist or proximal third of the scaphoid interrupt the blood supply to the proximal pole; this may lead to avascular necrosis. Despite adequate immobilization, only 60% to 70% of proximal-third fractures unite (Figure 18-9). One can expect a union rate of up to

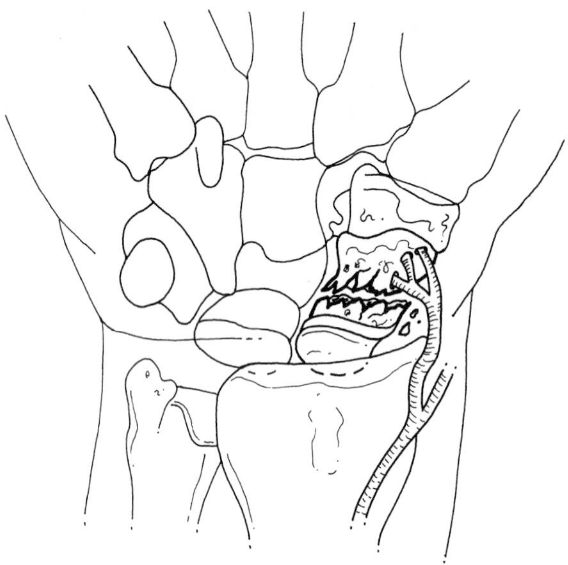

FIGURE 18-8 Eighty percent of the blood supply to the scaphoid is via branches of the radial artery. These enter distally and dorsally so that the blood supply is retrograde, from distal to proximal. Fractures through the waist or proximal third of the scaphoid interrupt the blood supply to the proximal pole. This may lead to nonunion and avascular necrosis.

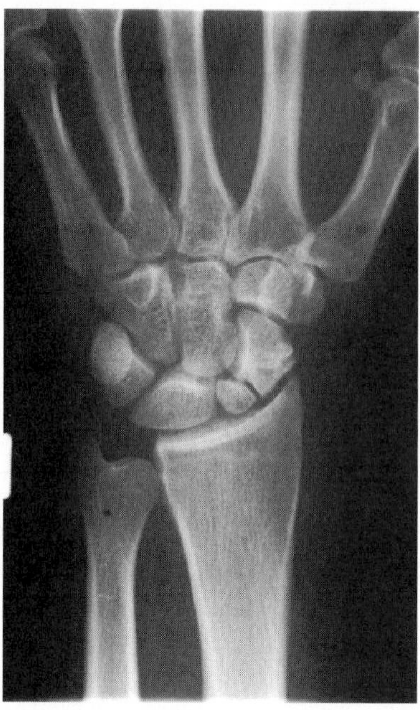

FIGURE 18-9 Nonunion of the proximal third of the scaphoid. The bone edges at the fracture site are rounded indicating a nonunion. This frequently is accompanied by a painful wrist and possible instability. Note that the scaphoid articulates with five bones: radius, lunate, capitate, trapezium, and trapezoid.

100% in nondisplaced fractures, 65% in angulated fractures, and 45% in displaced fractures. Revascularization has been reported with fracture healing.

Suspected Scaphoid Fractures without Radiographic Evidence

If a scaphoid fracture is clinically suspected, the affected extremity should be protected in a short arm thumb spica cast or splint and the patient reevaluated in approximately 2 weeks. If at that time the patient is nontender and the radiographs remain negative, immobilization may be terminated. If, however, the patient is tender and the radiograph remains negative without signs of bony resorption at the fracture site, continue the immobilization and obtain a bone scan. This is the most sensitive but least specific test. If the bone scan is positive, tomograms or computed tomography (CT) scans may be used to further delineate the injury. If the bone scan is negative, a scaphoid fracture is unlikely. Flexion/extension tomograms or CT scans may also be of assistance. For patients who require an early return to their usual activities, the diagnosis can be confirmed after the first 48 hours using a tomogram or CT scan.

Fracture Nonunion and Carpal Instability

Scaphoid nonunion has been associated with an increased risk of wrist degenerative changes and carpal collapse. This is true even in the presence of an asymptomatic nonunion and is related to the role of the scaphoid as a link between the proximal and distal carpal rows (*see* Figure 18-9). Stress is concentrated in the scaphoid, and late displacement of the nonunion may occur. This leads to progressive arthritis of the radioscaphoid, scaphocapitate, and capitolunate joints. The final result is known as scapholunate advanced collapse.

Associated Injuries

There may be concomitant radial styloid or distal radius fractures or carpal ligament injuries. Concomitant lunate or perilunate dislocations, capitate fractures, and distal radius fractures should be aggressively sought because they result from a higher-energy trauma and require different treatment than an isolated scaphoid fracture.

Weight Bearing

The involved extremity should be non-weight bearing. The patient should avoid supporting the body's weight by using a walker or cane or when pushing off from a chair or bed with the affected arm. A platform walker or cane may be used if necessary because the weight is borne more proximally at the elbow.

Gait

The role of reciprocating arm swing as a balancing and stabilizing force is affected by a cast. This is usually not a major concern.

TREATMENT

Treatment: Early to Immediate (Day of Injury to One Week)

BONE HEALING

Stability at fracture site: No bony stability, although ligamentous stability may be present.

Stage of bone healing: Inflammatory phase. The fracture hematoma is colonized by inflammatory cells, and débridement of the fracture begins.

X-ray: No callus. Fracture line is visible.

Orthopaedic and Rehabilitation Considerations

Physical Examination

Assess complaints of pain, swelling, and paresthesia. Check capillary refill and sensation, as well as the active and passive range of motion of the digits. Trim the cast just proximal to the distal palmar crease volarly and to the metacarpophalangeal prominences dorsally to allow for free interphalangeal and metacarpophalangeal motion. Dependent edema should be treated by elevation or, when severe, removal and reapplication of the cast or splint.

Dangers

Although rare with isolated scaphoid fractures, compartment syndrome and acute compression neuropathy do occur. If these are suspected, compartment pressures should be measured. If elevated, fasciotomies should be performed. Median nerve compression may occur when a scaphoid fracture with concomitant lunate dislocation is present. In this situation, immediate reduction of the lunate should be performed; median nerve release may also be required, if the nerve does not show recovery.

Radiography

Anteroposterior, lateral, and oblique wrist films should be checked for step-off, displacement, and angulation.

Weight Bearing

No weight bearing is allowed on the affected extremity.

Range of Motion

Active and passive range-of-motion exercises are prescribed to the digits (i.e., interphalangeal and metacarpophalangeal joints) except the thumb, because it is in a cast. Active-assistive range-of-motion exercises are prescribed to the shoulder for patients in a long arm cast.

Muscle Strength

Isometric exercises are prescribed to the deltoid, biceps, and triceps; these are done inside the cast.

Functional Activities

The patient should use the uninjured arm for grooming, feeding, and self-care. The patient may need assistance with these activities. The patient is instructed to don the shirt or blouse with the involved extremity first and doff it from the uninvolved extremity first. If in a long arm cast, the patient drapes the shirt or blouse over the involved extremity first.

Elderly patients who use a walker for ambulation are instructed in the use of a hemiwalker or a quad cane. They can also use a platform walker on the affected side to avoid bearing weight on the wrist.

Methods of Treatment: Specific Aspects

Cast

At this time, most nonoperative scaphoid fractures are in a long arm thumb spica cast. Suspected fractures not visualized on plain radiographs may be maintained in a short arm thumb spica cast.

Open Reduction and Internal Fixation

Postoperative scaphoid fractures are protected in a short arm thumb spica cast. If the patient is in a short arm cast, gentle active elbow range of motion is allowed in flexion and extension. Avoid supination and pronation to prevent stress at the fracture site.

Prescription

DAY ONE TO ONE WEEK

Precautions Avoid supination and pronation of the elbow.

Range of Motion

Thumb—None (immobilized).

Wrist—None (immobilized).

Elbow—None if immobilized in a long arm cast. If in a short arm cast, gentle active elbow flexion and extension.

Digits—Gentle active range of motion.

Shoulder—Gentle active and active-assistive range of motion.

Strength

Thumb—No strengthening exercises.

Wrist—No strengthening exercises.

Elbow—No strengthening exercises.

Shoulder—Isometric exercises to deltoid, biceps, and triceps.

Functional Activities One-handed activities. Uninvolved extremity used in self-care and dressing.

Weight Bearing No weight bearing on the affected extremity.

Treatment: Two weeks

BONE HEALING

Stability at fracture site: None to minimal.

Stage of bone healing: Beginning of reparative phase. Osetoprogenitor cells differentiate into osteoblasts, which lay down woven bone.

X-ray: No callus. Resorption at fracture site may be seen.

Orthopaedic and Rehabilitation Considerations

Physical Examination

Assess complaints of pain, swelling, and paresthesia. Check capillary refill and sensation, as well as the active and passive range of motion of the digits. Dependent edema should be treated with elevation. Remove and reapply the cast or splint if swelling is severe.

For suspected but unconfirmed fractures, the cast should be removed to examine the snuff box and to determine whether compression in the box or of the first digit elicits pain. Obtain radiograph out of plaster.

Dangers

Compression neuropathy may occur as a result of swelling in a tight cast.

Radiography

Anteroposterior, lateral, and oblique wrist films should be checked for step-off, displacement, and angulation. Postoperative radiographs should be compared to the initial treatment films. If there were no initial radiographic findings, the cast should be removed for these follow-up films. Pay special attention to any indication of K-wire loosening.

Bone resorption indicates an earlier fracture. If no fracture is noted on plain film but the clinical examination remains suspicious, a bone scan should be ordered.

Weight Bearing

No weight bearing is allowed on the affected extremity.

Range of Motion

Digit pain and swelling usually decreases by this time. Continue active and passive range of motion of the digits and active-assistive range of motion of the shoulder.

Muscle Strength

Continue isometric exercises to the biceps, deltoid, and triceps.

Functional Activities

The patient continues one-handed activities and may need assistance with self-care, grooming, and dressing.

Methods of Treatment: Specific Aspects

Cast

Most nonoperative scaphoid fractures are in a long arm thumb spica cast.

Open Reduction and Internal Fixation

Postoperative scaphoid fractures still require protection in a short arm spica cast. Casts should be changed to allow suture removal. Patients should be examined for possible damage to the sensory branch of the radial nerve (dorsal approach) or the palmar cutaneous branch of the median nerve (volar approach). Continue shoulder, elbow, and digit range of motion.

Prescription

TWO WEEKS

Precautions Avoid supination and pronation at the elbow.

Range of Motion

Thumb—None (immobilized).

Wrist—None (immobilized).

Elbow—None if immobilized in a long arm cast. If in a short arm cast, gentle active elbow flexion and extension.

Digits—Active and passive range of motion.

Shoulder—Active and active-assistive range of motion.

Strength

Thumb—No strengthening exercises.

Wrist—No strengthening exercises.

Elbow—No strengthening exercises.

Shoulder—Isometric exercises to deltoid, biceps, and triceps.

Functional Activities The patient uses the uninvolved extremity for personal hygiene and self-care.

Weight Bearing No weight bearing on the affected extremity.

Treatment: Four to Six Weeks

BONE HEALING

Stability at fracture site: Bridging callus indicates stability.

Stage of bone healing: Reparative phase. Lamellar bone deposition begins.

X-ray: Callus is not seen because there is no periosteum. This is a membranous bone. Trabecular bone may be visible.

Orthopaedic and Rehabilitation Considerations

Physical Examination

An examination out of plaster should be performed at approximately 6 weeks. Check for bony tenderness. Check the range of active and passive motion at the shoulder, elbow, and digits. Check for reflex sympathetic dystrophy, which is characterized by trophic changes, vasomotor disturbances, hyperesthesia, pain, and tenderness out of proportion to the stage of fracture healing. If discovered, this will require aggressive therapy. Regardless of the presence or absence of tenderness, a short arm thumb spica should be reapplied if there is no radiographic evidence of union.

Radiography

Anteroposterior, lateral, and oblique wrist films out of plaster should be checked for step-off, displacement, and angulation. Look for bridging trabecular bone indicated by disappearance of the fracture line. If rigid fixation was used, less bridging callus is visible, and the progression of bony union should be followed by the disappearance of the fracture line.

Weight Bearing

No weight bearing is allowed on the affected extremity.

Range of Motion

At the end of 6 weeks, the long arm cast should be removed and a short arm spica cast applied. Gentle active range-of-motion exercises in flexion and extension are given to the elbow joint. The elbow may be quite stiff secondary to immobilization. Supination and pronation are still restricted to help prevent motion at the fracture site. Continue active and active-assistive range-of-motion exercises to the shoulder and digits.

Muscle Strength

Continue isometric exercises to the biceps, triceps, and deltoid. At the end of 6 weeks, isotonic exercises are prescribed to the elbow and shoulder in flexion and extension and to the shoulder in adduction and abduction.

Functional Activities

The patient continues one-handed activities, because the forearm and wrist are still in a cast.

Methods of Treatment: Specific Aspects

Cast

Nonoperative scaphoid fractures require further protection with a short arm thumb spica cast. The elbow may be stiff secondary to immobilization, and active-assistive range of motion is provided to supplement active range of motion.

Open Reduction and Internal Fixation

If there is radiographic evidence of bone healing at 6 weeks, the short arm cast is removed. Gentle active range-of-motion exercises are prescribed to the wrist in flexion and extension. No passive exercises are given at this time. Because the thumb is free, gentle active opposition and flexion/extension exercises are prescribed to the thumb.

Hydrotherapy or fluidotherapy may be helpful in decreasing stiffness and discomfort during the range-of-motion exercises.

K-wires may be removed after 6 weeks and a short arm thumb spica cast applied for another 6 weeks.

Herbert screw fixation is not removed unless it is protruding.

Prescription

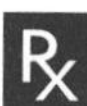

FOUR TO SIX WEEKS

Precautions Avoid passive range of motion to thumb and wrist.

Range of Motion

Wrist and thumb—If short arm cast is removed (open reduction and internal fixation), gentle active range of motion to the wrist and thumb in flexion, extension, and thumb opposition. Hydrotherapy to improve the range of motion.

Elbow—Gentle active range of motion in flexion extension (long arm cast removed) and short arm cast applied. No supination/pronation.

Shoulder—Active and passive range of motion.

Digits—Active and passive range of motion.

Strength

Elbow—Isotonic exercises in flexion

Shoulder—Extension, shoulder adduction/abduction

Functional Activities The patient needs assistance in self-care and dressing and uses the uninvolved extremity for self-care and personal hygiene.

Weight Bearing No weight bearing on the affected extremity.

Treatment: Eight to Twelve Weeks

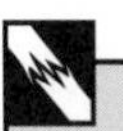

BONE HEALING

Stability at fracture site: Stable.

Stage of bone healing: Remodeling phase. Woven bone is replaced by lamellar bone. The process of remodeling takes months to years.

X-ray: Fracture line begins to disappear with reconstitution of trabecular bone pattern.

Orthopaedic and Rehabilitation Considerations

Physical Examination

Perform the examination out of plaster. Check the wrist for bony tenderness (palpate in the snuff box, because the scaphoid forms its base). Check the range of active and passive motion of the affected extremity at the shoulder, elbow, and digits. Check for reflex sympathetic dystrophy.

Dangers

No change.

Radiography

Check radiographs out of plaster for step-off, displacement, or angulation; examine for trabecular bone pattern and the disappearance of the fracture line. If the fracture is still visible, consider recasting for an additional 6 weeks. If avascular necrosis of the proximal pole has occurred, it appears more dense than the other carpal bones. If the fracture is healed even with avascular necrosis, remove the cast.

Weight Bearing

Weight bearing is allowed after 12 weeks if the fracture is healed and the range of motion and strength of the wrist have been restored.

Range of Motion

At the end of 12 weeks, if the fracture has healed, the short arm cast is removed. Gentle active range-of-motion exercises are prescribed to the wrist in flexion, extension, and ulnar and radial deviation. The wrist joint is quite stiff after being immobilized for 12 weeks, and initially the range of motion may be very limited and painful. Fluidotherapy or hydrotherapy can be prescribed to decrease the discomfort at the wrist during the range-of-motion exercises. The thumb may also be quite stiff because it was held in extension. Gentle active range-of-motion exercises are prescribed to the metacarpophalangeal and interphalangeal joints of the thumb. Gentle supination and pronation exercises are started at the elbow. Active-assistive to passive exercises in flexion and extension are prescribed to the elbow. Continue shoulder, elbow, and digit range-of-motion exercises.

Muscle Strength

At the end of 12 to 18 weeks, strengthening exercises are prescribed to the long flexors and extensors of the hand in the form of ball-squeezing or putty exercises. This is to improve grip strength. Continue isotonic exercises to the shoulder and elbow. The patient can hold a 2-lb weight in the hand and lift it against gravity to improve elbow flexion and strengthen the biceps. Holding the weight, the patient can abduct and adduct the shoulder to improve the strength of shoulder girdle muscles.

Functional Activities

The patient is instructed in using the involved extremity for stabilization purposes at the end of 12 weeks and can start to use it for grooming and self-care as well.

No lifting, pushing, or pounding activities are allowed at this time.

Gait

Tandem swing of the involved extremity is restored.

Methods of Treatment: Specific Aspects

Cast

If the fracture is clinically and radiographically healed, no further casting is required, a bivalved cast may be used as a splint, or a thumb spica splint may be prescribed for continued protection. Upon commencing aggressive rehabilitation exercises, the patient may receive relief from splinting for the first few weeks. If the fracture is not united, a delayed union is present, and a short arm thumb spica cast should be applied. If the fracture is not united by 18 weeks, a nonunion is present and surgical repair with bone grafting may be necessary. If there is evidence of trabecular bone formation but union is not complete, continue the cast for another 6 weeks and then reevaluate. If there is no evidence of callus formation, other therapeutic options may need to be considered, such as electrical stimulation/pulsed electromagnetic field (PEMF) or bone grafting.

Open Reduction and Internal Fixation

These patients have already started therapy, and it should be advanced.

If full range of motion is not restored at the wrist and thumb, passive range of motion is instituted. Progressive resistive exercises with weights to the elbow and wrist musculature is prescribed to improve strength.

K-wires were removed after 6 weeks. These patients should remain in a thumb spica cast for 3 full months from the date of surgery. The cast may then be discontinued and occupational therapy commenced if there is clinical and radiographic evidence of healing. With Herbert screw fixation, the cast can be removed at 6 weeks and active range of motion begun at the wrist.

Prescription

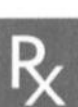

EIGHT TO TWELVE WEEKS

Precautions Avoid heavy lifting.

Range of Motion Cast is removed after 12 weeks. Gentle active range of motion to wrist and digits and metacarpophalangeal and interphalangeal joints of thumb.

With open reduction and internal fixation, active, active-assistive, and passive range of motion to the wrist and thumb to maximize full range of motion.

Strength

Wrist—After 12 weeks, active resistive exercises to long flexors and extensors of thumb and wrist.

Elbow—Resistive exercises to elbow flexors, extensors, supinators, and pronators.

Functional Activities Patient uses the involved extremity for stabilization purposes and certain self-care activities.

Weight Bearing Weight bearing is allowed after 12 weeks.

Treatment: Twelve to Sixteen Weeks

BONE HEALING

Stability at fracture site: Stable.

Stage of bone healing: Remodeling phase. Woven bone is replaced by lamellar bone. The process of remodeling takes months to years.

X-ray: Fracture line begins to disappear. There is reconstitution of the trabecular bone pattern.

Orthopaedic and Rehabilitation Considerations

Physical Examination

Perform the examination out of plaster. Check the wrist for bony tenderness and range of motion. Tenderness in the snuff box may indicate a nonunion. Check the range of active and passive motion of the affected extremity at the shoulder, elbow, and digits. Check for reflex sympathetic dystrophy, which may still develop.

Dangers

No change.

Radiography

Check radiographs out of plaster for step-off, displacement, or angulation; examine for callus and the disappearance of the fracture line. If the fracture is still visible, consider obtaining additional studies such as plain tomography or a CT scan to further evaluate the fracture. If avascular necrosis of the proximal pole has occurred, it appears more dense than the other carpal bones.

Weight Bearing

Full weight bearing is allowed.

Range of Motion

Range-of-motion exercises are prescribed to the wrist, digits, thumb, and elbow. If the movement is limited, active-assistive to passive range-of-motion exercises are prescribed. Fluidotherapy or hydrotherapy can be prescribed to reduce the discomfort of tissue stretching and aid in obtaining a full range of motion.

Muscle Strength

Progressive resistive exercises are prescribed to the extremity. The patient can use his or her uninvolved extremity to offer resistance.

Functional Activities

Patients are encouraged to work on improving their grip and grasp strength and to use the involved extremity for all activities of self-care, grooming, feeding, writing, opening doors, and placing and turning keys in doors.

Methods of Treatment: Specific Aspects

Cast

Patients who have previously demonstrated healing should advance in their therapy. If there is evidence of callus formation but union is not complete, continue the cast with monthly follow-up to evaluate healing. If the fracture line is still visible and there is no evidence of callus formation, other therapeutic options such as electrical stimulation or bone grafting should be considered.

Open Reduction and Internal Fixation

These patients have already started therapy, and it should advance. Injuries treated with K-wires (which were removed after 6 weeks) should remain in a thumb spica cast for 3 full months. If there is then clinical and radiographic evidence of healing, the cast should be discontinued and occupational therapy commenced.

Herbert screws do not have to be removed unless they are protruding or causing difficulty. They do not need casting at this point.

Prescription

Twelve to Sixteen Weeks

Precautions None if fracture is healed.

Range of Motion Active-assistive, passive range of motion of wrist and thumb.

Strength Active-resistive to progressive-resistive exercises to the wrist and thumb.

Functional Activities Involved extremity is used for all self-care activities.

Weight Bearing Full weight bearing is allowed.

LONG-TERM CONSIDERATIONS

If the fracture is not united after 18 weeks of nonoperative treatment, open reduction and bone grafting should be performed.

Malunion with humpback deformity results in decreased extension and grip strength; however, this clinical outcome should be accepted and no further surgical treatment undertaken.

Obtaining union is the best way to avoid instability and resulting painful arthritis.

IMMEDIATE TO ONE WEEK

	Cast	*Open Reduction and Internal Fixation*
Stability	None.	Stability afforded by fixation only.
Orthopedics	Long arm cast for known fracture; short arm cast for suspected fracture without radiographic evidence.	Short arm cast.
	Trim cast to distal palmar crease volarly and to metacarpophalangeal (MCP) prominences dorsally to allow free finger and MCP motion.	Trim cast to distal palmar crease volarly and to MCP prominences dorsally to allow free finger and MCP motion. Short arm cast should be trimmed proximally if impingement occurs with elbow flexion
	Treat dependent edema with elevation.	Treat dependent edema with elevation.
Rehabilitation	Active and passive range-of-motion exercises to the digits, except for the thumb, which is immobilized.	Active and passive range-of-motion exercises to the digits, except for the thumb, which is immobilized.
	Active and active-assistive range-of-motion exercises to the shoulder.	Active and active-assistive range-of-motion exercises to the elbow and shoulder.
	Isometric exercises to the biceps, triceps, deltoid.	Isometric exercises to the biceps, triceps, and deltoid.
		Limit supination and pronation.

TWO WEEKS

	Cast	*Open Reduction and Internal Fixation*
Stability	None to minimal.	Stability mainly afforded by fixation, with minimal contribution from organization at fracture site.
Orthopedics	Long arm cast for known fracture. Remove short arm cast used for suspected fracture and reexamine patient. May obtain bone scan (preferable) or computed tomography if continued pain over snuff-box with radiographs that remain negative.	Change short arm cast for suture removal. Trim cast to allow free finger, metacarpophalangeal (MCP), and elbow motion. Treat dependent edema with elevation.
Rehabilitation	Active and passive range-of-motion exercises to the digits, except for the thumb, which is immobilized. Active and active-assistive range-of-motion exercises to the shoulder. Isometric exercises to the biceps, triceps, and deltoid.	Active and passive range-of-motion exercises to the digits, except for the thumb, which is immobilized. Active and active-assistive range-of-motion exercises to the elbow and shoulder. Limit supination and pronation.

FOUR TO SIX WEEKS

	Cast	*Open Reduction and Internal Fixation*
Stability	Bridging callus indicates stability.	Stability afforded by fixation and bridging callus.
Orthopedics	Change long arm cast to short arm cast. Trim cast to allow for free finger, metacarpophalangeal (MCP), and elbow motion.	Remove short arm cast at 6 weeks if radiographically healed. Use wrist splint for protection.
Rehabilitation	Continue active and passive range-of-motion exercises to the digits, except for the thumb, which is still immobilized. Active and active-assistive range-of-motion exercises to the shoulder and elbow. Limit supination and pronation.	Advance therapy with gentle active range-of-motion exercises of the wrist and gentle active opposition and flexion/extension exercises to the thumb. No passive exercises. Continue active and active-assistive range-of-motion exercises to the elbow and shoulder.

EIGHT TO TWELVE WEEKS

	Cast	*Open Reduction and Internal Fixation*
Stability	Stable.	Stable.
Orthopedics	Remove short arm cast at 10 to 12 weeks if radiographically and clinically healed. May use wrist splint initially for protection. Fracture should be completely healed by 12 weeks. Consider electrical stimulation/pulsed electromagnetic field if no evidence of union by 8 weeks. If no progression to union by 12 to 14 weeks, consider surgical intervention with bone grafting.	May use wrist splint for protection. Consider electrical stimulation/pulsed electromagnetic field if no progression to union by 8 weeks.
Rehabilitation	Advance therapy with gentle active range-of-motion exercises of the wrist and gentle active opposition and flexion/extension exercises of the thumb. Continue active and active-assistive range-of-motion exercises to the elbow and shoulder. Start gentle supination/pronation exercises to the elbow. May begin grip strengthening (ball squeezing and putty) at 10 weeks.	Continue gentle active, active-assistive, and passive range-of-motion exercises of the wrist and gentle active opposition and flexion/extension exercises of the thumb. Continue active and active-assistive range-of-motion exercises to the elbow and shoulder. May begin grip strengthening (ball squeezing and putty) at 10 weeks.

TWELVE TO SIXTEEN WEEKS

	Cast	*Open Reduction and Internal Fixation*
Stability	Stable.	Stable.
Orthopedics	Should be healed. Consider electrical stimulation/pulsed electromagnetic field or surgery if no progression to union.	Should be healed. Consider electrical stimulation/pulsed electromagnetic field if no progression to union.
Rehabilitation	Range-of-motion exercises to all digits, wrist, elbow, and shoulder. In addition to active and active-assistive range-of-motion exercises, passive exercises used to achieve full motion. Grip strengthening with squeeze ball or putty. Progressive resistive exercises to wrist and thumb. Use 2-pound weights and increase for strengthening of biceps and shoulder girdle. Fluidotherapy or hydrotherapy reduces discomfort.	Range-of-motion exercises to all digits, wrist, elbow, and shoulder. In addition to active and active-assistive range-of-motion exercises, passive exercises used to achieve full motion. Grip strengthening with squeeze ball or putty. Progressive resistive exercises to wrist and thumb. Use 2-pound weights and increase for strengthening biceps and shoulder girdle. Fluidotherapy or hydrotherapy reduces discomfort.

BIBLIOGRAPHY

Amadio PC, Taleisnik J. Fractures of the carpal bones. In: Green DP, ed. *Operative Hand Surgery,* Vol. 1, 3rd ed. New York: Churchill Livingston, 1993, pp. 799–860.

Cooney WP III, Linscheid RL, Dobyns JH. Fractures and dislocations of the wrist. In: Rockwood CA, ed. *Fractures in Adults,* Vol. 1, 3rd ed. Philadelphia: J.B. Lippincott, 1991, pp. 638–647.

Cooney WP III, Dobyns JH, Linscheid RL. Fractures of the scaphoid: a rationale approach to management. *Clin Orthop Rel Res,* 149:90–97, 1980.

Gelberman RH, Menon J. The vascularity of the scaphoid bone. *J Hand Surg,* 5:508–513, 1980.

Gelberman RH, Wolock BS, Siegel DB. Fractures and nonunions of the carpal scaphoid. *J Bone Joint Surg,* 71A:1560–1565, 1989.

Gellman H, Caputo RJ, Carter V, et al. Comparison of short and long thumb-spica casts for nondisplaced fractures of the carpal scaphoid. *J Bone Joint Surg,* 71A:354–357, 1989.

Herbert TJ, Fischer WE. Management of the fractured scaphoid using a new bone screw. *J Bone Joint Surg,* 66B:114–123, 1984.

Jupiter JB. Scaphoid fractures. In: *Hand Surgery Update.* Rosemont, IL: American Academy of Orthopaedic Surgeons, 1996, pp. 77–84.

Kerluke L, McCabe SJ. Nonunion of the scaphoid: a critical analysis of recent natural history studies. *J Hand Surg,* 18A:1–3, 1993.

Lindstrom G, Nystrom A. Natural history of scaphoid non-union, with special reference to asymptomatic cases. *J Hand Surg,* 17B:697–700, 1992.

Ruby L. Fractures and dislocations of the carpus. In: Browner BD, ed. *Skeletal Trauma,* Vol. 2, 1st ed. Philadelphia: W.B. Saunders, 1992, pp. 1025–1062.

Tiel-Van Buul MM, Van Beek EJ, Borm JJ, et al. The value of radiographs and bone scintigraphy in suspected scaphoid fracture: a statistical analysis. *J Hand Surg,* 18B:403–406, 1993.

CHAPTER *Nineteen*

Metacarpal Fractures

DEREK A. KRAM, MD

VASANTHA L. MURTHY, MD

INTRODUCTION

Definition

Metacarpal fractures involve the metacarpal head, neck, shaft, or base and can be intraarticular or extraarticular (Figures 19-1, 19-2, and 19-3). Intraarticular fractures involve either the head or the base of the metacarpal bones.

Metacarpal fractures are classified as stable or unstable. Stable fractures are impacted with little or no displacement and are usually isolated metacarpal shaft fractures. Unstable fractures usually are com-

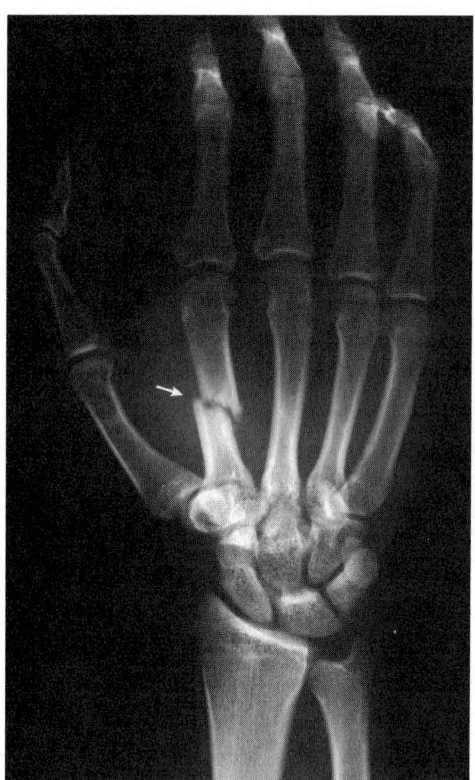

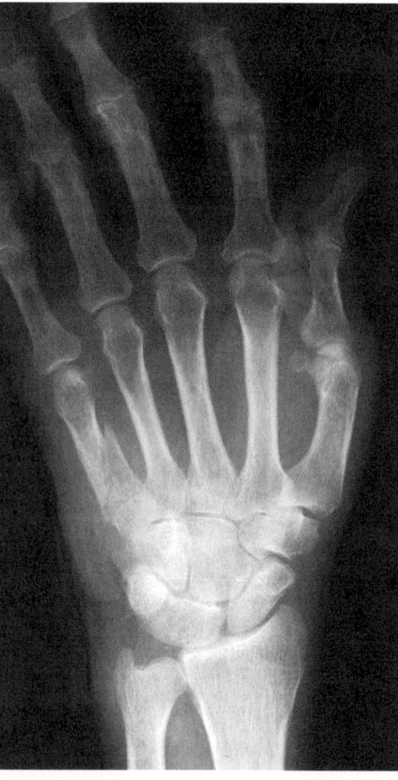

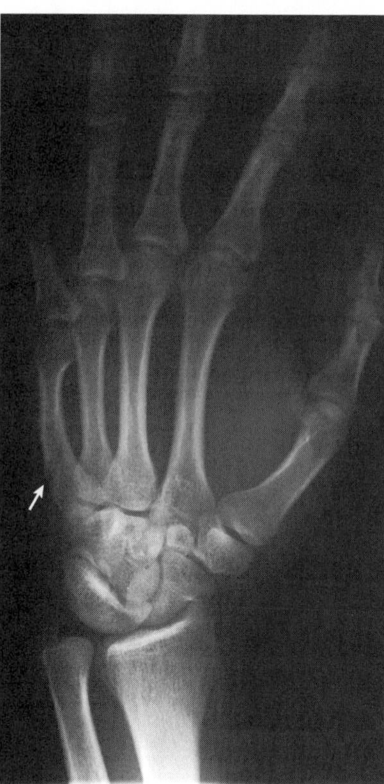

FIGURE 19-1 *(above, left)* Anteroposterior radiograph of the hand showing extraarticular fracture of the shaft of the second metacarpal.

FIGURE 19-2 *(above, middle)* Oblique fracture of the shaft of the fifth metacarpal in an elderly patient. This was initially treated with splint immobilization.

FIGURE 19-3 *(above, right)* Fracture of the base of the shaft of the fifth metacarpal.

minuted, displaced, oblique, or spiral and are often multiple.

Specific metacarpal fractures have the following special eponyms:

- *Two-part intraarticular* fractures of the base of the first metacarpal are known as Bennett's fractures (Figures 19-4 and 19-4A).
- *Three-part intraarticular* fractures of the base of the first metacarpal are known as Rolando's fractures (Figures 19-5 and 19-6).

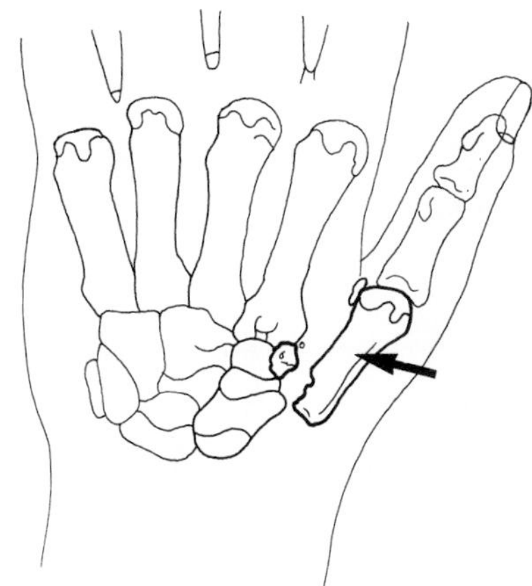

FIGURE 19-4 Bennett's fracture involving the base of the first metacarpal. This intraarticular fracture is best treated with percutaneous pinning.

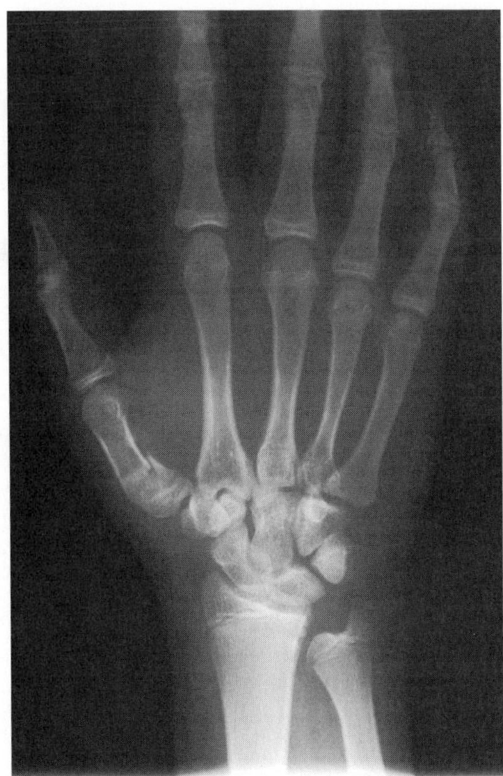

FIGURE 19-4A Fracture of the base of the first metacarpal. This is extraarticular, in contrast to the Bennett's fracture.

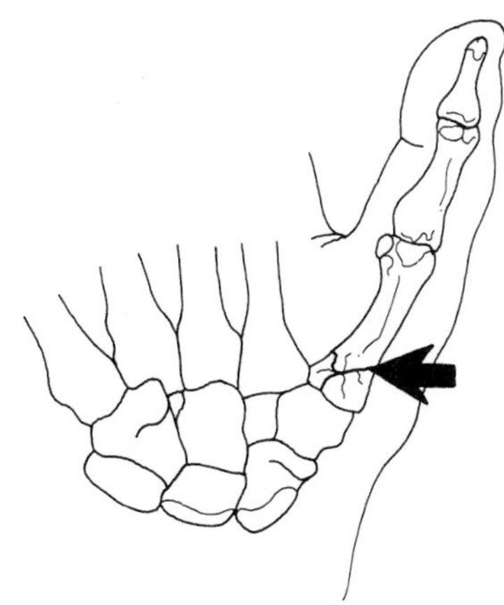

FIGURE 19-5 Intraarticular comminuted fracture of the base of the first metacarpal (Rolando's fracture).

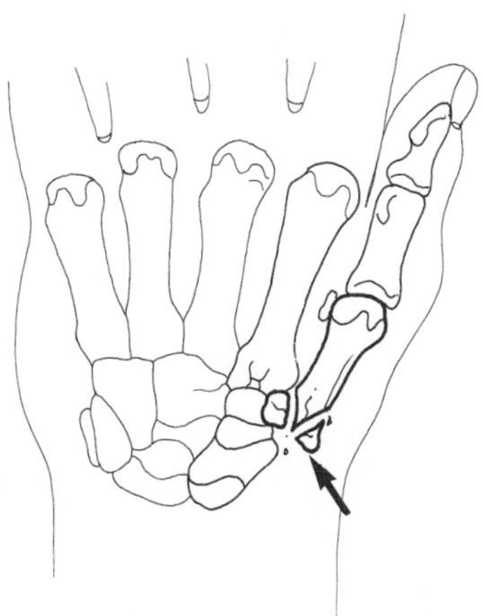

FIGURE 19-6 Comminuted fracture of the base of the first metacarpal (Rolando's fracture). It is best treated with open reduction and pin fixation.

- *Three-part intraarticular* fractures of the base of the fifth metacarpal are known as reverse-Rolando's fractures.
- Fractures of the fifth metacarpal neck are known as boxer's fractures (Figures 19-7A, 19-7B, 19-8, and 19-9).

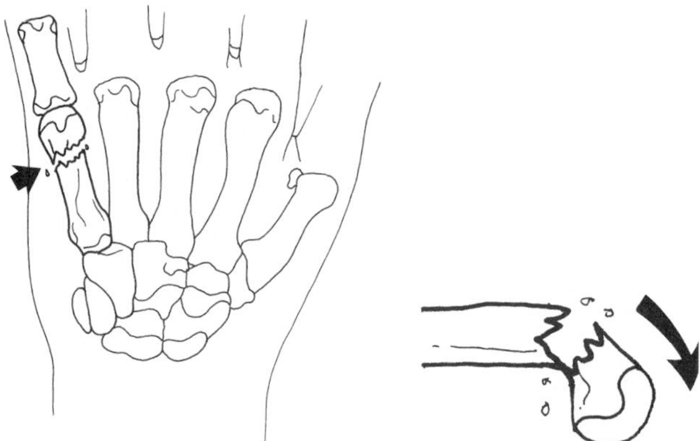

FIGURE 19-7A *(above, left)* Fracture of the base of the fifth metacarpal (boxer's fracture). There is palmar displacement of the distal end of the fracture. Boxer's fractures are frequently treated with casting, although if the angulation is great, reduction is necessary and pinning may be appropriate.

FIGURE 19-7B *(above, right)* Lateral view. Palmar placement of the distal portion of the fracture.

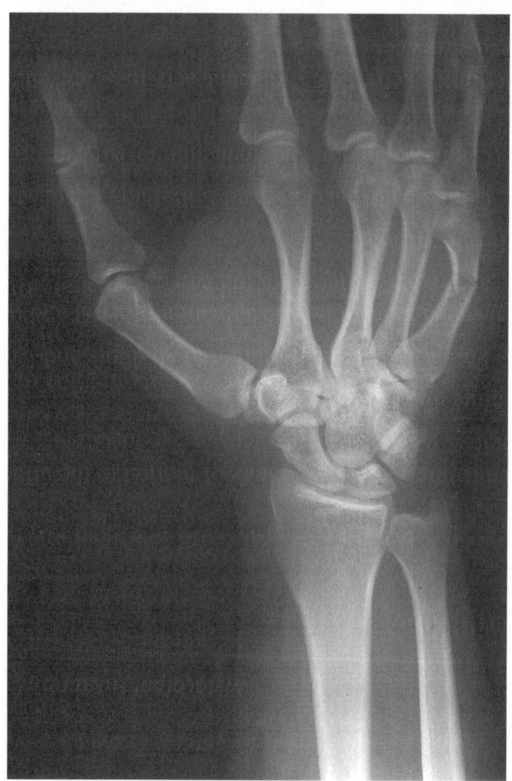

FIGURE 19-8 Boxer's fracture with angulation. The fracture is caused by striking a hard object with the very mobile fifth metacarpal.

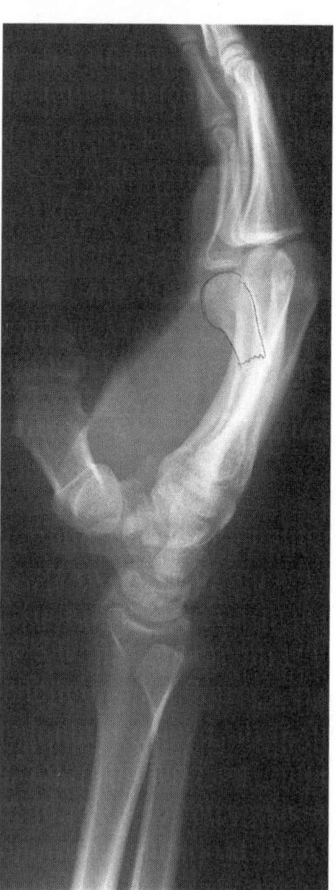

FIGURE 19-9 Boxer's fracture requiring closed reduction and fixation. There is marked angulation of the distal end of the fifth metacarpal.

Mechanism of Injury

Most metacarpal fractures are caused by direct trauma to the hand.

Treatment Goals

Orthopaedic Objective

Alignment

No degree of rotational deformity is acceptable. If the fracture is intraarticular, the articular step-off must be less than 1 to 2 mm. For metacarpal *neck* fractures, *apex* dorsal angulation of 10 degrees for the second digit, 20 degrees for the third digit, 30 degrees for the fourth digit, and 40 degrees for the fifth digit is acceptable. The fourth and fifth metacarpals are more mobile than the second and third and are able to compensate for a greater degree of deformity. For metacarpal *shaft* fractures, *apex* dorsal angulation of 30 degrees for the first digit, 10 degrees for the second and third digits, and 20 degrees for the fourth and fifth digits is acceptable (see Appendix).

Stability

Stability is best achieved when bony congruity is restored and there is no risk of displacement during finger motion.

Rehabilitation Objectives

Range of Motion

Restore full range of motion to the wrist and digits (Tables 19-1 and 19-2).

TABLE 19-1 ***Interphalangeal Joint Motion***

	Proximal interphalangeal	Distal interphalangeal	Thumb interphalangeal
Flexion	0–100°	0–70°	0–80°
Extension	0–7°	0–8°	0–5°

Finger motion is primarily in flexion and extension.

Abduction and adduction are limited and occur only at the metacarpophalangeal joints.

Functional range of motion: there is little leeway in range of motion of the digits, in contrast to other joints. Loss of motion at the distal and proximal interphalangeal and metacarpophalangeal joints results in loss of function to varying degrees, such as grasp, dexterity, and pinch.

TABLE 19-2 ***Metacarpophalangeal Joint Motion***

	Index, long, ring, and little	Thumb
Flexion	0–90°	0–80°
Extension	0–5°	0°

Flexion at the metacarpophalangeal (MP) joint increases in almost linear fashion from the index to the little finger.

Extension at the MP joints is approximately equal for all digits.

Abduction and adduction occur only at the MP joints and are limited.

Any loss of motion of the MP and distal and proximal interphalangeal joints results in loss of function to varying degrees, such as grasp, dexterity, and pinch.

The clinical measurement of joint motion, American Academy of Orthopaedic Surgeons. Edited by W.B. Greene and J.D. Heckman, 1994, pp. 45.

Muscle Strength

Restore the preinjury strength of the muscles that supply the hand and digits. These muscles include the interossei and lumbricals, the long and short flexors and extensors of the digits, and the hypothenar and thenar muscles.

Maintain the strength of the muscles within the cast. These muscles include:

Interossei and lumbricals
Long and short flexors of the digits
Extensors of the digits
Hypothenar and thenar muscles
Flexor carpi ulnaris and flexor carpi radialis
Extensor carpi ulnaris and extensor carpi radialis

Functional Goals

Reestablish power grip, grasp, and pincer grip.

Expected Time of Bone Healing

Usually, 4 to 6 weeks are required for bony union. However, immobilizing the metacarpophalangeal and interphalangeal joints for more than 3 to 4 weeks is associated with an increased risk of stiffness, and therefore an earlier return to motion is recommended.

Expected Time of Rehabilitation

Six to 12 weeks.

Methods of Treatment

Cast/Splint

Biomechanics: Stress-sharing device.

Mode of Bone Healing: Secondary, with callus formation.

Indications: A cast or splint is the treatment of choice for stable fractures, including metacarpal shaft and neck fractures. It is also used for extraarticular basal metacarpal fractures, intraarticular basal fractures of the second through fourth metacarpals, and severely comminuted metacarpal head fractures. The affected digit is often buddy taped to an adjacent digit to help maintain alignment early and improve range of motion later. The wrist should be maintained in the cast in approximately 30 degrees of extension, the metacarpophalangeal joints in 60 to 90 degrees of flexion, and the proximal and distal interphalangeal joints in approximately 5 to 10 degrees of flexion to maintain taut (elongated) collateral ligaments and prevent posttreatment stiffness.

Closed Reduction and Percutaneous Pinning

Biomechanics: Stress-sharing device.

Mode of Bone Healing: Secondary, with callus formation.

Indications: This is the treatment of choice for unstable metacarpal neck fractures, unstable metacarpal shaft fractures, and most intraarticular basal fractures of the first and fifth metacarpals. Different methods of percutaneous pinning include intramedullary pin fixation, transfixation to adjacent metacarpals, and crossed Kirschner wires. The pins can be cut off beneath the skin or allowed to protrude through the skin, depending on the surgeon's preference. Pins are usually kept in place for 3 to 4 weeks, during which the affected metacarpal usually is immobilized in a cast or splint to reduce the risks of pin loosening and pin infection (Figures 19-10, 19-10A, 19-10B, 19-10C, and 19-10D).

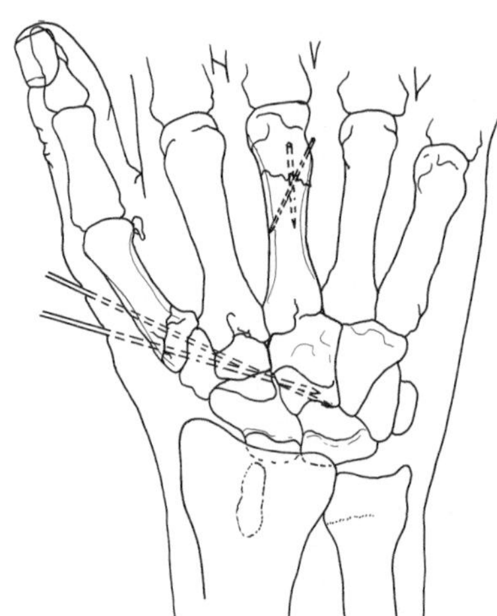

FIGURE 19-10 Closed reduction and percutaneous pinning of fractures of the base of the first metacarpal and the shaft of the third metacarpal. The base of the third metacarpal may be transfixed with an intramedullary pin or crossed Kirschner wires. Dual pinning of the base of the first metacarpal fracture provides stability and prevents rotation at the fracture site. After surgery, a cast or splint is used to keep the pin from loosening.

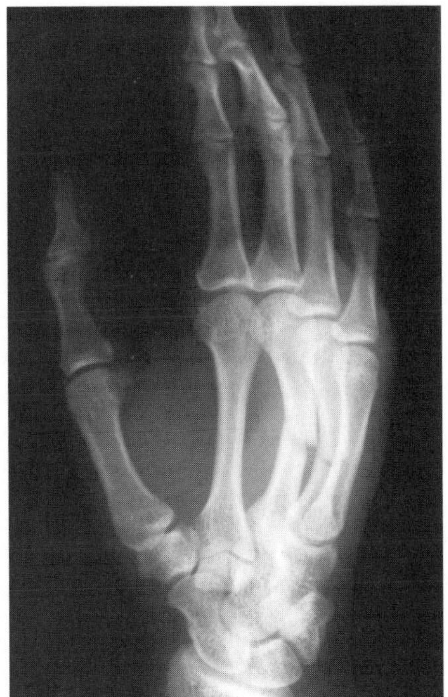

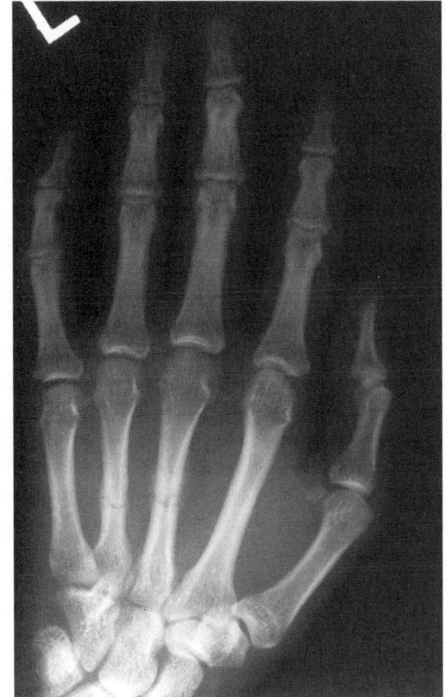

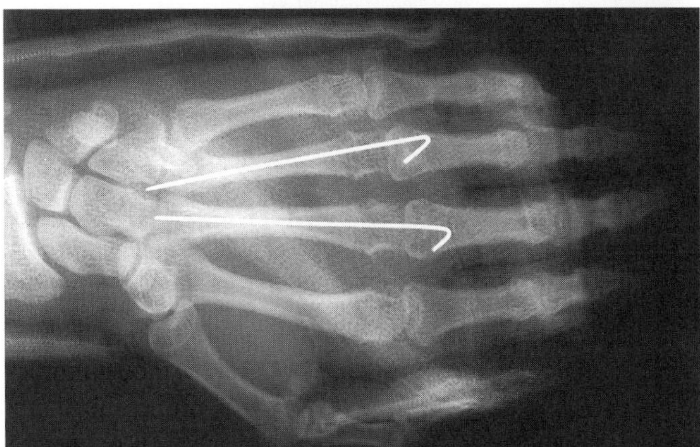

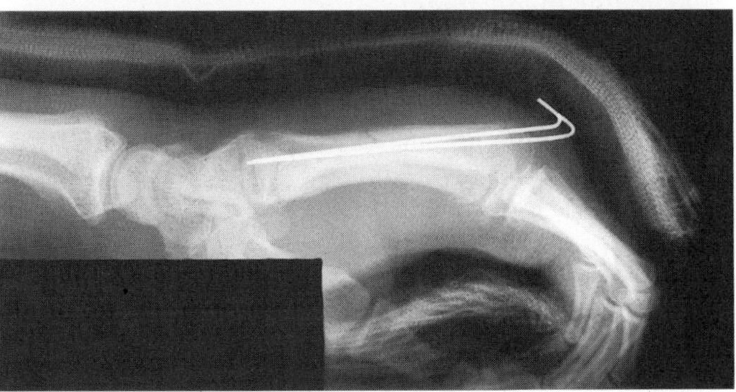

FIGURE 19-10A *(above, left)* Fractures of the shafts of the third and fourth metacarpals with dorsal angulation.

FIGURE 19-10B *(left)* Fractures of the shafts of the third and fourth metacarpals treated with closed reduction and percutaneous fixation (anterior/posterior view). Courtesy of Dr. Roy Kulick, Albert Einstein College of Medicine, Bronx, NY.

FIGURE 19-10C *(left, bottom)* Fractures of the shafts of the third and fourth metacarpals treated with percutaneous fixation. They are treated postoperatively with a splint or cast for approximately 6 weeks. Courtesy of Dr. Roy Kulick, Albert Einstein College of Medicine, Bronx, NY.

FIGURE 19-10D *(above)* Fractures of the shafts of the third and fourth metacarpals after 6 weeks. Pins have been removed. Note the callus formation.

Open Reduction and Internal Fixation

Biomechanics: Stress-shielding device with plate fixation. Stress-sharing device with pin fixation.

Mode of Bone Healing: Primary, when solid fixation is achieved. Secondary, with pin fixation or when solid fixation is not achieved.

Indications: This treatment is used for metacarpal shaft fractures and intraarticular basal metacarpal fractures in which the reduction cannot be maintained by closed means and for metacarpal head fractures in which there is minimal comminution and the articular surface can be restored. It is rarely used for metacarpal neck fractures. For shaft fractures in which rigid fixation is achieved, early range of motion of the digits is encouraged. For shaft fractures without rigid fixation, however, and for intraarticular basal fractures and head fractures, the affected metacarpal is initially immobilized in a cast or splint for 3 to 4 weeks (Figure 19-11).

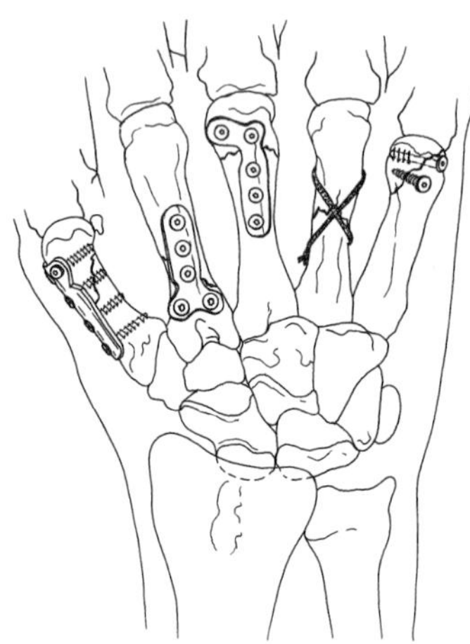

FIGURE 19-11 Fractures of the metacarpal shaft may be fixed with plates or screws. This is best done when reduction cannot be maintained by closed means and for metacarpal head fractures in which there is minimal comminution and the articular surface can be restored.

Closed Reduction and Functional Bracing

Biomechanics: Stress-sharing device.

Mode of Bone Healing: Secondary, with callus formation.

Indications: These braces are placed after closed reduction in stable fractures, usually of the metacarpal shaft, to provide three-point fixation of the fracture while allowing motion of the metacarpophalangeal and proximal and distal interphalangeal joints. The braces are difficult to apply properly as well as to maintain for the required period of treatment, and thus are used infrequently. However, they also can be used later in the treatment after a cast or splint is removed. This method is not discussed further in this chapter.

External Fixation

Biomechanics: Stress-sharing device.

Mode of Bone Healing: Secondary, with callus formation.

Indications: External fixation is used for open fractures or severely comminuted fractures not amenable to closed reduction or internal fixation. It is used rarely and is not discussed further in this chapter.

Special Considerations of the Fracture

Age

Elderly patients are at greater risk for development of joint stiffness secondary to the fracture and its treatment.

Articular Involvement

Fractures involving the articular surface require an anatomic reduction to minimize the risk of decreased range of motion and the development of degenerative changes. This is especially true for intraarticular basal fractures of the first and fifth metacarpals (*see* Figures 19-4, 19-5, and 19-6).

Location

Metacarpal shaft fractures involving the first, fourth, and fifth digits can heal with moderate angulation without undue effects because of the hypermobility of these digits. The more proximal the fracture is along the shaft, the less angular deformity can be accepted. Thus, more angular deformity is permitted in the neck region of the metacarpals. Most metacarpal neck and shaft fractures result in apex dorsal angulation. This is due to the dorsal and volar interosseous muscles that arise from the metacarpal shafts, leading to flexion of the metacarpophalangeal joints and extension of the interphalangeal joints.

Associated Injury

Collateral Ligament Injury

This may occur secondary to the primary injury or, most often, to treatment. External plaster immobilization of the metacarpophalangeal joints must be maintained in 60 to 90 degrees of flexion to keep the collateral ligaments elongated. If flexion is not maintained, the collateral ligaments shorten during immobilization, causing the patient difficulty in flexing the metacarpophalangeal joint adequately after the immobilization device is removed. Conversely, the interphalangeal joints must be maintained relatively extended to keep the collateral ligaments elongated. This prevents shortening of the collateral ligaments during immobilization and prevents difficulty achieving interphalangeal joint extension after the immobilization device is removed.

Soft-Tissue Injury

Many fractures involving the metacarpals are due to crushing injuries or penetrating trauma, which can be associated with soft-tissue injury and edema. Scarring may occur in the intrinsic musculature of the hand as well as in the gliding portion of the tendons, either secondary to the direct trauma or due to the treatment (e.g., pins may spear these structures during placement). This scarring may result in residual stiffness.

Open Fractures

Any lacerations associated with metacarpal head or neck fractures should be considered open fractures, especially when a human bite injury is suspected. These injuries should be treated with aggressive irrigation and débridement and intravenous antibiotics because they have a high risk of infection.

Weight Bearing

The involved hand should be non-weight bearing. The patient should avoid supporting the body's weight using a walker or cane, or during push-off from a chair. If the involved extremity must be used for weight bearing during ambulation, a platform walker may be used so that no weight is borne by the involved hand.

Gait

Arm swing in tandem with the opposite extremity is affected, especially if an arm sling is used to elevate the extremity during the initial phase of treatment.

TREATMENT

Treatment: Early to Immediate (Day of Injury to One Week)

BONE HEALING

Stability at fracture site: None.

Stage of bone healing: Inflammatory phase. The fracture hematoma is colonized by inflammatory cells, and débridement of the fracture begins.

X-ray: No callus.

Orthopaedic and Rehabilitation Considerations

Physical Examination

Pay special attention to complaints of pain, paresthesia, and cast discomfort as an indicator of compartment syndrome. Check for *swelling* (dependent edema as well as discoloration of skin are common, with resultant sausage-shaped digits). If swelling is noted, instruct the patient to elevate the extremity and perform retrograde massage (milking the edema from the fingertips toward the palm). Check for any rotational deformity of the digits, which is not acceptable and requires realignment and placement of fixation devices.

Dangers

The patient should be warned of the possibilities of residual decreased grip strength and dorsal prominence along the metacarpal shaft with decreased metacarpophalangeal joint prominence. The patient should also be informed of possible degenerative changes if the injury involves an articular surface. In addition, the patient should be informed of the possibilities of prolonged swelling and development of reflex sympathetic dystrophy.

Radiography

Check radiographs for loss of correction (see Appendix for acceptable values).

Weight Bearing

The patient should not bear weight on the affected hand. A platform walker can be used as needed.

Range of Motion

If rigid fixation is achieved, *active* range of motion of the affected digit is allowed once the wounds appear to be healing. No active-assisted or passive range of motion is allowed. If rigid fixation is *not* achieved, however, no range of motion of the affected digit is allowed at this stage. Active range of motion of the nonsplinted digits is encouraged to prevent stiffness and swelling. Active range of motion of the ipsilateral elbow and shoulder is also encouraged to prevent stiffness, especially if the affected extremity is placed in a sling.

Muscle Strength

Once the swelling and pain subside, the patient can perform isometric exercises in abduction, adduction, flexion, and extension with the nonsplinted fingers to maintain intrinsic muscle strength.

Functional Activities

The patient may use the uninvolved extremity for self-care, hygiene, feeding, grooming, and dressing. The patient is instructed in donning clothes on the involved arm first and doffing clothes from the uninvolved arm first. Patients with lower extremity ailments who must use crutches, a cane, or a walker need a walker with a platform attachment because weight bearing on the affected hand is not allowed.

Gait

There is diminished arm swing if the patient is in a sling or cast.

Methods of Treatment: Specific Aspects

Cast/Splint

Trim the cast to allow visualization of the tip of the injured digit and the adjacent buddy-taped digit to evaluate capillary refill. Check the cast padding and cast edges and evaluate for any skin breakdown at the edges. Check for any cast softening and repair as needed.

Closed Reduction and Percutaneous Pinning

Evaluate the pin sites for discharge, erythema, or skin tenting. Instruct the patient in proper pin care. Clean the pin sites with peroxide- or povidone–iodine-soaked swabs as needed. If the pin sites appear infected, depending on the severity, give the patient oral antibiotics or admit the patient for intravenous antibiotics and possible débridement. Release any skin tenting. Pay special attention to complaints of pain, paresthesia, or pin discomfort because these could indicate a pin skewed a nerve or tendon. The affected digit and an adjacent buddy-taped digit are often splinted and should be evaluated for capillary refill, adequate cast padding, and cast softening.

Open Reduction and Internal Fixation

Evaluate the wound for erythema, discharge, or fluctuance. If any signs of infection are present, aggressive therapy is recommended, including intravenous antibiotics and possible débridement. The affected digit and an adjacent buddy-taped digit are often splinted and should be evaluated as described previously for capillary refill, adequate cast padding, and cast softening.

Prescription

DAY ONE TO ONE WEEK

Precautions No passive range of motion.

Range of Motion Active range of motion to nonsplinted digits.

Muscle Strength Isometric exercises prescribed within the cast of the nonsplinted fingers.

Functional Activities Uninvolved extremity used in self-care and personal hygiene.

Weight Bearing None.

Treatment: Two Weeks

BONE HEALING

Stability at fracture site: None to minimal.

Stage of bone healing: Beginning of reparative phase. Osteoprogenitor cells differentiate into osteoblasts that lay down woven bone.

X-ray: No callus.

Orthopaedic and Rehabilitation Considerations

Physical Examination

Check for any rotational deformity of the affected digits, which requires realignment and the placement of fixation devices as needed. Check for swelling and range of motion of the nonsplinted digits. Apply retrograde massage and aggressive range-of-motion exercises as needed to nonsplinted digits.

Dangers

Make sure that the splint maintains the metacarpophalangeal joints in 60 to 90 degrees of flexion and the interphalangeal joints relatively extended to reduce collateral ligament shortening during immobilization, because such shortening results in decreased range of motion of the splinted digits.

Radiography

Check radiographs for callus as well as for loss of correction (see Appendix for acceptable values). Loss of reduction usually occurs within the first 2 weeks.

Weight Bearing

The patient should not bear weight on the affected hand. A platform walker can be used as needed.

Range of Motion

If rigid fixation is achieved, continue active range of motion of the affected digit. If rigid fixation is not achieved, however, no range of motion of the affected digit is allowed. Active, active-assisted, and passive range of motion of the nonsplinted digits and the elbow and shoulder are performed to decrease swelling and stiffness.

Strength

Continue isometric exercises to the intrinsic muscles of the nonsplinted digits.

Functional Activities

The patient still uses the uninvolved extremity for self-care, hygiene, feeding, grooming, and dressing. During two-handed activities, the patient may start using the nonsplinted digits of the involved extremity for stabilization purposes.

Gait

There usually is diminished arm swing if the patient is in a cast or sling.

Methods of Treatment: Specific Aspects

Cast/Splint

Trim the cast to allow visualization of the tip of the injured digit and the adjacent buddy-taped digit to evaluate capillary refill. Check the cast padding and cast edges and evaluate for any skin breakdown at the edges. Check for any cast softening and repair as needed.

Closed Reduction and Percutaneous Pinning

Evaluate the pin sites for erythema, discharge, or skin tenting. Treat any problems encountered as needed. Pay special attention to complaints of pain, paresthesia, or pin discomfort because these could indicate a skewed nerve or tendon. If the affected digit and an adjacent digit are splinted, evaluate as described previously for capillary refill, adequate padding, and cast softening.

Open Reduction and Internal Fixation

Remove the cast and evaluate the wound for erythema, discharge, or fluctuance. Aggressively treat any signs of infection with oral or intravenous antibiotics, débridement, or removal of hardware. Remove the sutures. Replace the cast if needed.

Prescription

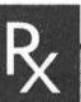

Two Weeks

Precautions No passive range of motion to the affected digit.

Range of Motion

1. If rigid fixation is achieved, active range of motion to the affected digit.
2. Active, active-assistive, and passive range of motion to nonsplinted digits.

Muscle Strength Isometric exercises to the intrinsic muscles of nonsplinted digits.

Functional Activities Uninvolved extremity used in self-care and personal hygiene.

Weight Bearing None.

Treatment: Four to Six Weeks

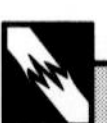

Bone Healing

Stability at fracture site: With bridging callus, the fracture is usually stable; confirm with physical examination.

Stage of bone healing: Reparative phase. Once the callus is observed bridging the fracture site, the fracture is usually stable. However, the strength of the callus, especially with torsional load, is significantly lower than that of woven bone. This requires continued protection of bone (if not further immobilization) to avoid refracture. Further organization of the callus and formation of lamellar bone begins.

X-ray: Bridging callus is visible. With increased rigidity, less bridging callus is noted, and healing with endosteal callus predominates. Fracture line is less distinct.

Orthopaedic and Rehabilitation Considerations

Physical Examination

Metacarpal shaft fractures of the thumb usually require 6 weeks of plaster immobilization. Most other metacarpal fractures require only 3 to 4 weeks of immobilization. Examination at this stage is performed out of plaster. Check the affected metacarpal for stability and tenderness, and check the entire digit for range of motion.

Dangers

Check for reflex sympathetic dystrophy (characterized by trophic changes, vasomotor disturbances, hyperesthesia, and pain out of proportion to the stage of fracture healing). If present, this requires aggressive occupational hand therapy.

Radiography

Check radiographs, taken out of plaster, for callus as well as for loss of correction (see Appendix for acceptable values).

Weight Bearing

The patient should not bear weight on the affected hand unless the fractured metacarpal is completely nontender, with no motion at the fracture site, and callus is seen on the radiograph.

Range of Motion

Full active range of motion to all digits and the wrist is instituted. Fluidotherapy, paraffin, or hydrotherapy can begin to diminish the patient's pain during joint mobilization. After 6 weeks, gentle passive range of motion can be added to the program to improve range and decrease stiffness in the joints. This is important because metacarpophalangeal and interphalangeal motion is central to grip and grasp activities.

Muscle Strength

Emphasis is placed on grip and grasp. The patient is instructed in gentle ball-squeezing and Silly Putty exercises to reestablish the flexor strength of the digits and improve the interphalangeal joint motion.

Functional Activities

The patient is encouraged to resume bimanual activities, using the involved extremity for self-care, hygiene, feeding, grooming, and dressing. Avoid lifting and pushing.

Gait

Arm swing is usually reduced because of stiffness even though the cast has been removed.

Methods of Treatment: Specific Aspects

Cast/Splint

If there is no tenderness or motion at the fracture site, and abundant callus can be seen on radiography, remove the cast. Consider protective splinting for 1 to 2 additional weeks if the patient is unreliable or if further support is needed. A night splint also may be helpful, especially after aggressive rehabilitation exercises have begun.

If tenderness or motion is present at the fracture site, or if inadequate callus is seen on radiography, the splint or cast should be replaced. A removable splint is recommended to allow for early gentle range-of-motion exercises to limit future mobility deficits. The patient should then be evaluated at 2-week intervals until stability of the fracture is noted, at which time more aggressive rehabilitation and less splinting are necessary.

Closed Reduction and Percutaneous Pinning

Percutaneous pins are usually removed at 3 to 4 weeks. Pin sites should be evaluated for erythema or discharge, and any problems encountered should be treated as necessary. After removal of the pins, casting or splinting should be continued for another 1 to 2 weeks, especially if the patient is unreliable or if further support is needed. Casting is discontinued when tenderness and motion at the fracture site are absent and abundant callus is visualized on radiography. Night splinting may be helpful for the first few weeks, especially after aggressive rehabilitation exercises have begun.

Open Reduction and Internal Fixation

Evaluate the wound for erythema or discharge, and treat any problems as necessary. If there is no tenderness or motion at the fracture site and abundant callus or the disappearance of the fracture line is seen on radiography, remove the cast. A protective splint is often used for 1 to 2 additional weeks if the patient is unreliable or further support needed. Night splinting may also be helpful, especially after aggressive rehabilitation exercises have begun. If tenderness and motion are present at the fracture site, or if inadequate callus or the fracture line is seen on radiography, a removable splint is often placed to allow for gentle range-of-motion exercises. The patient should then be evaluated at 2-week intervals until stability of the fracture is noted, signifying that more aggressive rehabilitation and less time in a splint are necessary.

Prescription

FOUR TO SIX WEEKS

Precautions No passive range of motion to the affected digit.

Range of Motion

1. Full active range of motion to all digits and wrist.
2. Active pronation and supination of wrist and ulnar and radial deviation of the wrist.

Muscle Strength

1. Gentle ball-squeezing and Silly Putty exercises.
2. Gentle adduction and abduction resistive exercises of the digits.

Functional Activities Bimanual activities are encouraged at 6 weeks.

Weight Bearing None.

Treatment: Six to Eight Weeks

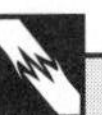

BONE HEALING

Stability at fracture site: With bridging callus, the fracture is usually stable; confirm with physical examination.

Stage of bone healing: Reparative phase. Once the callus is observed bridging the fracture site, the fracture is usually stable. However, the strength of the callus, especially with torsional load, is significantly lower than that of woven bone. This requires continued protection of bone (if not further immobilization) to avoid refracture. Further organization of the callus and formation of lamellar bone begins.

X-ray: Bridging callus is visible. With increased rigidity, less bridging callus is noted, and healing with endosteal callus predominates. Fracture line is less distinct.

Orthopaedic and Rehabilitation Considerations

Physical Examination

Check the affected metacarpal for stability and tenderness, and check the entire digit for range of motion. Pay special attention to the patient's comments on his or her activity level, noting any functional disabilities or decreased grip strength.

Dangers

Check for the resolution of reflex sympathetic dystrophy.

Radiography

Check radiographs, taken out of plaster, for callus and the disappearance of the fracture line. Evaluate for malunion (see Appendix for acceptable values), delayed union, and nonunion.

Weight Bearing

The patient may progressively increase weight bearing on the involved extremity, as tolerated.

Range of Motion

Active, active-assisted, and passive range of motion of all digits is encouraged, with fluidotherapy instituted to aid joint mobilization. Active-assistive and passive range of motion of the wrist in all planes is also encouraged. Ulnar and radial deviation are important for functional activities.

Muscle Strength

Continue with resistive exercises to the digits. Kneading, ball- or sponge-squeezing, and bead-threading exercises are performed to improve grasp and pincer grip.

Functional Activities

The patient uses the affected extremity for all activities. Elderly patients can hold a regular cane and bear weight on the affected extremity during ambulation.

Gait

The patient's arm swing should gradually increase. The aim is to normalize the arm swing pattern.

Methods of Treatment: Specific Aspects

Cast/Splint

Remove the cast, if this has not already been done. Examine for tenderness and motion at the fracture site.

Closed Reduction and Percutaneous Pinning

Remove the cast, if this has not already been done. Examine for tenderness and motion at the fracture site. Night splinting may still be useful while aggressive rehabilitation exercises are performed.

Open Reduction and Internal Fixation

Remove the cast, if this has not already been done. Examine for tenderness and motion at the fracture site. Night splinting may still be useful while aggressive rehabilitation exercises are performed.

Prescription

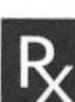

SIX TO EIGHT WEEKS

Precautions None.

Range of Motion Active, active-assistive, and passive range of motion to all digits.

Muscle Strength Active-resistive exercises to all digits and wrist.

Functional Activities The patient uses affected extremity for self-care and personal hygiene.

Weight Bearing Full weight bearing as tolerated.

Treatment: Eight to Twelve Weeks

BONE HEALING

Stability at fracture site: Stable.

Stage of bone healing: Remodeling phase. Woven bone is replaced with lamellar bone. The process of remodeling takes months to years for completion.

X-ray: Abundant callus is seen and the fracture line begins to disappear; with time, there will be reconstitution of the medullary canal. Metaphyseal areas do not produce as much callus as diaphyseal regions.

Orthopaedic and Rehabilitation Considerations

Physical Examination

Check the range of motion of all digits, the wrist, elbow, and shoulder.

Dangers

Check for resolution of reflex sympathetic dystrophy.

Radiography

Check radiographs for malunion, delayed union, and nonunion. If abundant callus or the disappearance of the fracture line was seen on a previous radiograph, it is *not* necessary to take new radiographs.

Weight Bearing

The patient should be able to bear full weight on the affected hand.

Range of Motion

The patient should have full range of motion of the digits and thumb as well as the wrist, elbow, and shoulder.

Muscle Strength

Resistive exercises to the digits can be continued and a home program given to improve or maintain the strength.

Functional Activities

The patient uses the affected extremity for all activities.

Gait

The patient's arm swing is normal now.

Prescription

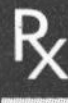

EIGHT TO TWELVE WEEKS

Precautions None.

Range of Motion Full active and passive range of motion to all digits and wrist.

Muscle Strength Progressive resistive exercises to the digits and wrist.

Functional Activities The involved extremity is used in all activities to tolerance.

Weight Bearing Full weight bearing.

LONG-TERM CONSIDERATIONS AND PROBLEMS

The patient needs to be warned of possible future degenerative joint disease (which is an increased risk with any intraarticular fracture), decreased range of motion, residual deformity, decreased grip strength, and prolonged swelling secondary to the injury. The patient should be informed that to limit residual stiffness, motion is usually begun before complete bony union has occurred, which places the fracture at risk of displacing or losing its proper alignment.

APPENDIX

Acceptable Values

1. Metacarpal head fractures
   A. Articular step-off/displacement of less than 1 to 2 mm
   B. Conventional tomography or computed tomography scan might assist in further evaluation of these fractures.
2. Metacarpal neck fractures
   A. No rotational deformity is accepted.
   B. Apex dorsal angulation of 10 degrees (second digit), 20 degrees (third digit), 30 degrees (fourth digit), and 40 degrees (fifth digit) is accepted. The metacarpal neck angle is normally 15 degrees, however, which must be taken into consideration when evaluating the dorsal angulation at the fracture site.
3. Metacarpal shaft fractures
   A. No rotational deformity is accepted.
   B. Dorsal angulation of 30 degrees (first digit), 10 degrees (second and third digits), and 20 degrees (fourth and fifth digits) is accepted.
4. Basal metacarpal fractures
   A. No rotational deformity is accepted.
   B. If intraarticular, articular step-off/displacement of less than 1 to 2 mm.
   C. Conventional tomography and a computed tomography scan might assist in further evaluation of these fractures. Comparison views are strongly recommended.

IMMEDIATE TO ONE WEEK

	Splint	Closed Reduction and Percutaneous Pinning	Open Reduction and Internal Fixation
Stability	None.	None.	None.
Orthopaedics	Trim splint to allow visualization of the tip of the injured digit and the adjacent buddy-taped digit.	Evaluate pin sites and tendon functions as well as any open wounds that require management. If splinted, treat as for splint instructions.	Perform wound care for any incisions or open wounds. If splinted, treat as per splint instructions.
Rehabilitation	No range of motion of the splinted digits is allowed. Active, active-assisted, and passive range of motion of the nonsplinted digits as well as the ipsilateral elbow and shoulder is encouraged. Isometric exercises of the nonsplinted digits are encouraged. The affected hand is not used for weight bearing.	No motion of the affected digit is allowed. Active, active-assistive and passive range of motion of the nonsplinted digits, as well as the ipsilateral elbow and shoulder is encouraged. Isometric exercises of the nonsplinted digits are encouraged. The affected hand is not used for weight bearing.	If rigid fixation is achieved, active range of motion of the affected digit is allowed once the wound permits. If rigid fixation is not achieved, no motion of the affected digit is allowed. Active, active-assisted, and passive range of motion of the nonsplinted digits as well as the ipsilateral elbow and shoulder is encouraged. Isometric exercises of the nonsplinted digits are encouraged. The affected hand is not used for weight bearing.

TWO WEEKS

	Splint	Closed Reduction and Percutaneous Pinning	Open Reduction and Internal Fixation
Stability	None to minimal.	None to minimal.	None to minimal.
Orthopaedics	Trim cast to allow visualization of the tip of the injured digit and the adjacent buddy-taped digit.	Evaluate pin sites and tendon functions as well as any open wounds that require wound management. If splinted, treat as per splint instructions.	Remove sutures and perform wound care for any open wounds. If splinted, treat as per splint instructions.
Rehabilitation	No range of motion of the splinted digits is allowed. Active, active-assisted, and passive range of motion of the nonsplinted digits as well as the ipsilateral elbow and shoulder is continued. Isometric exercises of the nonsplinted digits are continued. The affected hand is not used for weight bearing.	No motion of the affected digit is allowed. Active, active-assistive and passive range of motion of the nonsplinted digits as well as the ipsilateral elbow and shoulder is encouraged. Isometric exercises of the nonsplinted digits are encouraged. The affected hand is not used for weight bearing.	If rigid fixation is achieved, active range of motion of the affected digit is allowed. If rigid fixation is not achieved, no motion of the affected digit is allowed. Active, active-assisted, and passive range of motion of the nonsplinted digits as well as the ipsilateral elbow and shoulder is continued. Isometric exercises of the nonsplinted digits are continued. The affected hand is not used for weight bearing.

FOUR TO SIX WEEKS

	Splint	Closed Reduction and Percutaneous Pinning	Open Reduction and Internal Fixation
Stability	Partial to complete.	Partial to complete.	Partial to complete.
Orthopaedics	If nontender, no motion at fracture site, and abundant callus on radiograph, discontinue splint. May consider protective splinting or night splinting for additional 1 to 2 weeks.	Pins are removed, and splint is usually applied for additional 1 to 2 weeks. Pin sites should still be evaluated for evidence of infection.	Perform wound care as needed. If nontender, no motion at fracture site, and disappearance of fracture line seen on radiograph, discontinue splint. May consider protective splinting or night splinting for additional 1 to 2 weeks.
Rehabilitation	Full active range of motion to all digits and the wrist is instituted. After 6 weeks, gentle passive range of motion to the digits and wrist. Digit flexor strengthening is encouraged. Continue motion to ipsilateral elbow and shoulder. Weight bearing is allowed on the affected hand once the fracture is healed.	Same as for splint.	Same as for splint.

SIX TO EIGHT WEEKS

	Splint	Closed Reduction and Percutaneous Pinning	Open Reduction and Internal Fixation
Stability	Stable.	Stable.	Stable.
Orthopaedics	Discontinue splint.	Discontinue splint.	Discontinue splint.
Rehabilitation	Active, active-assisted, and passive range of motion of all digits, as well as ipsilateral wrist, elbow, and shoulder is encouraged. Resistive exercises to the digits are continued. Weight bearing on the affected hand is allowed.	Same as for splint.	Same as for splint.

EIGHT TO TWELVE WEEKS

	Splint	Closed Reduction and Percutaneous Pin	Open Reduction and Internal Fixation
Stability	Stable.	Stable.	Stable.
Orthopaedics	No splint needed.	No splint needed.	No splint needed.
Rehabilitation	All activity is allowed.	All activity is allowed.	All activity is allowed.

BIBLIOGRAPHY

Black DM, Mann RJ, Constine R, Daniels AU. Comparison of internal fixation techniques in metacarpal fractures. *J Hand Surg [Am]*, 10:466–472, 1985.

Diwaker HN, Stothard J. The role of internal fixation in closed fractures of the proximal phalanges and metacarpals in adults. *J Hand Surg [Br]*, 11:103–108, 1986.

Ferraro MD, Coppola A, Lippman K, Hurst LC. Closed functional bracing of metacarpal fractures. *Orthop Rev*, 12:49–56, 1983.

Foster RJ, Hastings H II. Treatment of Bennett, Rolando, and vertical intraarticular trapezial fractures. *Clin Orthop*, 214:121–129, 1987.

Green DP, Rowland SA. Fractures and dislocations in the hand. In: Rockwood CA Jr, Green DP, Bucholz RW, eds. *Fractures in Adults*, 3rd ed, Vol 1. Philadelphia: J.B. Lippincott, 1991, pp. 484–500.

Hall RF. Treatment of metacarpal and phalangeal fractures in noncompliant patients. *Clin Orthop*, 214:31–36, 1987.

Jupiter JB, Belsky MR. Fractures and dislocations of the hand. In: Browner BD, Jupiter JB, Levine AM, Trafton PG, eds. *Skeletal Trauma*, Vol 2. Philadelphia: W.B. Saunders, 1992, pp. 925–976.

Lamb DW, Abernethy PA, Raine PAM. Unstable fractures of the metacarpals: a method of treatment by transverse wire fixation to intact metacarpals. *Hand*, 5:43–48, 1973.

McKerrell J, Bowen V, Johnston G, Zondervan J. Boxer's fractures: conservative or operative management? *J Trauma*, 27:486–490, 1987.

Melone CP. Rigid fixation of phalangeal and metacarpal fractures. *Orthop Clin North Am*, 17:421–435, 1986.

Pellegrini VD Jr. Fractures at the base of the thumb. *Hand Clin*, 4: 87–101, 1988.

Pritsch M, Engel J, Farin I. Manipulation and external fixation of metacarpal fractures. *J Bone Joint Surg Am*, 63:1289–1291, 1981.

Ruggeri S, Osterman AL, Bora FW. Stabilization of metacarpal and phalangeal fractures in the hand. *Orthop Rev*, 9:107–110, 1980.

Stern PJ. Fractures of the metacarpals and phalanges. In: Green DP, ed. *Operative Hand Surgery*, Vol 1. New York: Churchill Livingstone, 1993, pp. 695–758.

Wright TA. Early mobilization in fractures of the metacarpals and phalanges. *Can J Surg*, 11:491–498, 1968.

CHAPTER *Twenty*

Phalangeal Fractures

DEREK A. KRAM, MD

VASANTHA L. MURTHY, MD

INTRODUCTION

Definition

Phalangeal fractures include proximal, middle, and distal phalanx fractures and are classified as intraarticular or extraarticular and as stable or unstable.

Articular fractures involve the base or the condyles of the phalanx and are subdivided into the following types: *avulsion fractures* with attached collateral ligaments, *shaft fractures* that extend into the joint, and fractures secondary to compressive loads. *Extra-articular fractures* are diaphyseal or involve the neck of the phalanx (Figure 20-1).

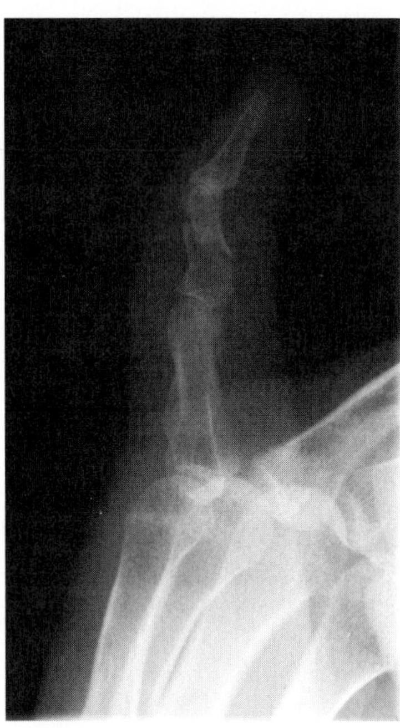

FIGURE 20-1 A diaphyseal fracture of the middle phalanx of the small or fifth finger. It is extraarticular.

Stable phalangeal fractures are impacted with little or no displacement. They are usually isolated transverse fractures. Unstable phalangeal fractures are usually comminuted, displaced, oblique, or spiral. Multiple fractures in the same digit also lead to instability.

Mechanism of Injury

Most phalangeal fractures are caused by direct trauma to the hand.

Treatment Goals

Orthopaedic Objectives

Alignment

No degree of rotational or angulatory deformity is acceptable. If the fracture is intraarticular, the articular step-off must be less than 1 to 2 mm.

Stability

Stability is best achieved when bony congruity is restored and no risk of displacement exists during finger motion.

Rehabilitation Objectives

Range of Motion

Restore full range of motion to the digit and hand (Tables 20-1 and 20-2).

TABLE 20-1 *Interphalangeal Joint Motion*

	Proximal interphalangeal	Distal interphalangeal	Thumb interphalangeal
Flexion	0–100°	0–70°	0–80°
Extension	0–7°	0–8°	0–5°

Finger motion is primarily in flexion and extension.

Abduction and adduction are limited and occur only at the metacarpophalangeal joints.

Functional range of motion: there is little leeway in range of motion of the digits, in contrast to other joints. Loss of motion at the distal and proximal interphalangeal and metacarpophalangeal joints results in loss of function to varying degrees, such as grasp, dexterity, and pinch.

TABLE 20-2 *Metacarpophalangeal Joint Motion*

	Index, long, ring, and little	Thumb
Flexion	0–90°	0–80°
Extension	0–5°	0°

Flexion at the metacarpophalangeal (MP) joint increases in almost linear fashion from the index to the little finger.

Extension at the MP joints is approximately equal for all digits.

Abduction and adduction occur only at the MP joints and are limited.

Any loss of motion of the MP joints results in loss of function to varying degrees, such as grasp, dexterity, and pinch.

Muscle Strength

Restore the preinjury strength of the muscles that supply the hand and digits. These muscles include the interossei and lumbricals, the long and short flexors and extensors of the digits, and the hypothenar and thenar muscles.

Maintain the strength of the muscles within the cast. These may include:

Interossei and lumbricals
Long and short flexors of the digits
Extensors of the digits
Hypothenar and thenar muscles
Flexor carpi ulnaris and flexor carpi radialis
Extensor carpi ulnaris and extensor carpi radialis

Functional Goals

Reestablish power grip, grasp, pincer grip, and key pinch.

Expected Time of Bone Healing

Usually, 3 to 6 weeks is required for bony union. However, immobilizing the metacarpophalangeal and interphalangeal joints for more than 3 to 4 weeks is associated with an increased risk of residual stiffness, and therefore early range of motion is recommended. In phalangeal fractures, bone healing as observed on radiography lags behind clinical bone healing. It can take 10 to 12 weeks for bony union to be visualized on radiographs.

Expected Duration of Rehabilitation

Six to 12 weeks.

Methods of Treatment

Buddy Taping

Biomechanics: Stress-sharing device.

Mode of Bone Healing: Secondary, with callus formation.

Indications: The treatment of choice for stable fractures, including nondisplaced and impacted fractures and distal phalanx tuft fractures, this treatment method involves taping the involved digit to an adjacent uninvolved digit. Buddy taping allows for early range-of-motion exercises and subsequent improved range of motion. A drawback is the possibility of stiffness developing in the digit that was previously uninvolved (Figure 20-2).

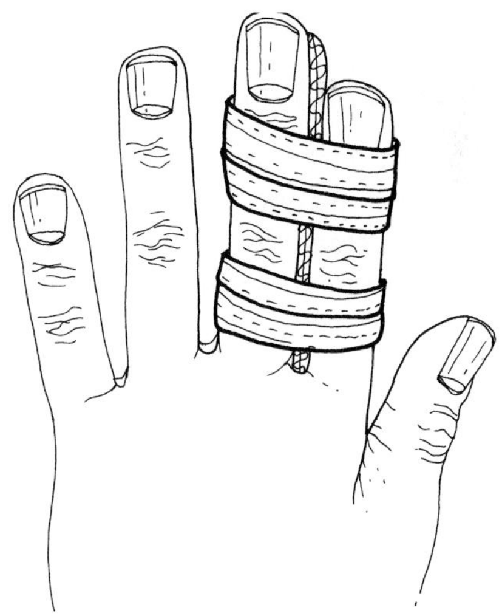

FIGURE 20-2 Buddy taping, the treatment of choice for stable fractures, including nondisplaced and impacted fractures and distal phalangeal tuft fractures, entails taping the involved digit to the adjacent uninvolved digit. This method of treatment allows for early range-of-motion exercises.

Closed Reduction and Application of Cast or Splint

Biomechanics: Stress-sharing device.

Mode of Bone Healing: Secondary, with callus formation.

Indications: This is the treatment of choice for displaced transverse fractures that are stable after closed reduction, as well as for stable dorsal fracture/dislocations of the proximal interphalangeal joint. The involved digit is usually buddy taped to an adjacent digit and a splint is placed. If the proximal phalanx is involved, a cast or splint is placed with the wrist in 30 degrees of extension, the metacarpophalangeal joints in 60 to 90 degrees of flexion, and the interphalangeal joints in 5 to 10 degrees of flexion. Dorsal fracture/dislocations of the proximal interphalangeal joint usually require an extension block dorsal splint after closed reduction.

Closed Reduction and Percutaneous Pinning

Biomechanics: Stress-sharing device.

Mode of Bone Healing: Secondary, with callus formation.

Indications: This is the treatment of choice for displaced transverse fractures that are unstable after closed reduction, for comminuted fractures, for condylar fractures, and for oblique or spiral fractures.

Open Reduction and Internal Fixation

Biomechanics: Stress-shielding device for screw fixation; stress-sharing device for pin fixation.

Mode of Bone Healing: Primary, when solid fixation is achieved; secondary, with pin fixation or when solid fixation is not achieved.

Indications: This treatment is recommended for comminuted articular fractures or highly unstable oblique or spiral fractures. However, because there is lack of adequate subcutaneous tissue in the digits, this treatment method is fraught with wound and healing complications and is not usually suggested. It is not discussed further in this chapter (Figures 20-3, 20-4, 20-5, 20-6, 20-7, 20-8, 20-9, 20-10, 20-11, and 20-12).

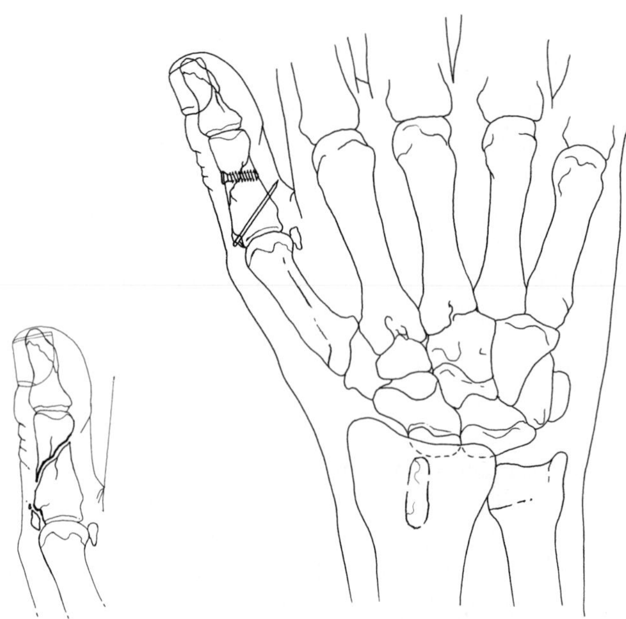

FIGURE 20-3 *(above, left)* Oblique fracture of the shaft of the proximal phalanx of the thumb as well as an avulsion fracture involving the articular surface of the proximal end of the middle phalanx.

FIGURE 20-4 *(above, right)* Screw fixation for the unstable oblique fracture of the shaft of the proximal phalanx of the thumb. There is pin fixation of the articular fragment of the proximal phalanx.

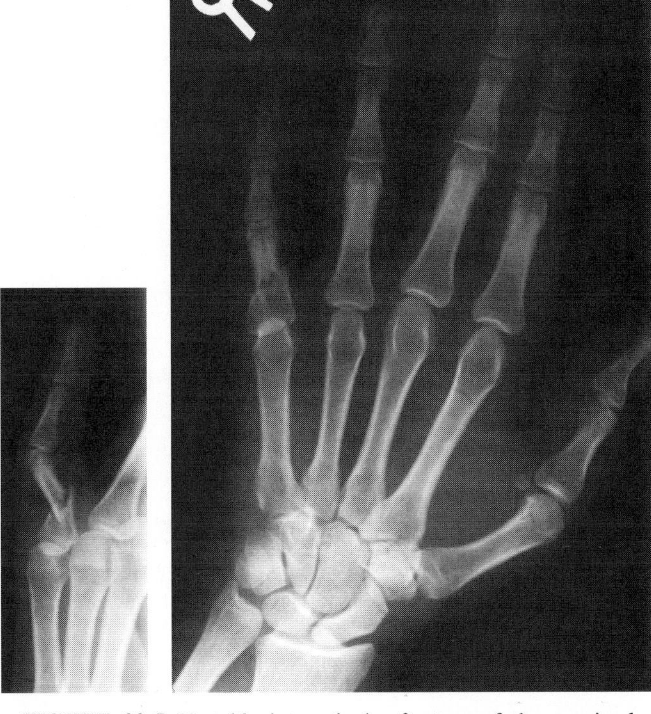

FIGURE 20-5 Unstable intraarticular fracture of the proximal phalanx of the small finger.

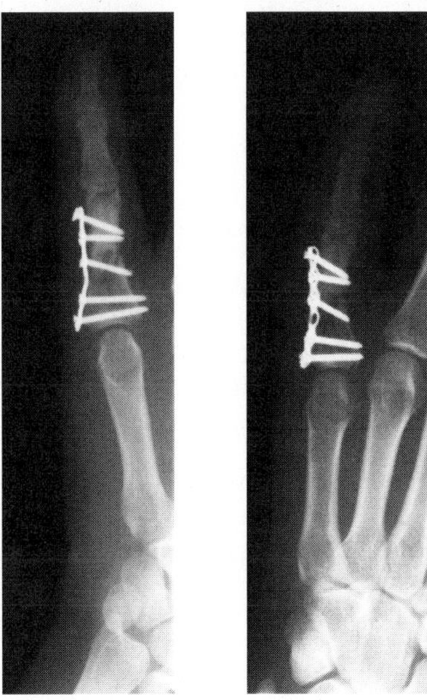

FIGURE 20-6 Intraarticular comminuted unstable fracture of the proximal phalanx. This fracture is treated with a mini-plate and screw fixation to restore length and alignment. In addition, the articular surfaces are now congruous. The fixation is rigid.

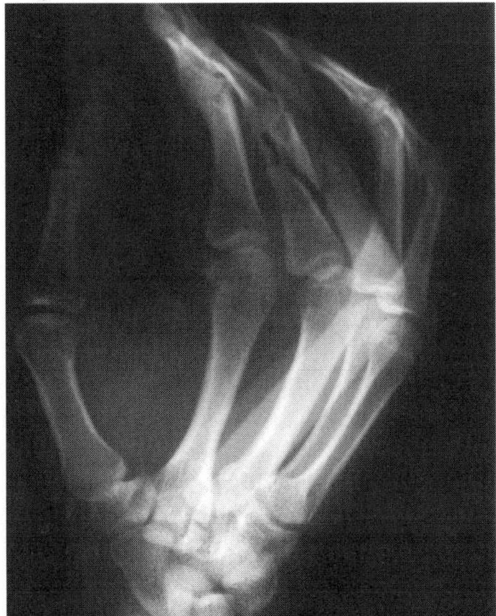

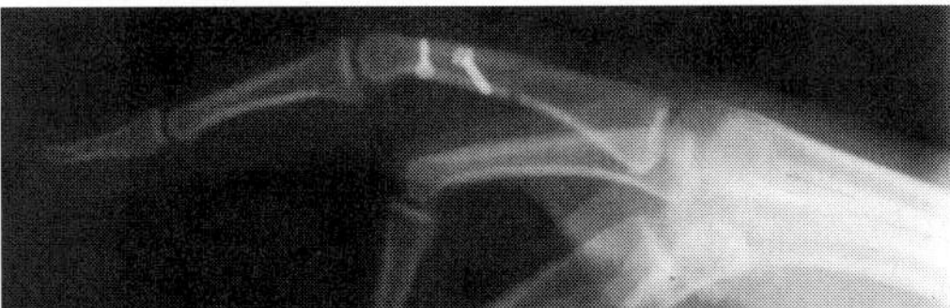

FIGURE 20-7 *(left)* Unstable spiral oblique fracture of the proximal phalanx of the long finger (extraarticular).

FIGURE 20-8 *(above)* Fracture of the proximal phalanx of the long finger treated with mini-lag screw fixation. This maintains the length of the phalanx and prevents rotation. The fixation is rigid, so a splint is not necessary. There is no callus formation.

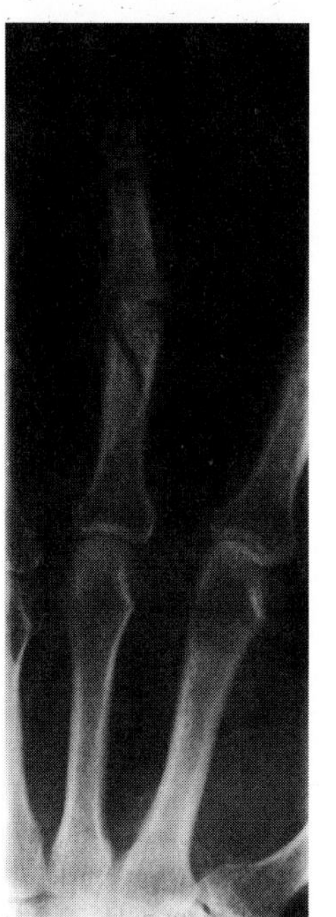

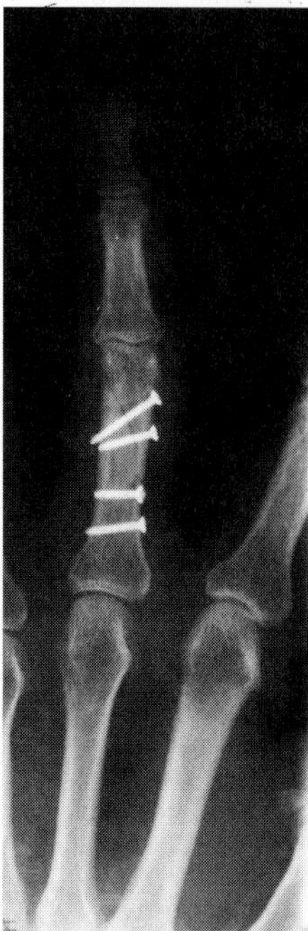

FIGURE 20-9 *(above, left)* Spiral oblique fracture of the proximal phalanx of the middle finger.

FIGURE 20-10 *(above, right)* Spiral oblique fracture of the proximal phalanx of the middle finger treated with mini-lag screw fixation. This holds the length of the bone to prevent shortening of the proximal phalanx and rotation of the bone fragments. The fixation is rigid, so a splint is not necessary. There is no callus formation. Start motion immediately as tolerated. No passive motion is allowed.

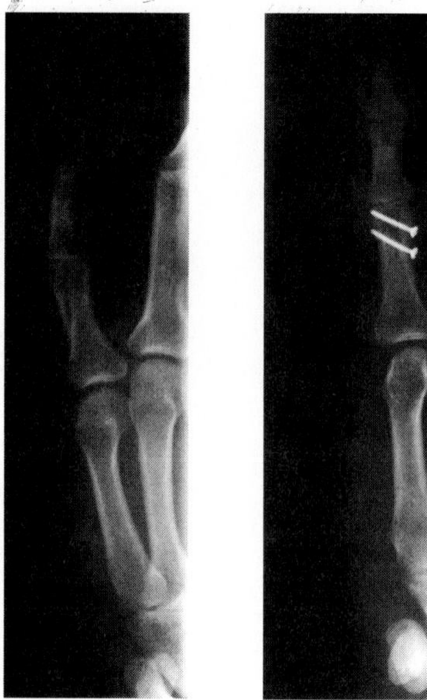

FIGURE 20-11 *(above, left)* Spiral oblique fracture of the proximal phalanx of the small finger. This is accompanied by shortening. The fracture is unstable.

FIGURE 20-12 *(above, right)* Fracture of the proximal phalanx treated with mini-lag screw fixation to restore length and alignment. A splint may be required for a few days after surgery to control swelling and pain. The patient should move the finger actively at will once the splint is removed.

External Fixation

Biomechanics: Stress-shielding device.

Mode of Bone Healing: Primary, unless a solid fixation is not achieved, in which case secondary healing also occurs.

Indications: This treatment is usually reserved for open or comminuted fractures that are not amenable to open reduction and internal fixation. It is not discussed further in this chapter.

Traction

Biomechanics: Stress-sharing device.

Mode of Bone Healing: Secondary, with callus formation.

Indications: Various types of traction have been used in the past, including skin and skeletal. However, many complications have arisen and therefore traction is not recommended. It is not discussed further in this chapter.

Special Considerations of the Fracture

Age

Elderly patients are at greater risk for development of joint stiffness secondary to the fracture and its treatment.

Articular Involvement

Fractures involving the articular surface require anatomic reduction to minimize subsequent decreased range of motion and degenerative changes. For comminuted fractures in which anatomic reduction cannot be achieved, early range-of-motion exercises are instituted to decrease the risk of stiffness.

Location

Diaphyseal proximal phalanx fractures usually have an apex that is palmer angulated secondary to an imbalance of muscle pull. The interosseous muscle inserts into the base of the proximal phalanx, and thereby flexes the proximal fracture fragment. The distal fracture fragment is then pulled into hyperextension by the central slip of the finger extensor tendon, which inserts on the base of the middle phalanx. This hyperextension is accentuated by the extrinsic muscles pulling on the extensor hood. This muscle imbalance leads to a loss of interphalangeal extension and secondary flexion contracture of the interphalangeal joints. These complications can be prevented by achieving skeletal realignment and maintaining the skeletal length.

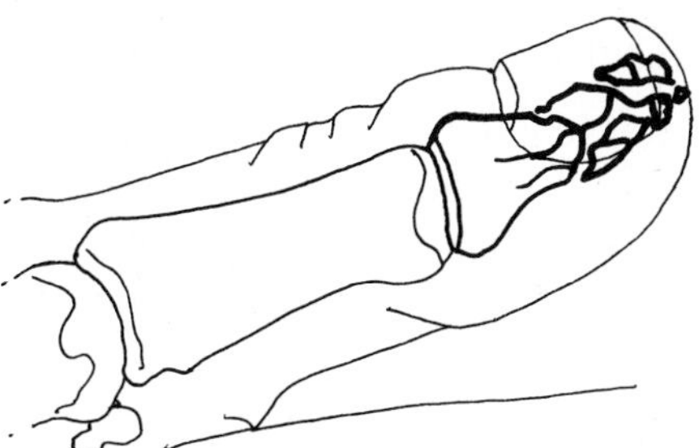

FIGURE 20-13 A tuft crush injury of the distal phalanx of the thumb. This is associated with nail bed laceration and subungual hematoma.

Associated Injury

Collateral Ligament Injury

This may occur from either the primary injury or treatment. The primary injury is usually due to partial avulsion of the volar plate from the middle phalanx. It is treated with buddy taping for 4 to 6 weeks or by splinting the proximal interphalangeal joint in 50 to 60 degrees of flexion for 2 to 3 weeks. Collateral ligament injuries to the second digit are usually surgically repaired, especially in young people, because they are usually accompanied by gross instability. Collateral ligament injury after treatment is usually secondary to improper immobilization. External plaster immobilization of the metacarpophalangeal joints must be maintained in 60 to 90 degrees of flexion to keep the collateral ligaments elongated. If the flexion is not maintained, the collateral ligaments will shorten during immobilization. This causes the patient difficulty in achieving adequate metacarpophalangeal joint flexion after the immobilization device is removed. Conversely, the interphalangeal joints must be maintained in relative extension (except in volar plate injuries, as described previously) to keep the collateral ligaments elongated. This prevents shortening of the collateral ligaments during immobilization, and prevents difficulty achieving interphalangeal joint extension after the immobilization device is removed.

Nail Bed Injury

Many distal phalanx fractures, especially tuft crush injuries, are associated with nail bed lacerations. If a subungual hematoma involves more than 25% of the nail bed, the nail should be removed and the hematoma evacuated. The nail bed should be repaired with absorbable suture (Figure 20-13).

Open Fracture

Any lacerations associated with phalangeal fractures should be considered open fractures, especially when a human bite injury is suspected. These should be treated with aggressive irrigation and débridement and with intravenous or oral antibiotics.

Mallet Fracture

Mallet fractures are distal interphalangeal joint flexion deformities secondary to loss of the extensor mechanism of the distal phalanx, due to either soft-tissue or bony injury. The treatment of soft-tissue interruptions or small avulsion fractures is closed splinting of the distal interphalangeal joint in hyperextension for 6 to 8 weeks. This is followed by night splinting for another 4 to 6 weeks. If the bony avulsion fracture is displaced more than 2 to 3 mm, or involves more than one third of the articular surface, open reduction and internal fixation of the extensor mechanism is recommended (Figure 20-14).

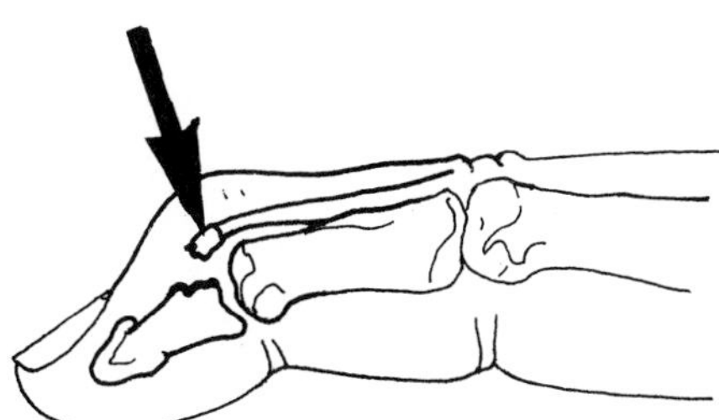

FIGURE 20-14 Mallet finger fracture. The extensor tendon avulses a fragment of bone from the proximal end of the proximal fragment, resulting in loss of extensor mechanism of the distal phalanx.

Rupture of the Flexor Digitorum Profundus Tendon

The flexor digitorum profundus tendon can be avulsed from the base of the distal phalanx, requiring open reduction and internal fixation of the avulsed tendon to achieve functional range of motion of the distal interphalangeal joint.

Boutonnière Deformity

This deformity results from disruption of the extensor mechanism, specifically from rupture of the central slip dorsally or a dorsal avulsion fracture from the base of the middle phalanx. This loss of effective extensor function at the proximal interphalangeal joint leads to volar displacement of the lateral bands. There is resulting flexion of the proximal interphalangeal joint with compensatory hyperextension of the distal interphalangeal joint. Acutely, this is treated by splinting the proximal interphalangeal joint in extension and allowing distal interphalangeal joint motion for 4 to 6 weeks. Occasionally, a boutonnière injury associated with a significantly displaced avulsion fracture requires open reduction and internal fixation (Figure 20-15).

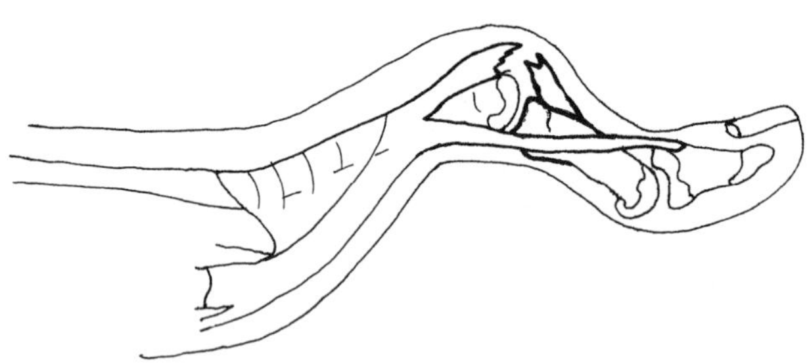

FIGURE 20-15 Boutonnière deformity. There is disruption of the extensor mechanism, with rupture of the central slip dorsally or a dorsal avulsion fracture from the base of the middle phalanx. This loss of extensor function at the proximal interphalangeal joint leads to volar displacement of the lateral bands, resulting in flexion of the proximal interphalangeal joint and compensatory hyperextension of the distal interphalangeal joint.

Proximal Interphalangeal Fracture/Dislocation

These are subdivided into three types. Type I is a hyperextension injury with volar plate avulsion but with a congruous articular surface remaining. Type II is a dorsal dislocation of the middle phalanx, where volar plate avulsion is accompanied by articular incongruity. Type III is an actual fracture/dislocation with either less than one third of the articular surface involved, leading to a stable situation after closed reduction, or greater than one third of the articular surface involved, leading to instability after closed reduction.

Types I and II and stable type III injuries require 4 to 6 weeks of immobilization with buddy taping (to allow early active range of motion) and a dorsal extension block splint in approximately 20 to 30 degrees of flexion (to prevent hyperextension). From 3 to 6 weeks, the extension block is gradually decreased to allow full range of motion by 6 weeks. Unstable type III fractures require open reduction and internal fixation of the articular fragment.

Weight Bearing

No weight should be borne on the involved digit. It should not be used for push-off or to grasp a cane or walker.

Gait

Arm swing in tandem with the opposite extremity usually is not affected, unless an arm sling is used for extremity elevation during the initial stage of treatment.

TREATMENT

Treatment: Early to Immediate (Day of Injury to One Week)

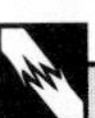

BONE HEALING

Stability at fracture site: None.

Stage of bone healing: Inflammatory phase. The fracture hematoma is colonized by inflammatory cells, and débridement of the fracture begins.

X-ray: No callus; fracture line is visible.

Orthopaedic and Rehabilitation Considerations

Physical Examination

Pay special attention to complaints of pain, paresthesia, and cast discomfort as indicators of compartment syndrome, although this is rare with phalangeal fractures. Check for swelling; if noted, instruct the patient to elevate the extremity and perform retrograde massage (milk the edema from the fingertip toward the palm). Check for any rotational or angulatory deformity of the digit, which is not acceptable and requires realignment and placement of fixation devices as needed.

Dangers

The patient should be warned of the possibility of stiffness and the residual loss of grip strength, as well as possible degenerative changes if the injury involves an articular surface. Also, the patient should be informed that tuft fractures are notorious for long-term residual pain, despite clinical union. In addition, the patient should be informed of the possibility of prolonged swelling and the development of reflex sympathetic dystrophy.

Radiography

Check radiographs for loss of correction. No rotational or angulatory deformity is acceptable because this may impair the extensor and flexor mechanisms.

Weight Bearing

The patient should not bear weight on the involved digit. It should not be used for push-off or to grasp a cane or walker.

Range of Motion

For all stable fractures amenable to buddy taping, full active range of motion is encouraged. For unstable fractures requiring splints or operative fixation, no range of motion of the splinted joints is allowed at this stage. Active range of motion of the nonsplinted joints of the affected digit, as well as all other digits and the ipsilateral wrist, elbow, and shoulder, is encouraged to prevent stiffness.

Muscle Strength

The patient can perform isometric exercises of abduction, adduction, flexion, and extension with the nonsplinted fingers to maintain intrinsic muscle strength.

Functional Activities

The patient is instructed in using the uninvolved hand for self-care, hygiene, feeding, grooming, and dressing. The patient should don clothes on the involved arm first and doff clothes from the uninvolved arm first.

Methods of Treatment: Specific Aspects

Buddy Taping

Make sure there is adequate padding and no skin maceration between the fractured and adjacent digit. To prevent skin maceration and possible secondary infection, the patient is instructed to change the tape and padding at least twice a week. Evaluate the active range of motion of the affected digit.

Cast/Splint

Trim the cast to allow visualization of the tip of the injured digit to evaluate capillary refill. Check the cast padding and cast edges and evaluate for any skin breakdown at the edges. Check for any cast/splint softening and repair as needed. The patient may perform isometric exercises of the flexors, extensors, and ulnar and radial deviators of the wrist within the cast.

Closed Reduction and Percutaneous Pinning

Evaluate the pin or wound sites for drainage, erythema or skin tenting. Instruct the patient in proper pin care. Clean the pin sites with peroxide-soaked or povidine–iodine-applied swabs as needed. If pin sites appear infected, give the patient oral antibiotics or admit the patient for intravenous antibiotics and possible débridement, depending on the severity. Release any skin tenting. Pay special attention to complaints of pain, paresthesia, or pin discomfort because these could indicate a skewed nerve or tendon.

Prescription

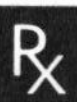

DAY ONE TO ONE WEEK

Precautions No range of motion to the digit if the *fracture is unstable.*

Range of Motion Active range of motion to the unaffected digits and to the fractured digit if the fracture is stable.

Muscle Strength Isometric exercises to the intrinsic muscles of the nonsplinted fingers.

Functional Activities The uninvolved extremity used for self-care and personal hygiene.

Weight Bearing None.

Treatment: Two Weeks

BONE HEALING

Stability at fracture site: None to minimal.

Stage of bone healing: Beginning of reparative phase. Osteoprogenitor cells differentiate into osteoblasts that lay down woven bone.

X-ray: None to early callus; fracture line is visible.

Orthopaedic and Rehabilitation Considerations

Physical Examination

Check for any rotational or angulatory deformity of the affected digit, which requires realignment and the placement of fixation devices as needed. Check for swelling and the range of motion of the nonsplinted digits, applying retrograde massage and aggressive range-of-motion exercises as needed.

Dangers

If the fracture is splinted across the wrist, make sure that the splint maintains the metacarpophalangeal joints in 60 to 90 degrees of flexion and the interphalangeal joints relatively extended to reduce the collateral ligament shortening during immobilization. Collateral ligament shortening results in decreased range of motion of the affected digits.

Radiography

Check radiographs for loss of correction. No degree of angulatory or rotational deformity is acceptable.

Weight Bearing

The patient should not bear weight on the involved digit.

Range of Motion

Full active range of motion is encouraged in all buddy-taped digits. In injuries requiring splinting, active range of motion is encouraged to all nonsplinted joints of the affected digit, as well as all other digits and the wrist, elbow, and shoulder.

Muscle Strength

Continue isometric exercises of the intrinsic muscles of the nonsplinted digits. Continue isometric exercises of the ulnar and radial deviators, flexors, and extensors within the cast.

Functional Activities

The patient continues to use the uninvolved hand for self-care.

Methods of Treatment: Specific Aspects

Buddy Taping

Check that adequate padding lies between the fractured digit and the adjacent digit and ensure the skin between them is not macerated. The tape and padding should be changed at least twice a week. Evaluate the active range of motion of the affected digit.

Cast/Splint

Trim the cast to allow visualization of the tip of the injured digit to evaluate capillary refill. Check the cast padding and cast edges and evaluate for any skin breakdown at the edges. Check for any cast/splint softening and repair as needed. Continue performing isometric exercises to the ulnar and radial deviators, flexors and extensors within the cast.

Closed Reduction and Percutaneous Pinning

Evaluate the pin or wound sites for drainage, erythema, or skin tenting and treat appropriately. Pay special attention to complaints of pain, paresthesia, or pin discomfort because these could indicate a skewed nerve or tendon.

Prescription

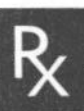

TWO WEEKS

Precautions No range of motion to the splinted joint.

Range of Motion Active range of motion to all nonsplinted joints and digits.

Muscle Strength Isometric strengthening exercises to the intrinsic muscles.

Functional Activities The uninvolved extremity used for self- care.

Weight bearing None.

Treatment: Four to Six Weeks

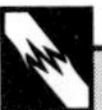

BONE HEALING

Stability at fracture site: With bridging callus the fracture is usually stable; confirm with physical examination.

Stage of bone healing: Reparative phase. Further organization of the callus and formation of lamellar bone begins. However, the strength of the callus, especially with torsional load, is significantly lower than that of lamellar bone. It may require further protection of bone (if not further immobilization) to avoid refracture.

X-ray: Bridging callus is visible. With increased rigidity, less bridging callus is noted, and healing with endosteal callus predominates. Fracture line is less distinct.

Orthopaedic and Rehabilitation Considerations

Physical Examination

Most phalangeal fractures require 3 to 4 weeks of buddy taping or immobilization. Examination at this stage is performed out of the splint, if one was used. Check the affected phalanx for stability and tenderness and the entire digit for range of motion.

Dangers

Any trophic changes or pain and tenderness out of proportion to the stage of fracture healing may signify reflex sympathetic dystrophy, which requires aggressive occupational therapy.

Radiography

Radiographs should be taken without any external immobilization device in place. Check radiographs for correction. Look for callus and the disappearance of the fracture line; these usually lag behind clinical healing and may not be radiographically observed for 10 to 12 weeks.

Weight Bearing

The affected digit can begin progressively to bear weight, as tolerated.

Range of Motion

If there is no tenderness or motion at the fracture site, full active range of motion to all digits is instituted. Hydrotherapy can be used to aid joint mobilization while reducing pain. Active-assistive and passive range-of-motion exercises can begin on the affected digit at 6 weeks. Continue the rest of the range-of-motion exercises to other digits, wrist, and elbow.

Muscle Strength

Emphasis is placed on improving grip and grasp. The patient is instructed in gentle ball-squeezing and Silly Putty exercises to reestablish the flexor strength of the digits and improve interphalangeal joint motion. Continue isometric exercises as before. Isotonic exercises of the intrinsic musculature, flexors, and extensors of the digits and wrist also aid in improving the range of motion.

Functional Activities

The patient is encouraged to resume bimanual activities, using the involved extremity for self-care, hygiene, feeding, grooming, and dressing.

Methods of Treatment: Specific Aspects

Buddy Taping

If there is no tenderness or motion at the fracture site, remove the buddy tape. If tenderness or motion is present at the fracture site, reapply the buddy tape.

Cast/Splint

If there is no tenderness or motion at the fracture site, remove the cast. Protective splinting or buddy taping for 1 to 2 additional weeks may be considered if the patient is unreliable or if further support is needed. Night splinting may also be helpful, especially after aggressive rehabilitation exercises have begun.

If tenderness or motion is present at the fracture site, the splint or cast can be replaced. Often, however, a removable splint or buddy taping is used to allow gentle active range-of-motion exercises and avoid future mobility deficits. Because of prolonged immobilization, range of motion of the digits and wrist may be limited. Active-assistive range-of-motion exercises are initiated to improve the range. Hydrotherapy or fluidotherapy may be quite helpful in decreasing the discomfort. The patient should be evaluated at 2-week intervals until stability of the fracture is noted, signifying that more aggressive rehabilitation and less splinting are necessary.

Closed Reduction and Percutaneous Pinning

Pins are usually removed at 3 to 4 weeks. After pin removal, continue casting or splinting for 1 to 2 weeks. Subsequently, a removable splint or buddy taping is used to allow for gentle active range-of-motion exercises to limit future mobility deficits. The splinting or buddy taping is continued until there is no tenderness or motion at the fracture site. Night splinting may be helpful after this, especially after aggressive rehabilitation exercises have begun.

Prescription

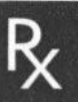

Four to Six Weeks

Precautions No passive range of motion to the affected joint.

Range of Motion Full active and active-assistive range of motion to all digits.

Muscle Strength Isometric and isotonic exercises to the flexors, extensors, abductors, and adductors of the digit.

Functional Activities Bimanual activities using the involved extremity are encouraged for self-care.

Weight bearing Weight bearing as tolerated by the patient.

Treatment: Six to Eight Weeks

Bone Healing

Stability at fracture site: With bridging callus, the fracture is usually stable. However, the strength of this callus, especially with torsional load, is significantly lower than that of normal lamellar bone. Confirm with physical examination.

Stage of bone healing: Reparative phase. Further organization of the callus and formation of lamellar bone begins.

X-ray: Bridging callus is visible. With increased rigidity, less bridging callus is noted, and healing with endosteal callus predominates. Fracture line is less distinct.

Orthopaedic and Rehabilitation Considerations

Physical Examination

Check the affected phalanx for stability and tenderness and the entire digit for range of motion. Pay special attention to the patient's comments on his or her activity level or any functional disabilities, especially decreased grip strength.

Dangers

Check for the resolution of reflex sympathetic dystrophy.

Radiography

Check radiographs for callus and the disappearance of the fracture line. Evaluate for malunion (any angulatory or rotational deformity), delayed union and nonunion. Note that radiographic healing usually lags behind clinical healing, and it is not absolutely necessary to obtain radiographs if the fracture is clinically stable.

Weight Bearing

The affected digit can be used for weight bearing, as tolerated.

Range of Motion

Active, active-assisted, and passive range of motion of all digits is encouraged, with hydrotherapy used to aid joint mobilization. Most patients should now have full range of motion of the affected digit. If the patient is treated with casting or splint, active-assistive to passive range of motion is prescribed.

Muscle Strength

Continue resistive exercises to the digits. The patient offers resistance to flexion, extension, abduction, and adduction using his or her uninvolved hand. The patient should continue ball-squeezing and Silly Putty exercises to improve grip strength.

Functional Activities

The patient uses the affected extremity for all activities.

Methods of Treatment: Specific Aspects

Buddy Taping

The taping should be removed if this has not already been done. Examine for tenderness and motion at the fracture site.

Cast/Splint

Remove the splint, if this has not already been done. Examine for tenderness and motion at the fracture site. Night splinting or buddy taping may still be useful while aggressive rehabilitation exercises are performed as described previously.

Closed Reduction and Percutaneous Pinning

Remove the splint, if this has not already been done. Examine for tenderness and motion at the fracture site. Night splinting or buddy taping may still be useful while aggressive rehabilitation exercises are performed as described previously.

Prescription

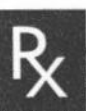

SIX TO EIGHT WEEKS

Precautions Night splint is used if necessary.

Range of Motion Active, active-assistive, and passive range of motion to all digits.

Muscle Strength Gentle resistive exercises to all digits.

Functional Activities The involved extremity is used for self-care.

Weight Bearing Full weight bearing.

Treatment: Eight to Twelve Weeks

BONE HEALING

Stability at fracture site: Stable.

Stage of bone healing: Remodeling phase. Woven bone is replaced with lamellar bone. The process of remodeling takes months to years for completion.

X-ray: Abundant callus is seen, and the fracture line begins to disappear; there is reconstitution of the medullary canal. Metaphyseal areas do not produce as much callus as diaphyseal regions.

Orthopaedic and Rehabilitation Considerations

Physical Examination

A patient who was nontender with full range of motion, and had evidence of fracture healing on previous examination does not need to be seen at this time. All others should be seen, and the digit should be checked for tenderness and range of motion.

Dangers

Check for the resolution of reflex sympathetic dystrophy.

Radiography

Check radiographs for callus and the disappearance of the fracture line. Evaluate for malunion, delayed union, and nonunion.

Weight Bearing

The affected digit can be used for weight bearing.

Range of Motion

The patient should now have full range of motion of the affected digit.

Muscle Strength

The affected muscles are all strengthened with resistive exercises. Resistive exercises to the digits and wrist can continue with increasing weights to offer resistance.

Functional Activities

The patient uses the affected extremity for all activities.

Prescription

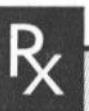

EIGHT TO TWELVE WEEKS

Precautions None.

Range of Motion Full active and passive range of motion to all digits.

Muscle Strength Progressive resistive exercises to all digits with increasing weights.

Functional Activities The affected extremity used for self-care.

Weight Bearing Full weight bearing.

LONG-TERM CONSIDERATIONS AND PROBLEMS

The patient needs to be warned about possible future degenerative joint disease (an increased risk with intraarticular fractures), decreased range of motion, residual deformity, decreased grip strength, and prolonged swelling secondary to injury.

The patient should be informed that to limit residual stiffness, motion is begun before complete bony union, which places the fracture at risk of displacing or losing its proper alignment.

IMMEDIATE TO ONE WEEK

	Buddy Taping	*Splint*	*Closed Reduction and Percutaneous Pinning*
Stability	None.	None.	None.
Orthopaedics	Evaluate for adequate padding and any skin maceration.	Trim splint to allow visualization of the tip of the injured digit and the adjacent buddy-taped digit.	Evaluate pin sites and tendon function as well as any open wounds. If splinted, trim splint to allow proper visualization of the tip of the injured digit and adjacent buddy-taped digit.
Rehabilitation	Active range of motion of the affected and taped digits is encouraged. Active range of motion of all nontaped digits as well as the ipsilateral wrist, elbow, and shoulder is also encouraged. Isometric exercises to all nontaped digits. The involved digit is non-weight bearing.	No range of motion of the splinted joints is allowed. Active range of motion of all nonsplinted joints on the affected digits as well as all other digits and the ipsilateral wrist, elbow, and shoulder is encouraged. Isometric exercises to all nonsplinted digits. The involved digit is non-weight bearing.	No range of motion of the pinned/splinted joints is allowed. Active range of motion of all nonsplinted joints on the affected digits as well as all other digits and the ipsilateral wrist, elbow, and shoulder is encouraged. Isometric exercises to all nonsplinted digits. The involved digit is non-weight bearing.

TWO WEEKS			
	Buddy Taping	*Splint*	*Closed Reduction and Percutaneous Pinning*
Stability	None to minimal.	None to minimal.	None to minimal.
Orthopaedics	Evaluate for adequate padding and any skin maceration.	Trim splint to allow visualization of the tip of the injured digit and the adjacent buddy-taped digit.	Evaluate pin sites and tendon function as well as any open wounds. If splinted, trim splint to allow proper visualization of the tip of the injured digit and adjacent buddy-taped digit.
Rehabilitation	Active range of motion of all digits as well as ipsilateral wrist, elbow, and shoulder is continued. Isometric exercises to all nontaped digits and the wrist. The involved digit is non-weight bearing.	No range of motion of the splinted joints is allowed. Active range of motion of all nonsplinted joints on the affected digits as well as all other digits and the ipsilateral wrist, elbow, and shoulder. Isometric exercises to all nonsplinted digits and the wrist are continued. The involved digit is non-weight bearing.	Same as for splint.

FOUR TO SIX WEEKS			
	Buddy Taping	*Splint*	*Closed Reduction and Percutaneous Pinning*
Stability	Partial to complete.	Partial to complete.	Partial to complete.
Orthopaedics	If nontender with no motion at fracture site, discontinue buddy taping.	If nontender with no motion at fracture site, discontinue splint.	Pins are removed, and splint or buddy taping can be applied for additional 1 to 2 weeks.
Rehabilitation	Active range of motion of all digits as well as ipsilateral wrist, elbow, and shoulder is continued. Active-assisted and passive range-of-motion exercises can begin on the affected digit at 6 weeks. Digit flexor strengthening is encouraged. Affected digit can begin progressively to bear weight.	Active range of motion to the affected joint begins. Active range of motion of all unaffected joints on the affected digits as well as all other digits and the ipsilateral wrist, elbow, and shoulder is continued. Digit flexor strengthening is encouraged. Affected digit can begin progressively to bear weight.	Same as for splint.

SIX TO EIGHT WEEKS			
	Buddy Taping	***Splint***	***Closed Reduction and Percutaneous Pinning***
Stability	Stable.	Stable.	Stable.
Orthopaedics	Discontinue taping.	Discontinue splint.	Discontinue splint.
Rehabilitation	Active, active-assisted, and passive range of motion of all digits as well as ipsilateral wrist, elbow, and shoulder is encouraged. Resistive exercises to the digit are continued. Weight bearing on the affected digit is allowed.	Same as for buddy taping.	Same as for buddy taping.

EIGHT TO TWELVE WEEKS			
	Buddy Taping	***Splint***	***Closed Reduction and Percutaneous Pinning***
Stability	Stable.	Stable.	Stable.
Orthopaedics	No taping needed.	No splint needed.	No splint needed.
Rehabilitation	Full range-of-motion and progressive resistive exercises with increasing weights are prescribed.	Same as buddy taping.	Same as buddy taping.

BIBLIOGRAPHY

Abouna JM, Brown H. The treatment of mallet finger: the results in a series of 148 consecutive cases and a review of the literature. *Br J Surg*, 55:653–667, 1968.

Belsky MR, Eaton RG, Lane LB. Closed reduction and internal fixation of proximal phalangeal fractures. *J Hand Surg [Am]*, 9: 725–729, 1984.

DaCruz DJ, Slade RJ, Malone W. Fractures of the distal phalanges. *J Hand Surg [Br]*, 13:350–352, 1988.

Diwaker HN, Stothard J. The role of internal fixation in closed fractures of the proximal phalanges and metacarpals in adults. *J Hand Surg [Br]*, 11:103–108, 1986.

Green DP, Rowland SA. Fractures and dislocations in the hand. In: Rockwood CA Jr, Green DP, Bucholz RW, eds. *Fractures in Adults*, Vol 1, 3rd ed. Philadelphia: J.B. Lippincott, 1991, pp. 441–484.

Hall RF. Treatment of metacarpal and phalangeal fractures in noncompliant patients. *Clin Orthop*, 214:31–36, 1987.

Hastings H II, Carroll C IV. Treatment of closed articular fractures of the metacarpophalangeal and proximal interphalangeal joints. *Hand Clin*, 4:503–528, 1988.

Jupiter JB, Belsky MR. Fractures and dislocations of the hand. In: Browner BD, Jupiter JB, Levine AM, Trafton PG, eds. *Skeletal Trauma*, Vol 2. Philadelphia: W.B. Saunders, 1992, pp. 925–949, 976–1014.

McCue FC, Abbott JL. The treatment of mallet finger and boutonierre deformities. *Virginia Medical*, 94:623–628, 1967.

Melone CP. Rigid fixation of phalangeal and metacarpal fractures. *Orthop Clin North Am*, 17:421–435, 1986.

Reyes FA, Latta LL. Conservative management of difficult phalangeal fractures. *Clin Orthop*, 214:23–30, 1987.

Ruggeri S, Osterman AL, Bora FW. Stabilization of metacarpal and phalangeal fractures in the hand. *Orthop Rev*, 9:107–110, 1980.

Stern PJ. Fractures of the metacarpals and phalanges. In: Green DP, ed. *Operative Hand Surgery*, Vol 1. New York: Churchill Livingstone, 1993, pp. 695–758.

Wright TA. Early mobilization in fractures of the metacarpals and phalanges. *Can J Surg*, 11:491–498, 1968.

CHAPTER Twenty-one

Femoral Neck Fractures

KENNETH W. TAYLOR, MD

VASANTHA L. MURTHY, MD

INTRODUCTION

Definition

A femoral neck fracture is a fracture occurring proximal to the intertrochanteric line in the intracapsular region of the hip (Figures 21-1A, 21-1B, 21-1C, 21-1D, 21-2, and 21-3).

Mechanism of Injury

Most femoral neck fractures in the elderly are spontaneous or caused by low-energy trauma. This population is subject to senile osteoporosis (type II), which causes weakness in both the cortical and trabecular bone of the femoral neck and predisposes it to fracture. In younger patients, high-energy trauma is necessary

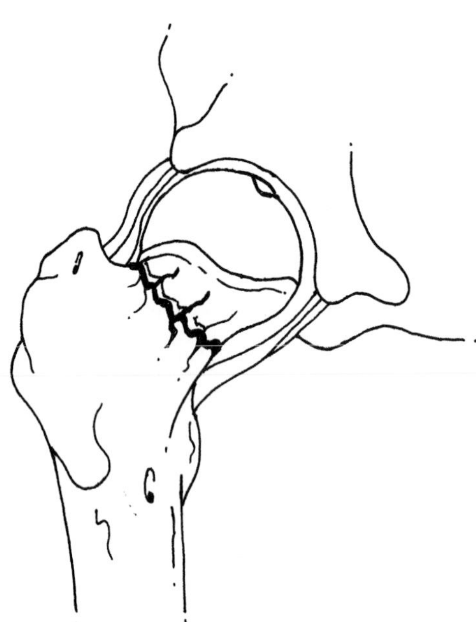

FIGURE 21-1A Femoral neck fracture classified as Garden's type 1: an incomplete impacted femoral neck fracture in valgus position. All femoral neck fractures are intracapsular.

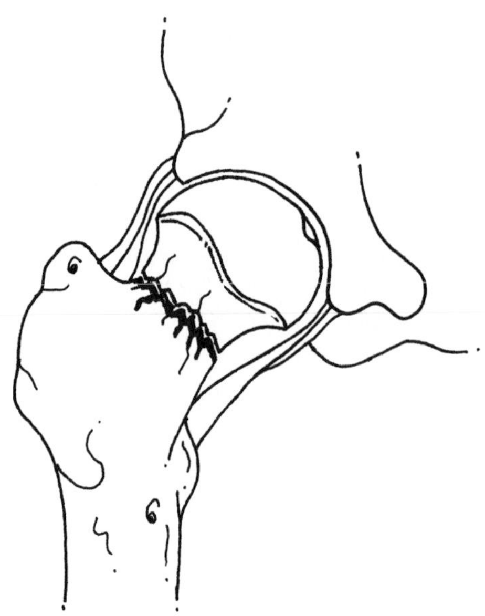

FIGURE 21-1B Garden's type 2: nondisplaced complete femoral neck fracture.

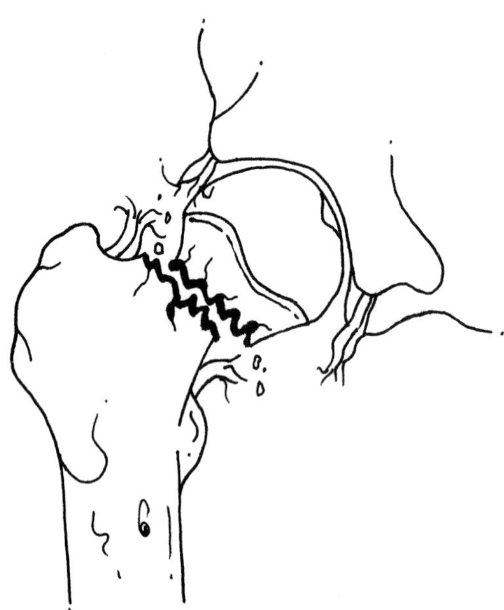

FIGURE 21-1C Garden's type 3: displaced femoral neck fracture in varus position. There is often disruption of the joint capsule.

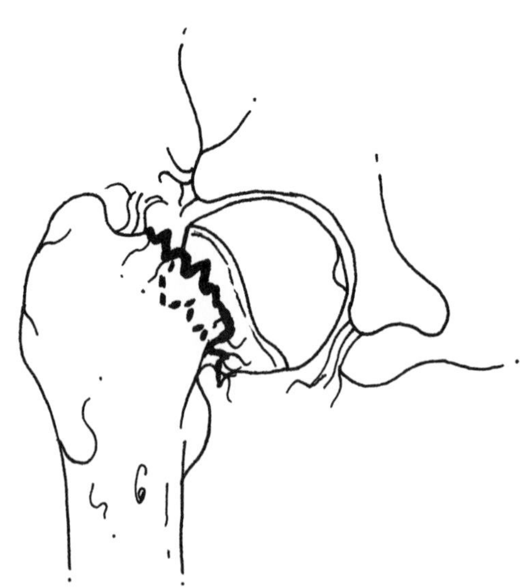

FIGURE 21-1D Garden's type 4: completely displaced femoral neck fracture. It has the poorest prognosis. The femoral head may go on to avascular necrosis. In older patients, this fracture is usually treated with a endoprosthesis (*see* Figure 21-6).

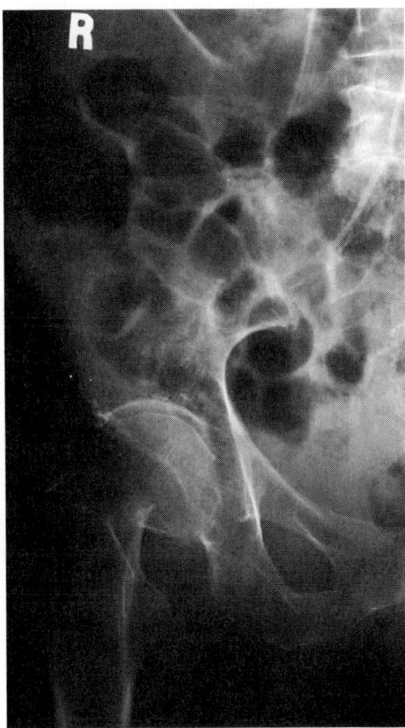

FIGURE 21-2 Subcapital femoral neck fracture at the proximal end of the neck. This fracture is displaced and in varus position (Garden's type 3).

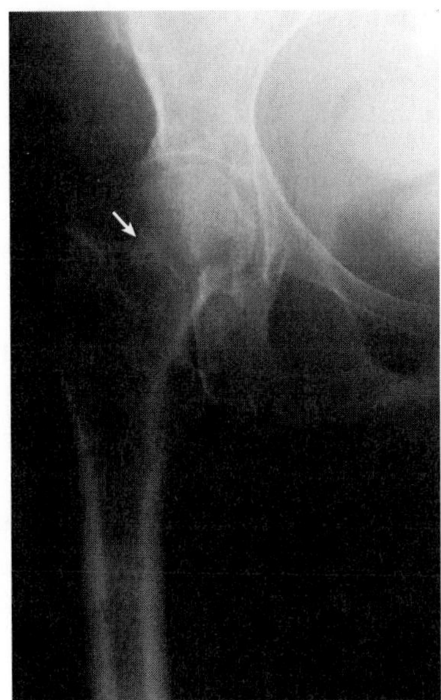

FIGURE 21-3 Subcapital fracture of the femoral neck impacted and in valgus position (Garden's type 1).

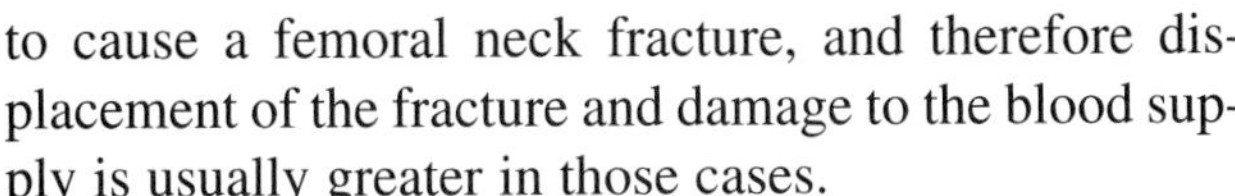

to cause a femoral neck fracture, and therefore displacement of the fracture and damage to the blood supply is usually greater in those cases.

Treatment Goals

Orthopaedic Objectives

Alignment

Restore fragments to their correct anatomic position for unstable hip fractures. Maintain alignment in nondisplaced or impacted stable fractures. Satisfactory alignment after reduction of an unstable fracture should have no more than 15 degrees of valgus and 10 degrees of anterior posterior angulation.

Stability

Compress the fracture fragments with lag screws to restore cortical and cancellous contact (*see* Figure 21-4). Replace the femoral head in the elderly patient with an unstable fracture to achieve immediate stability (Figures 21-3A, 21-3B, and 21-3C).

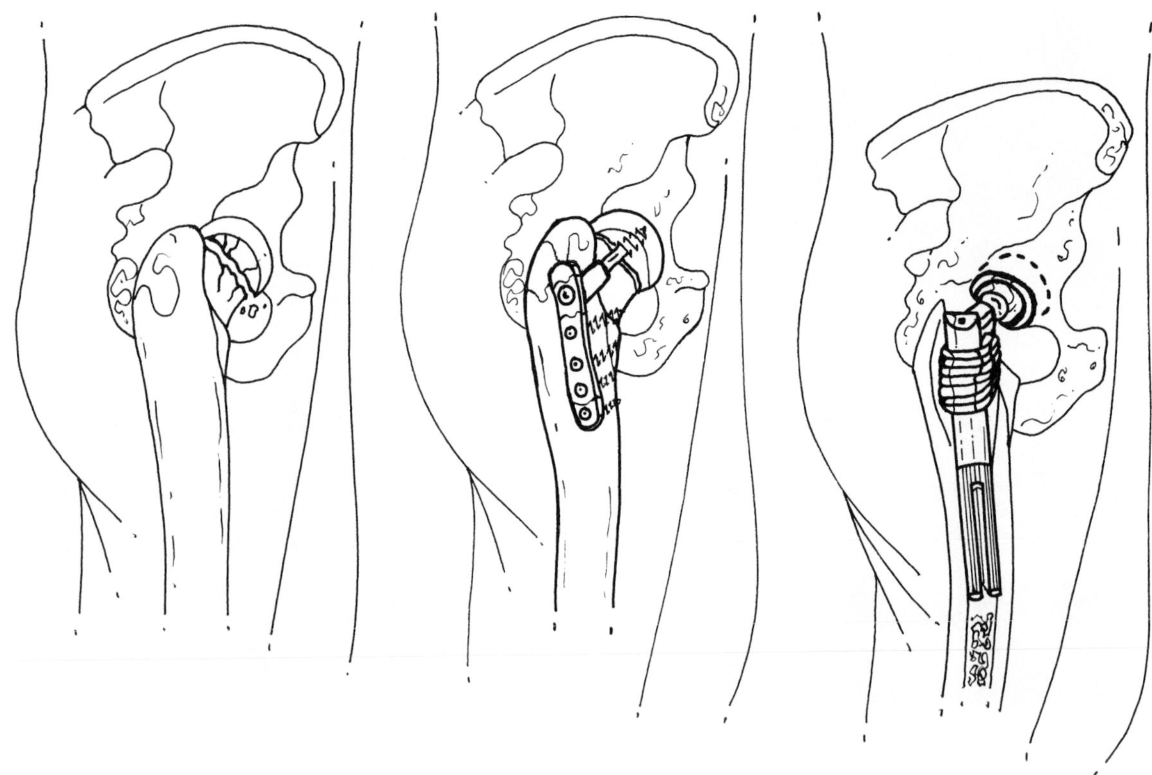

FIGURE 21-3A *(above, left)* Subcapital fracture of the femoral neck.

FIGURE 21-3B *(above, middle)* Fracture fixed with a screw and side plate to compress the fracture in an attempt to restore cortical and cancellous contact.

FIGURE 21-3C *(above, right)* To achieve immediate stability, the femoral head and neck are replaced in an elderly patient with an unstable fracture.

Rehabilitation Objectives

Range of Motion

Improve and restore range of motion of the knee and hip (Table 21-1).

TABLE 21-1 *Range of Motion of Knee and Hip*

Motion	Normal	Functional
Knee		
Flexion	130–140°	110°
Extension	0°[a]	0°[a]
Hip		
Flexion	125–128°	90–110°
Extension	0–20°	0–5°
Abduction	45–48°	0–20°
Adduction	40–45°	0–20°
Internal rotation	40–45°	0–20°
External rotation	45°	0–15°

[a]"Zero" indicates measurement from neutral position.

Muscle Strength

Improve the strength of the muscles that are affected by the fracture.

Gluteus medius: hip abductor, most important for post-operative stability.
Iliopsoas: hip flexor.
Gluteus maximus: hip extensor.
Adductor magnus, longus, and brevis: hip adductors.
Quadriceps: knee extensor, especially the lateralis, because it is exposed during surgery.
Hamstrings: knee flexor (two-jointed muscle). Assists in hip extension.

Functional Goals

Normalize the patient's gait pattern. Achieve 90 degrees hip flexion for proper sitting position.

Expected Time of Bone Healing

Twelve to 16 weeks.

Expected Duration of Rehabilitation

Fifteen to 30 weeks.

Methods of Treatment

Closed or Open Reduction and Internal Fixation

Biomechanics: Stress-sharing device.

Mode of Bone Healing: Primary in nondisplaced, impacted, or anatomically reduced fractures.

Indications: Fractures that are impacted, nondisplaced, or adequately reduced in patients younger than 65 years of age should be internally fixed (*in situ*) with multiple parallel cannulated screws or pins. A compression screw and side plate and an additional antirotation screw may be used for basicervical fractures (to prevent the loose head from spinning on the screw) that have a comminuted lateral cortex or severe osteoporosis (Figures 21-4 and 21-5).

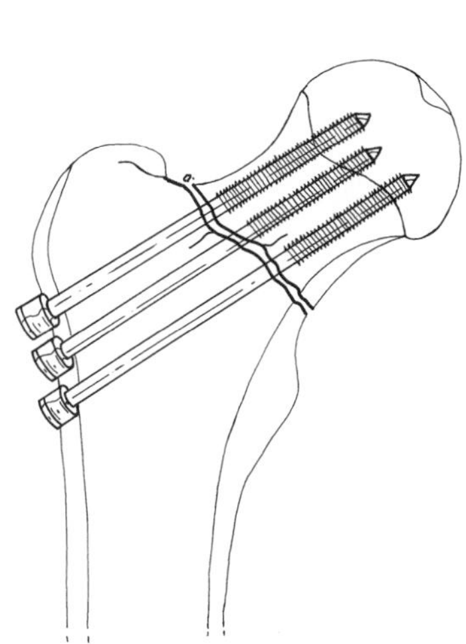

FIGURE 21-4 Multiple parallel cannulated screws for internal fixation of a Garden's type 1 fracture. Fractures that are adequately reduced in patients younger than 65 years of age are treated with internal fixation *in situ*.

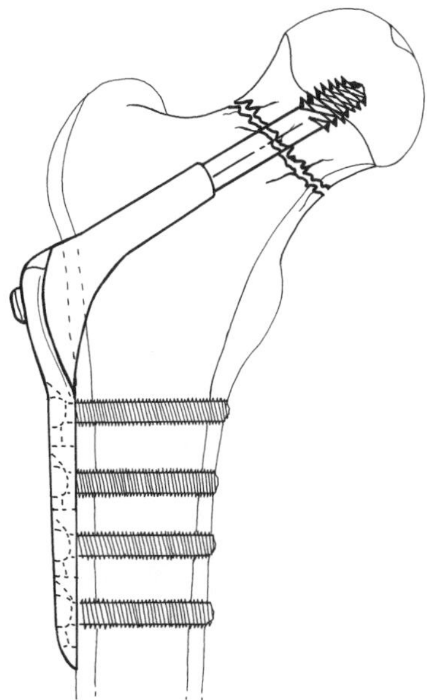

FIGURE 21-5 Compression screw and slide fixation. This is an alternative to multiple parallel cannulated screws. An additional proximal antirotational screw may be used to prevent the loose head from spinning on the screw.

Prosthetic Replacement of the Femoral Head

Biomechanics: Stress-bearing device.

Mode of Bone Healing: None.

Indications: A fixed unipolar (Austin-Moore or Thompson type) or bipolar endoprosthesis may be used to treat an unstable displaced fracture when a satisfactory reduction cannot be achieved and the patient is older than 65 years of age. Other indications include cases in which rheumatoid, degenerative, or malignant disease has caused preexisting articular damage (Figures 21-6, 21-7, and 21-8).

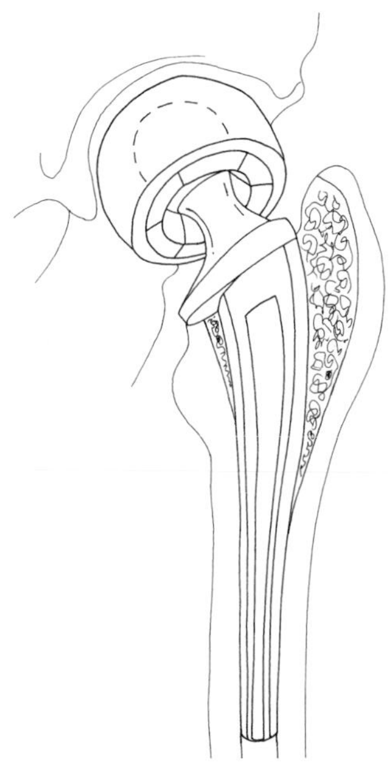

FIGURE 21-6 Bipolar endoprosthesis for treatment of an unstable displaced femoral neck fracture. This is frequently used in patients older than 65 years of age when satisfactory reduction cannot be achieved.

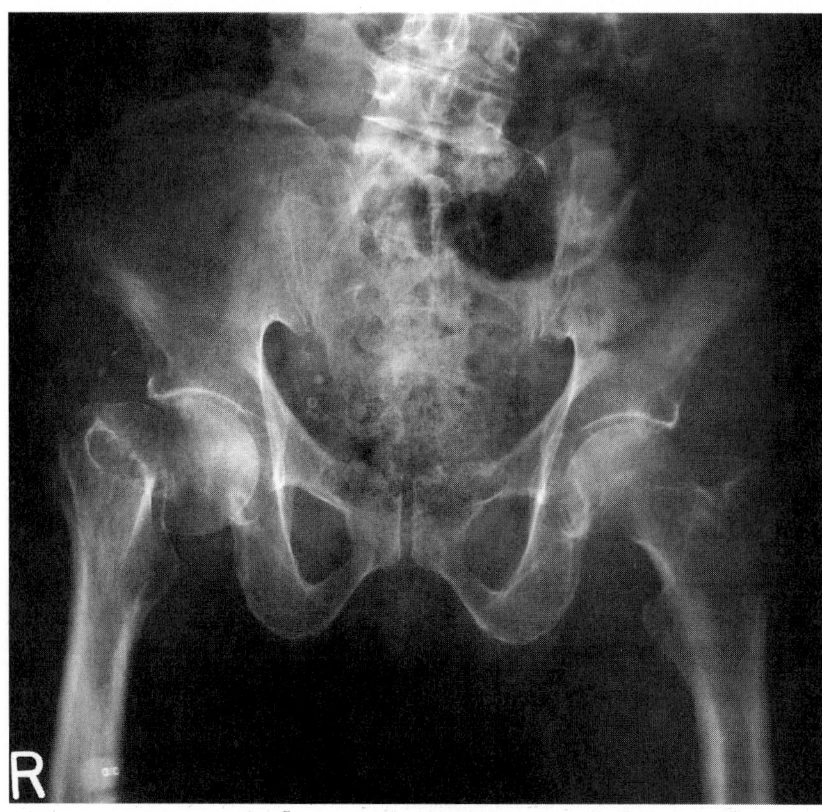

FIGURE 21-7 Garden's type 4: femoral neck fracture, completely displaced, in an older patient.

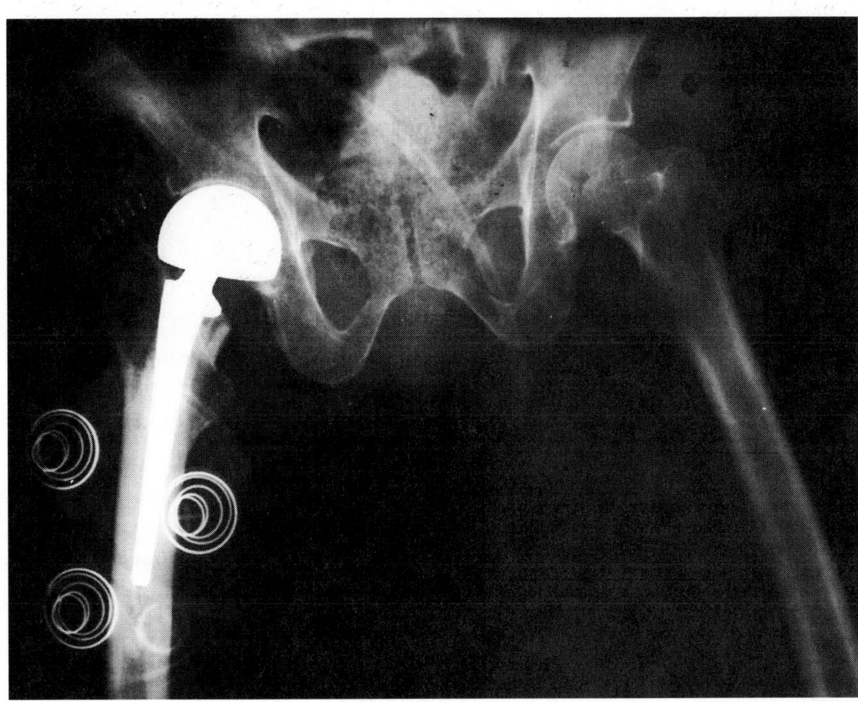

FIGURE 21-8 Bipolar endoprosthesis replacement of the fractured femoral neck during the immediate postoperative period. Note the drains and staples in place.

Special Considerations of the Fracture

These fractures have a high rate of nonunion and avascular necrosis because of the disruption of the blood supply to the femoral head. There is no periosteum in this area, and therefore all healing occurs through the endosteum. In addition, the fracture is bathed in synovial fluid, which dissolves the fibrin clot formed at the fracture site and retards healing.

Thromboembolic disease is a risk for all patients. Venous pooling may occur before surgery in patients whose surgery is delayed and may also occur after surgery in patients who are not rapidly mobilized and ambulated. Symptoms of pulmonary embolism include sudden chest pain and shortness of breath. The use of pneumatic and elastic stockings when patients are immobile, combined with early mobilization, helps reduce the risk of this condition.

Associated Injury

In osteopenic patients, fractures of the wrist, shoulder, and ribs may occur in a fall that causes a femoral neck fracture.

Weight Bearing

Weight bearing varies with the stability of the reduction achieved and the method of fixation. All patients should begin early mobilization out of bed and ambulation with an appropriate degree of weight on the affected extremity with a walker (see Figures 7-11, 7-12, and 7-13).

Stable fractures (nondisplaced or impacted) may be weight bearing as tolerated after they are pinned. (Some surgeons prefer to use toe touch or partial weight bearing.)

Unstable fractures (those requiring reduction or manipulation) are usually kept non-weight bearing after surgery. This is also done for patients with severe osteopenia.

Gait

Serial evaluation of leg length must be performed and shoe lift prescribed for the rare case of a significant leg-length discrepancy of greater than 3/4 inch. A progressive leg-length discrepancy after stabilization of the fracture may represent loss of correction of the fracture.

Stance Phase

The stance phase constitutes 60% of the gait cycle.

Heel Strike

The *gluteus maximus* is a strong hip extensor. It prevents jackknifing at the hip on heel strike and acts as a hip stabilizer. Because it crosses the fracture site, the muscle may be weakened and, on rare occasions, may cause a gluteus maximus lurch. If the posterior approach is used, the lower half of the muscle is incised. The *vastus lateralis* contracts concentrically (shortens) to achieve full knee extension at heel strike. It is partially incised proximally for nail and plating. This may weaken the muscle and full knee extension may not be achieved at heel strike because of weakness and pain (*see* Figure 6-1).

Foot-Flat

The *quadriceps* muscle goes through eccentric contraction (elongation) to control knee flexion in a smooth fashion from heel strike to foot-flat. The knee is flexed throughout the rest of the gait cycle. The *rectus femoris* is a two-jointed muscle that crosses the hip and knee joints. It may shorten with immobilization. This may cause a flexion contracture of the hip or decrease knee flexion. The *vastus lateralis* is partially incised during surgical approach, and retraction during surgery may weaken the muscle. This may shorten the foot-flat phase. Because of muscle injury, gait may be painful when the vastus lateralis contracts (*see* Figure 6-2).

Mid-Stance

Weight bearing at the fracture site is increased as double stance diminishes and ends. This increase in stress may be painful and cause an antalgic (painful) gait.

The *iliopsoas* muscle contracts to flex the hip and advance the limb during forward propulsion and allows the pelvis to rotate over the femur for limb advancement. The iliopsoas crosses the fracture site and may be weakened. The patient may take short steps to decrease the excursion of the muscle. The *gluteus medius* may be slightly weakened because it crosses the fracture site. This muscle stabilizes the pelvis against the femur to prevent Trendelenburg gait.

The hip abductors are responsible for controlling pelvic tilt during mid-stance. In fractures that are treated by endoprostheses, the length of the femoral neck must be restored or the pull of the gluteus medius will be weakened and lead to a Trendelenburg gait on the affected side. Abduction must be evaluated and strengthened as necessary (*see* Figure 6-3).

Abduction is also important to prevent dislocation of a hemiarthroplasty that was done through a posterior approach.

Push-off

Push-off is usually not affected (see Figures 6-4 and 6-5).

Swing Phase

The swing phase constitutes 40% of the gait cycle.

The iliopsoas is responsible for concentric contraction to power hip flexion (which shortens the leg to clear the ground) and advances the non–weight-bearing leg. This must be evaluated and strengthened as necessary once pain subsides. In addition, during the swing phase, the quadriceps functions to extend the knee to assist in acceleration. The advancement and rotation of the limb during the swing phase may be affected because of weakening of the iliopsoas muscle secondary to the fracture. This usually is not a major problem (see Figures 6-6, 6-7, and 6-8).

TREATMENT

Treatment: Early to Immediate (Day of Injury to One Week)

BONE HEALING

Stability at fracture site: No stability is present from bone healing. Partial bony stability is present in impacted femoral neck fractures. Immediate mechanical stability is present once the fracture is treated with screws except in severe osteopenia. Hemiarthroplasty treatment has full mechanical stability.

Stage of bone healing: Inflammatory phase. Fracture is colonized by inflammatory cells, and débridement of the fracture begins.

X-ray: No callus; fracture line is clearly visible. No periosteum is present; therefore, all healing is endosteal.

Orthopaedic and Rehabilitation Considerations

Physical Examination

Examine the wound for any erythema, edema, or discharge. Remove drains within 24 to 48 hours. Signs of infection should be treated locally and with systemic antibiotics. Persistent drainage may indicate a deep infection and require wound revision with incision and drainage in the operating room.

Compare the postoperative alignment of the repaired limb with the uninjured side. Evaluate capillary refill in the toes as well as motor and sensory function.

Sciatic neuropraxia is uncommon but may result from traction during fracture reduction, pressure from retraction during placement of an endoprosthesis, or inadequately padded bony prominences in slender patients.

Skin integrity must be assessed and carefully monitored until the patient returns to preoperative function. The rotational alignment of the limb may be assessed by the position of the knees and the length by the relation of the medial malleoli.

A significant leg-length discrepancy is uncommon and may be treated with a shoe lift. Measure the range of motion in the hip, knee, and ankle. Maintain and improve active and passive motion with early mobilization out of bed. This is the key to postoperative success in elderly patients. Pain secondary to operative trauma to the vastus lateralis and tensor fascia lata must be overcome through therapy. Explain to the patient that this is an intracapsular fracture and therefore has a risk of post-traumatic arthritis. Avascular necrosis and nonunion occur in less than 10% of cases after nondisplaced fractures. Displaced fractures have a much higher incidence of complications. Nonunion and avascular necrosis occur in up to one third of these fractures. These complications appear to depend most on the accuracy of the fracture reduction.

Dangers

Patients treated by hemiarthroplasty must avoid positioning the hip in adduction or internal rotation because this may dislocate the prosthesis. Care must be taken to prevent these positions during transfers, when turning in bed, and when using a bedpan or chair.

Note any shortness of breath or chest pain that might be secondary to pulmonary embolism or cardiac sources. Compression stockings are helpful in preventing deep vein thrombosis.

Hypovolemia may result from fracture hematoma and blood loss during surgery, and hemoglobin levels should be followed until they stabilize. Transfusion may be necessary for treatment or prophylaxis of myocardial ischemia.

Pressure ulcers may develop rapidly in patients who are nonambulators or who are allowed to be bed bound. Skin monitoring and proper positioning must be performed.

Radiography

Examine anteroposterior and lateral views for position and fixation of the fracture or endoprosthesis. The position of the screws must be evaluated for cut-out, which occurs in the anterior and superior region of the femoral head in very osteopenic bone. Cut-out leads to fracture collapse and varus deformity. In this case, the screws must be revised or weight bearing limited to prevent these consequences.

Weight Bearing

Closed or open reduction and internal fixation: Patients with impacted and rigidly fixed fractures may be out of bed and ambulating with partial to full weight on the affected extremity within the first week. Crutches or a walker and a three-point gait must be used (see Figure 6-17). Unstable fractures with posterior comminution and those requiring reduction must remain non-weight bearing to toe-touch weight bearing.

Endoprosthesis: Weight bearing as tolerated may begin within the first few days.

Range of Motion

Initially, active range of motion of the hip is quite painful secondary to injury and surgical trauma. The patient may resist range-of-motion activity. Once the pain and swelling subside in a few days, however, active range of motion of the hip is instituted.

Full extension of the knee may initially be painful because the vastus lateralis was surgically exposed.

Gentle active flexion/extension of the knee is performed.

The patient is instructed in full range of motion to the ankle.

Muscle Strength

Ankle isotonic exercises are prescribed to maintain the strength of the gastrocnemius-soleus group and dorsiflexor group. This also helps to pump blood up the lower extremity and minimize the risk of thrombophlebitis and deep vein thrombosis.

Once the pain has subsided, the patient is instructed in gluteal sets and quadriceps sets.

Functional Activities

Patients are taught to roll over onto their unaffected side and then raise themselves from bed. If that is not possible, they are taught to push themselves up with their upper extremities and gently raise themselves from bed. A pillow should be placed between the knees to prevent adduction and internal rotation and possible dislocation of the prosthesis and stress on the fracture site.

The patient dons pants on the affected extremity first and doffs them from the unaffected extremity first. Initially, the patient may need assistance with this and may prefer to wear only a robe because dressing is difficult.

The patient needs to use a raised toilet seat and chair to reduce hip flexion and needs assistance with lower extremity self-care.

Gait and Transfers

Gait depends on the patient's weight-bearing status. Assistive devices such as crutches or a walker may be needed for transfers and ambulation. If non-weight bearing, the patient is taught one-leg stand-pivot transfers and a two-point gait, in which the crutches and affected extremity act as one unit and the unaffected extremity as the other unit. Weight is borne on the crutches (*see* Figure 6-16).

The patient is taught to climb up stairs with the unaffected extremity first, followed by the affected extremity and crutches, and to descend stairs with the crutches and affected extremity first, followed by the unaffected extremity (see Figures 6-20, 6-21, 6-22, 6-23, 6-24, 6-25, 6-26, 6-27, 6-28, 6-29, 6-30, and 6-31).

Methods of Treatment: Specific Aspects

Closed or Open Reduction with Internal Fixation

If the fracture is rigidly fixed, the patient can bear partial weight on the affected extremity during ambulatory transfers and ambulation.

Prosthetic Replacement of the Femoral Head and Neck

During range-of-motion exercises, adduction past the midline and internal rotation are avoided to prevent prosthetic dislocation. A pillow is placed between the extremities when the patient is in bed.

Prescription

DAY ONE TO ONE WEEK

Precautions

Avoid passive range of motion.

Patients treated with endoprostheses avoid internal rotation and adduction past midline.

Range of Motion Active range of motion to hip and knee.

Muscle Strength

Isometric gluteal and quadriceps exercises.

Isotonic exercises to ankle.

Functional Activities Stand-pivot transfers and ambulation with assistive devices; raised toilet seat and chair.

Weight bearing Depending on procedure, either weight bearing as tolerated for stable impacted fractures or endoprostheses, or no weight bearing for unstable fractures that require reduction.

Treatment: Two Weeks

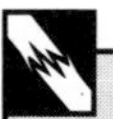

BONE HEALING

Stability at fracture site: Only minimal stability from bony healing. Partial bony stability is present in impacted femoral neck fractures. Immediate mechanical stability is present once the fracture is treated with screws except in severe osteopenia. Hemiarthroplasty treatment has full mechanical stability.

Stage of bone healing: Beginning of the reparative phase. Osteoprogenitor cells differentiate into osteoblasts that lay down woven bone.

X-ray: No callus is visible because healing is endosteal (internal). The fracture line is visible.

Orthopaedic and Rehabilitation Considerations:

Physical Examination

Sutures or skin staples should be evaluated and removed as necessary. Measure active and passive motion of the hip and particularly the knee. Decreased range of motion might be noted because of pain, swelling, or early adhesion between the vastus lateralis and the tensor fascia lata. Any edema of the lower leg should resolve with elevation of the extremity. Active range-of-motion exercises are given to the hip and knee. Reflex inhibition secondary to pain or muscle trauma may occur. Quadriceps strengthening exercises should be continued to help neutralize rotational forces. The patient should be encouraged to exercise and continue ambulation. Decreased knee range of motion requires therapy. Note any leg-length discrepancy and evaluate for a shoe lift as appropriate.

Dangers

See previous section (page 265).

Radiography

Examine anteroposterior and lateral views for angulation, cut-out, rotation, or gapping (opening) at the fracture site. Note the position of the hardware.

Weight Bearing

Closed or open reduction and internal fixation: Impacted and rigidly fixed fractures may continue with partial to full weight bearing on the affected extremity. Crutches or a walker and a three-point gait must be used (see Figure 6-17). Unstable fractures with posterior comminution and those that required reduction must remain non-weight bearing to toe-touch weight bearing.

Endoprosthesis: The patient may continue weight bearing as tolerated.

Range of Motion

Continue with active to active-assistive range-of-motion exercises to the hip and knee. Because the fracture is intracapsular, range-of-motion exercises are very important to avoid joint capsule tightness.

Continue with active range-of-motion exercises to the knee and ankle.

Muscle Strength

Continue with isometric exercises to the quadriceps and glutei group. Quadriceps strengthening exercises are important to help to neutralize rotational forces.

Functional Activities

See previous section.

When possible, patients are taught to roll over onto their unaffected side and then raise themselves from bed. If that is not possible, then they are taught to push themselves up with their upper extremities and gently raise themselves from bed. A pillow should be placed between the knees to avoid adduction and internal rotation.

The patient dons pants on the affected extremity first and doffs them from the unaffected extremity first.

The patient needs to use a raised toilet seat and chairs to reduce hip flexion.

Gait and Transfers

No significant changes. See previous section.

Methods of Treatment: Specific Aspects

Closed or Open Reduction and Internal Fixation

Continue with range-of-motion exercises.

Prosthetic Replacement of the Femoral Head and Neck

Avoid adduction and internal rotation to prevent prosthetic dislocation.

Prescription

Rx

Two Weeks

Precautions Avoid passive range of motion on fractures that have been reduced. Avoid internal rotation and adduction past midline on fractures treated with hemiarthroplasty.

Range of Motion Active, active-assistive range of motion to hip and knee.

Muscle Strength Isometric gluteal and quadriceps exercises.

Functional Activities Stand-pivot transfers and ambulation with assistive devices.

Weight Bearing Depending on procedure, either weight bearing as tolerated for stable impacted fractures or endoprostheses, or no weight bearing for unstable fractures that require reduction.

Treatment: Four to Six Weeks

Bone Healing

Stability at fracture site: Moderate stability from bone healing is present as endosteal callus bridges the fracture; correlate with physical examination. Mechanical stability from hardware or endoprosthesis is unchanged.

Stage of bone healing: Reparative phase. Osteoblasts continue to lay down woven bone. Once endosteal callus bridges the fracture site, some stability is present. However, the strength of this woven bone callus, especially with torsional load, is significantly lower than that of normal bone.

X-ray: No external callus is visible because healing is endosteal (internal) and composed of cartilage and fibrous tissue; this gradually becomes visible as it undergoes endochondral ossification.

Orthopaedic and Rehabilitation Considerations

Physical Examination

Measure the range of motion at the hip, knee, and ankle and encourage stretching exercises and strengthening as necessary.

Dangers

See previous section (page 265).

Radiography

Examine anteroposterior and lateral views for angulation, cut-out, rotation, or gapping at the fracture site. Note the position of the hardware. Look for any evidence of avascular necrosis or delayed healing. A bone scan may show decreased uptake in the femoral head in cases of avascular necrosis.

Weight Bearing

Closed or open reduction and internal fixation: Stable impacted and rigidly fixed fractures may continue with partial to full weight on the affected extremity. Crutches or a walker and three-point gait must be used (see Figure 6-17). Unstable fractures with posterior comminution and those that required reduction must remain non-weight bearing to toe-touch weight bearing.

Endoprosthesis: The patient may continue weight bearing as tolerated.

Range of Motion

By now, the patient should experience much less pain while ranging the hip actively and should achieve hip flexion up to 90 degrees. This is important for proper sitting position. Continue with active and active-assistive range-of-motion exercises to the hip and knee.

Muscle Strength

Hip abductors, flexors, and extensors should all be strengthened with isometric or isotonic strengthening exercises. Repeated active range of motion in flexion, extension, and abduction helps in strengthening the muscles. Quadriceps strengthening is continued.

Functional Activities

Bed mobility should be independent by now. The patient should be independent in dressing.

Gait and Transfers

Depending on weight-bearing status, the patient may need to use crutches during transfers and ambulation. Otherwise, no significant changes (see previous section).

Methods of Treatment: Specific Aspects

No significant changes. See previous section (page 267).

Prescription

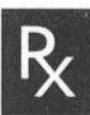

Four to Six Weeks

Precautions No passive range of motion on fractures that have been reduced. Avoid internal rotation and adduction past midline on fractures treated with hemiarthroplasty.

Range of Motion Active, active-assistive range of motion to hip and knee.

Muscle Strength Isometric and isotonic exercises to hip and knee.

Functional Activities Stand-pivot transfers and ambulation with assistive devices.

Weight Bearing Depending on procedure, either weight bearing as tolerated for stable impacted fractures or endoprostheses, or no weight bearing for unstable fractures that require reduction.

Treatment: Eight to Twelve Weeks

BONE HEALING

Stability at fracture site: Moderate stability from bone healing as endosteal callus bridges the fracture; correlate with physical examination. Mechanical stability from hardware or endoprosthesis is unchanged.

Stage of bone healing: Late reparative, early remodeling phase. Woven bone is being replaced by lamellar bone. Once callus bridges the fracture site, some stability is present. However, the strength of this callus, especially with torsional load, is significantly lower than that of normal bone.

X-ray: No external callus is visible because healing is endosteal (internal) and composed of cartilage and fibrous tissue; this gradually becomes visible as it undergoes endochondral ossification.

Orthopaedic and Rehabilitation Considerations

Physical Examination

Measure range of motion at the hip, knee, and ankle and encourage stretching exercises and strengthening as necessary.

Dangers

No significant changes. See previous sections.

Radiography

Examine anteroposterior and lateral views for angulation, cut-out, rotation, or gapping at the fracture site. Note the position of the hardware. Look for any evidence of avascular necrosis or delayed healing.

Weight Bearing

Closed or open reduction and internal fixation: Stable impacted and unstable rigidly fixed fractures should all be advanced to weight bearing as tolerated by this time. Assistive devices such as crutches or a walker may be used as necessary.

Endoprosthesis: The patient may continue weight bearing as tolerated.

Range of Motion

Because the fracture site is more stable with moderate endosteal callus, passive range-of-motion exercises are instituted to the hip, if necessary. If limitations are noted in the hip, stretch the hip in extension/flexion.

Muscle Strength

The patient can start on isokinetic exercises at 12 weeks using Cybex or Nautilus machines to strengthen the quadriceps and the hip musculature. The patient should also continue with isometric exercises to the gluteal group of muscles. Resistive exercises can be instituted.

Functional Activities

The patient should be using the affected extremity during transfers and ambulation because it can bear more weight. At this time, fractures with posterior comminution can bear weight as tolerated. The patient may still need to use crutches or a walker. The use of a raised toilet seat and chairs should be minimized because the patient should have adequate hip flexion to use a regular toilet.

Gait

The patient is taught a four-point gait with crutches because he or she can bear more weight on the affected extremity (see Figures 6-18 and 6-19).

Methods of Treatment: Specific Aspects

Closed or Open Reduction and Internal Fixation

No significant changes, except that fractures with posterior comminution can bear weight as tolerated.

Prosthetic Replacement of Femoral Head and Neck

The patient should avoid excessive adduction and internal rotation.

Prescription

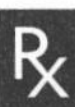

EIGHT TO TWELVE WEEKS

Precautions Avoid excessive adduction and internal rotation if an endoprosthesis is present.

Range of Motion Active, active-assistive, and passive range of motion to hip and knee.

Muscle Strength Isotonic and isokinetic exercises to hip and knee. Progressive resistive exercises instituted.

Functional Activities Weight-bearing transfers and ambulation with assistive devices.

Weight Bearing Full weight bearing to weight bearing as tolerated.

Treatment: Twelve to Sixteen Weeks

BONE HEALING

Stability at fracture site: Significant stability is now present from bone healing as endosteal callus bridges the fracture; correlate with physical examination. Mechanical stability from hardware or endoprosthesis is unchanged.

Stage of bone healing: Remodeling phase. Woven bone is being replaced by lamellar bone. Once callus bridges the fracture site, some stability is present. However, the strength of this callus, especially with torsional load, is significantly lower than that of normal bone.

X-ray: No external callus is visible because healing is endosteal (internal) and composed of cartilage and fibrous tissue; this gradually becomes visible as it undergoes endochondral ossification. Fracture line is obliterated.

Orthopaedic and Rehabilitation Considerations

Physical Examination

Measure the range of motion at the hip, knee, and ankle and encourage stretching exercises and strengthening as necessary. The patient should have hip and knee flexion greater than 90 degrees to be able to sit comfortably.

Dangers

The joint capsule is healed by now, and the risk of hemiarthroplasty dislocation is reduced. However, avascular necrosis of an intact femoral head may be developing.

Radiography

Examine anteroposterior and lateral views for angulation, cut-out, rotation, or gapping at the fracture site. Note the position of the hardware. Look for any evidence of avascular necrosis or delayed healing.

Weight Bearing

Closed or open reduction and internal fixation: Stable impacted and unstable reduced and rigidly fixed fractures should all be advanced to weight bearing as tolerated by this time. Assistive devices such as crutches or a walker may be used as necessary.

Endoprosthesis: The patient may continue weight bearing as tolerated.

Range of Motion

The range of motion of the hip and knee should be within normal range.

Muscle Strength

Exercise machines like Nautilus or Cybex can be used to strengthen the muscles in young patients who have had femoral neck fractures. Progressive resistive exercises using weights are also instituted to strengthen the muscles. As the weight and repetitions increase, the muscle strength also increases.

Gait

Emphasis should be placed on normalization of the gait pattern.

If the hip abductors are weak, the patient may have a Trendelenburg gait with pelvic tilt (see Figure 6-11).

Methods of Treatment: Specific Aspects

No change.

Prescription

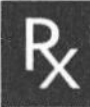

TWELVE TO SIXTEEN WEEKS

Precautions Avoid excessive adduction if an endoprosthesis is present.

Range of Motion Full active and passive range of motion to hip and knee.

Strength Isokinetic and isotonic exercises and progressive resistive exercises.

Functional Activities Patient is independent in transfers and ambulation without assistive devices.

Weight Bearing Full weight bearing.

LONG-TERM CONSIDERATIONS AND PROBLEMS

Avascular necrosis of the femoral head may require prosthetic replacement if it becomes symptomatic and causes pain.

Nonunion may require prosthetic replacement of the femoral head and neck.

Leg-length discrepancy is rare, but may be a long-term problem requiring a shoe lift.

Prominent and painful screws, pins, and plates may require removal.

IMMEDIATE TO ONE WEEK

	Internal Fixation	Hemiarthroplasty
Stability	Partial bony stability is present in impacted femoral neck fractures. Immediate mechanical stability is present once the fracture is treated with hardware, except cases of severe osteopenia.	Full mechanical stability.
Orthopaedics	Examine wounds. Remove drains when appropriate. Deep vein thrombosis (DVT) prophylaxis. Check blood count.	Examine wounds. Remove drains when appropriate. DVT prophylaxis. Check blood count. Maintain abduction pillow when the patient is seated or supine to prevent dislocation of the prosthesis.
Rehabilitation	Isometric gluteal and quadriceps exercises. Isotonic ankle exercises. General conditioning and strengthening exercises.	Same as for internal fixation.

TWO WEEKS

	Internal Fixation	Hemiarthroplasty
Stability	Partial bony stability is present in impacted femoral neck fractures. Immediate mechanical stability is present once the fracture is treated with hardware, except in cases of severe osteopenia.	Full mechanical stability.
Orthopaedics	Examine wounds. Remove sutures or staples. Deep vein thrombosis (DVT) prophylaxis.	Examine wounds. Remove sutures or staples. DVT prophylaxis. Maintain abduction pillow when the patient is seated or supine to prevent dislocation of the prosthesis.
Rehabilitation	Active and active-assistive range of motion to the hip, knee, and ankle. Isometric gluteal and quadriceps strengthening exercises. Stand/pivot transfers and ambulation with appropriate assistive devices.	Same as for internal fixation.

FOUR TO SIX WEEKS

	Internal Fixation	Hemiarthroplasty
Stability	Moderate stability is present from bone healing as endosteal callus bridges the fracture.	Unchanged.
Orthopaedics	Examine radiograph for healing and hardware position.	Maintain abduction pillow when the patient is seated or supine to prevent dislocation of the prosthesis.
Rehabilitation	Unchanged.	Unchanged.

EIGHT TO TWELVE WEEKS

	Internal Fixation	Hemiarthroplasty
Stability	Moderate additional stability at fracture from endosteal callus is now present.	Unchanged.
Orthopaedics	Examine radiograph for healing, hardware position, and possible avascular necrosis.	Maintain voluntary abduction to prevent dislocation of the prosthesis.
Rehabilitation	Isometric and isotonic to the hip and knee.	Same as for internal fixation.

TWELVE TO SIXTEEN WEEKS

	Internal Fixation	Hemiarthroplasty
Stability	Significant additional stability at fracture from endosteal callus.	Unchanged.
Orthopaedics	Examine radiograph for healing, hardware position, and possible avascular necrosis.	Maintain voluntary abduction to prevent dislocation of the prosthesis.
Rehabilitation	Isometric and isotonic to the knee and hip. Full weight bearing.	Same as for internal fixation.

BIBLIOGRAPHY

Anderson LD, Hamsa WR Jr, Waring TL. Femoral-head prostheses: a review of three hundred and fifty-six operations and their results. *J Bone Joint Surg Am*, 46:1049–1065, 1964.

Barnes R, Brown JT, Garden RS, et al. Subcapital fractures of the femur: a prospective review. *J Bone Joint Surg Br*, 58:2–24, 1976.

Bray TJ, Smith-Hoefer E, Hooper A, et al. The displaced femoral neck fracture: internal fixation versus bipolar endoprosthesis—results of a prospective, randomized comparison. *Clin Orthop*, 230:127–140, 1988.

Cassebaum WH, Nugent G. Predictability of bony union in displaced intracapsular fractures of the hip. *J Trauma*, 3:421–424, 1963.

Christie J, Howie CR, Armour PC. Fixation of displaced subcapital femoral fractures: compression screw fixation versus double divergent pins. *J Bone Joint Surg Br*, 70:199–201, 1988.

DeLee JC. Fractures and dislocations of the hip. In: Rockwood CA Jr, Green DP, Bucholz RW, eds. *Fractures in Adults*, Vol 2, 3rd ed. Philadelphia: J.B. Lippincott, 1991, pp. 1481–1651.

Garden RS. Malreduction and avascular necrosis in subcapital fractures of the femur. *J Bone Joint Surg Br*, 53:183–197, 1971.

Harper WM, Barnes MR, Gregg PJ. Femoral head blood flow in femoral neck fractures: an analysis using intraosseous pressure measurement. *J Bone Joint Surg Br*, 73:73–75, 1991.

Koval KJ, Zukerman JD. Hip fractures: I. overview and evaluation and treatment of femoral-neck fractures. *Journal of the American Academy of Orthopedic Surgeons*, 2:141–149, 1994.

Miller CW. Survival and ambulation following hip fracture. *J Bone Joint Surg Am*, 60:930–934, 1978.

Scheck M. The significance of posterior comminution in femoral neck fractures. *Clin Orthop*, 152:138–142, 1980.

Swiontkowski MF. Intracapsular hip fractures. In: Browner BD, Jupiter JB, Levine AM, Trafton PG, eds. *Skeletal Trauma,* Vol 2. Philadelphia: W.B. Saunders, 1992, pp. 1369–1442.

CHAPTER *Twenty-two*

Intertrochanteric Fractures

KENNETH W. TAYLOR, MD

STANLEY HOPPENFELD, MD

CONTRIBUTIONS BY MARK A. THOMAS, MD

INTRODUCTION

Definition

An intertrochanteric fracture is a fracture occurring between the greater and lesser trochanters along the intertrochanteric line, outside of the hip joint capsule (Figure 22-1; *see* Figure 22-4).

Mechanism of Injury

Falls occurring in patients with senile and postmenopausal osteoporosis account for most of these fractures. High-energy trauma may cause this type of fracture in younger patients; in this situation, an intertrochanteric fracture may accompany a femoral shaft fracture.

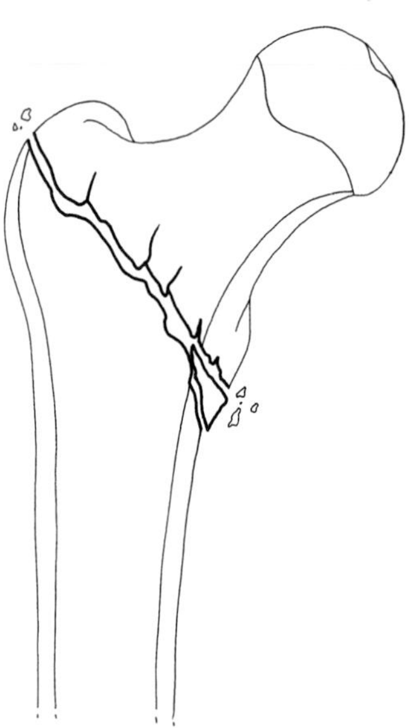

FIGURE 22-1 Intertrochanteric fracture of the femur. The fracture extends from the greater trochanter to the lesser trochanter.

Treatment Goals

Orthopaedic Objectives

Alignment

Restore the neck-shaft angle (normal = 127 degrees; Figures 22-2A and 22-2B).

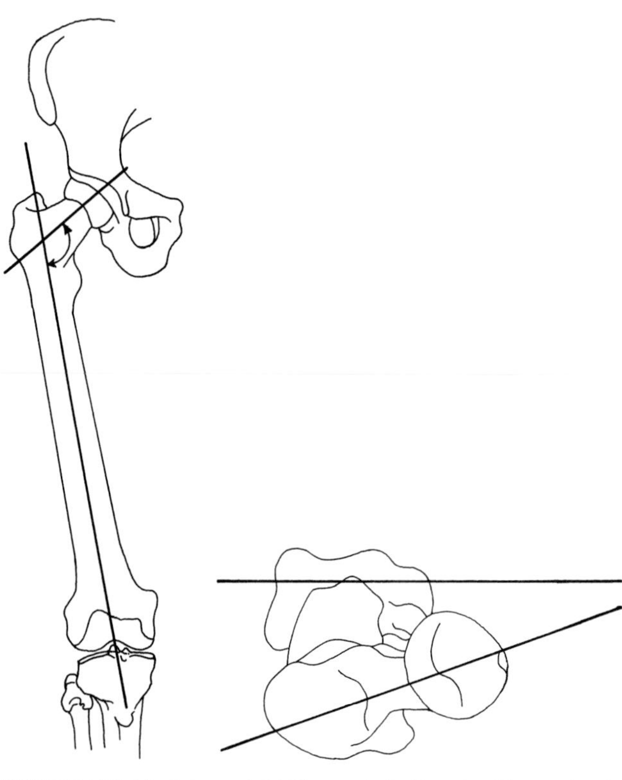

FIGURE 22-2A *(above, left)* The next shaft angle. The anatomic axis of the femur intersects the anatomic axis of the neck, forming an angle of 127 degrees.

FIGURE 22-2B *(above, right)* Angle of inclination. The anatomic neck of the femur is angulated anteriorly 12 to 15 degrees in relationship to a line drawn through the femoral condyles.

Stability

Restore the medial buttress, also known as the calcar femoralis.

Rehabilitation Objectives

Range of Motion

Restore and improve range of motion of the hip to enable the patient to sit properly (90 degrees flexion) and climb stairs. Full extension of the hip is required to avoid gait deviations, excessive lumbar lordosis, and back pain when standing. Maintain full range of motion of the *knee* and *ankle* (Table 22-1).

TABLE 22-1 *Ranges of Motion of Hip*

Motion	Normal	Functional
Flexion	0–120°	0–110°
Extension	0–20°	
Abduction	0–45°	0–20°
Adduction	0–45°	
Internal rotation	0–45°	0–20°
External rotation	0–45°	

Muscle Strength

Restore and maintain the strength of muscles that cross the hip joint and effect hip joint functions.

Hip extensor: gluteus maximus
Hip abductor: gluteus medius
Hip flexor: iliopsoas
Hip adductors: adductors magnus, longus, and brevis. Avoid strengthening the adductor group of muscles until the fracture is stable because they stress the fracture site and any implant (sliding hip screw)
Knee extensor and hip flexor: quadriceps (rectus femoris, two-joint muscle)
Knee flexor and hip extensor: hamstrings (biceps femoris, two-joint muscle)

Note that the joints at either end of a two-joint muscle cannot achieve full range of motion at the same time, making this muscle more susceptible to shortening.

Functional Goals

Normalize gait pattern and achieve a proper sitting position.

Expected Time of Bone Healing

Twelve to 15 weeks.

Expected Duration of Rehabilitation

Fifteen to 20 weeks.

The treatment of choice is a sliding hip screw. Rehabilitation principles are therefore based on this mode of treatment (*see* Figure 22-3).

Methods of Treatment

Sliding Hip Screw (Nail and Plate)

Biomechanics: Stress-sharing device.
Mode of Bone Healing: Secondary.
Indications: Fixation of the fracture allows for early mobilization of the patient and is therefore the treatment of choice. The sliding action of the screw in the barrel of the plate creates dynamic compression of the fracture on weight bearing. This maintains a large area of contact between the proximal and distal fracture fragments and aids healing. In reverse oblique and very comminuted fractures, many surgeons medially displace the distal fragment on the proximal one. An osteotomy is performed to notch the distal fragment and allow the proximal fragment to impact onto it. This restores apposition of the fracture fragments by creating a medial buttress (Figures 22-3, 22-4, and 22-5).

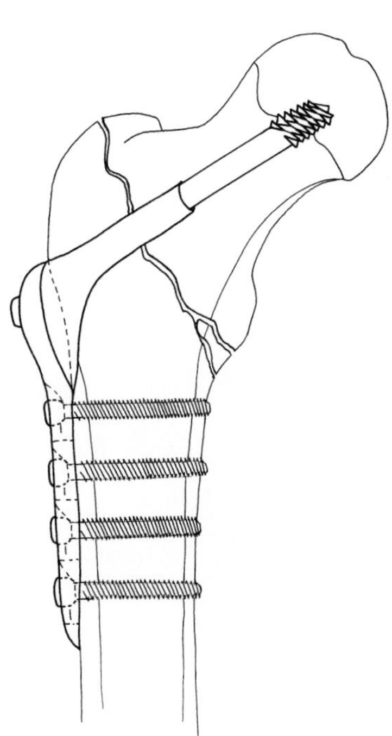

FIGURE 22-3 Internal fixation of an intertrochanteric fracture using a dynamic hip screw, which provides compression across the fracture site. The smooth portion of the screw slides through the barrel of the fixation to allow impaction of the fracture site.

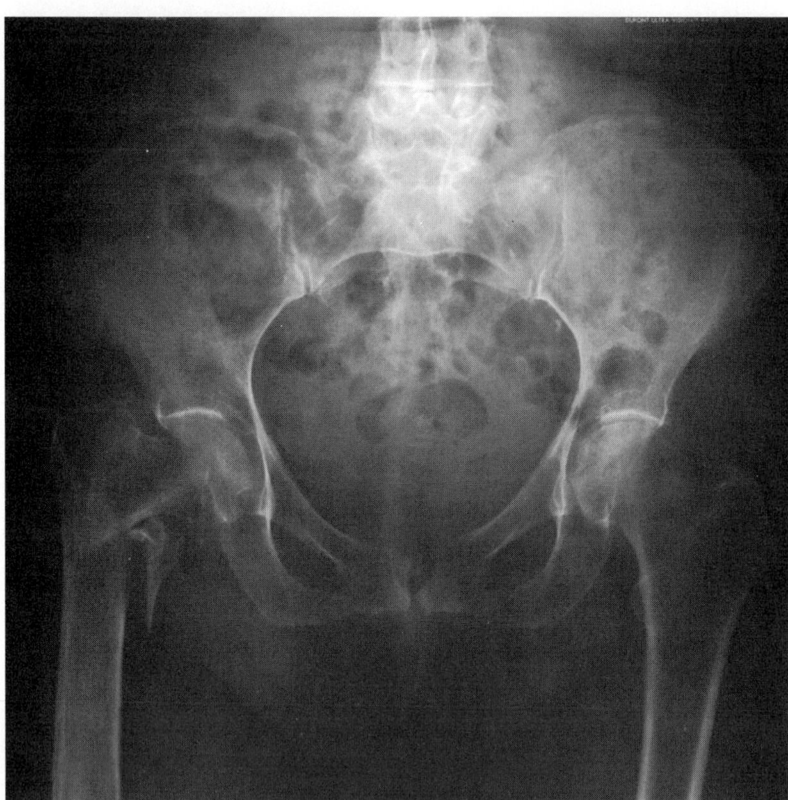

FIGURE 22-4 Intertrochanteric fracture of the right hip in an adult female patient. There is fracture comminution in the intertrochanteric region and shortening of the femur compared with the opposite side.

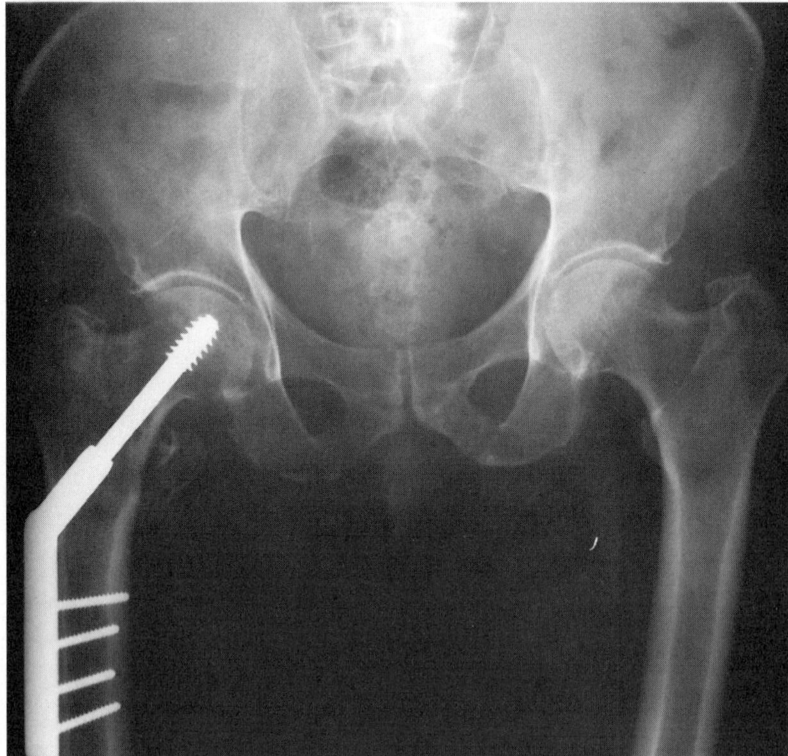

FIGURE 22-5 Sliding hip screw nail provides internal fixation and maintenance of reduction of an intertrochanteric fracture with restoration of length. The neck shaft angle has been restored to approximately 127 degrees. This fixation is stable; early weight bearing may begin.

Skeletal Traction

Biomechanics: Stress-sharing device.
Mode of Bone Healing: Secondary.
Indications: Terminally ill and nonambulatory patients who are incapable of enduring open reduction and internal fixation with a sliding hip screw may be treated using Buck's traction. Patients are maintained in traction until the fracture has become sticky and less painful, at which point they may undergo mobilization to a seated position. Because shortening, external rotation, and varus deformity are likely consequences of this treatment, it should be reserved for severely ill patients. Complications of prolonged bed rest such as venous pooling and thrombosis, urinary tract infection, and pressure ulcers are other pitfalls. This method of treatment is not discussed further in this chapter.

Special Considerations of the Fracture

The bone is cancellous and has a rich vascular supply, as do metaphyseal regions. This accounts for both a high union rate and extensive fracture hematoma. Intertrochanteric fractures are commonly described according to the number of fragments or parts present (e.g., the proximal fragment, distal fragment, greater trochanter, and lesser trochanter). The stability of trochanteric fractures depends on the restoration of the posteromedial buttress through reduction and fixation. If this can be accomplished, the fracture pattern is classified as *stable*. Such a fracture usually has minimal comminution and normal obliquity (extending in the same direction as the intertrochanteric line from superolateral to inferomedial). An *unstable* fracture has a comminuted medial buttress or reverse obliquity (extending perpendicular or skewing [oblique] to the intertrochanteric line from superomedial to inferolateral). This fracture is at risk for collapse or varus malunion.

Associated Injury

Because intertrochanteric fractures are extracapsular, the fracture hematoma may be large but still hidden in the thigh. The preoperative and postoperative hemodynamic status should be followed until stable hemoglobin levels are maintained. In cases of intertrochanteric fracture, osteopenic patients must also be evaluated for concomitant fractures of the wrist, shoulder, and ribs that may have occurred during a fall. Check for head injuries in cases of high-energy or multiple injuries.

Weight Bearing

The opportunity for early weight bearing is one of the advantages of fixation with a sliding hip screw. As soon as the acute pain subsides, most patients are able to bear weight as tolerated, using assistive devices. Less stable fractures may occasionally require limited weight bearing or non-weight bearing. This is discussed in the treatment sections. Assistive devices such as walkers are initially used for safety and stability.

Gait

Stance Phase

The stance phase constitutes 60% of the gait cycle.

Heel Strike

The *gluteus maximus* is a strong hip extensor. It prevents jackknifing at the hip on heel strike, and acts as a hip stabilizer. Because it crosses the fracture site, the muscle may be weakened and, on rare occasions, cause gluteus maximus lurch (*see* Figure 6-10). The *vastus lateralis* contracts concentrically (shortens) to achieve full knee extension at heel strike. It is partially incised proximally for nail and plating. This may weaken the muscle and full knee extension may not be achieved at heel strike secondary to weakness and pain (*see* Figure 6-1).

Foot-Flat

The *quadriceps* muscle goes through eccentric contraction (elongation) to control knee flexion in a smooth fashion from heel strike to foot-flat; to allow for early flexion of the knee, it is flexed throughout the rest of the gait cycle. The *rectus femoris* is a two-joint muscle that crosses the hip and knee joints. It shortens with immobilization. This may cause a flexion contracture of the hip or decrease knee flexion. The *vastus lateralis* is partially incised during the surgical approach, and retraction during surgery may further weaken the muscle. This may shorten foot-flat. Because of muscle injury, gait may be painful when the muscle contracts (*see* Figure 6-2).

Mid-Stance

Weight bearing at the fracture site is increased as double stance diminishes and ends. This increase in stress may be painful and cause an antalgic (painful) gait.

The *iliopsoas* muscle contracts to flex the hip and advance the limb during forward propulsion and allows the pelvis to rotate over the femur for limb advancement. The iliopsoas crosses the fracture site and may be weakened. The patient may take short steps to decrease pull on the muscle. The *gluteus medius* may be slightly weakened because it crosses the fracture site. This muscle stabilizes the pelvis against the femur to prevent Trendelenburg gait (*see* Figure 6-3).

Push-off

Push-off is usually not affected (*see* Figure 6-4).

Swing Phase

The swing phase constitutes 40% of the gait cycle. It usually is not affected. However, the iliopsoas is weakened and may require strengthening (*see* Figures 6-6, 6-7, and 6-8).

TREATMENT

Treatment: Early to Immediate (Day of Injury to One Week)

Bone Healing

Stability at fracture site: None.

Stage of bone healing: Inflammatory phase. The fracture hematoma is colonized by inflammatory cells, and débridement of the fracture begins.

X-ray: No callus; the fracture line is visible.

Orthopaedic and Rehabilitation Considerations

Physical Examination

Alignment of the repaired limb must be compared with the uninjured side. Rotation may be assessed by noting the position of the patella. Length may be assessed by comparing the medial malleoli. Leg-length discrepancies are common. If they are significant or increase as the fracture impacts with weight bearing, they are treated with a shoe lift at a later date.

Wounds must be examined for any erythema, edema, or discharge. Drains should be removed within 48 to 72 hours. Infection should be treated both locally and with systemic antibiotics. Persistent drainage may indicate a deep infection and require wound revision by incision and drainage in the operating room.

Dangers

Common dangers are *thromboembolic* events. Note any shortness of breath or chest pain that might indicate pulmonary embolism. *Hypovolemia* may be present if there is extensive fracture hematoma or operative blood loss; hemoglobin levels should be followed until they stabilize, usually by the fourth postoperative day. Transfusion may be necessary to correct the blood loss and as prophylaxis for myocardial ischemia. *Pressure ulcers* may develop rapidly in patients who are nonambulators or who remain in bed. Skin monitoring and proper positioning must be performed.

Radiography

Examine anteroposterior and lateral views for position of the fracture and hip screw. The fracture should become slightly impacted on itself with continued weight bearing (*see* Figure 22-5). When this occurs, the screw will slide through the barrel. However, when the threads of the screw slide down to the neck of the barrel, further impaction is prevented. When this occurs with a fracture that still shows a gap, consideration must be given to exchanging the plate for one with a shorter barrel. The position of the screw must be evaluated for cut-out from the femoral head or neck. This condition occurs in the anterior and superior region of the femoral head in very osteopenic bone. Impending cut-out is recognized on radiography by migration of the screw toward the anterior superior region of the head. This has the potential to lead to fracture collapse and varus deformity. In such instances, the screw must be revised or weight bearing limited to avoid these consequences.

Weight Bearing

Weight bearing as tolerated begins within the first few days for fractures that have a restored posteromedial buttress and good purchase of the screw within the femoral head. For reverse oblique, pathologic, and severely comminuted fractures, the patient begins partial or toe-touch weight bearing, or remains nonweight bearing depending on the security of fixation and bone stock. Assess the fracture with serial radiographs as weight bearing is advanced.

Range of Motion

Hip: If fixation of the fracture is stable, start gentle active range-of-motion at the hip in flexion, extension, and abduction. The tensor fascia lata and vastus lateralis are cut for surgical exposure. Adduction and internal rotation can be painful because of stretching of tensor fascia lata. If the fracture involves the greater trochanter, gluteus medius contraction is painful. If the lesser trochanter is involved, iliopsoas muscle contraction is painful.

Knee: The knee is actively ranged. Extension may be painful and limited secondary to involvement of the vastus lateralis.

Ankle: Active range-of-motion exercises may be given for the ankle and foot in all planes to prevent tightness at the ankle joint. The patient should draw the alphabet with the foot.

Muscle Strength

Knee: Knee strength should be improved with isometric quadriceps exercises.

Hip: The hip extensors should be strengthened with isometric gluteal sets. Avoid strengthening the adductors because this may stress the fracture site.

Ankle: Isotonic exercises may be performed at the ankle joint to maintain strength and motion and to help decrease the chance of thrombosis by increasing venous blood flow.

Functional Activities

If weight-bearing is as tolerated on the affected extremity, the patient can use that extremity during transfers from bed to chair. To assume a sitting position for transfers, the patient usually comes to sit on the same side of the bed as the fractured limb. The affected leg is then dangled off the bed and the patient sits up. If the patient cannot do this, a leg lifter can be used. Transfers are taught using a leg lifter (see page 53) to support the affected limb and swing it over the side of the bed to assume a sitting position. The arms are then used to push off from the bed or chair to a standing position (rather than grasping a walker and attempting to pull up, which could cause the walker to topple over). Assistive devices like crutches or a walker may be used for support once the patient is erect (*see* Figures 7-10 and 7-11). If the patient is non-weight bearing, stand-pivot transfers on the good leg are taught. A raised seat is helpful to reduce stresses on the hip (*see* Figure 7-5). The patient can also use the unaffected limb for transfers if he or she does not feel comfortable or experiences pain on the affected side.

Bathrooms should be equipped with a raised toilet seat to reduce the hip flexion required to sit and stand up. This will reduce pain and the force of muscle contractions.

If possible, the patient should try to roll onto his or her unaffected side and push up into a sitting position and get out of bed on the unaffected side. If that is not possible, the patient is instructed to push himself or herself up with the upper extremities to come to a sitting position, or use a bed trapeze. Once in a seated position, the patient pivots with the unaffected extremity first, followed by the affected extremity. This allows the patient to get out of bed. If the patient feels comfortable using the affected extremity, he or she can do so during bed mobility and transfers.

Pants should be donned on the involved extremity first and doffed from the uninvolved extremity first. This produces less stress and movement at the fracture site. Assistance of a pants puller or family member may be helpful.

Gait

Depending on weight-bearing status, a two- or three-point gait is taught using crutches or a walker (*see* Figures 6-16 and 6-17). If non-weight bearing, the patient is taught stand-pivot transfers and a two-point gait, in which the crutches and affected extremity act as one unit and the unaffected extremity acts as the other unit. Weight is borne on the crutches.

The patient is taught to climb up stairs by advancing the unaffected extremity first, followed by the affected extremity and crutches (*see* Figures 6-20, 6-21, and 6-22). Descending stairs is done with the affected extremity and crutches first, followed by the unaffected extremity (*see* Figures 6-23, 6-24, and 6-25). Patients should be checked carefully for ambulatory stability. Stair walking may need to be delayed until the patient's pain level is reduced.

Methods of Treatment: Specific Aspects

Because the sliding hip screw is the treatment of choice, the general rehabilitation principles discussed are based on that treatment. Open reduction and internal fixation with a sliding hip screw and plate allows for controlled impaction of the fracture with ambulation. Therefore, fracture impaction must be serially evaluated to ensure stability and avoid screw cut-out from the femoral head and neck. Impaction may be facilitated by increasing plate angles and is limited by the distance between the plate barrel and screw threads. Therefore, if screws shorter than 80 mm are used, a short barrel plate should be considered. Screw placement is also important. For maximal strength, the screw should be slightly posterioinferior to the center of the femoral head and within 1 cm of the subchondral bone.

Prescription

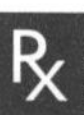

DAY ONE TO ONE WEEK

Precautions Avoid passive range of motion.

Range of Motion Gentle active range-of-motion exercises to hip and knee in flexion, extension, abduction, and adduction.

Muscle Strength Isometric exercises to glutei and quadriceps.

Functional Activities

Stand-pivot transfers if non-weight bearing. If weight bearing, the affected extremity is used during transfers. A raised toilet seat is used to decrease hip flexion.

For ambulation, use a two- or three-point gait depending on weight-bearing status, using assistive devices.

Weight Bearing Weight bearing as tolerated for stable fractures. Toe-touch to partial or non-weight bearing for unstable fractures.

Treatment: Two Weeks

BONE HEALING

Stability at fracture site: None to minimal.

Stage of bone healing: Beginning of reparative phase. Osteoprogenitor cells differentiate into osteoblasts that lay down woven bone.

X-ray: None to very early callus; fracture line is visible. Bone in the metaphyseal region has very thin periosteum and does not form an abundant external callus.

Orthopaedic and Rehabilitation Considerations:

Physical Examination

Sutures or skin staples should be evaluated and removed as necessary. Measure active and passive motion of the hip and particularly the knee. Decreased range of motion might be noted secondary to pain, swelling, or early adhesion between the vastus lateralis and the tensor fascia lata. Any edema of the lower leg should resolve with elevation of the extremity. Note any leg-length discrepancy and evaluate for a shoe lift as appropriate.

Dangers

Same as those that occur from the day of injury to one week. See previous section.

Radiography

Examine radiographs for loss of correction and position of the sliding hip screw in the femoral head. Look for any signs of screw migration or cut-out. Follow the radiographs for impaction of the fracture site and sliding of the hip screw in the barrel of the plate. No further impaction can occur once the threads are in contact with the barrel.

Weight Bearing

Continue weight bearing as tolerated in fractures that have a restored medial buttress and good purchase of the screw in the femoral head. Patients with reverse oblique, pathologic, and severely comminuted fractures should begin partial or toe-touch weight bearing or remain non-weight bearing; depending on the security of fixation and bone stock, assess the fracture with serial radiographs as weight bearing is advanced. Use assistive devices as needed.

Range of Motion

Range of motion at the hip, knee, and ankle should be continued to achieve 90 degrees of hip flexion when the knee is flexed. Continue active range-of-motion exercises to the knee and ankle. Decreased knee range of motion requires active and active-assistive range-of-motion exercises. Reflex inhibition of the quadriceps secondary to pain or muscle trauma may occur.

Muscle Strength

Continue isometric exercises.

Repeated movement in various planes not only improves joint range of motion but strengthens the muscles in an isotonic manner.

Quadriceps strengthening exercises should continue to help to neutralize the natural rotational forces on the limb. The patient should be encouraged to exercise and continue ambulation.

Functional Activities

Depending on weight-bearing status, the patient continues stand-pivot transfers or uses the affected extremity for transfers. The patient still needs to use assistive devices such as crutches, a walker, and a raised toilet seat.

Gait

Continue a two- or three-point gait on hard surfaces and stairs using assistive devices (*see* Figures 6-16 and 6-17). The gait pattern depends on weight-bearing status.

When ascending stairs, the patient leads with the unaffected extremity, descending stairs with the affected extremity (*see* Figures 6-20, 6-21, 6-22, 6-23, 6-24, and 6-25).

Methods of Treatment: Specific Aspects

See previous section (pages 279 and 280).

Prescription

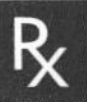

TWO WEEKS

Precautions Avoid standing on the affected leg without support. Avoid passive range of motion.

Range of Motion Active range of motion to hip and knee. Achieve 90 degrees flexion at hip.

Muscle Strength Isometric exercises to glutei, quadriceps, and hamstrings.

Functional Activities

Depending on weight bearing, the patient performs stand-pivot transfers or uses the affected extremity during transfers.

For ambulation, use two- or three-point gait with assistive devices.

Weight Bearing Depending on procedure, weight bearing as tolerated. Non-weight bearing to partial weight bearing, to toe-touch for unstable fractures.

Treatment: Four to Six Weeks

BONE HEALING

Stability at fracture site: With a bridging callus, the fracture is usually stable; confirm with physical examination.

Stage of bone healing: Reparative phase. Once callus is observed bridging the fracture site, some stability is present. However, the strength of this callus, especially with torsional load, is significantly lower than that of normal bone.

X-ray: Bridging callus is beginning to be visible. Endosteal callus may predominate in the metaphyseal region and the fracture line should become less visible.

Orthopaedic and Rehabilitation Considerations

Assess joint range of motion and strength.

Physical Examination

Measure range of motion of the hip, knee, and ankle, and encourage stretching and strengthening exercises as necessary.

Dangers

No significant change from previous section.

Increased postural sway may result in an increased risk of falling.

Avoid torsional stress across the fracture site. This occurs with extremes of motion and weight bearing such as when getting out of a car.

Radiography

Examine radiographs for loss of correction and position of the sliding hip screw in the femoral head. Look for any signs of screw cut-out or avascular necrosis. Check the position of the screw in relation to the barrel of the plate. Check for impaction at the fracture site and sliding of the hip screw in the barrel of the plate.

Weight Bearing

Continue weight bearing as tolerated in fractures that have a restored medial buttress and good purchase of the screw in the femoral head. Patients with reverse oblique, pathologic, and severely comminuted fractures should begin partial or toe-touch weight bearing or remain non-weight bearing depending on the security of fixation and available bone stock. Assess the fracture with serial radiographs as weight bearing is advanced. Use assistive devices as needed.

Range of Motion

Range of motion should be full at the hip, knee, and ankle. If muscle shortening is noted, active-assistive range-of-motion exercises may be used to stretch the muscle. Gentle passive stretching may be performed when the fracture site is stable. If these exercises are necessary, the assistance of a therapist should be obtained. Full knee extension should be achieved at this stage because the vastus lateralis is healed.

Muscle Strength

Continue isometric exercises. When hip joint motion is well tolerated, strengthening exercises may be advanced to progressive resistive exercises of the quadriceps, hamstrings, abductors, adductors, iliopsoas, and glutei. If pain persists, modalities like moist heat and hydrotherapy can be used.

Functional Activities

The patient should use the affected extremity more now. Once 90 degrees flexion at the hip is achieved, a raised toilet seat is no longer needed. Instruct the patient to use the affected limb and increase weight bearing to tolerance. Encourage independence in activities of daily living.

Gait

Continue a two- or three-point gait as before (*see* Figures 6-16 and 6-17). Watch for structural limb shortening; if it is present, a shoe lift may be needed. Work on static balance and weight shifting. Concentrate on gait training. Postural sway and risk of falling decrease with strengthening and training. The patient may still need ambulatory assistive devices depending on weight-bearing status.

Methods of Treatment: Specific Aspects

No change. See previous section (pages 279 and 280).

Prescription

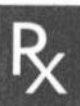

FOUR TO SIX WEEKS

Precautions Avoid torsion or twisting at the fracture site.

Range of Motion Active, active-assistive range of motion to hip and knee.

Muscle Strength Isometric exercises to glutei, quadriceps, and hamstrings. Active resistive exercises to quadriceps, glutei, and hamstrings, if motion is well tolerated.

Functional Activities Depending on weight bearing, stand-pivot transfers or weight bearing as tolerated on the affected extremity during transfers. Ambulation with assistive devices.

Weight Bearing Weight bearing as tolerated for stable fractures. Partial to non-weight bearing to toe-touch for unstable fractures.

Treatment: Eight to Twelve Weeks

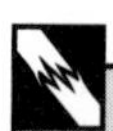

BONE HEALING

Stability at fracture site: Stable.

Stage of bone healing: Early remodeling phase. Woven bone is being replaced with lamellar bone in the cortex. The process of remodeling takes months to years to complete.

X-ray: Abundant callus has formed and the fracture line begins to disappear. The medullary canal and metaphyseal region begin to be reconstituted.

Orthopaedic and Rehabilitation Considerations

Physical Examination

Observe the patient's gait for any functional disability. Continue to assess joint range of motion and strength.

Dangers

No change. See previous sections. Torsional load and balance are less problematic.

Radiography

Examine radiographs for loss of correction and maintenance of the sliding hip screw position in the femoral head. Look for any signs of screw cut-out or avascular necrosis. Check the position of the screw in relation to the barrel of the plate. Follow radiographs for impaction of the fracture site and sliding of the hip screw in the barrel of the plate.

Weight Bearing

Advance weight bearing as tolerated in fractures that have a restored medial buttress and good purchase of the screw in the femoral head. Patients with reverse oblique, pathologic, and severely comminuted fractures should all be weight bearing as tolerated by this time. The patient may use assistive devices as needed.

Range of Motion

Range of motion of the hip, knee, and ankle should be full at this point. If not, institute passive range of motion and gentle stretch.

Muscle Strength

Instruct the patient to perform progressive resistive exercises of the lower extremities to increase muscle strength of the hip and knee. The patient can use weights in increasing gradation as strength improves. The number of repetitions of the exercises should also be increased. If the patient is young and cardiopulmonary capacity allows, and the fracture has good callus formation, isokinetic and isotonic exercises to the hip and knee can be prescribed to improve the strength through the use of Cybex and Kinetron machines.

Functional Activities

Encourage the patient to stop using assistive devices. In reverse oblique and severely comminuted fractures, the patient is still weight bearing as tolerated and needs assistive devices for ambulation and transfers. Patients with healed fractures should begin to negotiate stairs in a normal fashion, step over step.

Gait

A normal gait pattern with heel strike, foot-flat, mid-stance, heel-off, and push-off stages should gradually evolve (*see* Figures 6-1, 6-2, 6-3, 6-4, and 6-5). If this does not occur, gait training should address the specific abnormalities of gait. Wean the patient from crutches and canes.

Methods of Treatment: Specific Aspects

No change. See previous section (pages 279 and 280).

Prescription

EIGHT TO TWELVE WEEKS

Precautions None.

Range of Motion Continue active, active-assistive range of motion. Start passive range of motion and stretching to hip and knee.

Muscle Strength Progressive resistive exercises to hip and knee.

Functional Activities The patient uses involved extremity with weight bearing as tolerated or full weight bearing during transfers and ambulation. Weaning from assistive devices.

Weight Bearing Full.

LONG-TERM CONSIDERATIONS AND PROBLEMS

Orthopaedic Considerations

Nonunion is a rare occurrence, often associated with loss of fixation. If nonunion occurs, it may be treated by restoring rigid fixation and bone grafting.

Rehabilitation Considerations

A shortened limb caused by impaction of the fracture may be treated with a shoe lift if the discrepancy results in a limp or in back pain. This may occur with shortening of 1 inch or greater.

Patients are often unsteady or have some imbalance from weakness. If this unsteadiness does not respond to strengthening and balancing exercises, the patient may need to use a cane. If the patient is unstable with a cane, a quad cane or walker might be needed.

Gait deviations may occur secondary to pain or muscle weakness. Antalgic gaits are usually secondary to prominent hardware. An abductor lurch gait (Trendelenburg gait) may also occur if the greater trochanter was fractured and displaced.

IMMEDIATE TO ONE WEEK

	Internal Fixation
Stability	Partial bony stability may be initially present because of impaction of cancellous surfaces. This occurs only in fractures amenable to fixation in a near-anatomic position. Otherwise, there is no early bony stability at the fracture site other than that provided by the sliding hip screw and plate.
Orthopaedics	Examine wounds and remove drains when appropriate. Deep vein thrombosis prophylaxis. Check blood count.
Rehabilitation	Isometric gluteal and quadriceps exercises. Isotonic ankle exercises. General conditioning and strengthening exercises. Stand/pivot transfers if non-weight bearing, otherwise learn to use affected extremity cautiously for transfers. Most patients are weight bearing as tolerated.

TWO WEEKS

	Internal Fixation
Stability	Unchanged
Orthopaedics	Examine wounds. Remove sutures or staples. Deep vein thrombosis prophylaxis.
Rehabilitation	Active and active-assistive range of motion to the hip, knee, and ankle. Transfer training and ambulation with appropriate assistive devices.

FOUR TO SIX WEEKS

	Internal Fixation
Stability	Stability is gradually increased by formation of endosteal and bridging callus.
Orthopaedics	Examine radiograph for healing and hardware position and impaction of the fracture with weight bearing. Watch for any evidence of migration or cut-out of the lag screw.
Rehabilitation	Active, active-assistive range of motion to the hip, knee and ankle. Isometric exercises to the glutei and quadriceps. Active resistive exercises to the hip and knee if motion is well tolerated.

EIGHT TO TWELVE WEEKS

	Internal Fixation
Stability	Moderate additional stability at fracture from callus.
Orthopaedics	Examine for any leg length discrepancy that might develop as the fracture continues to become impacted and heal, and provide shoe lift if significant.
Rehabilitation	Progressive resistive exercises to the hip and the knee. Begin to wean from assistive devices. Isotonic and isokinetic exercises to the hip and knee musculature.

TWELVE TO SIXTEEN WEEKS

	Internal Fixation
Stability	Significant additional stability at fracture from callus.
Orthopaedics	Unchanged.
Rehabilitation	Unchanged.

BIBLIOGRAPHY

Apel DM, Patwardhan A, Pinzur MS, et al. Axial loading studies of unstable intertrochanteric fractures of the femur. *Clin Orthop*, 246:156–164, 1989.

Den Hartog BD, Bartal E, Cooke F. Treatment of the unstable intertrochanteric fracture: effect of the placement of the screw, its angle of insertion, and osteotomy. *J Bone Joint Surg Am*, 73: 726–733, 1991.

Desjardins AL, Roy A, Paiement G, et al. Unstable intertrochanteric fracture of the femur: a prospective randomized study comparing anatomical reduction and medial displacement osteotomy. *J Bone Joint Surg Br*, 75:445–447, 1993.

Dimon JH III, Hughston JC. Unstable intertrochanteric fractures of the hip. *J Bone Joint Surg Am*, 49:440–450, 1967.

Hopkins CT, Nugent JT, Dimon JH III. Medial displacement osteotomy for unstable intertrochanteric fractures: twenty years later. *Clin Orthop*, 245:169–172, 1989.

Kaufer H, Matthews LS, Sonstegard D. Stable fixation of intertrochanteric fractures: a biomechanical evaluation. *J Bone Joint Surg Am*, 56:899–907, 1974.

Koval KJ, Zukerman JD. Hip fractures: II. evaluation and treatment of intertrochanteric fractures. *Journal of the American Academy of Orthopedic Surgeons*, 2:150–156, 1994.

Levy RN, Capozzi JD, Mont MA. Intertrochanteric hip fractures. In: Browner BD, Jupiter JB, Levine AM, Trafton PG, eds. *Skeletal Trauma*, Vol 2. Philadelphia: W.B. Saunders, 1992, pp. 1443–1484.

Meislin RJ, Zuckerman JD, Kummer FJ, et al. A biomechanical analysis of the sliding hip screw: the question of plate angle. *J Orthop Trauma*, 4:130–136, 1990.

Mulholland RC, Gunn DR. Sliding screw plate fixation of intertrochanteric femoral fractures. *J Trauma*, 12:581–591, 1972.

Wolfgang GL, Bryant MH, O Neill JP. Treatment of intertrochanteric fracture of the femur using sliding screw plate fixation. *Clin Orthop*, 163:148–158, 1982.

CHAPTER Twenty-three

Subtrochanteric Femur Fractures

KENNETH W. TAYLOR, MD

VASANTHA L. MURTHY, MD

INTRODUCTION

Definition

Subtrochanteric fractures occur between the lesser trochanter and the adjacent proximal third of the femoral shaft. They may extend proximally to the intertrochanteric region (Figures 23-1 and 23-2).

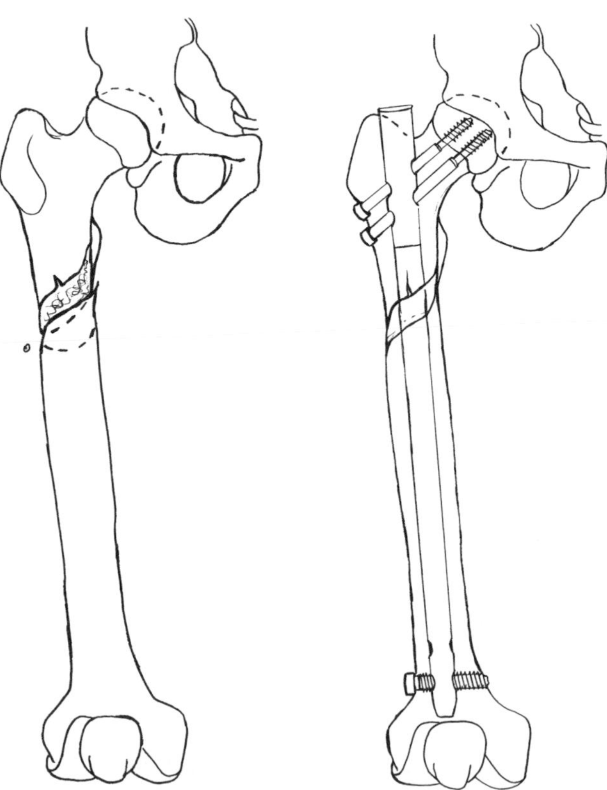

FIGURE 23-1 *(above, left)* Subtrochanteric fractures occur between the lesser trochanter and the adjacent proximal third of the femoral shaft. The fracture may extend proximally to the intertrochanteric region.

FIGURE 23-2 *(above, right)* Subtrochanteric fracture treated with a femoral nail that is locked proximally with two parallel screws and distally (static locking). The locking mechanism provides control of the rotation of the proximal and distal fragments.

Mechanism of Injury

These fractures may result from high-energy trauma in young patients or from distal extension of intertrochanteric fractures in elderly patients.

Treatment Goals

Orthop]aedic Objectives

Alignment

Restore rotation so that the femoral head and neck are anteverted 15 to 20 degrees relative to the shaft.

Stability

Restore continuity of the medial buttress (calcar) and its ability to withstand compressive load.

Rehabilitation Objectives

Range of Motion

Improve and restore hip range of motion (sitting in a chair requires 90 degrees of flexion).

Maintain knee and ankle range of motion (Table 23-1).

TABLE 23-1 *Range of Motion of Hip*

Motion	Normal	Functional[a]
Flexion	125–128°	90–110°
Extension	0–20°	0–5°
Abduction	45–48°	0–20°
Adduction	40–45°	0–20°
Internal rotation	40–45°	0–20°
External rotation	45°	?0–15°

[a]These are estimates of the functional range of motion.

Muscle Strength

Improve the strength of the following muscles:

Quadriceps: knee extensors; especially the vastus lateralis, which is incised during surgery. The rectus femoris portion of the muscle is also a hip flexor.

Hamstrings: knee flexor and secondary hip extensor.
Gluteus medius: hip abductor.
Gluteus maximus: hip extensor.
Tensor fascia lata: hip external rotator and abductor.
Adductor magnus: hip adductor. Do not strengthen this muscle because it stresses the fracture site and the implants.

Functional Goals

Restore normal gait pattern and independent ambulation.

Expected Time of Bone Healing

Twelve to 16 weeks.

Expected Duration of Rehabilitation

Sixteen to 20 weeks.

Methods of Treatment

Intramedullary Rod

Biomechanics: Partial stress-shielding device due to proximal and distal interlocking mechanism.

Mode of Bone Healing: Secondary.

Indications: Interlocking intramedullary devices are the treatment of choice for most subtrochanteric femur fractures. They must always be proximally interlocked to provide control of rotation, angulation, and length. This allows for early mobilization of the patient and minimizes the complications associated with prolonged bed rest. A standard intramedullary nail may be used only when the lesser trochanter is not involved in the fracture pattern, because the proximal interlocking screws gain purchase in this region. A fracture that includes the lesser trochanter must be treated with a reconstruction-type nail. This device has proximal interlocking screws that traverse the femoral neck and gain purchase into the femoral head (Figures 23-3, 23-4, 23-5, 23-6, and 23-7).

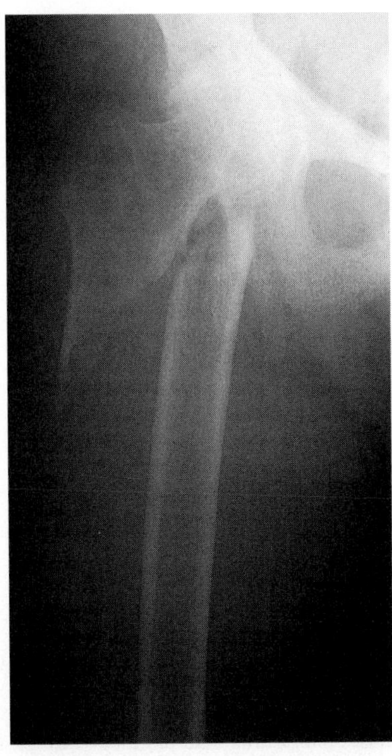

FIGURE 23-3 Displaced subtrochanteric fracture in an elderly patient. Note the shortening and overlap of the distal fragment on the proximal fragment.

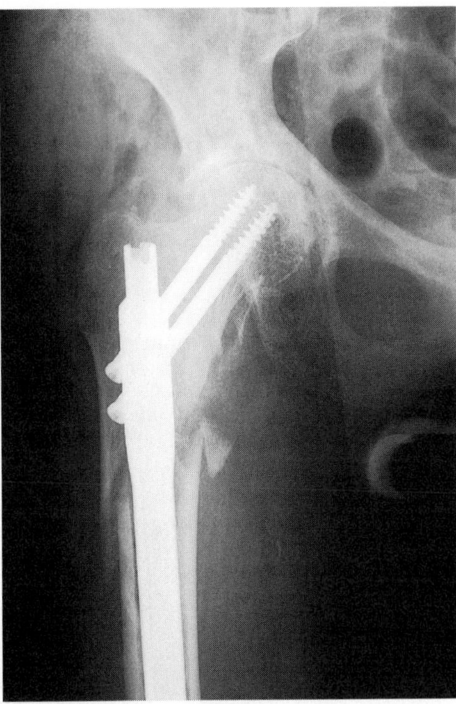

FIGURE 23-4 Subtrochanteric fracture fixed with an intermedullary rod with proximal locking screws that provide control of rotation, angulation, and length. This allows for the patient's early mobilization and minimizes complications associated with prolonged bed rest.

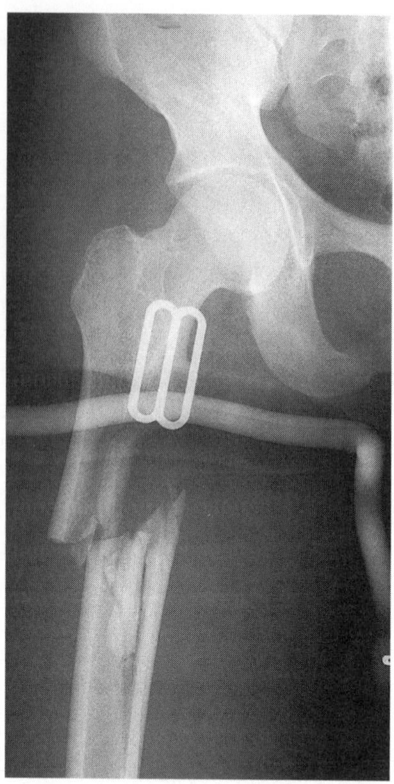

FIGURE 23-5 High-energy subtrochanteric fracture with marked comminution and displacement at the fracture site. Early treatment consisted of a Thomas splint, which can be seen overlying the fracture area.

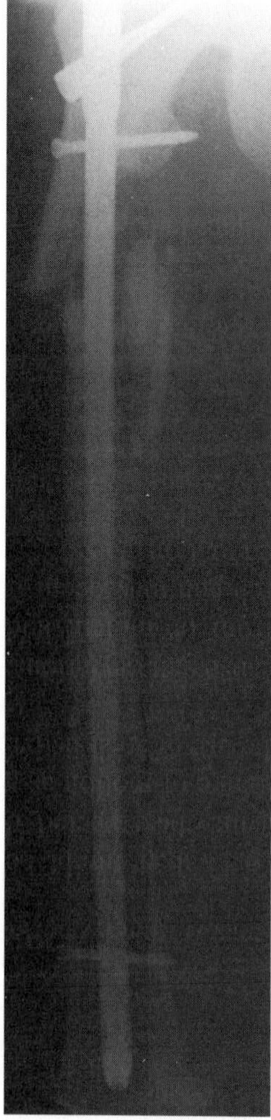

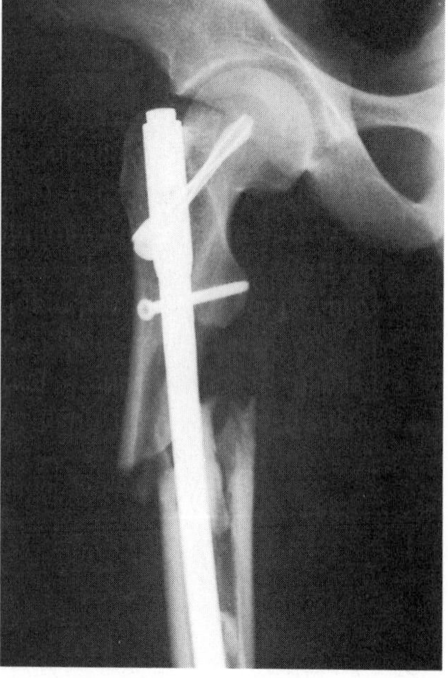

FIGURE 23-6 *(far left)* High-energy comminuted subtrochanteric fracture treated with an intramedullary rod locked proximally and distally to prevent rotation of the proximal and distal fragments, shortening, and angulation at the fracture site. Because of the comminution and bone loss at the fracture site, early weight bearing is not allowed to prevent load transfer to the interlocking screws and early hardware failure. Weight bearing is limited to toe touch until cortical bone continuity is restored.

FIGURE 23-7 *(left)* Comminuted high-energy subtrochanteric fracture treated with an intramedullary rod and proximal locking screws (anteroposterior view).

Compression Screw and Side Plate

Biomechanics: Stress-shielding device.

Mode of Bone Healing: Primary in rigidly fixed fractures; secondary in extremely comminuted fractures and those with bone graft.

Indications: A 95-degree dynamic condylar plate maintains the length of a fracture by providing fixation above and below it. This prevents interfragmentary collapse and may be useful in restoring leg length in those young patients who sustain comminuted fractures. This device is also useful in fractures that extend into the piriformis fossa (the insertion point of femoral nails). When the comminution is severe enough to require the use of this device, consider applying bone graft to the medial buttress. Because the dynamic condylar plate is not commonly used, it is not discussed further in this chapter.

Sliding hip screws may be used in noncomminuted fractures with little extension below the lesser trochanter. It is not discussed further here (Figures 23-8, 23-9, and 23-10). See Chapter 22 for a detailed description of this device.

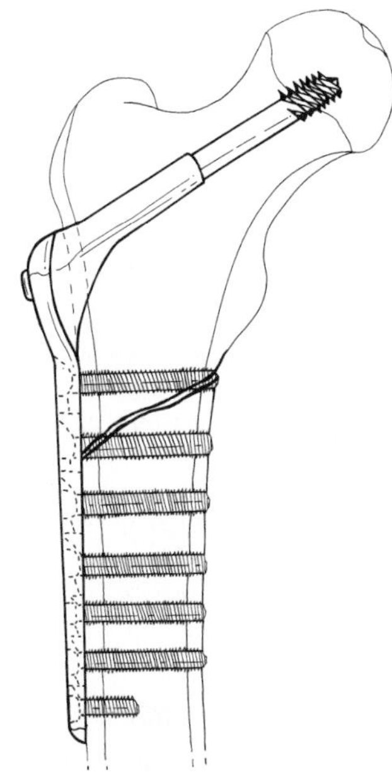

FIGURE 23-8 Subtrochanteric fracture treated with a sliding hip screw. This fixation is augmented with a bone graft along the medial side of the fracture, which provides for early healing of the medial side and prevents hardware failure.

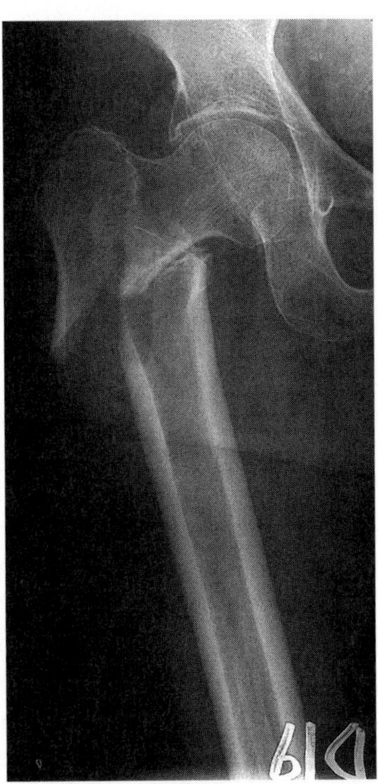

FIGURE 23-9 High subtrochanteric fracture. Note the angulation at the fracture site.

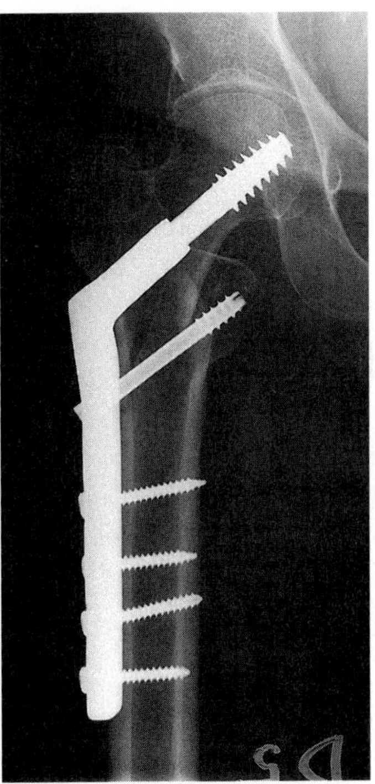

FIGURE 23-10 Subtrochanteric fracture treated with a sliding hip screw and locking screw into the lesser trochanter, augmented with a bone graft to the medial side.

Special Considerations of the Fracture

The subtrochanteric region of the femur is an area of high stress because of the combination of forces from gravity and muscle groups that insert on the proximal fragment. The compressive load on the medial cortex exceeds the tensile load laterally. This imbalance causes varus collapse. Cortical contact at the medial aspect of the femur must be restored for initial fracture stability. If comminution or bone loss has occurred, a bone graft may be necessary to restore this medial buttress.

Associated Injury

Unstable Hematoma

The subtrochanteric region has a rich blood supply and therefore a fracture may cause significant hemorrhage. This bleeding may be concealed in the soft tissues of the thigh; therefore, preoperative and postoperative hemodynamic status should be followed until stable hemoglobin levels are maintained.

Embolism

Baseline arterial blood gas measurements may be helpful because of the risk of fat or venous pulmonary emboli.

Fat emboli syndrome may occur within the first 72 hours after injury, causing sudden respiratory distress and hypoxia. Petechiae in the conjunctivae and axillae as well as tachypnea and tachycardia are signs of this condition.

Pulmonary venous embolism may occur after 72 hours of bed rest. Its symptoms are similar to those of fat emboli, except for the absence of petechiae. Early mobilization is possible with operative fracture fixation and helps to reduce the risk of this condition.

Weight Bearing

Comminuted fractures must be non-weight bearing to toe-touch weight bearing with assistive devices until cortical bone continuity has been restored. Weight bearing on fractures with comminution or bone loss transfers load to the interlocking screws and eventually causes hardware failure (*see* Figures 23-5, 23-6, and 23-7).

Noncomminuted fractures that have contact of proximal and distal fracture fragments may be full weight bearing as tolerated (*see* Figure 23-2).

Gait

Stance Phase

The stance phase constitutes 60% of the gait cycle.

Heel Strike

The gluteus maximus inserts into the subtrochanteric region of the femur and may be affected by the fracture pattern. It is a strong hip extensor and stabilizes the hip by controlling forward flexion at heel strike, thus preventing jackknifing. The *quadriceps* contracts concentrically to control the knee during heel strike and maintain knee extension. The muscle crosses over the fracture site and may have been contused during the initial trauma that led to the fracture. The *vastus lateralis* is commonly incised and mobilized during the surgical approach. The vastus intermedius and rectus are less involved than in a femoral shaft fracture (*see* Figure 6-1).

Foot-Flat

The *gluteus maximus* is still contracting at this phase. Patients may experience pain at the site of insertion if it was compromised by the fracture. The *quadriceps* contracts eccentrically to control the knee flexion from heel strike to foot-flat. This prevents buckling of the knee (*see* Figure 6-2).

Mid-Stance

The *gluteus medius* stabilizes the hip during midstance and prevents Trendelenburg gait by stabilizing the pelvis over the femur. This muscle may have been incised during the surgical approach for insertion of rods or nails. During mid-stance, there is significant stress on the fracture site when the pelvis rotates on the femur to advance the opposite extremity. Patients may experience pain secondary to weight bearing as the leg advances into single-limb support.

The *iliopsoas* contracts to flex the hip and advance the limb and allows the pelvis to rotate over the femur for limb advancement (*see* Figure 6-3).

Push-off

Push-off is usually not affected (*see* Figures 6-4 and 6-5).

Swing Phase

The swing phase constitutes 40% of the gait cycle.

Acceleration may be slowed because of quadriceps injury, which reduces the strength of this muscle as a knee extensor (*see* Figure 6-6).

Mid-swing may be prolonged. Quadriceps contractions, which bring the lower leg forward, may be weakened (*see* Figure 6-7).

Deceleration may be altered by impaired eccentric contraction of weakened hamstrings (*see* Figure 6-8).

TREATMENT

Treatment: Day One to One Week

BONE HEALING

Stability at fracture site: None.

Stage of bone healing: Inflammatory phase. The fracture hematoma is colonized by inflammatory cells and débridement of the fracture begins.

X-ray: No callus; fracture line is clearly visible.

Orthopaedic and Rehabilitation Considerations

Physical Examination

Examine the surgical wound and provide local care as necessary. Measure active and passive motion of the knee and hip. Decreased range of motion may result from pain, swelling, or early adhesion between the vastus lateralis and the tensor fascia lata. Any edema of the lower leg should resolve with elevation of the extremity. Active range-of-motion exercises are given for the hip and knee. Reflex inhibition of the quadriceps secondary to pain or muscle trauma may occur. Quadriceps strengthening exercises are instituted to help control the knee. The patient should be encouraged to exercise and begin early ambulation. Chronic swelling and mild pain may persist for several months up to a year. This should be explained to the patient. Decreased knee range of motion requires aggressive therapy. Note any leg-length discrepancy and evaluate for a shoe lift.

Dangers

Thromboembolic events are common dangers. Note any shortness of breath or chest pain that might be secondary to pulmonary embolism or cardiac sources.

Hypovolemia may result from fracture hematoma and operative blood loss. Hemoglobin levels should be monitored until stable. Occasional transfusions may be necessary for treatment or prophylaxis of myocardial ischemia.

Pressure ulcers may develop rapidly in nonambulatory or bed-bound patients, especially those with poor nutrition. Skin monitoring and proper positioning must be performed to prevent this complication.

Radiography

Examine anteroposterior and lateral views for angulation, shortening, rotation, or gaping at the fracture site. Note the position of hardware and the length of interlocking screws (*see* Figure 23-6).

Weight Bearing

Weight bearing must be adjusted to the fracture pattern.

Full weight bearing as tolerated may begin within the first few days as long as medial bone contact has been restored. Toe-touch to partial weight bearing should be initiated in fractures with extensive comminution and when the medial buttress required bone grafting (*see* Figure 23-7).

Protected weight bearing should also be used whenever a 95-degree hip screw is used because this device bears significant axial stress (*see* Figure 23-10).

Range of Motion

Because interlocked rods are the treatment of choice, the following discussion of rehabilitation pertains to that device.

Hip: Active range-of-motion exercises are prescribed as tolerated. Initially, range of motion might be decreased because of pain, swelling, or early adhesion between the vastus lateralis and the tensor fascia lata.

Knee: Full active knee range of motion is allowed and encouraged.

Muscle Strength

No strengthening exercises are given to the quadriceps or hamstrings at this time. Isometric gluteal sets and isotonic ankle exercises are prescribed to maintain strength. Adduction and abduction are not allowed because these motions place torque force on the fracture site.

Functional Activities

Weight bearing is allowed to tolerance if the medial cortex has been restored. If the fracture is comminuted, only toe-touch weight bearing is allowed and the patient is instructed in three-point crutch walking (*see* Figure 6-17). A walker or crutches should be used for support and stability during transfers. The patient is taught to negotiate stairs with crutches; elderly patients should use a railing in combination with a broad-based quad cane.

Patients are instructed in donning pants with the injured extremity first and doffing them from the uninjured extremity first. This avoids extremes of motion at the hip and thus prevents unnecessary stress at the fracture site.

A raised toilet seat is used initially to facilitate sitting. This reduces extreme hip flexion and the stress it creates on the fracture site.

Gait

Teach ambulation with a two- or three-point gait (*see* Figures 6-16 and 6-17). Crutches or walkers are used, depending on the patient's strength and weight-bearing status. Once the pain level is reduced and strength is improved, stair climbing may begin with careful supervision. The patient climbs up stairs with the unaffected extremity first, followed by the affected extremity and crutches, and descends with the affected extremity and crutches first followed by the unaffected extremity (*see* Figures 6-20, 6-21, 6-22, 6-23, 6-24, and 6-25).

Methods of Treatment: Specific Aspects

Because of their bending strength, femoral nails are able to support fractures in which reconstruction of the medial cortex is not possible. However, these devices are weakest in torsion. The interlocking screws are the mechanical weak link for both torsion and axial loading. These screws must therefore be watched closely during fracture healing.

Fractures treated by open reduction and internal fixation have a reduced blood supply because of surgical mobilization of the soft tissues and therefore often require a bone graft. Sliding hip screws and 95-degree screw–plate constructs are placed on the tension side of the bone. Therefore, these require reconstruction of the medial cortex to reduce tension on the plate and prevent the device from breaking (*see* Figure 23-10). As the reconstructed medial cortex heals, it absorbs compressive stresses on the medial side and thereby decreases tension laterally.

Prescription

DAY ONE TO ONE WEEK

Precautions No adduction and abduction to hip. No isometric exercises to quads and hamstrings.

Range of Motion Active range of motion to hip and knee in flexion and extension.

Muscle Strength Isometric exercises to glutei.

Functional Activities Weight bearing as tolerated or toe-touch weight bearing during transfers with assistive devices, and three-point gait with assistive devices.

Weight Bearing Weight bearing as tolerated on affected extremity in stable fractures treated with intramedullary nails. Toe-touch weight bearing in unstable fractures or those treated by open reduction and internal fixation.

Treatment Two Weeks

BONE HEALING

Stability at fracture site: None to minimal.

Stage of bone healing: Beginning of the reparative phase of fracture healing. Osteoprogenitor cells differentiate into osteoblasts that lay down woven bone.

X-ray: None to very early callus in the region below the lesser trochanter. No callus in the intertrochanteric region where the periosteum is thin, and healing is predominantly endosteal. Fracture line is visible.

Orthopaedic and Rehabilitation Considerations

Physical Examination

Sutures or skin staples should be evaluated and removed as indicated. Measure active and passive range of motion at the hip and the knee. Decreased range of motion might be noted secondary to pain, swelling, or early adhesion between the vastus lateralis and the tensor fascia lata. Any edema of the lower leg should resolve with elevation of the extremity. Active range-of-motion exercises are given to the hip and knee. Reflex inhibition of the quadriceps and hamstring muscles occurs secondary to pain. Quadriceps isometric strengthening exercises should start to help to stabilize the knee. The patient should be encouraged to exercise and continue ambulation. Decreased knee range of motion requires aggressive therapy. Compare the extremities, noting any further leg-length discrepancy, which may indicate loss of correction, and evaluate for a shoe lift as appropriate.

Dangers

Same as those that occur from day 1 to 1 week. See previous section.

Radiography

Examine anteroposterior and lateral views for angulation, shortening, rotation, or gaping at the fracture site. Note the position of hardware and the length of interlocking screws as well as any breakage of the screws.

Weight Bearing

Weight bearing as tolerated in fractures with cortical contact.

Toe-touch weight bearing with assistive devices is permitted in fractures with bone loss or comminution.

Range of Motion

Continue active range of motion to the hip. The patient should have full active hip range of motion. If not, active-assistive to gentle passive range of motion of the hip may be provided in flexion and extension. Continue knee range of motion.

Muscle Strength

Continue isometric gluteal strengthening exercises.

Isometric quadriceps and hamstring sets may be initiated at the end of 2 weeks. If there is persistent reflex inhibition, electrical stimulation can be considered.

Functional Activities

The patient needs the assistance of crutches or a walker during transfers for stability.

The patient may still need to use a raised toilet seat and chair both to decrease the stress on the fracture site and facilitate transfers. The patient may now shower because the staples are removed.

The patient should continue to don slacks with the injured extremity first and doff them with the uninjured extremity first. This technique places the least stress on the fracture site.

Gait

Continue a two- or three-point gait using crutches or a walker (*see* Figures 6-16 and 6-17). As the patient's pain level decreases, he or she is instructed to ascend stairs with the unaffected leg first, followed by the crutches and the affected leg, and to descend stairs with the affected leg and crutches first, followed by the unaffected leg (*see* Figures 6-20, 6-21, 6-22, 6-23, 6-24, and 6-25). Avoid torsion at the fracture site by preventing rotation of the affected extremity when the foot is planted.

Methods of Treatment: Specific Aspects

No change. See previous section (page 294).

Prescription

Two Weeks

Precautions Avoid torsional forces on fracture. Avoid excessive abduction or adduction.

Range of Motion Active, active-assistive to gentle passive range of motion to hip in flexion and extension.

Muscle Strength Isometric exercises to glutei, quadriceps, and hamstrings.

Functional Activities Toe-touch weight bearing or weight bearing as tolerated during transfers and three-point gait; weight bearing as tolerated or toe-touch weight bearing with assistive devices.

Weight Bearing Weight bearing as tolerated on affected extremity in stable fractures treated with intramedullary nails. Toe-touch weight bearing in unstable fractures or those treated by open reduction and internal fixation.

Treatment: Four to Six Weeks

Bone Healing

Stability at fracture site: Callus is beginning to bridge fracture fragments in the femoral region where thick periosteum is present, and endosteal healing is bridging the metaphyseal region where the periosteum is thin but intramedullary blood supply is rich. Unless bone loss or severe comminution is present, the fracture is usually stable; confirm with physical examination.

Stage of bone healing: Reparative phase. Osteoblasts continue to lay down woven bone. Once callus is observed bridging the fracture site, the fracture is usually stable. However, the strength of this callus, especially with torsional load, is significantly lower than that of normal bone.

X-ray: Bridging callus is beginning to be visible in the femoral shaft region. With increased rigidity of fixation, less bridging callus is noted, and healing with endosteal callus predominates. Fracture line is less visible in both the shaft and metaphyseal regions.

Orthopaedic and Rehabilitation Considerations

Physical Examination

Measure hip and knee range of motion and strength. Prescribe a shoe lift as necessary for limb-length inequality. Avoid torsional loading of the fracture (i.e., rotation of the leg with the foot planted).

Dangers

No change. See previous section (page 293).

Radiography

Examine anteroposterior and lateral views for angulation, shortening, rotation, or gaping at the fracture site. Note interlocking screw length and the position of hardware, and evaluate for possible migration of the rod.

Weight Bearing

Weight bearing may be as tolerated in stable fractures.

Toe-touch weight bearing with crutches or a walker and a three-point gait is permitted for unstable fractures with bone loss or comminution.

Range of Motion

Continue full active range of motion to the hip and knee.

Muscle Strength

Continue isometric quadriceps and gluteal sets. Initiate isometric hamstring exercises. This can be done in a sitting position with the patient digging the heel into the ground in slight (30-degree) knee flexion.

Functional Activities

The patient can begin using a quad cane at the end of 6 weeks if he or she is weight bearing as tolerated on the affected side. In the case of bone loss or comminution, a three-point gait with crutches or a walker is maintained because the patient is still restricted to toe-touch weight-bearing.

Continue precautions and restrictions in activities of daily living such as bathing, dressing, and transfers, avoiding rotation and torsional stress on the fracture site.

Gait

Continue a two- or three-point gait depending on weight-bearing status (*see* Figures 6-16 and 6-17).

Methods of Treatment: Specific Aspects

No changes. See the previous section (page 294).

Prescription

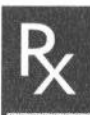

Four to Six Weeks

Precautions Avoid torsional forces on fracture site.

Range of Motion Active, active-assistive, passive range of motion to hip in flexion and extension. Active range of motion to hip in abduction and adduction.

Muscle Strength Isometric exercises to glutei, quadriceps, and hamstrings.

Functional Activities Toe-touch weight bearing or weight bearing as tolerated during transfers and ambulation with assistive devices.

Weight Bearing Weight bearing as tolerated on affected extremity in stable fractures treated with intramedullary nails. Toe-touch weight bearing in unstable fractures or those treated by open reduction and internal fixation.

Treatment: Eight to Twelve Weeks

BONE HEALING

Stability at fracture site: Stable.

Stage of bone healing: Early remodeling phase. Woven bone is being replaced with lamellar bone. The process of remodeling takes months to years for completion.

X-ray: Abundant callus in fractures with intact periosteum. Fracture line begins to disappear.

Orthopaedic and Rehabilitation Considerations

Physical Examination

Evaluate the patient's gait. Assess joint range of motion and strength. Evaluate for shortening of the fractured limb.

Dangers

No change. See previous sections.

Radiography

Examine anteroposterior and lateral views for angulation, shortening, rotation, or gaping at the fracture site. Consider bone grafting for fractures with bone loss or comminution of the medial buttress. Note the position of hardware and interlocking screws. Pay special attention to migration of the distal end of any nail that has been dynamized by removal of the distal screws.

Weight Bearing

Weight bearing may be as tolerated in stable fractures with cortical contact. In unstable fractures with bone loss or comminution, toe-touch weight bearing is permitted with assistive devices.

Range of Motion

Because the fracture is now stable, full active range of motion in all planes is allowed at the hip. If the patient still has decreased motion, active-assistive or passive range-of-motion exercises may be added.

Muscle Strength

Continue isometric gluteal, quadriceps, and hamstring muscles sets. Gentle resistive exercises to the quadriceps and hamstrings may be started at 10 weeks. Light weights starting at 5 pounds are used initially and resistance is increased gradually (2-pound increments) as allowed by pain and fracture healing. Hip abductors and adductors are now also strengthened by isometric contractions.

Functional Activities

The patient should continue a three-point gait with a quad cane for ambulation, depending on weight-bearing status. Most patients have advanced to full weight bearing by 12 weeks.

The patient should be able to dress without assistance and follow a normal dressing pattern. Raised seats may no longer be needed after 12 weeks.

Gait

Observe the patient's gait for limb shortening and treat with a shoe lift if necessary. The gait should evolve to a normal pattern with heel strike, foot-flat, midstance, heel off, and push-off (*see* Figures 6-1, 6-2, 6-3, 6-4, and 6-5). However, the amount of time spent in the stance phase may still be reduced if pain is present at the fracture site. Standing should be improved to allow dynamic unilateral balance and weight shifting onto one leg. Wean the patient off crutches and canes.

Methods of Treatment: Specific Aspects

Consider removing distal interlocking screws to dynamize any fracture that has a persistent fracture cleft and is healing slowly. This promotes bone healing by increasing cyclic loading.

Prescription

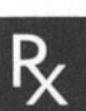

EIGHT TO TWELVE WEEKS

Precautions None.

Range of Motion Full range of motion in all planes to hip and knee.

Muscle Strength Gradual resistive exercises to hip and knee.

Functional Activities Weight bearing as tolerated or full weight bearing during transfers and ambulation with assistive devices.

Weight Bearing Almost all fractures have sufficient bone healing and callus to be full weight bearing as tolerated. Limited weight bearing should be necessary only for fractures with no callus present that are being considered for bone grafting.

Treatment: Twelve to Sixteen Weeks

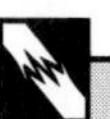

BONE HEALING

Stability at fracture site: Stable.

Stage of bone healing: Remodeling phase. Woven bone is being replaced with lamellar bone. The process of remodeling takes months to years for completion.

X-ray: Abundant callus is present and fracture line begins to disappear.

Orthopaedic and Rehabilitation Considerations

Physical Examination

No change. See previous sections (pages 293 and 296).

Dangers

No change. See previous section (page 293).

Radiography

Examine anteroposterior and lateral views for angulation, shortening, rotation, or gaping at the fracture. Consider bone grafting for fractures with bone loss or with comminution of the medial buttress. Note the position of hardware and evaluate for migration, breakage, and the position of the distal pole of any dynamized rod.

Weight Bearing

All fractures should be weight bearing as tolerated by this time.

Range of Motion

Full range of motion should be obtained in all planes. Gentle sustained passive stretch may be used to treat residual tightness in any muscle groups.

Muscle Strength

Start progressive resistive exercises as tolerated. Resistance is increased gradually depending on the patient's tolerance. The patient may start using Nautilus, Cybex, or other exercise equipment to help provide isotonic and isokinetic strengthening of all lower extremity muscle groups.

Functional Activities

The patient should be full weight bearing and decreasing the use of assistive devices for transfer and ambulation.

Gait

Emphasize gait training with a normal heel-strike and normal knee control during stance and swing phases.

Specific gait deviations such as the Trendelenburg gait may be addressed with focused strengthening of the abductors.

Methods of Treatment: Specific Aspects

Consider removing distal interlocking screws to dynamize any fracture that is healing slowly and has a persistent fracture cleft. This promotes healing by initiating cyclic loading of the fracture. Fractures that have already been dynamized or those treated by open reduction and internal fixation that have no visible callus should be treated with bone grafting to the medial femoral cortex.

Prescription

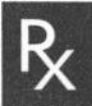

TWELVE TO SIXTEEN WEEKS

Precautions None.

Range of Motion Full range of motion in all planes to hip and knee.

Muscle Strength Progressive resistive exercises to hip and knee.

Functional Activities Full weight bearing during transfer and ambulation.

Weight Bearing Almost all fractures have sufficient bone healing and callus to be full weight bearing as tolerated. Limited weight bearing should be necessary only for fractures with no callus present that are being considered for bone grafting.

LONG-TERM CONSIDERATIONS AND PROBLEMS

Orthopaedic Considerations

Nonunion is a rare occurrence, often associated with loss of fixation. If nonunion occurs, it may be treated by restoring rigid fixation and bone grafting.

Rehabilitation Considerations

A shortened limb caused by bone loss, comminution, or impaction of the fracture may be treated with a shoe lift.

Patients are often unsteady or have some imbalance from weakness. If this unsteadiness does not rapidly improve with strengthening and gait training, the patient may need to use a cane. If the patient previously used a cane, a quad cane or walker might be needed. In general, elderly patients may be expected to lose some degree of strength and range of motion as a result of the fracture and require the use of an assistive device.

Muscle weakness or pain may cause gait deviations. Antalgic gaits may also result from prominent and painful hardware. An abductor lurch gait may occur if the greater trochanter was fractured and displaced.

IMMEDIATE TO ONE WEEK

	Intramedullary Rod	*Compression Screw and Side Plate*
Stability	None.	None.
Orthopaedics	Examine wounds.	Same as for intramedullary rod.
	Remove drains when appropriate.	
	Deep vein thrombosis prophylaxis.	
	Check blood count.	
Rehabilitation	Active range of motion to the hip and knee in the plane of flexion and extension. Isometric gluteal exercises. Transfer training.	Same as for intramedullary rod.

TWO WEEKS

	Intramedullary Rod	*Compression Screw and Side Plate*
Stability	None to minimal.	Same as for intramedullary rod.
Orthopaedics	Examine wounds.	Same as for intramedullary rod.
	Remove sutures or staples.	
	Consider deep vein thrombosis prophylaxis.	
Rehabilitation	Active and active-assistive range of motion to the hip, knee, ankle. Isometric gluteal, hamstring, and quadriceps strengthening exercises. Stand/pivot transfers on well leg to avoid torsional forces on fracture and ambulation with appropriate assistive devices. Weight bearing depends on fracture pattern.	Same as for intramedullary rod.

FOUR TO SIX WEEKS

	Intramedullary Rod	Compression Screw and Side Plate
Stability	Increasing stability is present as callus forms and bridges the fracture. Most fractures are stable by 6 weeks unless there is bone loss or severe comminution. Confirm stability with physical examination radiographs.	Same as for intramedullary rod.
Orthopaedics	Examine radiograph for healing and hardware position.	Same as for intramedullary rod.
Rehabilitation	Continue to increase active, active-assistive, and passive range of motion to hip in the flexion and extension plane and begin active adduction and abduction. Continue isometric exercises and increase weight bearing in accordance with fracture stability.	Same as for intramedullary rod.

EIGHT TO TWELVE WEEKS

	Intramedullary Rod	Compression Screw and Side Plate
Stability	Stable.	Same as for intramedullary rod.
Orthopaedics	Consider bone grafting any fracture with persistent gaping at the fracture site, especially if the medial buttress has had bone loss or severe comminution.	Same as for intramedullary rod.
Rehabilitation	Gradual resistive exercises may be started on the hip and knee. Most fractures should be weight bearing as tolerated. Begin to wean from assistive devices.	Same as for intramedullary rod.

TWELVE TO SIXTEEN WEEKS

	Intramedullary Rod	Compression Screw and Side Plate
Stability	Unchanged.	Unchanged.
Orthopaedics	Unchanged.	Unchanged.
Rehabilitation	Progressive resistive exercises to the hip and knee.	Same as for intramedullary rod.

BIBLIOGRAPHY

DeLee JC. Fractures and dislocations of the hip. In: Rockwood CA Jr, Green DP, Bucholz RW, eds. *Fractures in Adults*, Vol 2, 3rd ed. Philadelphia: J.B. Lippincott, 1991, pp. 1481–1651.

McKibbon B. The biology of fracture healing in long bones. *J Bone Joint Surg Br*, 60:150–161, 1978.

Russell TA, Taylor JC. Subtrochanteric fractures of the femur. In: Browner BD, Jupiter JB, Levine AM, Trafton PG, eds. *Skeletal Trauma*, Vol 2. Philadelphia: W.B. Saunders, 1992, pp 1485–1524.

Wiss DA, Matta JM, Sima W, et al. Subtrochanteric fractures of the femur. *Orthopedics*, 8:797–800, 1985.

Wu CC, Shih CH, Lee ZL. Subtrochanteric fractures treated with interlocking nailing. *J Trauma*, 31:326–333, 1991.

CHAPTER *Twenty-four*

Femoral Shaft Fractures

KENNETH W. TAYLOR, MD

VASANTHA L. MURTHY, MD

INTRODUCTION

Definition

A femoral shaft fracture is a diaphyseal fracture of the femur that does not extend into the articular or metaphyseal region (Figures 24-1, 24-2, and 24-3; *see* Figure 24-4).

Mechanism of Injury

High-energy trauma such as a motor vehicle accident is the cause of most femur fractures. These fractures are often associated with significant soft-tissue trauma and, at times, open wounds.

Low-energy trauma and indirect forces may cause fractures in elderly adults whose bones are osteopenic or weakened by tumors. Injuries of pathologic bone usually result from rotational or spiral forces and have less associated soft-tissue injury.

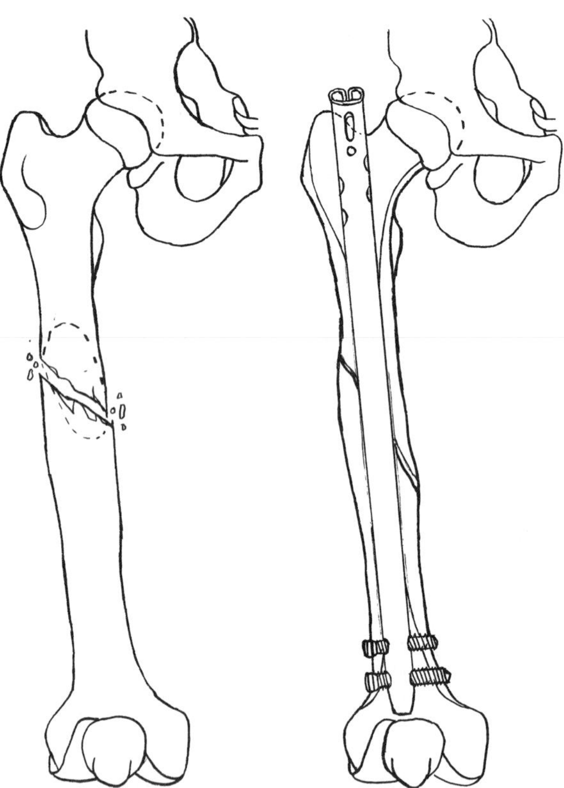

FIGURE 24-1 *(above, left)* Fracture of the femoral shaft. The diaphyseal fracture in the middle portion of the shaft does not extend to the articular or metaphyseal region.

FIGURE 24-2 *(above, right)* Oblique diaphyseal femur fracture fixed with a dynamically locked femoral rod with distal interlocking screws only. This allows control of the rotation of the distal fragment and provides for compression at the fracture site with weight bearing. Rotation control is provided by a tight fit between the isthmus of the femur and the femoral rod proximally.

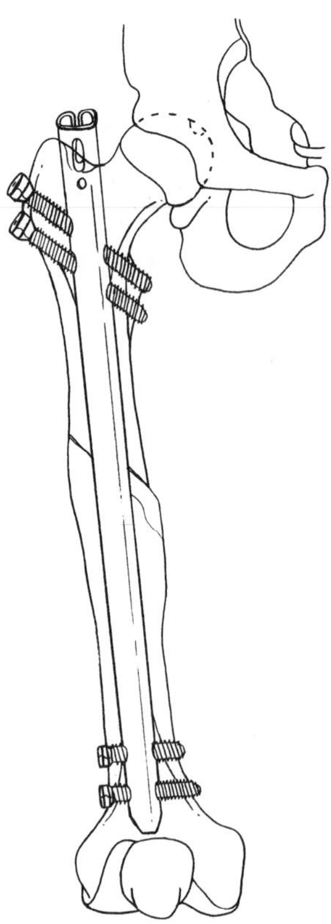

FIGURE 24-3 Oblique fracture of the femoral midshaft treated with a statically locked femoral rod. Rotation of the proximal and distal fragments is controlled with the interlocking screws. Early weight bearing is allowed.

Treatment Goals

Orthopaedic Objectives

Alignment

Restore rotation and length.

Stability

Restore cortical contact for axial stability.

Rehabilitation Objectives

Range of Motion

Restore and maintain full range of motion of the knee and hip (Table 24-1).

TABLE 24-1 *Ranges of Motion of Knee and Hip*

Motion	Normal	Functional
Knee		
Flexion	0–130 / 140°	110°
Extension	0°[a]	0°
Hip		
Flexion	125–128°	90–110°
Extension	0–20°	0–5°
Abduction	45–48°	0–20°
Adduction	40–45°	0–20°
Internal rotation	40–45°	0–20°
External rotation	45°	0–15°

[a]"Zero" indicates measurement from neutral position.

Muscle Strength

Improve the strength of the following muscles that are affected by the fracture:

Quadriceps: knee extensor
Hamstrings: knee flexor and secondary hip extensor

Functional Goals

Restore normal gait pattern.

Expected Time of Bone Healing

Four to 6 weeks until the fracture becomes sticky and shows early stability.

Twelve to 16 weeks until the fracture site is united.

Expected Duration of Rehabilitation

Twelve to 16 weeks.

Methods of Treatment

Intramedullary Nail Fixation

Biomechanics: Stress-sharing system if the nail is dynamically locked; partial stress shielding if it is statically locked.

Mode of Bone Healing: Secondary.

Indications: This method allows for early mobilization of the patient as well as early knee range of motion. It is therefore the treatment of choice and the most commonly used form of fixation for femoral shaft fractures. The anterior bow of the femur and femoral isthmus provide for an interference fit (a tight bony fit) when a rod is placed in its medullary canal. Interlocking proximal and distal to the fracture is necessary in fractures with unstable butterfly fragments or severe comminution. This creates static fixation and prevents shortening and loss of rotatory alignment. For transverse fractures and those with minimal comminution, the nail may be left unlocked at one end. This creates dynamic fixation and allows interfragmentary compression on weight bearing, which in turn stimulates healing (Figures 24-4, 24-5, 24-6, 24-7, 24-8, and 24-9).

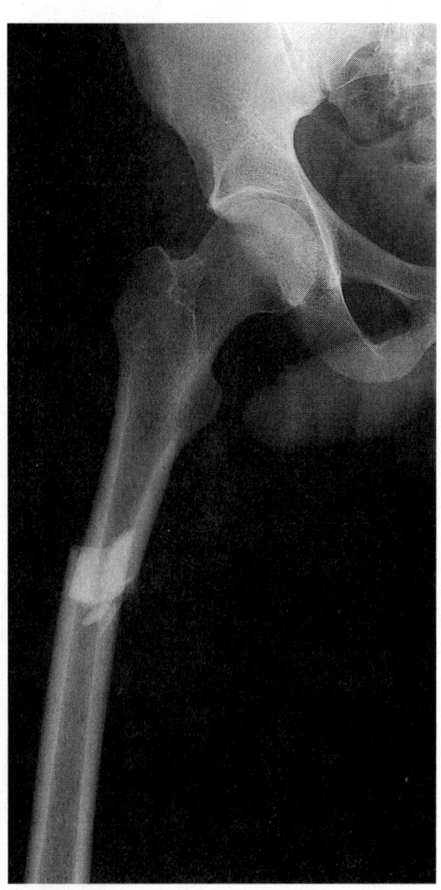

FIGURE 24-4 Transverse fracture of the femoral diaphysis. Note the shortening at the fracture site.

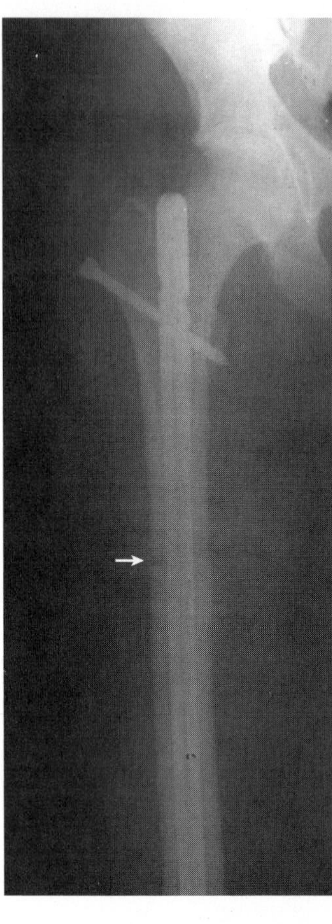

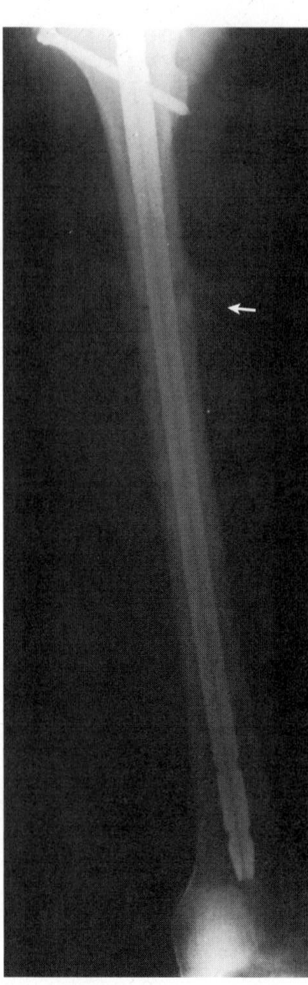

FIGURE 24-5 *(far left)* Transverse fracture of the femoral shaft treated with a proximally locked femoral nail.

FIGURE 24-6 *(left)* Healed transverse fracture of the femoral shaft treated with a dynamically locked intramedullary nail to allow impaction of the fracture site with weight bearing *(arrow)*. Note the callus formed at the fracture site.

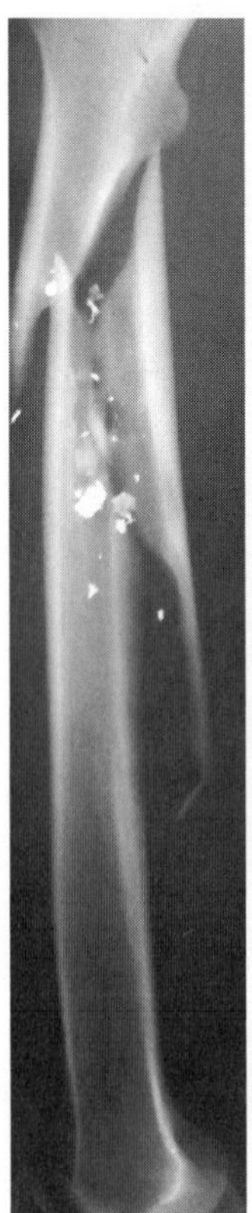

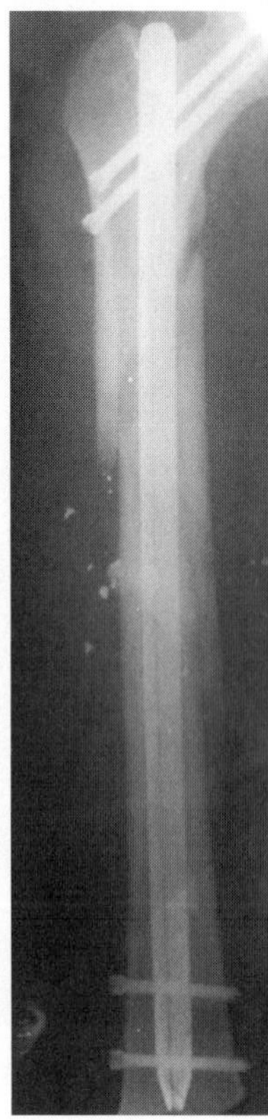

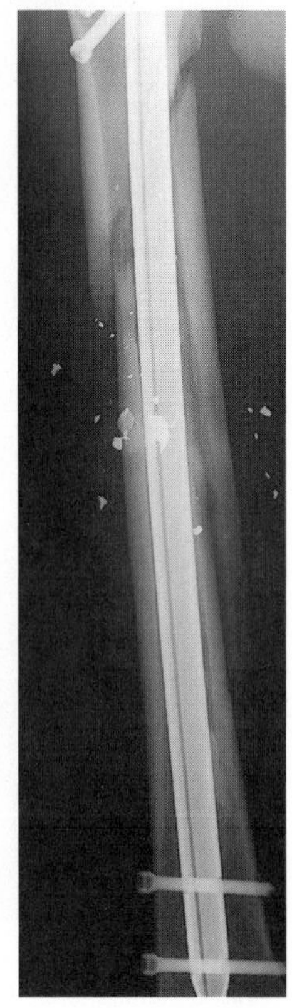

FIGURE 24-7 *(far left)* High-energy femoral shaft fracture secondary to a gunshot wound. Note the comminution at the fracture site and displacement with three large bony fragments.

FIGURE 24-8 *(middle left)* Spiral fracture of the femoral diaphysis with a large butterfly fragment treated with a statically locked femoral nail.

FIGURE 24-9 *(near left)* Spiral fracture of the femoral diaphysis with a large butterfly fragment fixed with a statically locked intramedullary nail. This allows early mobilization but only partial early weight bearing. High-energy fractures such as this may be associated with adherence of the quadriceps to the fracture site, affecting the glide mechanism of the quadriceps along the femoral shaft.

Open Reduction and Internal Plate Fixation

Biomechanics: Stress-shielding device.

Mode of Bone Healing: Primary.

Indications: This method of fixation is best for shaft fractures with periarticular or intraarticular extension, which precludes placement of an intramedullary nail. It is done by direct visualization of the fracture site and should provide anatomic reduction. For optimum fixation, the plate should be secured to the femur by eight cortical fixation points above and below the fracture site. When severe comminution is present, consider applying bone graft medially. This method allows the patient to be mobilized early, without weight bearing, despite the additional soft tissue trauma from surgical exposure. It is infrequently used in the treatment of femur fractures (Figure 24-10).

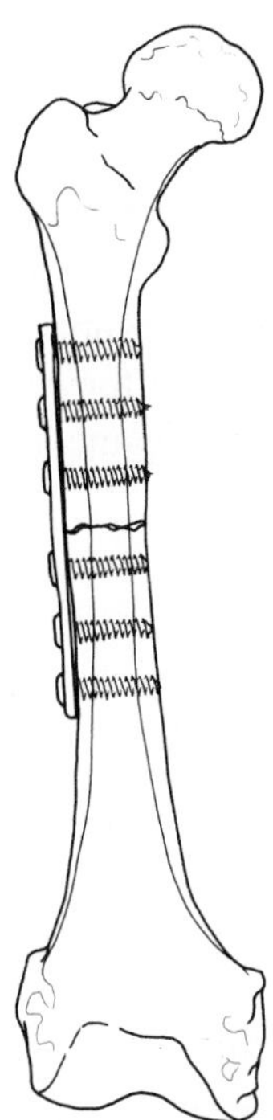

FIGURE 24-10 Transverse fracture of the femoral shaft with compression plate fixation, an unusual treatment for femur fractures. This allows the patient to be mobilized early, although weight bearing in the early postoperative period is not permitted.

External Fixation

Biomechanics: Stress-sharing device.

Mode of Bone Healing: Secondary.

Indications: External fixation is used in type III open fractures (those with a wound larger than 10 cm, contamination with severe soft-tissue injury and loss, and bone comminution) after intraoperative débridement of severely comminuted and displaced fractures. It allows for wound management without further trauma to injured soft tissues (Figure 24-11).

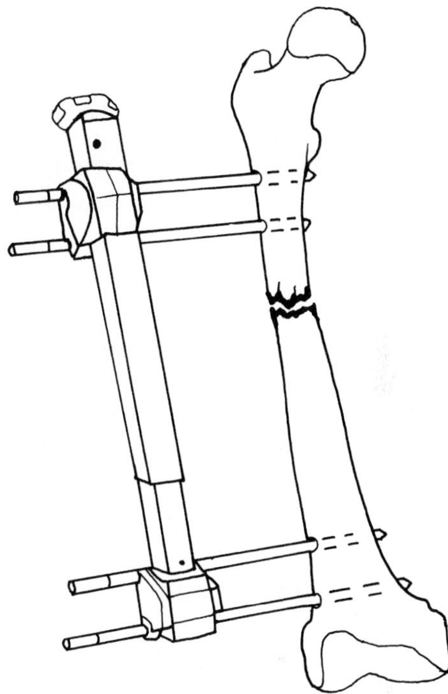

FIGURE 24-11 Transverse fracture of the femoral shaft treated with an external fixation device. External fixation of femur fractures is usually reserved for emergency treatment of unstable patients and severely contaminated wounds. Pins are placed through muscles, which may interfere with the quadriceps function.

A stable construct requires pins to be placed through the muscle. This may interfere with quadriceps function and impair knee range of motion. Fixators may be exchanged for definitive external or internal treatment methods after soft-tissue healing occurs. Aggressive pin care must be emphasized because pin tract infection precludes revision to an intramedullary nail after soft-tissue healing.

This form of treatment is not commonly used but is often helpful in complex fractures that extend into the knee joint or on both sides of the joint.

Skeletal Traction

Biomechanics: Stress-sharing device.

Mode of Bone Healing: Secondary.

Indications: Traction used to be the standard treatment for femoral shaft fractures; it has low infection rates but leads to knee stiffness and often malunion. In addition, traction requires prolonged hospitalization and frequent, time-consuming adjustments. The risk of morbidity from respiratory, integumentary, and hematologic complications is also increased with prolonged bed rest. Traction is used only as a temporizing treatment when an immediate operative procedure is not feasible and the definitive treatment must be delayed. This method of treatment is not discussed further in this chapter.

Special Considerations of the Fracture

Hemorrhage

Hematoma between the muscle fascia and subcutaneous tissue may result from direct blows. Displaced ends of the fracture may lacerate nerves, blood vessels, and muscles, altering motor function. They may create cavities that fill with hematoma. Serial hematocrits should be monitored until a stable value is obtained.

Embolism

Because of the risk of fat or pulmonary emboli, baseline arterial blood gas measurements should be considered on every patient with a long bone fracture.

Fat emboli syndrome may occur within the first 72 hours after injury, causing sudden respiratory distress and hypoxia. Petechiae in the conjunctiva and axillae as well as tachypnea and tachycardia are signs of this condition.

Venous pulmonary embolism may occur after 72 hours of bed rest or venous pooling. Its symptoms are similar to those of fat emboli, except for the absence of petechiae. Early mobilization, allowed by operative fracture fixation, can help to reduce the risk of this condition.

Associated Injury

Pelvic, hip, and knee radiographs should be obtained to rule out associated fractures that may have been overlooked because of significant pain from the femur fracture. Ipsilateral femoral neck fractures not uncommonly accompany femoral shaft fractures. When these are present, consideration should be given to treating these fractures with two devices. A retrograde femoral nail allows stabilization of the shaft fracture and leaves room proximally for fixation of the neck fracture with a dynamic hip compression screw. Some surgeons prefer to use reconstruction-type femoral nails.

Knee injuries are also commonly sustained in motor vehicle accidents. When the knee has impacted against the dashboard, it should be examined to rule out a posterior cruciate ligament rupture. It is important to evaluate the knee ligaments for stability after the fracture has been stabilized. Ligaments should be tested both during and after surgery.

Weight Bearing

A fracture treated with a dynamically locked nail may begin immediate weight bearing as tolerated to allow for compression of the fracture ends against each other and to stimulate healing. A statically locked nail may be treated similarly if minimal comminution is present (*see* Figures 24-4, 24-5, and 24-6).

Other fractures treated with a statically locked nail or open reduction and internal fixation may be toe-touch weight bearing to partially weight bearing, depending on comminution. This should continue for 6 to 8 weeks until bone healing takes stress off of the implants. If the reduction is stable and the cortices are in contact, the patient may walk immediately with full weight bearing. Axial loading of fractures without cortical continuity transfers the load to the interlocking screws, which eventually fatigue and fail. The comminuted area then collapses under the stress of the axial load (*see* Figures 24-7, 24-8, and 24-9).

Gait

The following muscles affected by the fracture are important during the gait cycle.

The *quadriceps muscle* and its fascia may become adherent to the fracture site, and the gliding mechanism may be affected. This causes pain during muscle contraction and alters the gait cycle because of the inability to achieve full knee extension (Figure 24-12).

The *hamstrings* may shorten because of the knee being held in flexion or possible loss of femoral length. This also prevents full knee extension when the hip is flexed.

Stance Phase

The stance phase constitutes 60% of the gait cycle.

Heel Strike

The *quadriceps* contracts concentrically to stabilize the knee at heel strike and maintain full knee extension. This can be quite painful because the quadriceps has had a contusion during the initial trauma that led to the fracture (Figure 24-13). The *hamstrings'* continued eccentric contraction (elongation) helps leg deceleration to heel strike. However, a contracted or shortened muscle prevents full knee extension (*see* Figure 6-1).

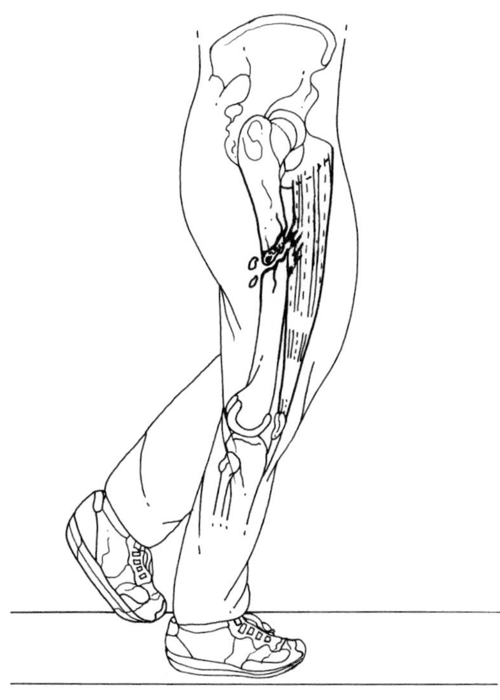

FIGURE 24-12 The quadriceps muscle and fascia may adhere to the fracture site and the glide mechanism may be affected, preventing full range of motion of the knee.

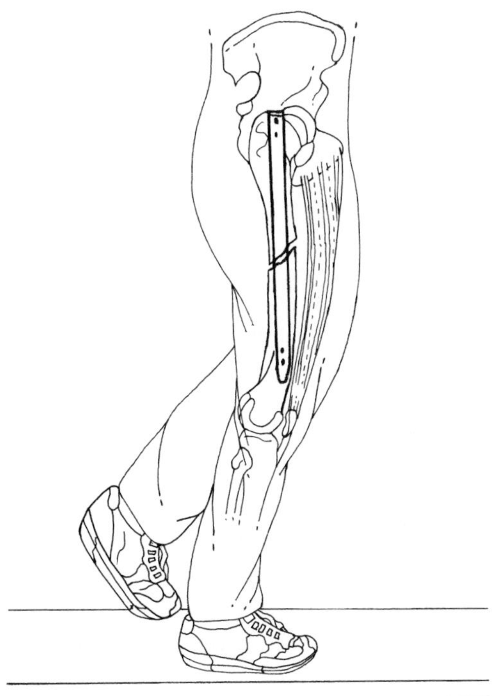

FIGURE 24-13 The quadriceps contracts concentrically during the stance phase to stabilize the knee. This can be quite painful because the quadriceps has been contused during the initial trauma.

Foot-Flat

The quadriceps contracts eccentrically to control knee flexion between heel strike and foot flat. This prevents buckling of the knee (*see* Figure 6-2).

Mid-Stance

The fracture site may be painful because the patient may be bearing weight through the affected limb in single-limb support (*see* Figures 6-3, 24-12, and 24-13).

Push-off

Push-off usually is not grossly affected (*see* Figures 6-4 and 6-5).

Swing Phase

The swing phase constitutes 40% of the gait cycle.

Acceleration

This phase may be slowed because of reduced quadriceps slide and force of concentric contraction (*see* Figure 6-6).

Deceleration

The hamstrings contract during this phase to decelerate the swinging leg, and also help hip extension along with the gluteus maximus. A contracted or shortened muscle may cause too rapid a deceleration and prevent the knee from becoming fully extended (*see* Figure 6-8).

TREATMENT

Treatment: Early to Immediate (Day of Injury to One Week)

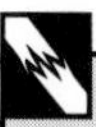

BONE HEALING

Stability at fracture site: None.

Stage of bone healing: Inflammatory phase. The fracture hematoma is colonized by inflammatory cells and débridement of the fracture begins.

X-ray: No callus; fracture line is clearly visible.

Orthopaedic and Rehabilitation Considerations

Physical Examination

Carefully assess complaints of pain, paresthesia, and swelling of the involved extremity. Evaluate for neuropathy, ischemia, or expanding thigh hematoma.

Grade the strength of the following foot muscle motions:

1. Dorsiflexion: deep peroneal nerve
2. Plantar flexion: tibial nerve
3. Big toe extension: deep peroneal nerve
4. Eversion: superficial peroneal nerve
5. Inversion: tibial nerve

The strength of these motions reflects the function of the tibial and peroneal divisions of the sciatic nerve.

Evaluate sensation as follows:

1. Superficial peroneal nerve: dorsum of foot
2. Deep peroneal nerve: web space (first and second toes)
3. Sural nerve: lateral border of foot
4. Tibial nerve: medial aspect of foot—plantar branches: sole of foot

Evaluate active and passive range of motion of the knee and hip joints.

Assess the alignment of the repaired limb compared with the uninjured side.

Dangers

Note any respiratory changes that might be secondary to fat embolism (first 3 days) or venous pulmonary embolism (after 3 days).

Radiography

Examine anteroposterior and lateral views for angulation, shortening, rotation, or cleft at the fracture site.

Weight Bearing

The possibility of weight bearing varies with the method of treatment. In general, weight bearing stimulates fracture healing and is allowed for fractures in which cortical contact and a stable fracture pattern can be reestablished. Specific aspects of weight bearing are discussed in each section under Methods of Treatment: Specific Aspects.

Range of Motion

Once the pain subsides, active range-of-motion exercises are prescribed to the hip, knee, and ankle. Initially, range of motion, especially of the knee, may be limited by edema and pain. To control edema, the patient is instructed to keep the leg elevated.

Muscle Strength

Instruct the patient in active ankle exercises (dorsiplantar flexion). The gastrocnemius acts as a venous pump and helps in preventing venous stasis and phlebitis. Dorsiplantar flexion exercises help to maintain the strength of the muscles and also retard plantar flexion contracture.

Isometric quadriceps strengthening exercises are instituted to help control the knee. Because the quadriceps spans the thigh, the patient may complain of pain when exercising the muscle.

Isometric exercises to the glutei group are taught to maintain strength.

Functional Activities

For bed mobility, the patient is instructed to roll to one side and use the upper extremities to push up into a seated position.

If weight bearing is allowed, the patient can use the affected limb for minimal support when performing ambulatory transfers between bed and chair with assistance. If non-weight bearing, the patient is instructed in stand-pivot transfers with the use of crutches.

A raised toilet seat is used to decrease hip flexion and reduce stress at the fracture site.

The patient is instructed in donning pants with the affected limb first and doffing them from the unaffected limb first to decrease stress at the fracture site.

Gait

The patient uses crutches or a walker for ambulation. If the patient is non-weight bearing, a two-point gait is taught in which the crutches advance as one unit followed by the unaffected extremity as the second unit (the patient hops; *see* Figure 6-16).

If the patient is allowed to bear weight as tolerated, then a three-point gait is taught (*see* Figure 6-17). The crutches go first, followed by the affected extremity (second) and the unaffected extremity (third).

The patient is not instructed in stair climbing until several days after injury.

Methods of Treatment: Specific Aspects

Intramedullary Nail Fixation

Measure active and passive motion of the hip and particularly the knee. Decreased range of motion might be noted secondary to pain or swelling. Any edema should be treated by elevating the extremity.

Active range-of-motion exercises are given to the hip and knee. Reflex quadriceps inhibition secondary to pain, muscle trauma, or knee effusion may occur. Quadriceps strengthening exercises are instituted to help neutralize rotational forces. The patient should be encouraged to exercise and begin early ambulation.

At this time, discuss the possibility that swelling and mild pain may persist for several months to a year. Decreased knee range of motion requires early, aggressive therapy to prevent adhesion and scarring. Note any leg-length discrepancy and evaluate for a shoe lift as appropriate. This should only occur with severe comminution or a segmental cortical defect.

With a statically locked nail, toe-touch to partial weight-bearing is allowed during ambulation and transfers (*see* Figure 24-3). Full weight bearing should be avoided to prevent femoral shortening at the fracture site. With a dynamically locked nail, weight bearing as tolerated is encouraged during ambulation and transfers (*see* Figure 24-2). If there is good cortical contact at the fracture site, the femur will not shorten.

Open Reduction and Internal Plate Fixation

Examine wounds and begin hip and knee range of motion. The patient is non-weight bearing to toe-touch weight bearing with crutches or a walker and a two-point gait. Plated fractures cannot tolerate the torsional and bending forces generated by weight bearing (*see* Figure 24-10).

External Fixation

Evaluate the wound for erythema, discharge, or purulence. Hydrotherapy may be needed for open wounds. Check pin sites for discharge, erythema, or skin tension and treat appropriately. Cleanse pin sites with peroxide or povidone–iodine solution. Release any skin tension. The patient should be able to perform aggressive routine pin care. Consider antibiotics if a pin site infection is evident. Fascia and muscle motion from therapy may lead to pin loosening. This can be corrected by slight advancement of the pins. Active range of motion should be instituted with strengthening exercises. The patient is allowed range of motion at both the hip and the knee with associated strengthening exercises. Until a callus is present, the patient should be instructed in non–weight-bearing ambulation with a walker or crutches and a two-point gait to avoid disruption of the fracture.

Placement of the pins through the quadriceps muscle may decrease the range of motion of the knee. Flexion is especially problematic because the muscle is pinned with the knee in extension. This muscle must be stretched. Ambulation and transfers are non-weight bearing with crutches (*see* Figure 24-11).

Prescription

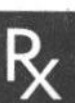

DAY ONE TO ONE WEEK

Precautions No passive range of motion to hip or knee. No rotation on a planted foot.

Range of Motion Active range of motion to hip and knee.

Muscle Strength Isometric exercises to quads and glutei.

Functional Activities Ambulatory stand-pivot transfers and ambulation with crutches.

Weight Bearing Depending on treatment, either toe touch or non-weight bearing for unstable fractures or those treated by plating or external fixator. Stable fractures may progress to full weight bearing as tolerated.

Treatment: Two to Four Weeks

BONE HEALING

Stability at fracture site: None to minimal.

Stage of bone healing: Beginning of reparative phase. Osteoprogenitor cells differentiate into osteoblasts that lay down woven bone.

X-ray: None to very early callus; fracture line visible.

Orthopaedic and Rehabilitation Considerations

Physical Examination

Carefully assess complaints of new or increasing pain, paresthesia, or swelling of the involved extremity. Pay special attention to drainage or other signs of infection at the surgical site. Remove sutures and staples at 2 weeks. Measure the range of motion and strength of the hip, knee, and ankle.

Assess the alignment and length of the repaired limb compared with the uninjured side.

Dangers

Same as those that occur from 1 day to 1 week. See previous section (page 308).

Radiography

Assess alignment and maintenance of correction and femoral length. Check for a cleft at the fracture site.

Weight Bearing

Continue weight bearing as allowed by fracture comminution and the method of fixation. See Methods of Treatment: Specific Aspects for specifics (pages 309–310).

Range of Motion

Continue active/active-assisted range of motion to the hip and knee. The patient is instructed to draw the alphabet with the foot to range the ankle fully.

It is important to achieve full knee flexion/extension as soon as possible. This helps prevent adhesion of the underside of the quadriceps to the fracture site.

If the patient is able to tolerate it, full passive range of motion is initiated. This is usually done with a pulley system while the patient is supine.

Initially, an extension lag of approximately 20 to 30 degrees is observed because of quadriceps and hamstring inhibition secondary to sympathetic effusion into the knee joint or trauma. This should have subsided by now to allow full range. If the knee is still swollen, range of motion is done in the seated position, with the foot sliding along the level surface of the floor (active range of motion) or with assistance from the other foot. This is gravity assisted or passive, depending on initiation of the movement, and it provides incomplete range of motion.

Muscle Strength

Straight leg raising exercises are started, depending on the patient's tolerance, to strengthen the quadriceps and hip flexion.

Repetition of knee flexion and extension not only improves the range of motion, but improves the strength of the quadriceps and hamstrings.

Continue with gluteal sets to improve the glutei strength.

Continue with ankle isotonic exercises.

Functional Activities

Continue with stand-pivot transfers using assistive devices.

The patient continues to don pants with the affected extremity first and doff them from the unaffected extremity first.

Gait

The patient may continue ambulation depending on weight-bearing status.

The patient is instructed to climb up the stairs with the unaffected extremity first, followed by the affected extremity and the crutches, and to descend stairs with the crutches and affected extremity first, followed by the unaffected extremity (*see* Figures 6-20, 6-21, 6-22, 6-23, 6-24, and 6-25).

Methods of Treatment: Specific Aspects

Intramedullary Nail Fixation

Continue active range of motion and strengthening exercises. Encourage the patient to continue aggressive physical therapy as tolerated.

Continue weight bearing as tolerated for fractures treated with a dynamically locked nail. Patients with unstable fractures treated with a statically locked nail should be non-weight bearing to partial weight bearing using crutches or a walker and a three-point gait. Stable fractures treated with this device may be advanced to full weight bearing as tolerated.

Open Reduction and Internal Plate Fixation

If the fracture is stable, advise the patient to advance to partial weight bearing with a cast brace. If it is unstable, continue non-weight bearing. Continue aggressive physical therapy and range of motion.

Continue non-weight bearing with crutches or a walker and a three-point gait (*see* Figure 6-17).

External Fixation

Assess for infection at the pin sites. Measure hip and knee range of motion. Continue range-of-motion and strengthening exercises to the quadriceps muscle. Advise the patient of possible leg shortening if there is severe comminution or bone loss. Stiffness of the knee joint, pain, and swelling at the fracture site may also occur and should be discussed.

Continue non-weight bearing using crutches or a walker and a three-point gait.

Prescription

Two Weeks to Four Weeks

Precautions Avoid rotation on the affected extremity with the foot planted.

Range of Motion Active, active-assistive range of motion to hip and knee, passive range of motion closer to 4 weeks.

Muscle Strength Isometric exercises to quads and glutei; straight leg raising.

Functional Activities Ambulatory stand-pivot transfers with crutches and ambulation with crutches.

Weight Bearing Depending on treatment, toe-touch to partial weight bearing for unstable fractures or those treated by plating or external fixator. Weight bearing as tolerated for stable fractures.

Treatment: Four to Six Weeks

Bone Healing

Stability at fracture site: With bridging callus, the fracture is usually stable; confirm with physical examination.

Stage of bone healing: Reparative phase. Once callus is observed bridging the fracture site, the fracture is usually stable. However, the strength of this callus, especially with torsional load, is significantly lower than that of normal bone.

X-ray: Bridging callus is beginning to be visible. With increased rigidity of fixation, less bridging callus will be noted, and healing with endosteal callus will predominate. The amount of callus formation is greater for diaphyseal than metaphyseal fractures. Fracture line is less visible.

Orthopaedic and Rehabilitation Considerations

Physical Examination

Assess all wounds and/or pin sites and treat appropriately. Measure hip and knee range of motion and strength. Prescribe a shoe lift for a significant leg-length discrepancy.

Dangers

No significant change. See previous section.

Radiography

Examine anteroposterior and lateral radiographs to confirm fixation, alignment, no rotation at the fracture site, and the position of hardware. To detect possible nail migration (backing out), pay special attention to the entry point of any nail that is proximally unlocked.

Weight Bearing

Continue weight bearing as allowed by fracture comminution and the method of fixation. See Methods of Treatment: Specific Aspects for specifics (pages 309–310).

Range of Motion

There should not be any limitations in range of motion at the knee and hip. Continue active/passive range-of-motion exercises.

Strength

Begin resistive exercises. Increase the strength of the quadriceps and hamstrings with increasing ankle weights. Begin with one set of 8 to 12 repetitions and progress to three sets. One-pound weights are initially used and gradually increased to two and then five pounds.

Functional Activities

Continue transfers according to the patient's weight-bearing status.

Gait

Continue with a two-point or three-point gait pattern according to the patient's weight-bearing status (*see* Figures 6-16 and 6-17).

Methods of Treatment: Specific Aspects

Intramedullary Nail Fixation

Assess complaints of pain, paresthesia, or swelling of the involved extremity (these should be decreasing). Examine the surgical site for any sign of infection. Avoid torsion loading. Continue active range of motion and strengthening exercises, emphasizing knee motion.

Weight Bearing. Continue weight bearing as tolerated for a fracture treated with a dynamically locked nail or a stable fracture treated with a statically locked nail. Partial weight bearing using crutches or a walker and a three-point gait should be continued for unstable fractures treated with statically locked nails.

Open Reduction and Internal Plate Fixation

Considerations are the same as for intramedullary nail fixation. See above.

Weight Bearing. Continue partial weight bearing or non-weight bearing.

External Fixation

All fixators should be removed by 4 to 6 weeks. Soft tissue defects should have healed or had skin coverage procedures, and the fracture site should be stable both radiologically and clinically. The patient may then be placed in a cast brace. If a segmental cortical defect is present a bone graft should be placed. If necessary, hydrotherapy may be used for cleansing the pin sites. Strengthening exercises to the quadriceps and hamstrings can be started when good callus formation is present.

Weight Bearing. Ambulation with partial weight bearing is started with crutches or a walker when the fixator is removed.

Prescription

FOUR TO SIX WEEKS

Precautions Avoid rotation on the affected extremity with the foot planted.

Range of Motion Active/passive range of motion to hip and knee.

Muscle Strength Resistive isotonic exercises and isometric exercises to the quads, hamstrings, and glutei.

Functional Activities Stand/pivot transfers and ambulation with crutches.

Weight Bearing Depending on treatment, partial weight bearing for unstable fractures and those treated with plating or external fixators. Full weight bearing for stable fractures.

Treatment: Eight to Twelve Weeks

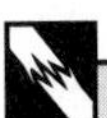

BONE HEALING

Stability at fracture site: Stable.

Stage of bone healing: Early remodeling phase. Woven bone is being replaced with lamellar bone. The process of remodeling will take months to years for completion.

X-ray: Abundant callus in fractures not rigidly fixed by plates. Fracture line begins to disappear; with time, there will be reconstitution of the medullary canal, except with an intramedullary nail.

Orthopaedic and Rehabilitation Considerations

Physical Examination

Examine the nail entry site for hardware prominence, which may limit hip motion. For any fracture that is healing slowly, consider removing proximal or distal interlocking screws to dynamize a statically locked nail. This will promote fracture healing. Assess for tenderness and motion at the fracture site.

Dangers

No significant changes. See previous section.

Radiography

Examine anteroposterior and lateral interval radiographs to confirm fixation, rotation, and the position of hardware. Carefully examine the entry point of any nail that is unlocked proximally. It may back out and become prominent.

Weight Bearing

Continue weight bearing as allowed by fracture comminution and the method of fixation.

Intramedullary nail fixation: Continue weight bearing as tolerated unless the fracture is not united, in which case consider another form of management such as a bone graft or exchanging the nail for a larger one.

Open reduction and internal plate fixation: If the fracture is clinically stable, the patient may begin full weight bearing. If pain is present at the fracture site on manual stress, the patient should continue or begin only partial weight bearing.

External fixation: If the patient is out of the fixator, partial weight bearing may begin. If the fixator is still in place, the patient should be non-weight bearing to partial weight bearing.

Range of Motion

No change. See previous section.

Muscle Strength

Continue with progressive resistive exercises to the quadriceps and hamstrings with an increasing number of repetitions.

Functional Activities

Once full weight bearing is achieved, the patient is gradually weaned from assistive devices for transfers and ambulation.

Gait

Concentrate on normalizing the gait pattern upon full weight bearing. Focus on heel strike, foot-flat, push-off, and toe-off (*see* Figures 6-1, 6-2, 6-3, 6-4, and 6-5). The fractured limb may be relatively lengthened secondary to decreased hip and knee flexion. Due to this relative lengthening, the patient either circumducts or hikes the hip on the involved side to clear the floor during the swing phase. Decreased knee flexion in the push-off phase (pre-swing) can delay toe-off, and a slight drag in the foot can be seen.

Watch for weight shifting and balance. When the patient was non-weight bearing or partially weight bearing, the balance was on the unaffected extremity. Once the patient is fully weight-bearing, weight-shifting and balance exercises are begun.

Methods of Treatment: Specific Aspects

Intramedullary Nail Fixation

Dynamize statically locked rods if a fracture cleft is still visible. This allows further impaction at the fracture site. Continue range of motion and strengthening exercises.

Open Reduction and Internal Plate Fixation

Continue range of motion and strengthening exercises. If union is delayed, consider other management options, such as a bone graft.

External Fixation

Remove the fixator if a callus is visible and consider a protective hinged orthosis. Continue range-of-motion and strengthening exercises.

Prescription

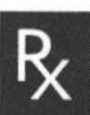

EIGHT TO TWELVE WEEKS

Precautions Avoid torsion loading of the femur.

Range of Motion Active/passive range of motion to hip and knee.

Muscle Strength Progressive resistive exercises to quads, hamstrings, and glutei.

Functional Activities Regular transfers. May need crutches for ambulation.

Weight Bearing Full weight bearing or weight bearing as tolerated for stable fractures. Partial weight bearing for unstable fractures.

Treatment: Twelve to Sixteen Weeks

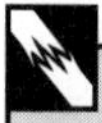

BONE HEALING

Stability at fracture site: Stable.

Stage of bone healing: Remodeling phase. Woven bone continues to be replaced with lamellar bone. The process of remodeling will take months to years for completion.

X-ray: Abundant callus in fractures not rigidly fixed by plates. Fracture line begins to disappear; with time, there will be reconstitution of the medullary canal, except with an intramedullary nail.

Orthopaedic and Rehabilitation Considerations

Physical Examination

Examine the nail entry site for hardware prominence, which may limit hip motion. Consider removing proximal or distal interlocking screws to dynamize any statically locked nail for slowly healing fracture. This will promote bone healing by impacting the fracture site. Assess any tenderness or motion at the fracture site. If present, consider a hinged orthosis. Patients may resume sports when the fracture is fully united and muscle strength and range of motion are again at their pre-injury levels.

Dangers

No change. See previous section.

Radiography

No change. See previous section.

Weight Bearing

Most patients should be weight bearing as tolerated at this time.

Range of Motion

Patients should have full range of motion at hip and knee by now. Continue with active and passive range of motion.

Muscle Strength

Isokinetic exercises to the quadriceps and hamstrings with the Cybex machine, can be instituted to increase strength.

Functional Activities

Patients are weight bearing as tolerated. They are instructed to bear weight on the affected extremity during transfers and ambulation. Assistive devices may still be needed. Attempt to wean the patient from these devices.

Gait

The patient should be full weight bearing. Concentrate on weight-shifting activities and on normalizing the gait pattern. The patient should be weaned from assistive devices for ambulation.

Methods of Treatment: Specific Aspects

No change. See previous section (pages 313–314).

Prescription

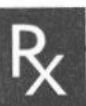

Twelve to Sixteen Weeks

Precautions None.

Range of Motion Active/passive range of motion to hip and knee.

Muscle Strength Progressive resistive exercises to quads, hamstrings, and glutei. Isokinetic exercises to the quadriceps and hamstrings.

Functional Activities Regular transfers. May need crutches for ambulation.

Weight Bearing Full weight bearing.

LONG-TERM CONSIDERATIONS AND PROBLEMS

Orthopaedic Considerations

Nonunion is a rare occurrence, usually associated with loss of fixation or delayed weight bearing and severe bone loss as seen in open fractures from high energy trauma. If nonunion occurs, first rule out infection. Then the fracture may be treated by restoring rigid fixation with a larger reamed femoral nail or by open reduction and internal fixation and bone graft.

Hardware may cause pain and removal should be considered if pain is localized to and correlated with radiographically prominent fixation devices. Femoral nails may be removed after one year if they protrude or cause pain. Interlocking screws may be removed for the same reason or if dynamization is necessary. Plates and screws may also be removed at one and a half to two years if they become sources of pain. If femoral nails or other hardware is removed, then partial weight bearing with crutches must be resumed for six weeks. A fracture may occur in the area formerly covered by the plate because the stress-shielding effect and poor blood supply weakens the bone beneath it in comparison to the adjacent bone.

The quadriceps muscle and fascia may become firmly adherent to the fracture site. This will reduce quadriceps glide on the femur causing pain and reduced flexion of the knee. A quadricepsplasty may be necessary to restore quadriceps glide and knee range of motion.

Rehabilitation Considerations

Hamstring shortening can reduce knee extension. Watch for knee flexion contractures, as the resting position for a swollen knee is approximately 30 degrees of flexion. If there is a 15-degree contracture, knee extension in deceleration (terminal swing), heel strike (initial contact), mid-stance, and push-off (mid-stance and terminal stance) will still be inadequate. A decrease in knee extension in deceleration (terminal swing) causes a shortening of step length. If the knee is not appropriately extended in mid-stance and push-off (mid-stance and terminal stance phases), the demand on quadriceps activity increases.

Limb-length shortening may occur in types III-B and III-C open fractures, and this can be treated with a shoe lift if the total leg-length discrepancy is less than 2 to 2.5 cm (see Chapter 9).

IMMEDIATE TO ONE WEEK

	Intramedullary Rod
Stability	No bony stability. Some mechanical stability from the strength of the metal rod. This stability is increased if the proximal and distal fracture fragments are in complete continuity, and decreased if comminution or bone loss is present.
Orthopaedics	Examine wounds.
	Remove drains when appropriate.
	Consider deep vein thrombosis prophylaxis (e.g., support stockings, compression boots, coumadin, heparin, low–molecular-weight heparin).
	Check blood count.
	Be aware of potential for fat emboli syndrome.
Rehabilitation	Active range of motion to the hip and knee in the plane of flexion and extension. Isometric gluteal and quadriceps exercises. Transfer training.

TWO WEEKS

	Intramedullary Rod
Stability	No to minimal bony stability. Otherwise unchanged.
Orthopaedics	Examine wounds. Remove sutures or staples. Consider deep vein thrombosis prophylaxis.
Rehabilitation	Active and active-assistive range of motion to the hip, knee, and ankle. Passive motion may begin near the end of this time. Isometric gluteal, hamstring, and quadriceps strengthening exercises. Stand/pivot transfers on well leg to avoid torsional forces on fracture and ambulation with appropriate assistive devices. Weight bearing depends on fracture pattern, but is usually as tolerated.

FOUR TO SIX WEEKS

	Intramedullary Rod
Stability	Increasing stability is present as callus forms and bridges the fracture. Most fractures are stable by 6 weeks unless there is bone loss or severe comminution. Confirm stability with physical examination and radiographs.
Orthopaedics	Examine radiograph for healing and hardware position. Observe for nail migration toward proximal or distal end if either is left without interlocking screws.
Rehabilitation	Continue to increase active, active-assistive, and passive range of motion to hip in the flexion and extension plane and begin active adduction and abduction. Begin light resistive exercises and increase weight bearing in accordance with fracture stability.

EIGHT TO TWELVE WEEKS

	Intramedullary Rod
Stability	Stable.
Orthopaedics	Consider bone grafting any fracture with persistent gaping at the fracture site, especially if there has been bone loss or severe comminution.
Rehabilitation	Progressive resistive exercises to the hip and knee. Most fractures should be weight bearing as tolerated. Begin to wean from assistive devices.

TWELVE TO SIXTEEN WEEKS

	Intramedullary Rod
Stability	Unchanged.
Orthopaedics	Unchanged.
Rehabilitation	Progressive resistive exercises to the hip and knee, including isokinetic exercises.

BIBLIOGRAPHY

Bucholz RW, Brumback RJ. Fractures of the shaft of the femur. In: Rockwood CA Jr, Green DP, Bucholz RW, eds. *Fractures in Adults*, Vol 2, 3rd ed. Philadelphia: J.B. Lippincott, 1991.

Johnson KD. Femoral shaft fractures. In: Browner BD, Jupiter JB, Levine AM, Trafton PG, eds. *Skeletal Trauma*, Vol 2. Philadelphia, W.B. Saunders, 1992, pp. 1525–1641.

McKibbon B. The biology of fracture healing in long bones. *J Bone Joint Surg Br*, 60:150–151, 1978.

Winquist RA: Locked femoral nailing. *Journal of the American Academy of Orthopedic Surgeons*, 1:95–105, 1993.

Winquist RA, Hansen ST Jr, Clawson DK: Closed intramedullary nailing of femoral fractures: a report of five hundred and twenty cases. *J Bone Joint Surg Am*, 66:529–539, 1984.

CHAPTER Twenty-five

Supracondylar Femur Fractures

DEREK A. KRAM, MD

VASANTHA L. MURTHY, MD

INTRODUCTION

Definition

A supracondylar femur fracture involves the distal aspect or metaphysis of the femur. This area includes the distal 8 to 15 cm of the femur. The fracture frequently involves articular surfaces.

Complex classification systems have been proposed for this fracture, all of which attempt to define the amount of comminution and the degree of displacement of the fracture fragments.

Müller's update of the AO classification system is widely accepted. This involves dividing the fractures into extraarticular (type A), unicondylar (type B), and bicondylar (type C) fractures. These are then subdivided into types 1 through 3 in each group. In progressing from type A to C, as well as subtypes 1 to 3, the severity of the fracture increases and the prognosis for a good result decreases (Figures 25-1, 25-2, 25-3, and 25-4).

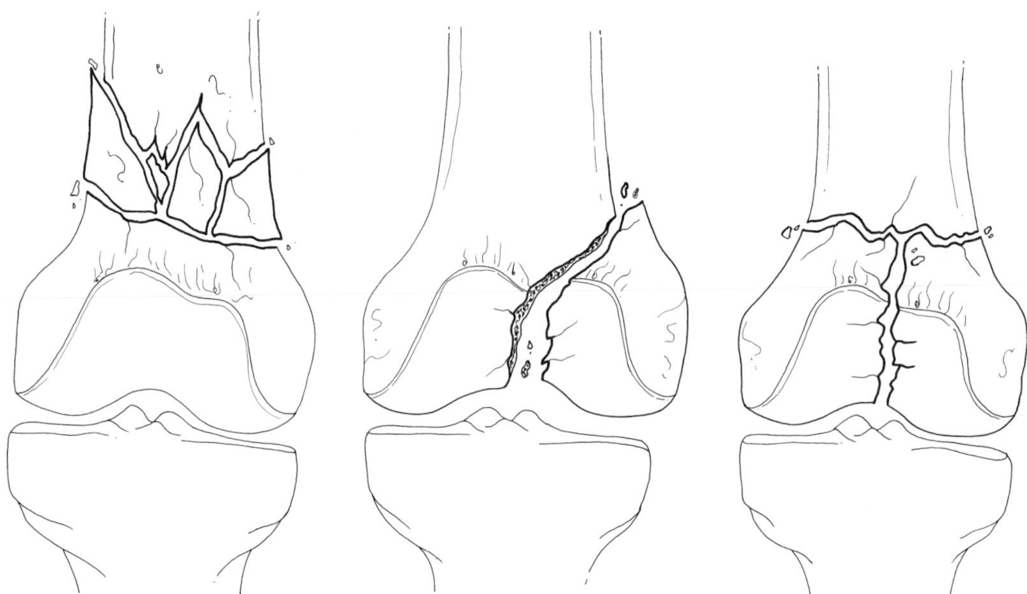

FIGURE 25-1 *(above, left)* Extraarticular supracondylar fracture of the femur within the metaphyseal region of the distal femur with comminution.

FIGURE 25-2 *(above, middle)* Intraarticular unicondylar fracture of the distal femur with displacement of one condyle.

FIGURE 25-3 *(above, right)* Intraarticular bicondylar fracture of the distal femur involving both condyles.

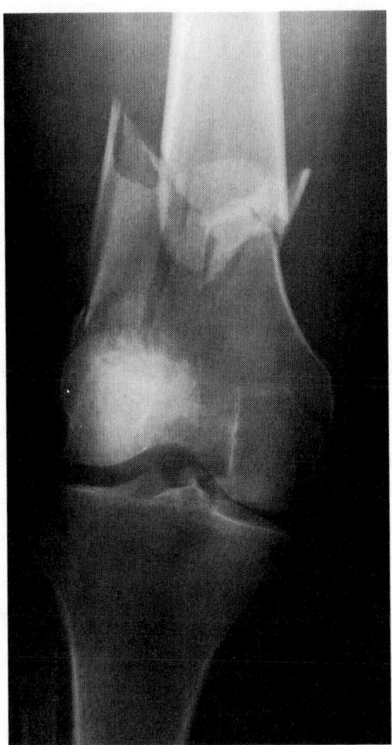

FIGURE 25-4 Extraarticular type A supracondylar femoral fracture within the metaphyseal region of the distal femur with comminution. Note the displacement of the metaphyseal region of the distal femur and shortening at the fracture site. This fracture requires open reduction and internal fixation.

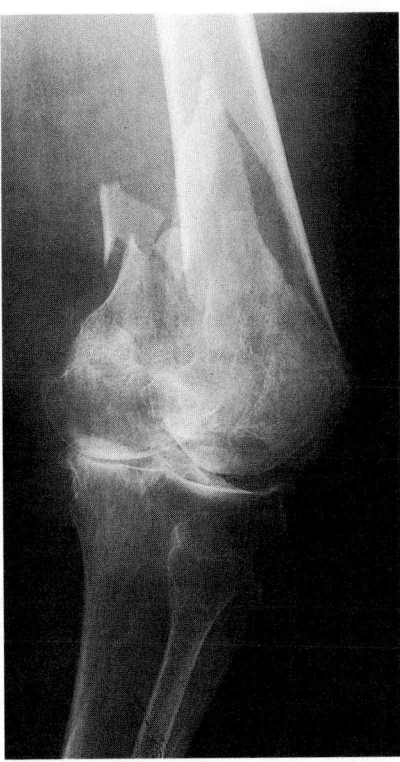

FIGURE 25-5 Supracondylar fracture of the femur in an elderly patient. This fracture usually results from low-energy trauma, such as a fall, and represents a bicondylar fracture of the distal femur. It requires open reduction and internal fixation.

Mechanism of Injury

In younger patients, this fracture is usually secondary to high-energy trauma, such as being struck by an automobile. These cases commonly have other associated injuries.

In elderly patients, this fracture is usually secondary to low-energy trauma, such as a simple fall. There are usually no other associated injuries in these cases (Figure 25-5).

Treatment Goals

Orthopaedic Objectives

Alignment

Restore alignment by minimizing any residual flexion/extension or varus/valgus angulation at the fracture site. Any articular step-off must be less than 1 to 2 mm in order to decrease or delay the risk of degenerative changes and allow for functional range of motion and normal gait.

Stability

Stability is best achieved by restoring bony congruity and using hardware to rigidly fix the fracture.

Rehabilitation Objectives

Range of Motion

Improve and restore range of motion of the knee, hip, and ankle (Table 25-1).

TABLE 25-1 *Range of Motion of Knee*

Motion	Normal	Functional
Flexion	0°–130°/140°	110°
Extension	0°–5°	

Muscle Strength

Improve and restore the strength of the following muscles:

Quadriceps, knee extensor
Hamstrings, knee flexor
Adductor magnus, longus and brevis group-hip adductors (attached to the femoral condyle)
Gastrocnemius, foot flexor (plantar), and knee flexor (two-joint muscle)

Functional Goals

Normalize gait pattern and achieve proper sitting position (knee flexion of 90 degrees).

Expected Time of Bone Healing

Twelve to 16 weeks.

Expected Duration of Rehabilitation

Fifteen to 20 weeks.

Methods of Treatment

Open Reduction and Internal Fixation

Biomechanics: Stress-shielding device and stress-sharing device. In most supracondylar femur fractures, especially those with significant comminution, rigid fixation is difficult to achieve. Therefore, stress sharing is present.

Mode of Bone Healing: Primary, if fixation is rigid; secondary, if rigid fixation is not achieved.

Indications: Open reduction and internal fixation is currently the method of choice for the treatment of these fractures. Commonly used fixator devices include the 95-degree condylar blade plate and the 95-degree dynamic compression screw. Also commonly in use are the condylar buttress plate and the retrograde supracondylar intramedullary nail. Devices that provide less rigid fixation and less optimal results, but are still used, include the Zickel supracondylar device, Ender's nail, and Rush pins. At the time of initial fixation, a bone graft is often placed to substitute for a bone deficit (Figures 25-6, 25-7, 25-8, 25-9, 25-9A, and 25-9B).

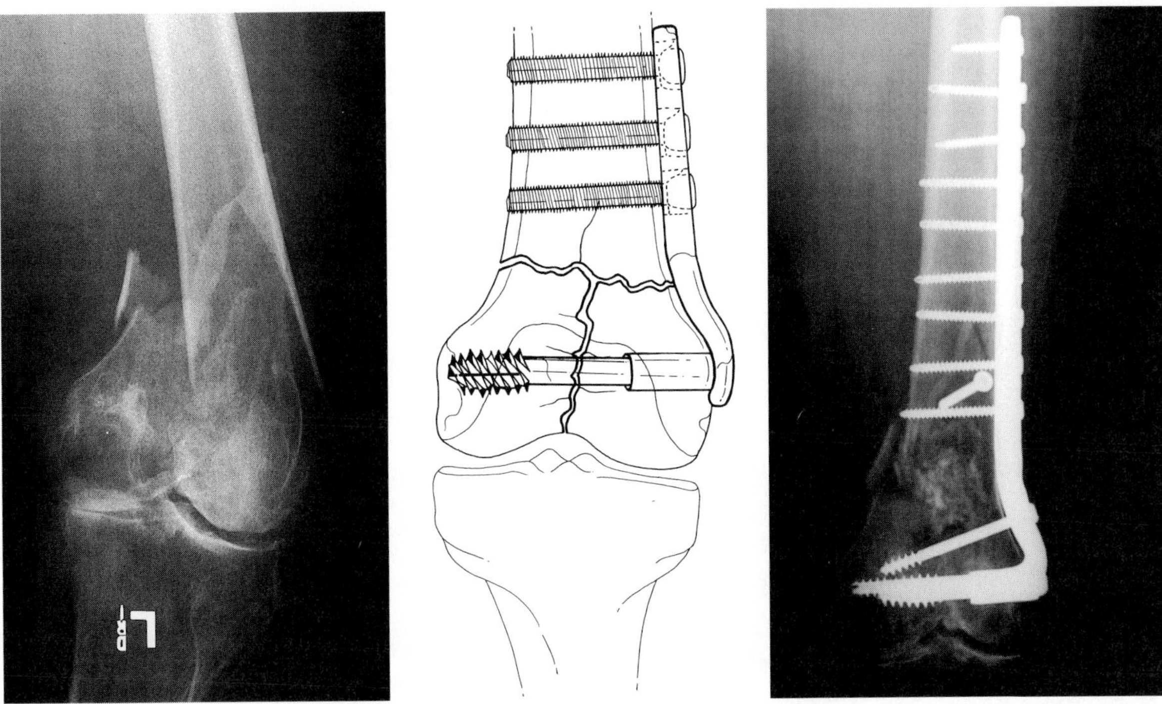

FIGURE 25-6 *(above, left)* Bicondylar fracture of the distal femur.

FIGURE 25-7 *(above, middle)* Bicondylar fracture of the distal femur treated with a 95-degree dynamic compression screw and plate.

FIGURE 25-8 *(above, right)* Bicondylar fracture of the distal femur, treated with a 95-degree dynamic compression screw and plate. Note the restoration of length with the use of the long plate device and filling of the metaphyseal defect with bone grafts. (Courtesy of Dr. Melvin Adler.)

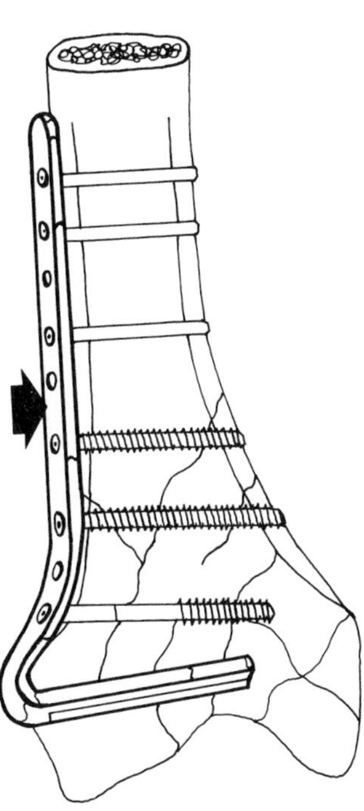

FIGURE 25-9 Comminuted intraarticular fracture of the distal femur involving both condyles treated with a 95-degree condylar blade plate.

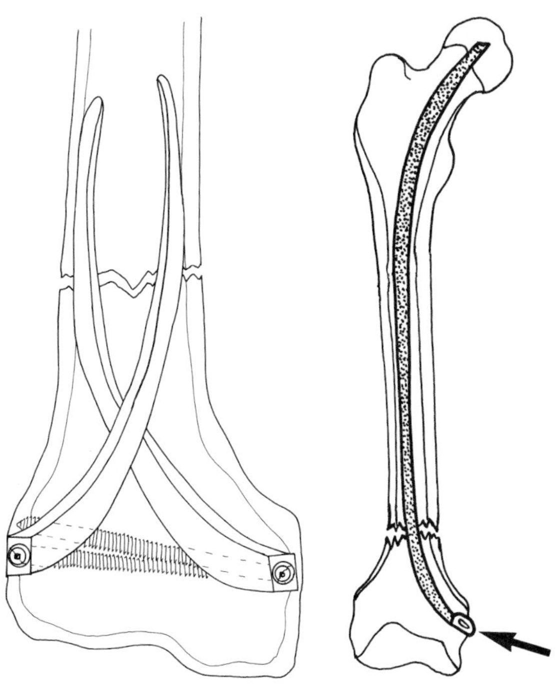

FIGURE 25-9A *(above, left)* Zickel supracondylar device. Used infrequently, this gives three-point fixation for supracondylar femoral fractures to provide stability.

FIGURE 25-9B *(above, right)* Ender's nail for the treatment of a supracondylar femoral fracture. This device does not provide rigid fixation and is not commonly used.

Casting or Traction

Biomechanics: Stress-sharing device.

Mode of Bone Healing: Secondary.

Indication: Treatments involving traction or casting are associated with a high risk of malunion, including varus, valgus, and rotational deformities. Additionally, treatment with traction requires a prolonged period of bed rest, with its associated risks of deep venous thrombosis, bed sores, urinary tract infections, and pulmonary compromise. This conservative treatment is indicated only for the management of severely comminuted fractures or for patients who are at high medical risk for any operative management. This method of treatment is not discussed in this chapter (Figures 25-10 and 25-11).

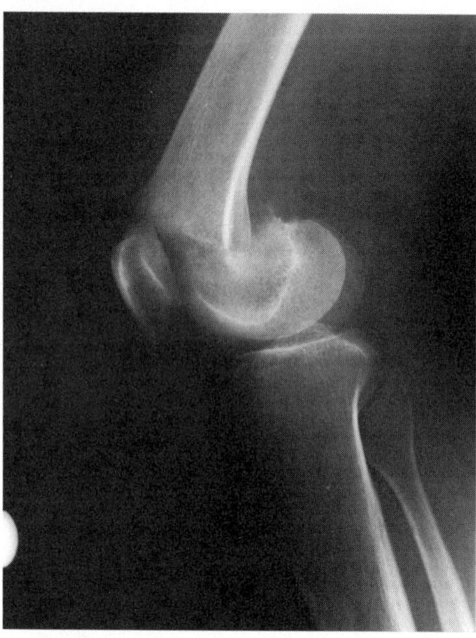

FIGURE 25-10 Extraarticular supracondylar fracture of the distal femur. Note the lack of metaphyseal comminution and the posterior displacement of the distal fragment.

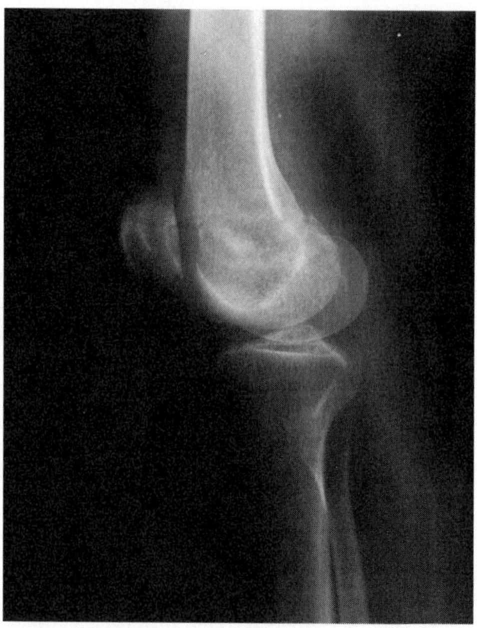

FIGURE 25-11 Closed reduction of a transverse extraarticular supracondylar femoral fracture with traction, performed under general anesthesia. Surprisingly, this fracture responded well to closed reduction and casting.

Special Considerations of the Fracture

Age

See Mechanism of Injury.

Bone Quality

Younger patients usually have good bone quality, allowing good purchase for orthopaedic fixation devices. Elderly patients, however, are often osteopenic, which makes fixation difficult.

Long-Term Sequelae

From the outset, the patient should be warned of possible degenerative joint disease (increased with intra-articular fracture), decreased knee range of motion, residual deformity and limp, and prolonged swelling secondary to the injury.

Associated Injuries

Vascular Injury

With highly comminuted fractures, especially those associated with high-energy trauma, the extremity should be carefully examined for signs of compartment syndrome or injury to the popliteal vessels. If there is any suspicion of injury to these vessels, further evaluation needs to include duplex studies or an angiogram.

Ligamentous Injury

It is not uncommon to find a concomitant ligamentous injury around the knee. However, it is difficult to evaluate ligamentous damage at the time of initial injury because of pain and fracture instability. After fracture stabilization, careful evaluation of these ligamentous structures should be undertaken and appropriate repair performed.

Weight Bearing

Typically, the patient is kept non-weight bearing for 3 months after the injury. This allows the relatively soft metaphyseal bone to heal and any bone graft to incorporate.

Gait Cycle

Stance Phase

Stance phase, constituting 60% of the gait cycle, is most affected by the fracture.

Heel Strike

The quadriceps contracts concentrically to bring the knee to full extension. However, a knee-flexion contracture may exist. The patellar groove may be disrupted and the glide mechanism of the patella in the groove may be affected, causing pain. The extensor mechanism that surrounds the knee joint may also be compromised. Occasionally the glide mechanism of the quadriceps is also involved, thus limiting terminal extension (*see* Figure 6-1).

Foot-Flat

Foot-flat is usually not affected; however, the quadriceps contracts eccentrically through elongation to keep the knee under slight tension. Muscle contraction may cause some pain (*see* Figure 6-2).

Mid-Stance

Full weight passes through the fracture site at mid-stance, because there is only single-limb support. Pain may be present (*see* Figure 6-3).

Push-Off

Push-off is usually not affected. The patella lies in the trochlear groove at this phase and may cause pain (*see* Figure 6-4).

Swing Phase

The swing phase constitutes 40% of the gait cycle. The quadriceps contract to cause acceleration of the tibia on the femur. The quadriceps glide mechanism is necessary to allow the knee to go to full extension before heel strike. The quadriceps may not be able to contract enough to achieve full extension (*see* Figures 6-6, 6-7, and 6-8).

TREATMENT

Treatment: Early to Immediate (Day of Injury to One Week)

BONE HEALING

Stability at fracture site: None.

Stage of bone healing: Inflammatory phase. The fracture hematoma is colonized by inflammatory cells, and débridement of the fracture begins.

X-ray: No callus.

Orthopaedic and Rehabilitation Considerations

Physical Examination

Initially, the most important aspect to check is the patient's neurovascular status. Check pulses and capillary refill, as well as sensation and active and passive range of motion of the extremity. (Do not perform passive range of motion of the knee unless absolutely rigid fixation has been achieved.) Check lower extremity compartments for softness and monitor compartment pressures if there is any suspicion of compartment syndrome. Additionally, check the wound for erythema or discharge that might indicate infection. If edema is present, the patient should be instructed to elevate the extremity properly.

Dangers

Look for compartment syndrome, especially when popliteal vessels are injured. Compartment syndrome is more common with high-energy trauma and is usually noted in the first few hours after injury.

Radiography

Check radiographs for varus, valgus, and rotational alignment at the fracture site, as compared to the unaffected knee. Also check for any displacement or loss of fixation. Because these fractures generally involve the metaphyseal region, which has a good blood supply, fracture healing usually occurs within the first 3 months after injury.

Weight Bearing

The patient is non-weight bearing on the affected extremity for 3 months.

Range of Motion

Gentle active range-of-motion exercises are prescribed to the knee, ankle, and hip. If fixation is not rigid, passive range-of-motion exercises are avoided. If ankle edema is present, the ankle is elevated to decrease swelling. Patients are encouraged to perform active range-of-motion exercises at the knee joint with the goal of full extension and 60 degrees to 90 degrees of knee flexion. Patients who are noncompliant or cannot follow orders are placed in a hinged-knee brace or cast brace to allow for protected range-of-motion exercises.

Muscle Strength

No strengthening exercises are prescribed at this point to avoid risk of fracture displacement.

Functional Activities

The patient is instructed in stand/pivot transfers using crutches or a walker, with no weight-bearing on the affected extremity. The patient dons pants with the affected extremity first and doffs them from the unaffected extremity first to decrease stress on the fracture site.

Gait

The patient is instructed in a two-point gait using crutches or a walker with no weight bearing on the affected extremity (placing the crutches first and then hopping to the crutches on level surfaces. *See* Figure 6-16). The patient ascends stairs with the uninvolved extremity first, followed by the fractured extremity and the crutches, and descends stairs with the crutches first, followed by the fractured extremity first and then the uninvolved extremity (*see* Figures 6-20, 6-21, 6-22, 6-23, 6-24, and 6-25).

Methods of Treatment: Specific Aspects

See Orthopaedic and Rehabilitation Considerations section (page 326).

Prescription

EARLY TO IMMEDIATE (DAY ONE TO ONE WEEK)

Precautions Avoid passive range of motion.

Range of Motion Active range of motion. Attempt full extension and 60 degrees to 90 degrees of flexion to the knee. Avoid passive range of motion.

Strength No strengthening exercises prescribed to the knee.

Functional Activities Non–weight-bearing stand/pivot transfers and non–weight-bearing ambulation.

Weight Bearing None.

Treatment: Two Weeks

Bone Healing

Stability at fracture site: None to minimal.

Stage of bone healing: Beginning of reparative phase. Osteoprogenitor cells differentiate into osteoblasts, which lay down woven bone.

X-ray: No callus to early callus; fracture line is visible.

Orthopaedic and Rehabilitation Considerations

Physical Examination

Check the wound for erythema or discharge, and remove staples or sutures. Evaluate for any crepitus or varus/valgus or sagittal angulation, which signifies loss of fixation. Check sensation, pulses, and capillary refill, especially if there was any previous neurovascular compromise.

Dangers

Loss of fixation is a risk. The risk of compartment syndrome at this point is small.

Radiography

Check radiographs for alignment at the fracture site. In particular, compare the affected knee to the unaffected knee for varus and valgus alignment and any rotational deformity. Also check for any displacement or loss of fixation.

Weight Bearing

The patient is kept non-weight bearing on the affected extremity for 3 months.

Range of Motion

Continue active range-of-motion exercises to the hip, knee, and ankle. If the fixation is rigid, active-assistive range-of-motion exercises are prescribed to the ankle to avoid stiffness and limitations in range of motion. The patient is instructed to draw the alphabet with the foot so that it is ranged in all planes.

Muscle Strength

Gluteal sets or isometric exercises are prescribed to maintain the strength of the hip musculature. Isometric exercise of the quadriceps may be prescribed when the patient is in bed, supine, with the knee in full extension. This is to avoid any pull on the fracture site and displacement of the fracture. Straight-leg–raising exercises are prescribed to strengthen the quadriceps.

Functional Activities

Continue with non-weight bearing on the affected extremity during stand/pivot transfers and ambulation. The patient uses crutches or a walker.

Gait

The patient continues to use a two-point gait with crutches, non-weight bearing on the affected side (*see* Figure 6-16).

Methods of Treatment: Specific Aspects

See Orthopaedic and Rehabilitation Considerations section (page 327).

Prescription

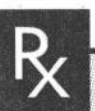

Two Weeks

Precautions Avoid passive range of motion.

Range of Motion Active range of motion 60 degrees to 90 degrees in flexion and full extension to the knee.

Strength (Knee) Isometric exercises to quadriceps in supine position and knee in full extension.

Functional Activities Non–weight-bearing ambulation and stand/pivot transfers.

Weight Bearing None.

Treatment: Four to Eight Weeks

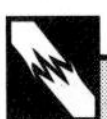

Bone Healing

Stability at fracture site: With bridging callus, the fracture is usually stable; confirm with physical examination.

Stage of bone healing: Reparative phase. Once callus is observed bridging the fracture site, the fracture is usually stable. The strength of this callus, especially with torsional load, however, is significantly lower than that of normal bone.

X-ray: Bridging callus is beginning to be visible. With increased rigidity of fixation, less bridging callus is noted and healing with endosteal callus predominates. The fracture line is less visible. A large amount of callus formation with a rigid fixation device indicates a lack of rigid fixation.

Orthopaedic and Rehabilitation Considerations

Physical Examination

Check the wound for erythema or discharge as signs of infection. Evaluate for any crepitus or angular deformities.

Dangers

Evaluate for loss of fixation, which is still a risk.

Radiography

Check radiographs for alignment and callus at the fracture site. Callus formation with a rigid fixation device indicates the lack of rigid fixation and therefore lack of primary bone healing. Compare the fracture to the unaffected knee for varus and valgus alignment and any rotational deformity. Also check for any displacement or loss of fixation.

Weight Bearing

The patient is kept non-weight bearing on the affected extremity for 3 months.

Range of Motion

Continue active range-of-motion exercises to the knee joint with the goal of full extension and flexion of 90 degrees or greater at this time. Continue full range-of-motion exercises to the hip and ankle. Gentle active-assistive exercises to the knee are prescribed if the fracture is stable. The patient can sit in a chair and slide the foot forward on the floor to allow at least 60 degrees in extension and backward to allow more than 90 degrees of flexion. These are called stool-scoot exercises.

Muscle Strength

Isometric exercise of the quadriceps and hamstrings are performed, as are ankle and gluteal isometric exercises.

Functional Activities

Continue stand/pivot transfers because the patient is still non-weight bearing on the affected extremity.

Gait

The patient continues to use a two-point gait with crutches, non-weight bearing on the affected side (*see* Figure 6-16).

Methods of Treatment: Specific Aspects

See Orthopaedic and Rehabilitation Considerations section (page 328).

Prescription

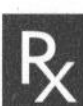

FOUR TO EIGHT WEEKS

Precautions No passive range of motion.

Range of Motion (Knee) Active range of motion greater than 90 degrees; active, active-assistive range of motion in flexion and extension, if the fracture is stable.

Strength (Knee) Isometric exercises to quadriceps and hamstrings.

Functional Activities Non–weight-bearing ambulation and stand/pivot transfers.

Weight Bearing None.

Treatment: Eight to Twelve Weeks

BONE HEALING

Stability at fracture site: Stable.

Stage of bone healing: Early remodeling phase. Woven bone is being replaced with lamellar bone. The process of remodeling takes months to years for completion.

X-ray: Abundant callus in fractures not rigidly fixed by plates. Fracture line begins to disappear. With time, there will be reconstitution of the medullary canal, except with an intramedullary nail.

Orthopaedic and Rehabilitation Considerations

Physical Examination

Check the wound for erythema or discharge and the limb for alignment or angular deformities.

Dangers

Loss of fixation is still a risk, although less so than before.

Radiography

Check radiographs for alignment and callus at the fracture site, as well as a decrease in size of the fracture lines. In particular, compare the fracture to the unaffected knee for varus and valgus alignment and any rotational deformity. Also check for any displacement or loss of fixation.

Weight Bearing

The patient is kept non-weight bearing on the affected extremity for 3 months.

Range of Motion

The patient should continue active and active-assistive range-of-motion exercises to the knee. By this time, more than 90 degrees flexion of the knee should be possible. Gentle passive range of motion may be allowed if there is any stiffness in the knee. The patient should continue full range of motion to the hip and ankle. Hydrotherapy helps relieve discomfort during range-of-motion exercises.

Muscle Strength

Patients should work on improving quadriceps and hamstring muscle strength with isometric exercises. Isotonic strengthening exercises also are prescribed. Repetitive isotonic exercises increase strength and improve range of motion.

Functional Activities

Because patients are non-weight bearing on the affected extremity, they should continue stand/pivot transfers using crutches or a walker.

Gait

The patient should continue a two-point gait using crutches or walker (*see* Figure 6-16).

Methods of Treatment: Specific Aspects

See Orthopaedic and Rehabilitation Considerations section (page 328).

Prescription

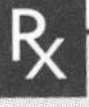

EIGHT TO TWELVE WEEKS

Precautions No aggressive passive range of motion.

Range of Motion (Knee) Active, active-assistive range of motion; gentle passive range of motion.

Strength (Knee) Isometric and isotonic exercises to quadriceps and hamstrings.

Functional Activities Non–weight-bearing ambulation and stand/pivot transfers.

Weight Bearing None.

Treatment: Twelve to Sixteen Weeks

BONE HEALING

Stability at fracture site: Stable.

Stage of bone healing: Woven bone is replaced with lamellar bone. The process of remodeling takes months to years for completion.

X-ray: Abundant callus, fracture line begins to disappear. With time, there will be resorption of the callus.

Orthopaedic and Rehabilitation Considerations

Physical Examination

Check the limb for alignment and angular deformities. Check the wound for erythema or discharge.

Radiography

Check radiographs for alignment and callus at the fracture site; in particular, compare to the unaffected knee for varus and valgus alignment and any rotational deformity. Also check for any displacement or loss of adequate fixation. If no callus is visualized and fracture lines are not disappearing, delayed union or nonunion can be diagnosed at approximately 4 to 5 months after injury. At this time, consideration should be given to other types of operative management, including bone grafting. This may even be performed as early as 6 weeks after injury, depending on the progression of healing.

Weight Bearing

As long as bone healing is progressing properly, weight bearing may be started, beginning with toe-touch ambulation and progressing to full weight bearing as tolerated by the patient.

Range of Motion

Because the fracture site is stable, with good callus formation, passive range-of-motion exercises to the knee can continue if joint stiffness is present. If full range of motion of the knee is not obtained by this time, active-assistive range of motion can be instituted to the patient's pain tolerance. Hydrotherapy may help relieve the discomfort during range-of-motion exercises.

Muscle Strength

Along with isometric exercises of the quadriceps, hamstrings, and gastrocnemius, isotonic exercises can be continued. Gentle resistance is applied to increase muscle strength. The resistance is progressively increased as are the numbers of repetitions. The use of a Cybex machine for isokinetic exercises may be helpful to strengthen the quadriceps and hamstring muscles. Because the resistance is variable and speed is constant, the muscle is exercised through the full range of motion.

Functional Activities

The patient is instructed in weight-bearing transfers on the affected extremity using crutches.

Gait

The patient is instructed to bear weight on the affected extremity during ambulation, beginning with toe-touch partial weight bearing and gradually progressing to full weight bearing. The patient may use a three-point or four-point gait, depending on the amount of weight borne on the affected extremity (*see* figures 6-17, 6-18, and 6-19). Patients who are on crutches progress to weight bearing with canes, then to full unassisted weight bearing during ambulation.

Methods of Treatment: Specific Aspects

See Rehabilitation and Orthopaedic Considerations section (page 329).

Prescription

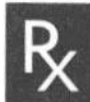

TWELVE TO SIXTEEN WEEKS

Precautions Do not be aggressive in passive range of motion.

Range of Motion (Knee) Active and passive range of motion; emphasize terminal extension to reduce extension lag.

Strength (Knee) Isometric, isotonic, and isokinetic exercises to quadriceps and hamstrings. Gentle progressive resistive exercises. Muscle strength 4+ or 5.

Functional Activities Partial weight bearing with crutches, progressing to full weight bearing during ambulation and transfers.

Weight Bearing Toe-touch to partial weight bearing progressing to full weight bearing.

Long-Term Considerations and Problems

At every stage of treatment, radiographs should be obtained to evaluate for loss of reduction, because a malunion may lead to shortening or rotational deformities and may hasten the onset of degenerative joint disease of the knee. Additionally, a loss of motion of the knee is common. Therefore, every attempt should be made to obtain rigid fixation, thus allowing the patient to begin range-of-motion exercises early in treatment.

Patients are not permitted to participate in sports, repetitive pounding activities, jogging, or jumping for 6 months from the time of injury.

IMMEDIATE TO ONE WEEK

	Open Reduction and Internal Fixation
Stability	None.
Orthopaedics	Perform wound care over incisions and in any open wounds.
Rehabilitation	No isometric or strengthening exercises prescribed for quadriceps.
	Gentle active range-of-motion exercises prescribed to hip, knee, ankle, and toes.

TWO WEEKS

	Open Reduction and Internal Fixation
Stability	None to minimal
Orthopaedics	Remove any sutures and continue wound care to any open wounds.
Rehabilitation	Isometric exercises prescribed for the glutei as well as the quadriceps when the knee is in full extension. Continue with active range-of-motion exercises to hip, knee, ankle, and toe.

FOUR TO SIX WEEKS

	Open Reduction and Internal Fixation
Stability	Partially stable.
Orthopaedics	Consider bone grafting if fracture cleft still present or collapse into varus or valgus.
Rehabilitation	Isometric exercises to the quadriceps and hamstrings as well as ankle and gluteal isometrics. Continue active and begin active-assistive range-of-motion exercises to hip, knee, ankle, and toes.

EIGHT TO TWELVE WEEKS

	Open Reduction and Internal Fixation
Stability	Stable.
Orthopaedics	Most fractures are completely healed; however, those with a persistent fracture cleft must be considered for bone grafting.
Rehabilitation	Continue isometric and isotonic exercises to the quadriceps and hamstrings. Continue active and active-assistive and begin passive range-of-motion exercises to knee, as well as the hip, ankle, and toes.

TWELVE TO SIXTEEN WEEKS

	Open Reduction and Internal Fixation
Stability	Stable.
Orthopaedics	If the fracture cleft is still present, consider bone grafting.
Rehabilitation	Use isometric, isotonic, and isokinetic exercises to quadriceps, hamstrings, and gastrocnemius. Gentle resistive can be started. Active, active-assistive, and passive range of motion exercises to hip, knee, ankle, and toes. Weight bearing is started, first with toe-touch ambulation and progressing to full weight bearing.

BIBLIOGRAPHY

Albert MJ. Supracondylar fractures of the femur. *J Am Acad Orthop Surg,* 5:163–171, 1997

Giles JB, DeLee JC, Heckman JD, Keever JE. Supracondylar-intercondylar fractures of the femur treated with a supracondylar plate and lag screw. *J Bone Joint Surg*, 64A:864–870, 1982.

Healy WL, Brooker AF Jr. Distal femoral fractures. Comparison of open and closed methods of treatment. *Clin Orthop,* 174:166–171, 1983.

Helfet DL. Fractures of the distal femur. In: Browner BD, Jupiter JB, Levine AM, Trafton P.G., eds. *Skeletal Trauma,* Vol. 2. Philadelphia: W.B. Saunders, 1992, pp. 1643–1683.

Lucas SE, Seligson D, Henry SL. Intramedullary supracondylar nailing of femoral fractures: a preliminary report of the GSH supracondylar nail. *Clin Orthop* 296:200–206, 1993.

Mooney V, Nickel VL, Harvey JP Jr, Nelson R. Cast-brace treatment for fractures of the distal part of the femur: a prospective controlled study of one hundred and fifty patients. *J Bone Joint Surg*, 52A:1563–1578, 1970.

Müller ME, Nazarian S, Koch P. Classification AO des Fractures. New York: Springer-Verlag, 1987.

Sanders R, Regazzoni P, Ruedi TP. Treatment of supracondylar-intercondylar fractures of the femur using the dynamic condylar screw. *J Orthop Trauma,* 3:214–222, 1989.

Schatzker J, Lambert DC. Supracondylar fractures of the femur. *Clin Orthop,* 138:77–83, 1979.

Wiss DA. Supracondylar and intercondylar fractures of the femur. In: Rockwood CA Jr, Green DP, Bucholz RW, eds. *Fractures in Adults,* Vol. 2, 3rd ed. Philadelphia: J.B. Lippincott, 1991, pp. 1778–1797.

Zickel RE, Hobeika P, Robbins DS. Zickel supracondylar nails for fracture of the distal end of the femur. *Clin Orthop*, 212:79–88, 1986.

CHAPTER *Twenty-six*

Patellar Fractures

DEREK A. KRAM, MD

STANLEY HOPPENFELD, MD

VASANTHA L. MURTHY, MD

INTRODUCTION

Definition

Patellar fractures are classified as either nondisplaced or displaced. Those that are less than 1 to 2 mm articular step-off or 3 mm of fragment separation displaced are considered nondisplaced fractures.

Patellar fractures may also be described as transverse, longitudinal, or comminuted (Figures 26-1 and 26-2).

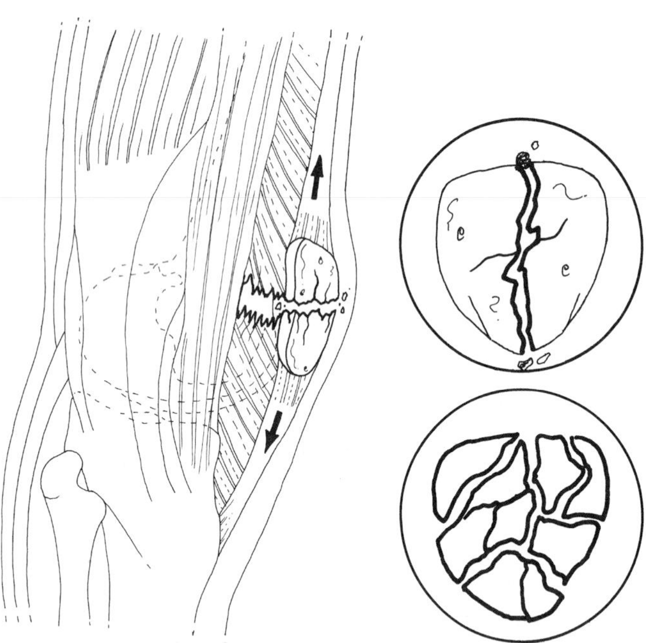

FIGURE 26-1 *(above, left)* Transverse patellar fracture with retinacular tear.

FIGURE 26-2 *(above, right)* Patellar fractures may be described as longitudinal or comminuted. These fractures are intraarticular.

Extraarticular patellar fractures involve the poles of the patella and are usually secondary to avulsion injuries.

Mechanism of Injury

A direct blow to the patella accounts for the majority of patellar fractures. Indirect force from a violent contraction of the quadriceps muscle can also result in a patellar fracture.

Treatment Goals

Orthopaedic Objectives

Alignment

1. Fracture displacement. Fractures displaced greater than 3 mm are usually associated with retinacular tears and a disruption of the extensor mechanism. If an extensor lag is present, open repair of the retinaculum should be performed.
2. Articular congruity. Any fracture with a step-off of greater than 2 mm on the articular surface should be considered significant. In such a case, open reduction should be performed to decrease the risk of future posttraumatic degenerative changes.

Stability

Stability is best achieved by restoring bony congruity and using hardware to rigidly fix the fracture.

Rehabilitation Objectives

Range of Motion

1. Restore full range of motion of the knee in flexion and extension to prevent extension lag.

2. Restore the rectus femoris (two-joint muscle) to its full length so as to achieve full range of motion of the hip and knee.
3. Maintain ligamentous flexibility, which may be reduced secondary to trauma and immobilization.

Muscle Strength

1. Improve the strength of the quadriceps muscle, which is an extensor of the knee, and the rectus femoris, also a flexor of the hip, which crosses two joints. The quadriceps may have sustained direct trauma from injury or sustained reflex inhibition. The vastus medialis is the first muscle affected and the last muscle to recover. Its oblique head is the stabilizer of the patella and prevents subluxation.
2. Improve the strength of the hamstring muscles, which are strong knee flexors.
3. Improve the quadriceps-hamstring balance.

Functional Goals

Normalize the gait pattern, especially in the stance phase. Undertake proprioceptive and sport-specific training.

Expected Time of Bone Healing

Eight to 12 weeks.

Expected Duration of Rehabilitation

Twelve to 15 weeks.

Methods of Treatment

Cast or Knee Immobilizer

Biomechanics: Stress-sharing device.

Mode of Bone Healing: Secondary.

Indications: This is the treatment of choice for nondisplaced patella fractures, including extraarticular fractures as long as the extensor mechanism remains intact. A cylinder cast is most often used, which allows full range of motion at the ankle. Examine the knee carefully for its ability to perform active extension. Loss of active extension signifies tearing of the retinacular mechanism, which requires an open repair. The choice of the knee immobilizer versus casting is made based on patient compliance; if the patient is noncompliant, a cast should be used. (The two modalities are discussed interchangeably in this chapter.) (*See* Figure 8-1A.)

Open Reduction and Internal Fixation

Biomechanics: Stress-shielding and stress-sharing depending on the device used.

Mode of Bone Healing: Primary, unless a solid fixation is not achieved, in which case secondary healing also occurs.

Indications: This is the method of choice for the treatment of comminuted and displaced fractures. The main goal of open reduction is to align the articular surface in the hope of decreasing posttraumatic degenerative changes. Any retinacular destruction is openly repaired (Figures 26-3, 26-4, 26-5, 26-6, and 26-7).

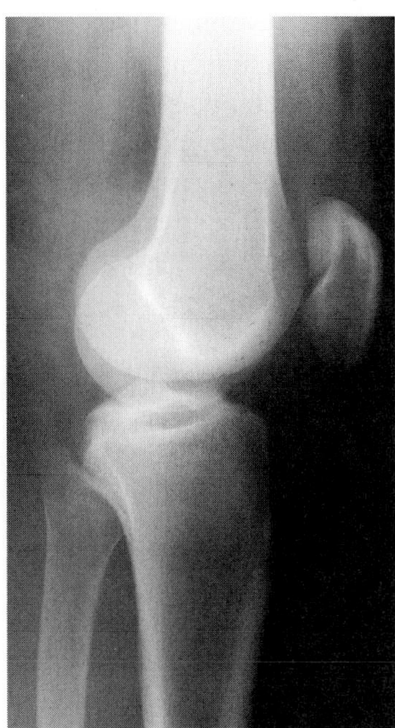

FIGURE 26-3 Transverse patellar fracture with intraarticular involvement.

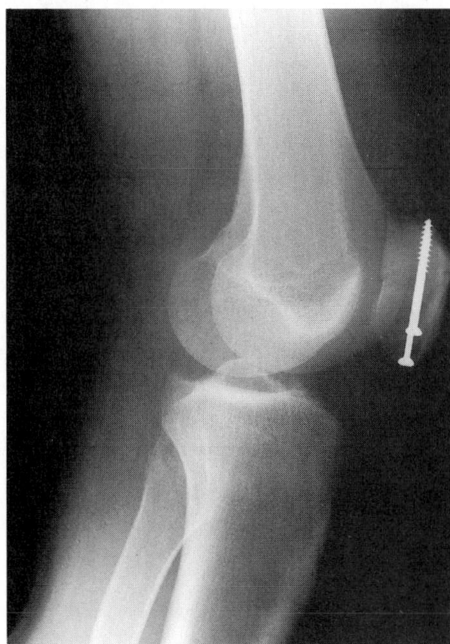

FIGURE 26-4 Transverse patellar fracture treated with lag screw fixation. This is a stress-shielding device unless solid fixation is not achieved.

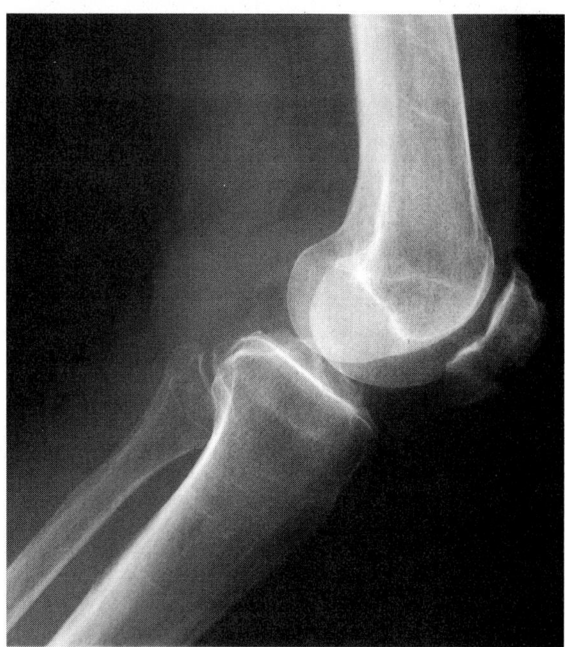

FIGURE 26-5 Transverse patellar fracture with displacement.

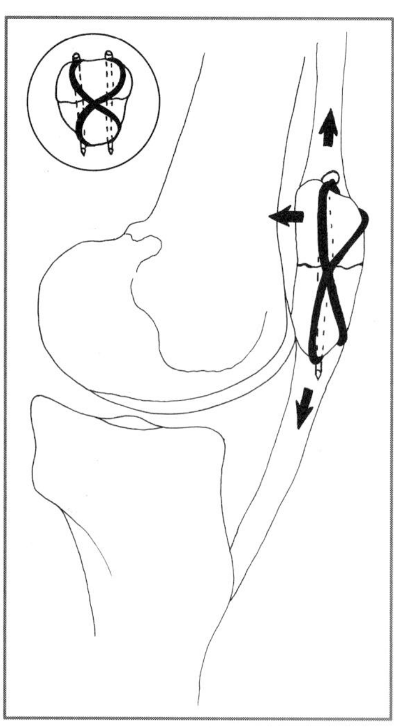

FIGURE 26-6 Transverse patellar fracture treated with tension band wiring. As the quadriceps muscle attempts to separate the fracture fragments, the wire tightens, forcing them back together.

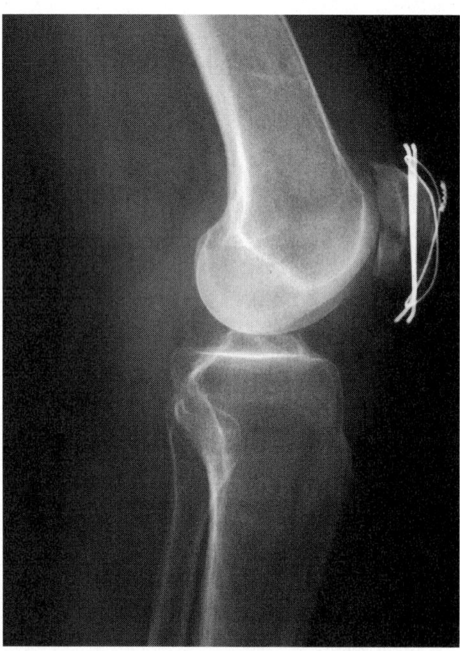

FIGURE 26-7 Tension band fixation for a transverse patellar fracture. The parallel wires control alignment and the tension band wire tightens with any attempt to distract the fracture. This is a stress-sharing device.

Partial/Total Patellectomy

If there is significant comminution that cannot be adequately repaired, partial patellectomy or total patellectomy is performed. However, the excision of the patella can lead to pain, loss of extensor strength, an extensor lag, and decreased range of motion of the knee. Following partial or total patellectomy, the extremity is immobilized in full extension for approximately 4 weeks. This allows tendon-to-bone healing (in case of partial patellectomy) or tendon-to-tendon healing (in case of total patellectomy). After 4 weeks, full active range of motion of the knee is begun with a gradual increase in the degree of flexion permitted.

Special Considerations of the Fracture

Bipartite Patella

Care should be taken not to mistake a bipartite patella for a patella fracture. The knee should be carefully examined for tenderness, and a comparison radiograph of the opposite extremity should also be obtained to assist in diagnosis.

Long-Term Sequelae

From the outset, the patient should be warned of the possibility of degenerative joint disease, decreased knee range of motion, permanent extensor lag, and prolonged swelling secondary to the injury.

Associated Injury

Retinacular Tear

In any patella fracture, the knee should be evaluated for its ability to perform active extension. Loss of this ability signifies a tear of the retinacular mechanism. Generally speaking, displaced fractures of the patella (greater than 3 mm of displacement) are associated with a tear of the extensor mechanism. Open repair of the patellar retinaculum should be undertaken in this circumstance. This may also help to prevent extensor lag.

Weight Bearing

Typically, the patient is allowed full weight bearing in a cast or knee immobilizer following the initial treatment, regardless of whether that treatment is casting or open reduction and internal fixation.

Gait Cycle

Stance Phase

The stance phase constitutes 60% of the gait cycle.

Heel Strike

The quadriceps maximally contracts concentrically to control knee extension. Tension is placed across the fracture line, which may cause pain. The patella rides in the patellar groove at the distal end of the femur. The patient may experience pain if there is step-off at the fracture site and surfaces are not smooth. If the quadriceps is weak, knee buckling occurs; the patient compensates by hyperextending and locking the knee to prevent falling (*see* Figure 6-1).

Foot-Flat

The quadriceps begins to contract in elongation to allow the beginning of flexion at the knee. The patient may experience pain as a result of quadriceps contraction (*see* Figure 6-2).

Mid-Stance

Mid-stance represents the single-leg support phase in which full weight bearing occurs. The knee is further flexed, and the patella may grind in the patellofemoral groove if the undersurface of the patella across the fracture site is uneven. Knee buckling may occur with quadriceps weakness (*see* Figure 6-3).

Push-Off

Push-off is usually not a problem, because the calf muscles dominate until the swing phase (*see* Figures 6-4 and 6-5).

Swing Phase

The swing phase constitutes 40% of the gait cycle.

Acceleration

The quadriceps contracts to bring the tibia forward on the femur. There may be patellofemoral grinding as the patella is pressed into the patellar groove. However, this is usually not as much of a problem as in the stance phase (*see* Figure 6-6).

Mid-Swing

This phase is usually not problematic because the hamstrings are contracting to slow the swing of the tibia (*see* Figure 6-7).

Deceleration

This phase is usually not problematic because the hamstrings are contracting to slow the swing of the tibia for heel strike (*see* Figure 6-8).

TREATMENT

Treatment: Early to Immediate (Day One to One Week)

BONE HEALING

Stability at fracture site: None.

Stage of bone healing: Inflammatory phase. The fracture hematoma is colonized by inflammatory cells, and débridement of the fracture begins.

X-ray: Fracture line is visible; no callus formation.

Orthopaedic and Rehabilitation Considerations

Physical Examination

Carefully assess complaints of pain, paresthesia, and cast discomfort. Check for swelling, especially around the ankle; if swelling is noted, instruct the patient to elevate the extremity. Evaluate neurovascular status by checking capillary refill, sensation, and active and passive range of motion of the ankle.

Dangers

Because this fracture commonly occurs secondary to a direct blow, extensive soft tissue injury can be present with swelling, hematoma, and even skin problems, particularly slough. Very little risk of compartment syndrome exists, unless there are associated injuries. Thrombophlebitis may result from the trauma.

Radiography

Check radiographs for loss of correction. If displacement greater than 2 to 3 mm or articular step-off greater than 1 to 2 mm is present, consider either another closed reduction and application of a cast if one is in place, or open reduction and internal fixation. If internal fixation has been performed, check for the position and possible breakage of fixation devices.

Weight Bearing

The patient is allowed full weight bearing in cast or knee immobilizer.

If the patient underwent open reduction with a stable internal fixation, a removable knee immobilizer is placed on the extremity during weight bearing. The immobilizer can be removed for performing active range-of-motion exercises to the knee in a sitting position. Weight bearing is not allowed while performing these exercises, because there may be uncontrolled flexion of the knee, disrupting the fixation devices and displacing the fracture.

Range of Motion

In patients treated with only a cast or knee immobilizer, no range of motion is allowed to the knee; in patients with open reduction and stable internal fixation, active range of motion is allowed. No passive range of motion is allowed.

Active range-of-motion exercises are begun at the hip and ankle in all planes. Initially, the hip may be sore after a fall. Hip flexion may be painful secondary to activation of the rectus femoris because it also flexes the hip. Straight leg raising is initiated as tolerated.

Muscle Strength

Isotonic exercises are prescribed to the dorsiflexors and plantar flexors of the ankle to prevent ankle stiffness and reduce the risk of thrombophlebitis.

Sets of gluteal exercises are prescribed to maintain the strength of the glutei group, which help to extend the hip and allow the patient to raise up from a chair.

Functional Activities

The patient is instructed in rolling over to one side and coming to a sitting position from a supine position by pushing up using the upper extremities.

As full weight bearing is allowed, the patient performs ambulatory transfers using the affected extremity. Initially, assistive devices such as crutches or a walker may be used for support during transfers because the patient may have pain and soreness.

The patient is instructed to don pants with the affected extremity first and doff them from the unaffected extremity first. This is the easiest way to dress without stressing the fracture site.

An elevated toilet seat is helpful for personal hygiene, because the knee cannot bend (*see* Figure 7-5).

Gait

Because the affected knee is kept in extension, the patient may have to circumduct the extremity or hip-hike to clear the floor. Initially, crutches or a walker may be used for support.

The patient ascends stairs with the unaffected extremity first, followed by the fractured extremity and the crutches, and descends stairs with the crutches first, followed by the fractured extremity and then the unaffected extremity (*see* Figures 6-20, 6-21, 6-22, 6-23, 6-24, and 6-25).

Methods of Treatment: Specific Aspects

Cast or Knee Immobilizer

Trim the cast around the thigh region and distally around the ankle. There should be abundant cast padding at the edges of the cast both proximally and distally. Be sure the cast does not rub over the malleoli. Also check for cast softening and repair appropriately. Decreased range of motion to the ankle might be noticed secondary to swelling or pain. If the patient is in a knee immobilizer, no range of motion of the knee is performed; straight leg raises can be performed with the cast or immobilizer on.

Open Reduction and Internal Fixation

Check the wound for erythema, discharge, or purulence, which could signify an infection. Once wounds appear benign, the patient can be placed in a cylinder cast or knee immobilizer, which should be checked for a good fit. If a cast is applied, check it for adequate padding at the proximal and distal edges and be sure it does not rub over the malleoli. Also check the cast for softening and repair appropriately. If a knee immobilizer is used, it can be removed for active range of motion of the knee as long as stable internal fixation was achieved.

Prescription

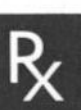

EARLY TO IMMEDIATE (DAY ONE TO ONE WEEK)

Precautions Avoid passive range of motion.

Range of Motion (Knee) None if in a cast.

If open reduction and stable internal fixation is achieved, active range of motion of the knee in a sitting position without weight bearing.

Strength No strengthening exercises prescribed to the knee.

Functional Activities Full weight bearing during transfers and ambulation using assistive devices.

Treatment: Two Weeks

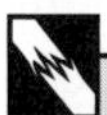

BONE HEALING

Stability at fracture site: None to minimal.

Stage of bone healing: Beginning of reparative phase. Osteoprogenitor cells differentiate into osteoblasts, which lay down woven bone.

X-ray: No callus; fracture line is visible.

Orthopaedic and Rehabilitation Considerations

Physical Examination

Carefully assess complaints of pain, paresthesia, and cast discomfort. Check for swelling, especially around the ankle; if swelling is present, instruct the patient to elevate the extremity. Check pins for prominence. Evaluate neurovascular status by checking capillary refill, sensation, and active and passive range of motion of the ankle. Range-of-motion evaluation of the knee is performed only if stable open reduction and internal fixation was performed.

Dangers

Assess the patient for loss of fixation and fracture displacement. Evaluate the skin for complications of the direct trauma, such as wound necrosis or slough.

Radiographs

Check radiographs for loss of correction. If displacement greater than 2 to 3 mm or articular step-off greater than 1 to 2 mm is present, consider either another closed reduction and application of cast or open reduction and internal fixation. If internal fixation has been performed, check for the position and possible breakage of fixation devices.

Weight Bearing

Full weight bearing is allowed in a cast or knee immobilizer.

Range of Motion

In patients treated with only a cast or knee immobilizer, no range of motion is allowed to the knee; in patients treated with open reduction and stable internal fixation, active range of motion to the knee is allowed in a sitting position. No passive range of motion is allowed, because this may disrupt the fracture site.

Continue active range of motion of the hip and ankle in all planes and continue straight-leg–raising exercises.

Muscle Strength

Continue isotonic exercises to the ankle in dorsiflexion and plantar flexion. Continue sets of gluteal exercises as before. Gluteus maximus strength is necessary for the patient to raise from a sitting to a standing position.

Functional Activities

Continue ambulatory transfers and full weight bearing with the cast or immobilizer on.

Gait

The patient may still need the crutches or a walker for ambulation with weight bearing on the affected extremity. The patient should ascend stairs with the unaffected extremity first, followed by the affected extremity and crutches, and descend stairs with the crutches first, followed by the affected extremity and then the unaffected extremity (*see* Figures 6-20, 6-21, 6-22, 6-23, 6-24, and 6-25).

Methods of Treatment: Specific Aspects

Cast

Trim the cast around the thigh region and distally around the ankle. Free motion of the ankle should be permitted. There should also be abundant padding at both edges of the cast, proximally and distally. Also, check for cast softening and repair appropriately. Straight leg raises are continued with the cast or immobilizer on.

Open Reduction and Internal Fixation

Remove the cast or knee immobilizer and check the wound for erythema, discharge, or purulence, which could signify infection. Remove staples or sutures. Subsequently replace the cast or knee immobilizer, ensuring that the cast is adequately padded proximally and distally. If a knee immobilizer is used, it can be removed for non–weight-bearing active range of motion to the knee if stable internal fixation was achieved.

Prescription

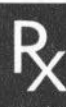

Two Weeks

Precautions Avoid passive range of motion.

Range of Motion (Knee) None.

If treated with open reduction and stable internal fixation, active knee flexion with no weight bearing.

Strength (Knee) None.

Functional Activities Full weight bearing during ambulation and transfers.

Treatment: Four to Six Weeks

Bone Healing

Stability at fracture site: None to minimal.

Stage of bone healing: Reparative phase. Osteoprogenitor cells differentiate into osteoblasts, which lay down woven bone.

X-ray: No callus; fracture line is less visible. Sesamoid bones produce minimal callus.

Orthopaedic and Rehabilitation Considerations

Physical Examination

Check the wound for erythema or discharge, which are possible signs of infection. Check whether pins are backing out or becoming prominent under the skin. Check active and passive range of motion of the knee.

Dangers

Evaluate the patient for loss of fixation and associated fracture displacement.

Radiography

Check radiographs for the presence of callus and the disappearance of the fracture line. Also check for any loss of fixation or associated displacement.

Weight Bearing

If the cast or knee immobilizer has been discontinued, the patient is allowed full weight bearing. If cast has been replaced, the patient is allowed full weight bearing in the cast. If a knee immobilizer is used, the patient is allowed full weight bearing while wearing it. The immobilizer can be removed to perform active range-of-motion exercises.

Range of Motion

The patient is instructed in active range-of-motion exercises to the knee as the cast is removed. If the fracture shows signs of healing, gentle active-assisted and passive range-of-motion exercises are also performed.

Muscle Strength

At the end of 6 weeks, the patient can start strengthening the quadriceps muscle. Gentle isometric exercises are prescribed. The patient actively extends the knee to perform isotonic exercises of quadriceps. Initially, no weights are used. The patient starts from 45 degrees of flexion to full extension (45 degrees to 0 degree) and then progresses from 90 degrees of flexion to full extension (90 degrees to 0 degree). The terminal 10 degrees of extension requires extra effort.

Stool-scoot exercises strengthen the hamstrings. The patient sits on a stool with knees flexed, then extends and flexes the knee with his or her foot on the floor. This improves the range of motion of the knee and strengthens the hamstring muscles.

Functional Activities

The patient can discontinue using crutches when independent and stable on stairs.

Gait

The patient continues to use the immobilizer for negotiating stairs. If the fracture is stable, the patient need not use the immobilizer for ambulation on level ground.

Methods of Treatment: Specific Aspects

Cast or Knee Immobilizer

If tenderness or motion is present at the fracture site, or if poor healing (inadequate callus) is seen radiographically, replace the cast. At this time, the fracture should be sticky enough that a knee immobilizer is adequate if the patient is compliant.

If there is no tenderness or motion at the fracture site, and if callus is present on x-ray film, discontinue the cast and the immobilizer. Continue active to active-assistive range of motion to the knee. However, the patient may use the immobilizer as a nighttime splint if the knee becomes tender from motion.

Open Reduction and Internal Fixation

If tenderness or motion at the fracture site or poor radiographic healing is present, replace the cast or knee immobilizer.

If there is no tenderness or motion at the fracture site and fracture line is disappearing on radiograph, discontinue the cast or knee immobilizer. However, if the knee becomes tender with motion, use the knee immobilizer as a temporary splint.

Prescription

FOUR TO SIX WEEKS

Precautions Maintain knee immobilizer if tenderness is present.

Range of Motion (Knee) Active range of motion in flexion/extension.

Strength (Knee) Isometric exercises to quadriceps and hamstrings.

At 6 weeks, isotonic exercises to quadriceps with active knee extension: 45 degrees to 0 degree and then from 90 degrees to 0 degree where 0 degree is full extension.

Functional Activities Full weight bearing during ambulation and transfers. Remove immobilizer for level ground walking if fracture is stable.

Treatment: Eight to Twelve Weeks

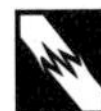

BONE HEALING

Stability at fracture site: Stable.

Stage of bone healing: Remodeling phase. Woven bone is being replaced with lamellar bone. The process of remodeling takes months to years for completion.

X-ray: Small amount of callus noted. Fracture line begins to disappear with time. Amount of callus formed is small, because this is a sesamoid bone.

Orthopaedic and Rehabilitation Considerations

Physical Examination

Check the wound for erythema or discharge, which are signs of possible infection. Check active and passive range of motion of the knee.

Dangers

Loss of fixation is still a risk, although less than before.

Radiography

Check radiographs for the presence of callus and disappearance of the fracture line. Also check for any loss of fixation or associated displacement.

Weight Bearing

The patient should progress to full weight bearing without any immobilization by this time, because the fracture is stable.

Range of Motion

The patient performs active and passive range-of-motion exercises to the knee. Initially, the knee may lack full flexion because of the immobilization. The patient may also have an extension lag secondary to weak quadriceps. Hydrotherapy decreases discomfort and pain during the exercises.

The patient can actively assist in flexing and extending the knee by using his or her uninvolved extremity to range the involved extremity. Hip and ankle range-of-motion exercises should continue.

Muscle Strength

Progressive resistive exercises are prescribed to improve the strength of the quadriceps and hamstrings. One- to two-pound weights are attached at the ankle initially, and the weights are gradually increased. The exercises are done in sets, with the number of sets being increased over time.

As the patient's strength increases, isokinetic exercises are also prescribed to strengthen the muscle. Plyometric closed-chain exercises can be instituted for sports activities, and their intensity can be increased gradually.

Gait

Emphasize normalization of the gait. Controlled elongation contraction of the quadriceps is necessary for heel strike to foot-flat during the stance phase.

Methods of Treatment: Specific Aspects

Cast or Knee Immobilizer

Discontinue the cast or knee immobilizer, if this has not already been done. Examine for tenderness and motion at the fracture site.

Open Reduction and Internal Fixation

Examine for tenderness and motion at the fracture site.

Prescription

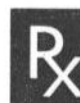

EIGHT TO TWELVE WEEKS

Precautions

Range of Motion (Knee) Active and passive range of motion. Patient may have extension lag secondary to quad weakness and immobilization.

Strength (Knee) Progressive resistive exercises to quadriceps and hamstrings with weights; isokinetic exercises using Cybex machine; plyometric closed chain exercises.

Functional Exercises Full weight bearing during ambulation and transfers without assistive devices.

LONG-TERM CONSIDERATIONS AND PROBLEMS

At every stage of treatment, radiographs should be checked for loss of correction, defined as persistence of greater than 1 to 2 mm of articular step-off or greater than 2 to 3 mm of displacement. If this occurs early in treatment before any operative procedure, casting can be performed again, but more likely open reduction and internal fixation will be necessary. If the loss of correction occurs after open reduction and internal fixation, possibly as a result of broken fixation devices, a revision of the procedure can be performed. If this is not successful, a partial or total patellectomy can be performed. On the other hand, the knee can simply be followed up for any future degenerative changes, which may manifest as pain with knee motion.

Quadriceps shortening can reduce knee extension. Watch for knee flexion contractures, because the resting position for a swollen knee is about 30 degrees and is not uncommon for a contracture. If there is a 15-degree contracture, then knee extension in terminal swing, initial contact, mid-stance, and terminal stance is inadequate. If there is a decrease in extension (in terminal swing), step length shortens. If the knee is not appropriately extended in the mid-stance and terminal stance phases, then there is an increase in the demand of quadriceps activity.

Chondromalacia patella may be present because of direct trauma to the cartilaginous undersurface of the patella. This may present long-term problems, especially in stair climbing when the patella is forced against the femur.

Reflex inhibition of the iliopsoas muscle is possible after surgery on the knee. Rehabilitation of the iliopsoas is needed if it has not recovered on the affected side.

IMMEDIATE TO ONE WEEK

	Cast	*Open Reduction and Internal Fixation*
Stability	None.	None.
Orthopaedics	Trim cast back so that it does not rub against malleoli. Elevate the extremity to decrease swelling.	Perform wound care over any incisions and in any open wounds.
Rehabilitation	No knee range of motion. Straight leg raises can be performed with the cast or knee immobilizer in place. Glutei sets are prescribed for the hips and isotonic exercises for the ankle. Weight bearing is allowed in the cast or immobilizer.	If stable internal fixation is achieved, active knee range of motion is allowed. No passive knee motion is allowed. Straight leg raises can be performed with the cast or knee immobilizer in place. Glutei sets are prescribed for the hips and isotonic exercises for the ankle. Weight bearing is allowed in the cast or immobilizer.

TWO WEEKS

	Cast	*Open Reduction and Internal Fixation*
Stability	None to minimal.	None to minimal.
Orthopaedics	Trim cast back and continue elevation when necessary to decrease swelling.	Remove sutures and continue wound care to any healing wounds.
Rehabilitation	No knee range of motion is allowed. Straight leg raises are continued with the cast or immobilizer in place. Glutei sets and ankle isotonic exercises are continued. Weight bearing is allowed in the cast or immobilizer.	If stable internal fixation is achieved, active knee range of motion is allowed. No passive knee motion is allowed. Straight leg raises are continued with the cast or knee immobilizer in place. Glutei sets and ankle isotonic exercises are continued. Weight bearing is allowed in the cast or immobilizer.

FOUR TO SIX WEEKS

	Cast	Open Reduction and Internal Fixation
Stability	Partially stable.	Partially stable.
Orthopaedics	If adequate callus is achieved and knee is nontender, discontinue the cast or immobilizer. If knee becomes tender from motion, immobilizer can be worn as nighttime splint.	Continue wound care as needed. If there is adequate fracture line disappearance and no tenderness discontinue the cast or immobilizer. If knee becomes tender from motion, immobilizer can be worn as nighttime splint.
Rehabilitation	Once cast is removed, active knee range of motion is allowed, progressing to active-assisted and passive range of motion. Quadriceps and hamstrings isometric and isotonic exercises are begun. Hip and ankle exercises are continued. Once cast is removed, full weight bearing is allowed.	Once cast or immobilizer is removed, active knee range of motion is progressed to active-assisted and passive range of motion. Quadriceps and hamstrings isometric and isotonic exercises are begun. Hip and ankle exercises are continued. Once immobilizer is removed, full weight bearing is allowed.

EIGHT TO TWELVE WEEKS

	Cast	Open Reduction and Internal Fixation
Stability	Stable.	Stable.
Orthopaedics	Discontinue cast or immobilizer, if not. already done	Continue wound care as needed. Discontinue cast or immobilizer, if not already done.
Rehabilitation	Active and passive range of motion to the knee is performed. Quadriceps and hamstrings exercises are continued, as are hip and ankle exercises. Full weight bearing is allowed.	Active and passive range of motion to the knee is performed. Quadriceps and hamstrings exercises are continued, as are hip and ankle exercises. Full weight bearing is allowed.

BIBLIOGRAPHY

Andrews JR, Hughston JC. Treatment of patellar fractures by partial patellectomy. *South Med J,* 70:800–813, 1977.

Dowd GSE. Marginal fratures of the patella. *Injury,* 14:287–291, 1982.

Huang LK, Chan KM, Chow YN, Leung PC. Fractures patella: operative treatment using the tension band principle. *Injury,* 16:343–347, 1985.

Jakobsen J, Christensen KS, Rasmussen OS. Patellectomy—a 20-year follow-up. *Acta Orthop Scand,* 56:430–432, 1985.

Johnson EE. Fractures of the patella. In: Rockwood CA Jr, Green DP, Bucholz RW, eds. *Fractures in Adults,* Vol. 2, 3rd ed. Philadelphia: JB Lippincott, 1991, pp. 1762–1777.

Levack B, Flannagan JP, Hobbs S. Results of surgical treatment of patellar fractures. *J Bone Joint Surg,* 67B:416–419, 1985.

Lotke PA, Ecker ML. Transverse fractures of the patella. *Clin Orthop,* 158:180–184, 1981.

Ma YZ, Zheng YF, Qu KF, Yeh Y. Treatment of fractures of the patella with percutaneous suture. *Clin Orthop* 191:235–241, 1984.

Sanders R. Patella fractures and extensor mechanism injuries. In: Browner BD, Jupiter JB, Levine AM, Trafton PG, eds. *Skeletal Trauma,* Vol. 2. Philadelphia: WB Saunders, 1992, pp. 1685–1716.

Stern RE, Harwin SF. Spontaneous and simultaneous rupture of both quadriceps tendons. *Clin Orthop,* 147:188–189, 1980.

CHAPTER Twenty-seven

Tibial Plateau Fractures

DEREK A. KRAM, MD

VASANTHA L. MURTHY, MD

INTRODUCTION

Definition

Tibial plateau fractures involve the proximal aspect or metaphysis of the tibia and frequently the articular surface as well. They are subdivided into six types by Schatzker (Figure 27-1 and *see* Figures 27-8 and 27-9):

1. Type I is a wedge or split fracture of the lateral tibial plateau.
2. Type II is a split depression fracture of the lateral plateau and involves an articular injury (Figure 27-2 and *see* Figures 27-10 and 27-11).
3. Type III is a pure depression fracture of the lateral plateau that also involves an articular injury (Figure 27-3).

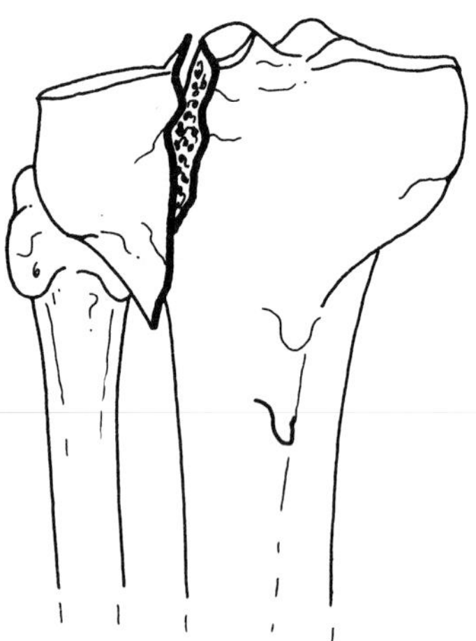

FIGURE 27-1 Split type I fracture of the lateral tibial plateau with displacement. Isolated split fractures generally occur in the younger patients.

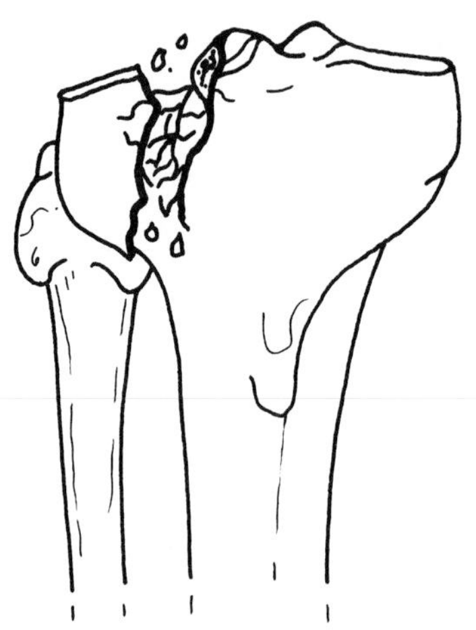

FIGURE 27-2 Type II fracture of the tibial plateau, a combination split and depression fracture of the lateral tibial plateau, where a portion of the articular surface is depressed.

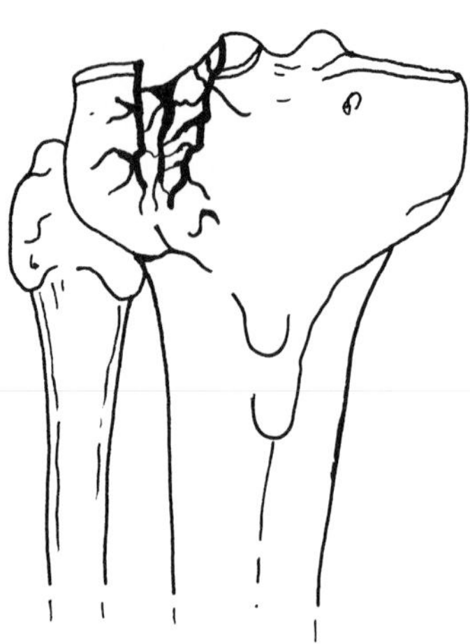

FIGURE 27-3 Type III depressed fracture of the lateral tibial plateau. Isolated depression fractures generally occur in older patients.

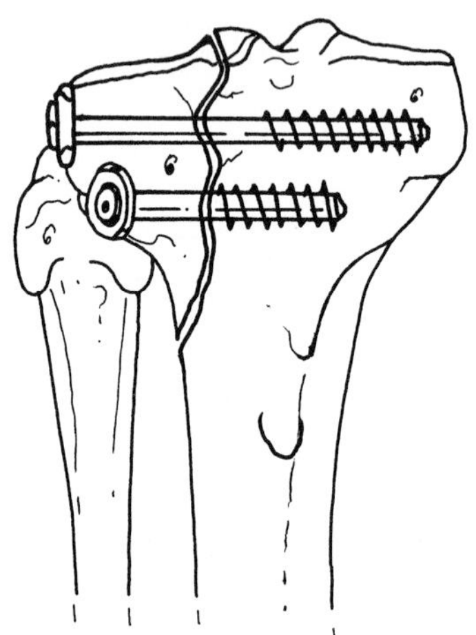

FIGURE 27-1A Type I split fracture of the lateral tibial plateau treated with cancellus screws and washers to provide compression across the fracture site. These fractures are to be kept non-weight bearing to prevent displacement of the split fragment in the soft metaphyseal bone.

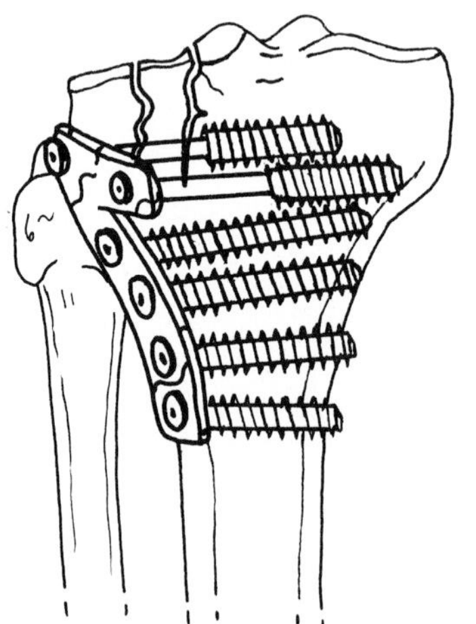

FIGURE 27-2A Type II plateau fracture treated with a buttress plate and screw fixation. The articular surface is elevated and the buttress plate prevents displacement of the split fragment. These fractures are kept non-weight bearing postoperatively to prevent depression of the articular surface.

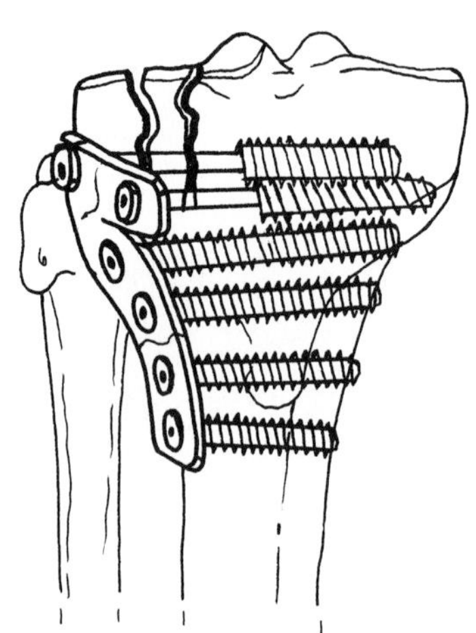

FIGURE 27-3A Type III tibial plateau fracture treated with buttress plate and screw fixation. The articular surface is elevated and the buttress plate is used to compress the fragments to prevent depression of the articular surface.

4. Type IV is a split depression fracture of the medial tibial plateau, often involving the intercondylar eminence and associated cruciate ligament. It is usually associated with an articular injury (Figure 27-4 and *see* Figures 27-12 and 27-13).
5. Type V is a bicondylar fracture involving both plateaus. It is also known as an inverted Y fracture and is usually associated with an articular injury (Figure 27-5).
6. Type VI is a fracture at the proximal tibial diaphyseal-metaphyseal junction (Figure 27-6).

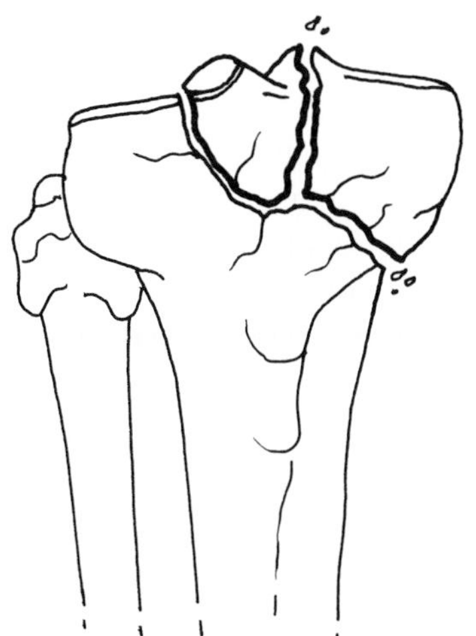

FIGURE 27-4 Type IV tibial plateau fracture. Fracture involving the medial tibial plateau may be split, depression, or split depression fractures. Type IV tibial plateau fractures are often associated with high-energy trauma and potential vascular injury.

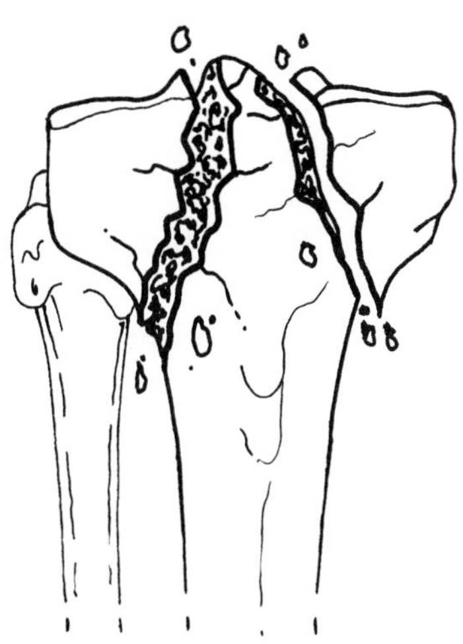

FIGURE 27-5 Type V tibial plateau fracture. Fracture involving both tibial plateaus (bicondylar fractures) are also known as inverted Y fractures.

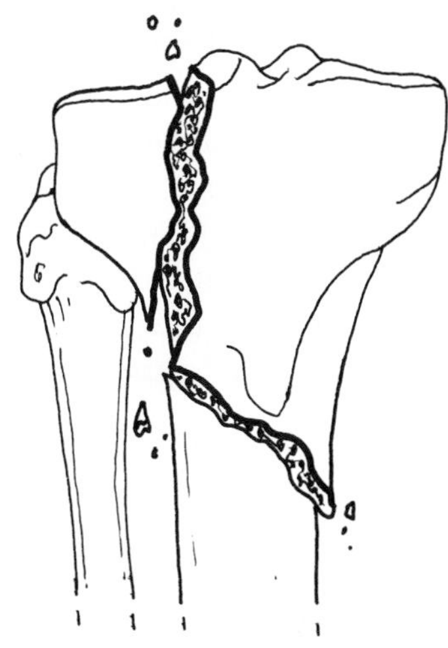

FIGURE 27-6 Type VI tibial plateau fracture. Fracture of either the medial or lateral tibial plateau with a second fracture line separating the metaphysis from the diaphysis. This fracture often involves high-energy trauma.

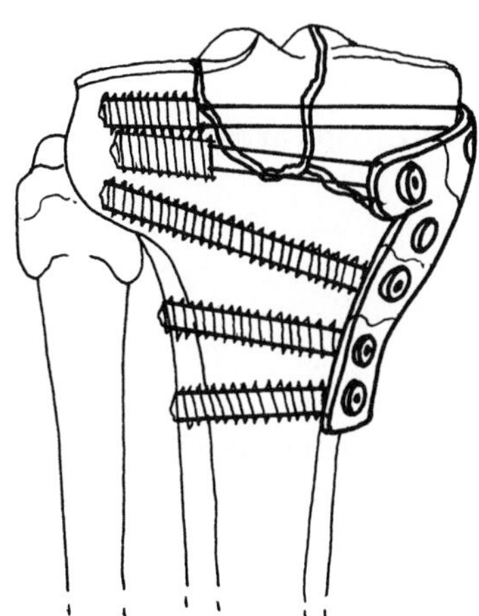

FIGURE 27-4A Type IV tibial plateau fracture treated with buttress plate and screw fixation.

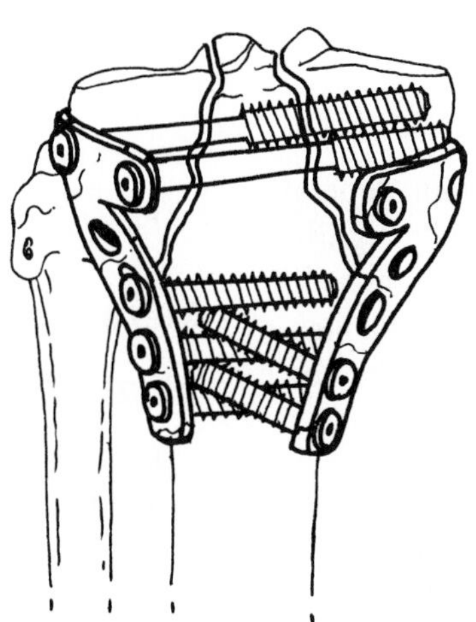

FIGURE 27-5A Type V tibial plateau fracture treated with buttress plates of both the medial and lateral plateaus. Fixation of this fashion involves extensive soft tissue stripping.

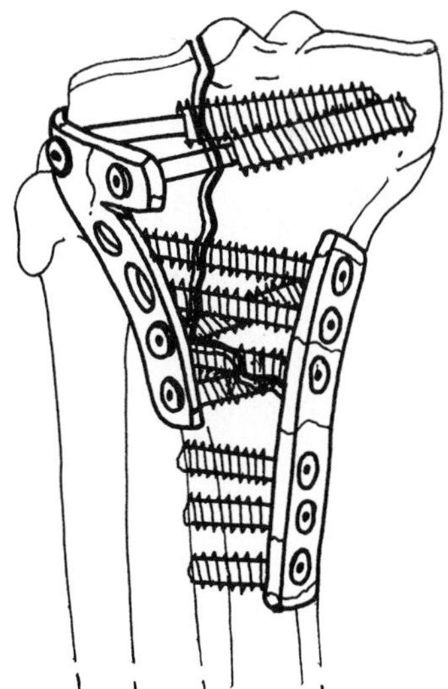

FIGURE 27-6A Type VI tibial plateau fracture treated with a lateral buttress plate and a compression plate fixation of the medial side for the diaphyseal metaphyseal fracture.

Tibial spines are located on the proximal surface of the tibia. Tibial spine fractures are classified and treated differently than plateau fractures. Type I and type II tibial spine fractures involve small and large degrees, respectively, of anterior tilt of the spine while still maintaining contact with the underlying tibia. Type III fractures involve complete disruption of the spine from the underlying tibia, with type III-A having no associated rotation of the fractured tibial spine and type III-B having an associated tibial spine rotation. Treatment involves placement of a long leg cast in extension for 6 weeks for types I, II, and III-A. All type III-B and any type I, II, or III-A fractures that cannot be brought into full extension require open reduction and internal fixation, usually with small fragment lag screws.

Mechanism of Injury

Tibial plateau fractures most commonly result from a medially directed force, resulting in a valgus deformity (the classic "bumper fracture"). They may also result from a laterally directed force (causing a varus deformity), an axial compressive force, or a combination of an axial force with either a medially or laterally directed force.

Young patients with relatively strong metaphyseal bone usually sustain pure split (type I) fractures. Older patients, however, with relatively weak metaphyseal bone, usually sustain depression fractures of varied types.

Treatment Goals

Orthopaedic Objectives

Alignment

Any fracture with greater than 4 mm of joint depression, if left unreduced, can be associated with significant varus or valgus deformity and instability as well as an increased risk of future degenerative changes. Therefore, these are often treated with open reduction and internal fixation.

Stability

Stability is best achieved when bony congruity is restored and the bone rigidly fixed with hardware.

Rehabilitation Objectives

Range of Motion

Restore full range of motion of the knee as early as possible to limit functional disability. Restore and maintain full range of motion of the ankle and hip (Table 27-1).

TABLE 27-1 *Range of Motion of Knee*

Motion	Normal	Functional
Flexion	130°–140°	0°–110°
Extension	0°–5°	

Muscle Strength

Improve and restore the strength of the following muscles:

Quadriceps: a powerful knee extensor.
Rectus femoris: a two-jointed muscle, crossing both the hip and knee, and thus flexing the hip.
Hamstrings: made up of the semimembranosus, semitendinosus, and biceps femoris. A group of muscles that function as primary knee flexors, spanning two joints and assisting hip extension.
Sartorius and gracilis: supporting the medial side of the knee, which is under considerable strain in gait as a result of the valgus angle between the femur and tibia. They are two-jointed muscles.
Gastrocnemius: a two-jointed muscle that functions as plantar flexor of the foot.

Functional Goals

Normalize the gait pattern and restore the stability of the knee during the stance phase.

Expected Time of Bone Healing

Ten to 12 weeks (as little as 8 weeks for type I fractures).

Expected Time of Rehabilitation

Fourteen to 20 weeks.

Methods of Treatment

Hinged Orthosis

Biomechanics: Stress-sharing device.
Mode of Bone Healing: Secondary.
Indications: This is the treatment of choice for split fractures of the lateral tibial plateau with no or minimal displacement, as well as for split depression fractures of the lateral tibial plateau with minimal or less than 3 mm of articular surface depression. These devices can be considered definitive treatment only if valgus or varus instability does not exceed 10 degrees and if no posterior wedge fracture is present. Additionally, a hinged orthosis can be used as definitive treatment in the management of severely comminuted fractures or in patients who are not good

candidates for operative management. After most open reduction and internal fixations, a hinged orthosis with a locked hinge on the affected side is often placed on the leg to help unload that side during healing (Figure 27-7).

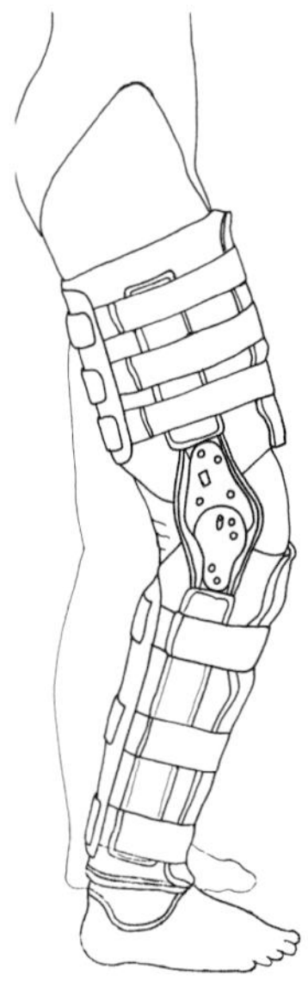

FIGURE 27-7 Hinged orthosis as a treatment for tibial plateau fractures. Patients are kept non-weight bearing.

Open Reduction and Internal Fixation

Biomechanics: Stress-shielding device.

Mode of Bone Healing: Primary, unless a solid fixation is not achieved, in which case secondary healing also occurs.

Indications: For fractures with marked displacement or greater than 3 mm of articular depression, fractures associated with greater than 10 degrees of varus or valgus angulation, posterior wedge fractures, fractures associated with trapped menisci, and fractures involving the medial plateau, open reduction and internal fixation is necessary to restore the articular surface and possibly repair or reposition the meniscus. The technique of articular reconstruction often involves the use of bone graft to the underlying metaphyseal bone and placement of a buttress plate or lag screws to maintain the reduction (Figures 27-8, 27-9, 27-10, 27-11, 27-12, 27-13 and *see* Figures 27-3, 27-4, 27-5, and 27-6).

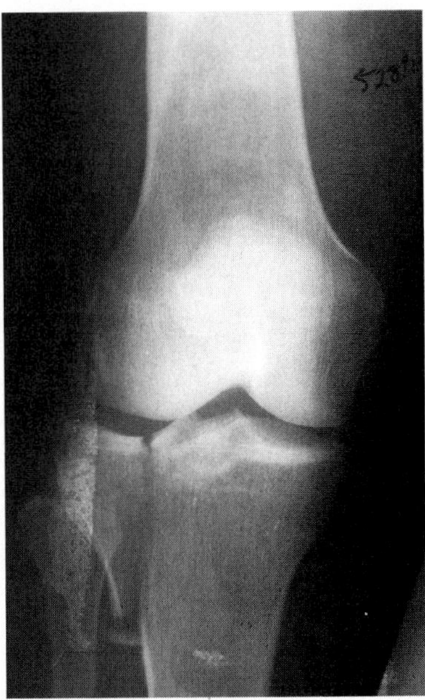

FIGURE 27-8 Type I tibial plateau fracture. Split fracture of the lateral tibial plateau with displacement.

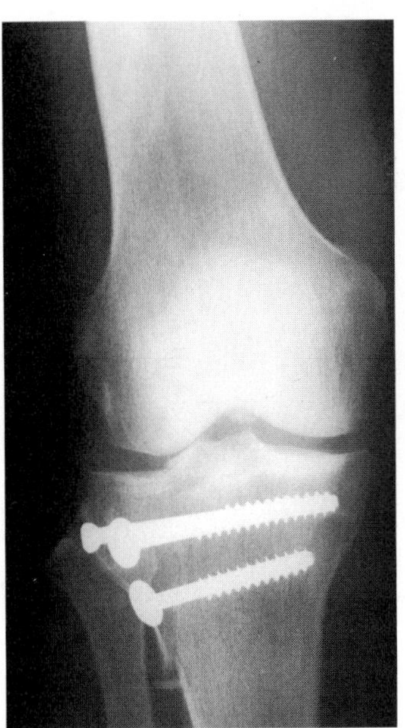

FIGURE 27-9 Type I lateral tibial plateau fracture treated with screw and washer fixation. Note restoration of the articular surface. To prevent depression of the split fragment, no weight bearing is allowed for 12 weeks.

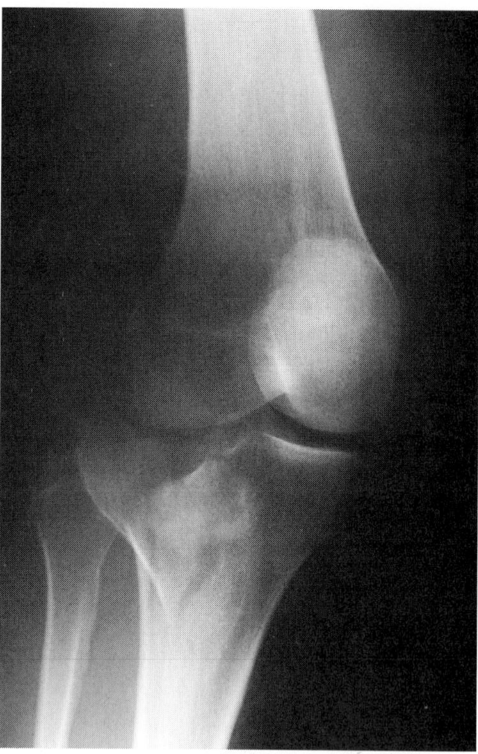

FIGURE 27-10 Type II tibial plateau fracture. Combination split and depression fracture of the lateral tibial plateau. Note the depression of the articular surface.

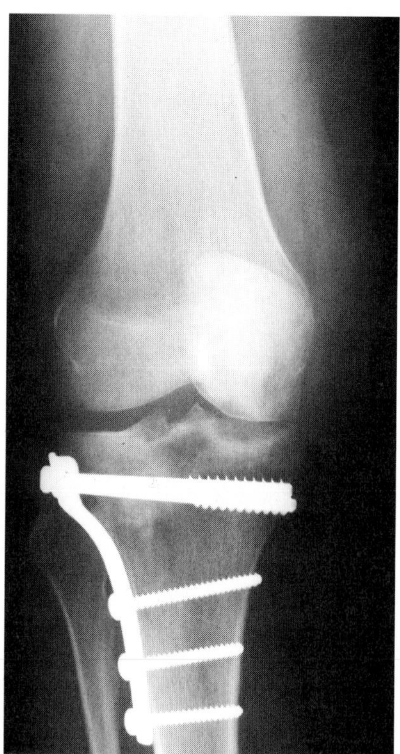

FIGURE 27-11 Type II tibial plateau fracture treated with buttress plate and screw fixation. Note the elevation of the tibial plateau with restoration of the articular surface.

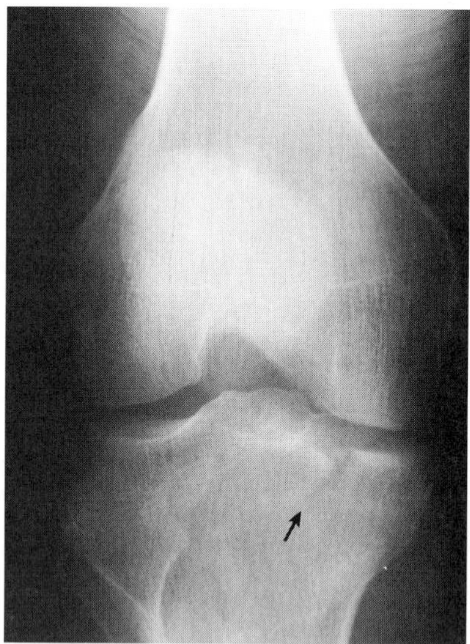

FIGURE 27-12 Type IV tibial plateau fracture. Split fracture of the medial tibial plateau.

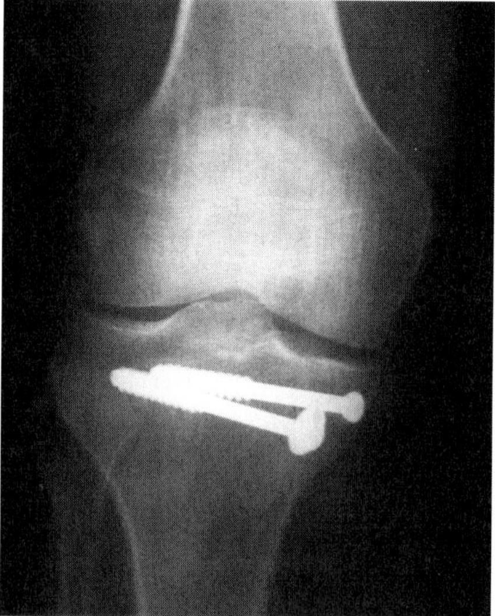

FIGURE 27-13 Type IV tibial plateau fracture treated with screw and washer fixation to prevent displacement of the split fragment.

External Fixation

Biomechanics: Stress-shielding device.

Mode of Bone Healing: Primary, unless a solid fixation is not achieved, in which case secondary healing also occurs.

Indications: External fixation is usually a temporizing measure. Open fractures of the tibial plateau are surgical emergencies, often requiring débridement and external fixation if adequate soft tissue coverage is not possible. The fixation often is placed across the knee and thus allows no knee motion. Newer "hybrid" fixator devices do not cross the knee and do allow knee motion. Once soft tissue healing occurs, a skin graft or flap and possible internal fixation can be placed, or the fixator can be replaced with a hinged orthosis.

Special Considerations of Fracture

Age

In elderly osteoporotic patients with marked loss of cancellous metaphyseal bone underlying a joint depression, the plateau is often difficult if not impossible to reconstruct. It is best to treat these cases nonoperatively initially; following fracture healing, evaluate the knee for stability and function. If it is unstable or functionally limited, arthroplasty can then be considered.

Location

Fractures of the medial plateau types IV through VI are generally associated with more extensive soft tissue injury, because a greater force is needed to cause those fractures. Repair of the soft tissue injury as well as reconstruction of the plateau is usually necessary. Fractures of the intercondylar eminence affect the function of the anterior cruciate ligament complex, leading to instability, and thus clearly indicate open reduction and internal fixation. Posterior wedge fractures lead to instability in the extended position, thus also requiring open reduction and internal fixation.

Injured Anatomy

Adequate radiographic evaluation of the fracture pattern using computed tomography, if necessary, and possibly magnetic resonance imaging to evaluate ligamentous and meniscal injury, is necessary before determining the final treatment.

Associated Injury

Fractures of the lateral plateau are often associated with injury to the medial collateral ligament complex or anterior cruciate ligament.

Fractures of the medial plateau are often associated with injuries to the lateral collateral ligament complex, the cruciates, the peroneal nerve, and possibly the popliteal artery. These fractures tend to be more unstable and are often associated with knee dislocations. Dislocations can realign before the initial examination and therefore may not be discovered during the examination.

All tibial plateau fractures should be carefully evaluated for subsequent development of compartment syndrome. The greater the energy absorbed during trauma, the more likely it is that there is extensive soft tissue injury.

Weight Bearing

Typically, the patient is kept non-weight bearing for 3 months after injury so that the relatively weak metaphyseal bone will heal and any bony graft can incorporate.

Gait Cycle

Stance Phase

Stance phase constitutes 60% of the gait cycle.

Heel Strike

The quadriceps contracts concentrically to bring the knee to full extension. Because the fracture is intraarticular, full knee extension may not be achieved and an antalgic gait may occur, reducing the duration of the stance phase. The ankle joint and the associated muscles are usually not affected (*see* Figure 6-1).

Foot-Flat

Foot-flat is usually not a problem, even though the quadriceps is contracting eccentrically (*see* Figure 6-2).

Mid-Stance

Full weight is borne through the tibial plateau at this phase. If the plateau surface is not smooth or is arthritic, pain ensues, causing an antalgic gait. The patient may hop off the extremity to reduce pain (*see* Figure 6-3).

Push-Off

Weight bearing is still within the joint, although it is reduced, and may be painful (*see* Figures 6-4 and 6-5).

Swing Phase

The swing phase is 40% of the gait cycle. It is usually not a problem, because weight is not borne through the joint (*see* Figures 6-6, 6-7, and 6-8).

TREATMENT

Treatment: Early to Immediate (Day of Injury to One Week)

BONE HEALING

Stability at fracture site: None.

Stage of bone healing: Inflammatory phase. The fracture hematoma is colonized by inflammatory cells, and débridement of the fracture begins.

X-ray: No callus.

Orthopaedic and Rehabilitation Considerations

Physical Examination

Initially, check the patient's neurovascular status by palpating pulses and checking capillary refill. Check sensation and active foot and ankle motion. Check lower extremity compartments for softness and monitor compartment pressures if there is any suspicion of compartment syndrome. Check wounds from the injury or from surgery for erythema or discharge; débridement should be performed or antibiotics given as needed. If edema is present, the patient should be instructed to elevate the extremity.

Dangers

Look for compartment syndrome, especially when the popliteal vessels have been injured. Compartment syndrome is more common with high-energy trauma and is usually noted in the first few hours after injury or surgery. Check for foot drop as a sign of peroneal nerve injury.

The patient must be advised that even minimally displaced or depressed fractures are at risk for future degenerative joint disease. The patient should be encouraged to work aggressively at obtaining adequate range of motion, because subsequent knee stiffness is a common complication. Also, the patient must be reminded to avoid bearing weight on the affected extremity for approximately 3 months, because any weight bearing may cause further displacement or depression of the fracture.

Radiography

If open reduction and internal fixation has not been performed, check radiographs for any loss of alignment or displacement of the fracture. Any significant displacement or loss of articular surface congruity, as well as posterior subluxation of the femur on the tibia, is an indication for open reduction and internal fixation. If the patient has had internal fixation, check for the proper position of hardware and for maintenance of correction.

Weight Bearing

The patient is kept non-weight bearing for 3 months.

Range of Motion

Early knee range of motion is the key to success. To minimize scar formation, adhesions, and ligamentous stiffness, active and active-assistive flexion/extension of the knee are allowed while protecting the knee from valgus and varus stress, once the initial pain has subsided. Usually this is done in a sitting position with the knee at the edge of the seat. Forty degrees to 60 degrees of flexion is allowed initially, increasing to 90 degrees of flexion after 1 week. Sometimes a continuous passive motion machine is used to maintain the range, depending on the stability of the fracture.

Active ankle dorsiflexion/plantar flexion is encouraged to maintain the range of motion, decrease stiffness, and reduce edema. The patient may be instructed to keep the extremity elevated to minimize fluid retention.

Muscle Strength

No strengthening exercises are prescribed at this time to avoid displacing fracture fragments. Once pain subsides, gentle ankle isotonics without resistance are prescribed. Sets of gluteal exercises are prescribed to maintain the strength of the glutei. These muscles are important for helping the patient raise from a sitting to a standing position.

Functional Activities

The patient should not bear weight on the affected side and is instructed to use crutches for transfers. The patient is taught to don pants on the affected extremity first and doff them from the unaffected extremity first.

Gait

The patient is taught a two-point non–weight-bearing gait using crutches, in which the crutches and affected extremity act as one unit and the unaffected extremity as the other unit (*see* Figure 6-16). The patient ascends stairs with the unaffected extremity first and descends stairs with the crutches and affected extremity first (*see* Figures 6-20, 6-21, 6-22, 6-23, 6-24, and 6-25). Elderly patients use a walker. Because it is difficult to ambulate in a non–weight-bearing manner with a walker (hopping), patients are allowed to toe touch on the affected extremity.

Methods of Treatment: Specific Aspects

Hinged Orthosis

Evaluate the hinged orthosis for adequate fit with the knee in all positions (*see* Figure 37-7).

Open Reduction and Internal Fixation

If the patient is in a hinged orthosis following surgery, evaluate the apparatus as above. The range of motion of the knee should be 0 degrees to at least 90 degrees. Strengthening exercises should be avoided to minimize the possibility of displacing the fracture. Continue ankle isotonic exercises and gluteal sets.

External Fixation

Check all the connecting bars for adequate tightness to ensure that alignment is maintained. The fixator can be adjusted as needed for any excess varus, valgus, anterior, or posterior displacement. If the fixator crosses the knee, no range of motion is possible. However, if a hybrid fixator is used and the condition of the soft tissue allows, active range of motion of the knee is permitted.

Prescription

DAY ONE TO ONE WEEK

Precautions No varus or valgus stress on knee; no passive range of motion.

Range of Motion Active and active-assistive flexion/extension: 40 degrees to 60 degrees of flexion allowed initially, increasing to 90 degrees of flexion after 1 week.

Strength No strengthening exercises to knee.

Functional Activities Non–weight-bearing stand/pivot transfers and ambulation with crutches.

Weight Bearing No weight bearing on the affected extremity.

Treatment: Two Weeks

BONE HEALING

Stability at fracture site: None to minimal.

Stage of bone healing: Beginning of reparative phase. Osteoprogenitor cells differentiate into osteoblasts, which lay down woven bone.

X-ray: None to early callus; fracture line is visible.

Orthopaedic and Rehabilitation Considerations

Physical Examination

Check the wounds for erythema or discharge, which indicate a possible infection that may require antibiotic therapy or possible surgical débridement.

Pay attention to complaints of pain, paresthesia, or symptoms of knee instability. Check capillary refill and sensation. Check the passive and active range of motion of the knee; flexion should be at least 90 degrees.

Dangers

There is a risk of fracture displacement or loss of fixation, which should be watched. At this point, the risk of compartment syndrome is small. Peroneal nerve injury is uncommon after the initial trauma.

Radiography

If open reduction and internal fixation has not been performed, check radiographs for loss of alignment or displacement of the fracture. Any significant displacement or loss of articular surface congruity, significant subluxation of the femur on the tibia, or any rotational or varus/valgus deformities are indications for open reduction and internal fixation. If the patient has had internal fixation, check for the proper position of hardware and for maintenance of correction. If correction is lost, the fixation may need to be revised (supplemental bone graft is often used).

Weight Bearing

The patient is kept non-weight bearing for 3 months.

Range of Motion

The patient should engage in active and active-assistive range-of-motion exercises, obtaining 0 degrees to at least 90 degrees of knee flexion. If the patient has not achieved the desired range of motion, emphasis should be placed on increasing the intensity and frequency of the exercise repetitions. Ankle dorsiflexion/plantar flexion is encouraged to maintain ankle motion and strength.

Muscle Strength

Isometric exercises to the quadriceps are started at the end of 2 weeks to prevent disuse atrophy and to maintain stability at the knee. If the patient complains of pain at the fracture site after exercising, he or she may be stressing the fracture site. The patient is to continue performing sets of gluteal exercises to maintain the strength of the hip extensors and ankle isotonics to maintain dorsiflexor/plantar flexor strength.

Functional Activities

The patient continues non-weight bearing transfers.

Gait

The patient continues two-point non–weight-bearing gait using crutches. In elderly patients, toe-touch with the affected extremity is allowed when they use a walker.

Methods of Treatment: Specific Aspects

Hinged Orthosis

Evaluate the hinged orthosis for adequate, snug fit with the knee in all positions. Adjust the orthosis to accommodate any increased range of motion.

Open Reduction and Internal fixation

If the patient is in a hinged orthosis following surgery, remove it and evaluate the wound for any erythema, discharge, or fluctuance. Remove sutures. Place a light, sterile dressing over the wound before applying a hinged orthosis.

External Fixation

Examine the patient's wounds and pin sites for erythema, drainage, or purulence. Check all the connecting bars for adequate tightness to ensure that alignment across the knee is maintained. The fixator can be adjusted as needed for any excess varus, valgus, anterior, or posterior displacement.

Prescription

Two Weeks

Precautions No varus or valgus stress on knee; no passive range of motion.

Range of Motion Active, active-assistive flexion/extension up to 90 degrees.

Strength Isometric exercises to the quadriceps.

Functional Activities Non–weight-bearing stand/pivot transfers and ambulation with crutches.

Weight Bearing Non–weight-bearing on affected extremity.

Treatment: Four to Six Weeks

Bone Healing

Stability at fracture site: With bridging callus, the fracture is usually stable; confirm with physical examination.

Stage of bone healing: Reparative phase. Once callus is observed bridging the fracture site, the fracture is usually stable. The strength of this callus, however, especially with torsional load, is significantly lower than that of normal bone.

X-ray: Bridging callus is beginning to be visible. With increased rigidity of fixation, less bridging callus is noted, and healing with endosteal callus predominates. The fracture line is less visible.

Orthopaedic and Rehabilitation Considerations

Physical Examination

Check any wounds for erythema or discharge, indicating a possible infection that may require antibiotic therapy with possible surgical débridement.

Pay attention to complaints of pain, paresthesia, or symptoms of knee instability. Check capillary refill and sensation. Check the passive and active range of motion of the knee; flexion should be at least 90 degrees.

Dangers

Fracture displacement and loss of fixation are still possible and should be excluded.

Radiography

Check radiographs for any loss of correction or displacement of the fracture, as well as any rotational or varus/valgus deformities. The fracture should be gaining some stability at this stage, and there should be evidence of a callus or the dissolution of the fracture line.

Weight Bearing

The patient is kept non-weight bearing for 3 months.

Range of Motion

The patient should engage in active and active-assistive range-of-motion exercises, obtaining 0 degrees to at least 90 degrees of knee flexion. At the end of 6 weeks, gentle passive range of motion is allowed to the knee if the desired range of motion has not been reached. Continue active and passive range-of-motion exercises to the ankle and hip.

Muscle Strength

Continue isometric exercises to the quadriceps and start isometric exercises to the hamstrings. Continue ankle isotonics to maintain the strength of the muscles around the ankle.

Functional Activities

Continue non–weight-bearing transfers.

Gait

The patient continues a two-point non–weight-bearing gait using crutches (*see* Figure 6-16).

Methods of Treatment: Specific Aspects

Hinged Orthosis

Evaluate the orthosis for adequate, snug fit with the knee in all positions. Adjust the orthosis to accommodate any increased range of motion.

Open Reduction and Internal Fixation

If the patient is in a hinged orthosis following surgery, remove it and evaluate the wound for any signs of infection. Replace the hinged orthosis and check the fit.

External Fixation

Check the wound and pin sites for any sign of infection. Unless the patient has a significant infection or soft tissue compromise, the fixator should be removed and a definitive procedure performed or a hinged orthosis placed. The longer the patient is in the external fixator, the greater the chance of infection. If the fixator crosses the knee, the less the chance of regaining functional knee range of motion. The goal is 0 degrees to 90 degrees of active knee flexion. Patients who are unable to achieve this range of motion require aggressive physical therapy. Hydrotherapy alleviates discomfort while exercising.

Prescription

Rx

Four to Six Weeks

Precautions No varus or valgus stress on knee; no passive range of motion.

Range of Motion Active and active-assistive range of motion to the knee.

Strength No strengthening exercises to the knee.

Functional Activities Non–weight-bearing transfers and ambulation with crutches.

Weight Bearing No weight bearing on affected extremity.

Treatment: Eight to Twelve Weeks

BONE HEALING

Stability at fracture site: Stable.

Stage of bone healing: Early remodeling phase. Woven bone is being replaced with lamellar bone. The process of remodeling takes months to years for completion.

X-ray: Abundant callus in fractures not rigidly fixed by plates. Fracture line begins to disappear; with time, the medullary canal will be reconstituted.

Orthopaedic and Rehabilitation Considerations

Physical Examination

Check any wounds for erythema or discharge, indicating a possible infection that may require antibiotic therapy or surgical dèbridement.

Pay attention to complaints of pain, paresthesia, or symptoms of knee instability. Check capillary refill and sensation. Check the passive and active range of motion of the knee; flexion should be at least 90 degrees.

Dangers

Fracture displacement and loss of fixation are still possible, although less likely than before.

Radiography

Check radiographs for any displacement or loss of correction. Look for callus and the disappearance of the fracture line.

Weight Bearing

If the callus is adequate and the fracture appears stable and if there is no collateral ligament tenderness or instability, the patient may begin partial weight bearing on crutches. This can progress as tolerated after physical examination and subsequent radiographs show maintenance of the fracture position.

Range of Motion

The patient should have full extension and at least 90 degrees of flexion. If not, aggressive range-of-motion exercises should be instructed, including active-assistive and passive range of motion.

Muscle Strength

Gentle resistive exercises are prescribed to the quadriceps, hamstrings, and ankle musculature. Initially, few repetitions are performed; the number of repetitions is increased gradually. At the end of 12 weeks, the patient can perform progressive resistive exercises if the callus is strong.

Functional Activities

If the callus is adequate, weight-bearing activities are started toward the end of 12 weeks. The patient may still need to use crutches or a walker for transfers and ambulation.

Gait

Once weight bearing resumes, the patient ambulates with a regular gait pattern. As motion and weight bearing progress, pain decreases and assistive devices are discarded.

Methods of Treatment: Specific Aspects

Hinged Orthosis

If there is no evidence of varus, valgus, anterior, or posterior instability and an adequate callus is present, the orthosis can be discontinued. Depending on the patient's reliability and need for support, he or she may require splinting in a removable knee immobilizer or locked hinged orthosis only while ambulating. This maintains varus/valgus stability while the soft tissue injuries continue to heal. If instability or collateral ligament tenderness is present, the orthosis should be continued for another 2 to 4 weeks and the patient kept non-weight bearing.

Open Reduction and Internal Fixation

If there is no evidence of varus, valgus, anterior, or posterior instability and there is adequate callus or dissolution of the fracture line, the orthosis can be discontinued. Depending on the patient's reliability and need for support, he or she may require splinting in a removable knee immobilizer or locked fracture brace only while ambulating. This maintains varus/valgus stability while the soft tissue injuries continue to heal. If instability or collateral ligament tenderness is present, the orthosis should be continued for another 2 to 4 weeks and the patient kept non-weight bearing.

External Fixator

Once the patient's definitive procedure is performed—either placement of a hinged orthosis or open reduction and internal fixation—follow the appropriate protocol as outlined. Always check the wound and pin sites for any evidence of infection.

Prescription

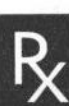

EIGHT TO TWELVE WEEKS

Precautions No varus or valgus stress.

Range of Motion Active, active-assistive, and passive range of motion to the knee.

Strength Gentle resistive exercises to the quadriceps and hamstrings.

Functional Activities Weight-bearing transfers and ambulation at the end of 12 weeks.

Weight Bearing Partial to full weight bearing at the end of 12 weeks.

Treatment: Twelve to Sixteen Weeks

BONE HEALING

Stability at fracture site: Stable.

Stage of bone healing: Remodeling phase. Lamellar bone replaces woven bone. The process of remodeling will take months to years for completion.

X-ray: Fracture line has disappeared.

Orthopaedic and Rehabilitation Considerations

Physical Examination

Check any wounds for erythema or discharge, indicating a possible infection that may require surgical débridement or antibiotic therapy. Check the passive and active range of motion of the knee; flexion should be at least 90 degrees.

Dangers

At this point, stiffness is the greatest danger. Aggressive therapy should have already been instituted to combat it.

Radiography

Check radiographs for any loss of correction or displacement of the fracture. Look for callus and the disappearance of the fracture line.

Weight Bearing

The patient is fully weight bearing and should be weaned off assistive devices.

Range of Motion

The patient should have full extension and at least 90 degrees of flexion.

Strength

Continue to increase the patient's muscle strength. Patients may be encouraged to use exercise machines to improve the strength in the quadriceps and hamstrings. Resistive exercises are increased progressively.

Functional Activities

The patient is weaned off assistive devices.

Gait

It is important to work on normalizing the gait pattern, with special emphasis on the stance phase.

Methods of Treatment: Specific Aspects

Hinged Orthosis

If the knee is stable and an adequate callus is present, the patient should bear weight as tolerated, initially locking the hinged orthosis but progressing from 0 degrees to 90 degrees of flexion (in the orthosis) as tolerated.

Open Reduction and Internal Fixation

If the knee is stable and an adequate callus is present or the fracture line has disappeared, the patient should bear weight as tolerated, initially locking the hinged orthosis but progressing to 0 degree to 90 degrees of flexion (in the orthosis) as tolerated.

External Fixation

Once the patient's definitive procedure is performed—either placement of a hinged orthosis or open reduction and internal fixation—follow the appropriate protocol as outlined earlier.

Prescription

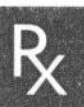

TWELVE TO SIXTEEN WEEKS

Precaution None.

Range of Motion Full active and passive range of motion to the knee.

Strength Progressive resistive exercises to the knee.

Functional Activities Full weight-bearing transfers and ambulation.

Weight Bearing Full weight bearing.

LONG-TERM CONSIDERATIONS AND PROBLEMS

At every stage of treatment, radiographs should be checked for loss of correction or displacement of the fracture, defined as any marked displacement or depression greater than 4 mm. If this occurs early in treatment (before any operative procedure), open reduction and internal fixation should be performed. If it occurs after an operative procedure, the operation should be revised.

Throughout treatment, the patient must be encouraged to attain active and passive knee range of motion of at least 0 degrees to 90 degrees. Aggressive physical therapy may be necessary to achieve the proper range of motion. Even so, the patient must be warned of possible future stiffness, as well as the risk for future degenerative disease associated with any articular injury.

IMMEDIATE TO ONE WEEK

	Cast Brace	*Open Reduction and Internal Fixation*	*External Fixation*
Stability	None.	None.	None.
Orthopaedics	Trim cast back to the metatarsophalangeal (MTP) joints to allow dorsi and plantar flexion of the toes. Elevate the lower extremity to decrease swelling.	Perform wound care over incisions and in any open wounds. Patient may be in cast brace after procedure, so treat as per instructions to left.	Evaluate pin sites and any open wounds that require wound management.
Rehabilitation	Active and gentle passive flexion/extension of the knee to 40° to 60° of flexion is allowed while protecting the knee from valgus and varus stress. No strengthening exercises are prescribed. Hip and ankle active and passive range of motion is allowed.	Same as for cast brace.	If fixator is "hybrid," then treat as per instruction for cast brace. If fixator crosses the knee, then no motion is allowed.

TWO WEEKS

	Cast Brace	*Open Reduction and Internal Fixation*	*External Fixation*
Stability	None to minimal.	None to minimal.	None to minimal.
Orthopaedics	Trim cast back and, continue elevation when necessary to decrease swelling.	Remove any sutures and continue wound care to any open wounds. If the patient is in cast brace, treat as per instructions for cast.	Evaluate pin sites and any open wounds which require wound management.
Rehabilitation	Active and gentle passive flexion/extension of the knee to at least 90° of flexion is allowed. No strengthening exercises are prescribed. Hip and ankle active and passive range of motion is continued.	Same as for cast brace.	If fixator is "hybrid," then treat as per instructions for cast brace. If fixator crosses the knee, then no motion is allowed.

FOUR TO SIX WEEKS

	Cast Brace	*Open Reduction and Internal Fixation*	*External Fixation*
Stability	Partially stable.	Partially stable.	Partially stable.
Orthopaedics	Trim and repair cast as needed. Adjust brace to allow increased range of motion	Evaluate wounds for any signs of infection. If in cast brace, treat as per instructions for cast brace.	Evaluate wound and pin sites for any signs of infection The fixator is usually removed by this stage and a definitive procedure is performed as a cast brace is applied.
Rehabilitation	Active and passive range of motion to at least 90° of knee flexion is allowed. No knee strengthening exercises are allowed. Continue with hip and ankle active and passive range of motion.	Same as for cast brace.	Same as for cast brace.

EIGHT TO TWELVE WEEKS

	Cast Brace	Open Reduction and Internal Fixation	External Fixation
Stability	Stable.	Stable.	Stable.
Orthopaedics	If adequate callus is formed and there is no instability, discontinue brace. Patient may require removable knee immobilizer or locked hinged orthosis only while ambulating.	Same as for cast brace.	Same as for cast brace.
Rehabilitation	Active, active-assistive and passive flexion/extension of the knee to at least 90° of flexion is allowed. Gentle resistive exercises are prescribed for the quadriceps, hamstrings, hip, and ankle musculature. Weight-bearing activities are started around the 12th week, usually with assistive devices.	Same as for cast brace.	Same as for cast brace.

TWELVE TO SIXTEEN WEEKS

	Cast Brace	Open Reduction and Internal Fixation	External Fixation
Stability	Stable.	Stable.	Stable.
Orthopaedics	The patient is usually weight bearing as tolerated, initially locking the hinged orthosis but progressing to 0° to 90° of flexion in the orthosis	Same as for cast brace.	Same as for cast brace.
Rehabilitation	Full active, active-assisted, and passive range of motion of the knee is allowed. Progressive resistive exercises are prescribed to the hip, knee, and ankle musculature. The patient is progressed to full weight bearing as tolerated.	Same as for cast brace.	Same as for cast brace.

BIBLIOGRAPHY

Apley AG. Fractures of the tibial plateau. *Orthop Clin North Am,* 10:61–74, 1979.

Blokker C, Roroabeck C, Bourne R. Tibial plateau fractures; an analysis of the results of treatment in 60 patients. *Clin Orthop,* 182:193–199, 1984.

Burri C, Bartzke G, Coldewey J, Muggler E. Fractures of the tibial plateau. *Clin Orthop,* 138:84–93, 1979.

Duwelius PJ, Connelly JF. Closed reduction of tibial plateau fractures: a comparison of functional and roentgenographic end results. *Clin Orthop,* 230:116–126, 1988.

Hohl M. Fractures of the proximal tibia and fibula. In: Rockwood CA Jr, Green DP, Bucholz RW, eds. *Fractures in*

Adults, Vol. 2, 3rd ed. Philadelphia: JB Lippincott, 1991, pp. 1725–1752.

Koval KJ, Helfet DL. Tibial plateau fractures: evaluation and treatment. *J Am Acad Orthop Surg,* 3:86–94, 1995.

Lachiewicz P, Funcik T. Factors influencing the results of open reduction and internal fixation of tibial plateau fractures. *Clin Orthop,* 259:210–215, 1990.

Moore T, Patzakis M, Harvey P. Tibial plateau fractures: definition, demographics, treatment rationale, and long-term results of closed traction management or operative reduction. *J Orthop Trauma,* 1: 97–119, 1997.

Schatzker J. Tibial plateau fractures. In: Browner BD, Jupiter JB, Levine AM, Trafton PG, eds. *Skeletal Trauma,* Vol. 2. Philadelphia: WB Saunders, 1992, 1745–1769.

Schatzker J, McBrown R, Bruce D. The tibial plateau fracture: the Toronto experience. *Clin Orthop,* 138:94–104, 1979.

Waddell J, Johnston D, Neidre A. Fractures of the tibial plateau: a review of 95 patients and comparison of treatment methods. *J Trauma,* 21:376–381, 1981.

CHAPTER *Twenty-eight*

Tibial Shaft Fractures

KENNETH W. TAYLOR, MD

VASANTHA L. MURTHY, MD

CONTRIBUTIONS BY STANLEY HOPPENFELD, MD

INTRODUCTION

Definition

A tibial shaft fracture is a diaphyseal fracture of the tibia that does not usually involve the articular or metaphyseal regions (Figures 28-1 and 28-2).

Mechanism of Injury

High-energy trauma from direct impact may result in transverse or comminuted fractures, which are often open. Low-energy indirect trauma from a twisting injury on a planted foot or a fall from a low height may cause a spiral or oblique fracture pattern.

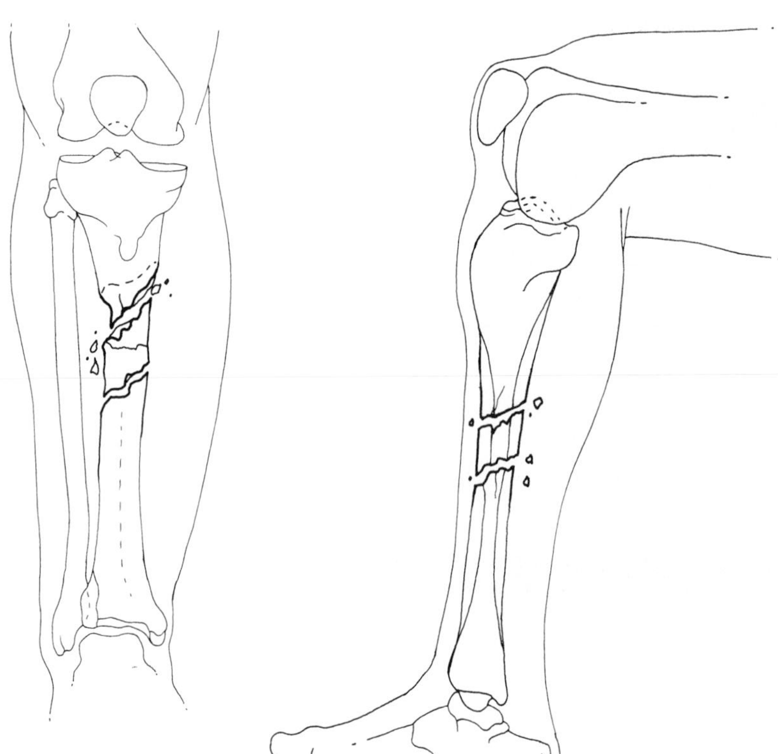

FIGURE 28-1 *(far left)* Segmental fracture of the tibial shaft.

FIGURE 28-2 *(left)* Segmental fracture of the tibial shaft without displacement (lateral view). The metaphyseal or articular regions are not involved.

Treatment Goals

Orthopaedic Objectives

Alignment

Restore length, angulation, and rotation and compare to the uninjured limb. Rotation may be best evaluated by comparison of the position of the second web space with the tibial tubercle.

Stability

Stability is best achieved by performing a reduction that restores bone congruity.

Rehabilitation Objectives

Range of Motion

Restore or maintain range of motion to the knee and ankle (Table 28-1).

TABLE 28-1 *Range of Motion of the Knee and Ankle*

Movement	Normal	Functional
Knee		
Flexion	0°–130°/140°	110°
Extension	0°	0°
Ankle		
Dorsiflexion	0°–25°	10°
Plantar flexion	0°–40°	20°

Muscle Strength

Improve the strength of the following muscles, which are affected as a result of the fracture and injury:

Dorsiflexors:
- Tibialis anterior
- Extensor hallucis longus
- Extensor digitorum longus

Plantar flexors:
- Gastrocnemius
- Soleus
- Flexor digitorum
- Flexor hallucis longus

Inverters:
- Tibialis posterior
- Tibialis anterior

Everters:
- Peroneus longus and brevis

Functional Goals

Normalize the gait pattern.

Expected Time of Bone Healing

Ten to 12 weeks.

Expected Duration of Rehabilitation

Twelve to 24 weeks.

Methods of Treatment

Cast

Biomechanics: Stress-sharing device.

Mode of Bone Healing: Secondary.

Indications: Long leg cast treatment is satisfactory for tibial shaft fractures with minimal comminution that are stable and acceptably aligned once immobilized. Relative criteria for stability include displacement less than 50% of the tibial width and shortening less than 1 cm. Alignment should restore rotation and angulation in all planes to within 5 degrees to 10 degrees of the uninjured tibia (Figures 28-3 and 28-4).

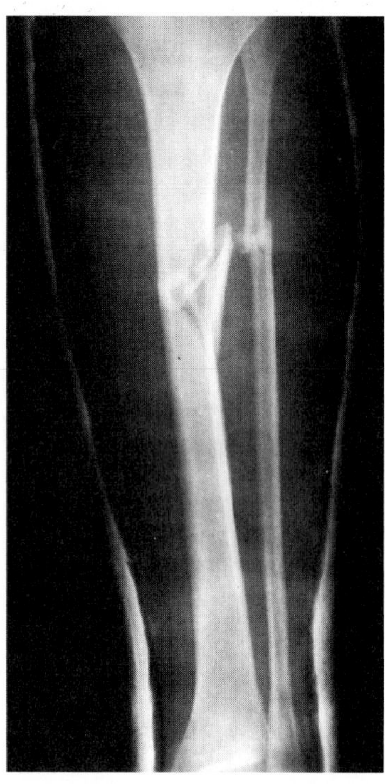

FIGURE 28-3 Fracture of the tibial shaft and fibula treated in a long leg cast. There is no displacement or angulation of the fracture site.

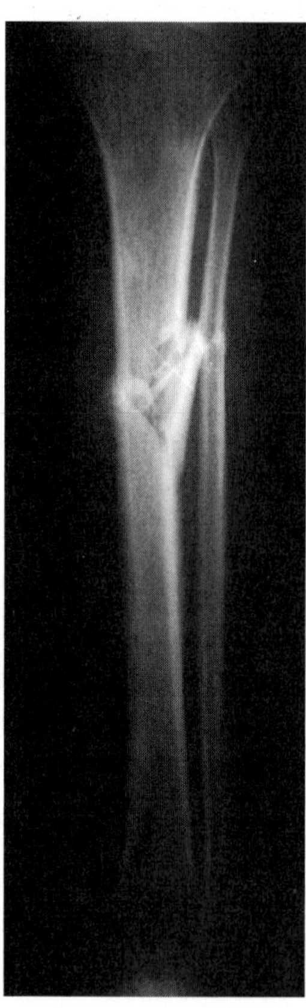

FIGURE 28-4 Healed fracture of the tibia and fibula 3 months after casting (anteroposterior view). The fracture site is stable; note the callus formation.

Intramedullary Rod

Biomechanics: The intramedullary rod is a stress-sharing device if the nail is dynamically interlocked; it is a partial stress-shielding device if the nail is statically interlocked.

Mode of Bone Healing: Secondary.

Indications: This treatment is the gold standard for unstable and segmental tibial fractures or those that cannot be adequately aligned and immobilized by non-operative means. The intramedullary rod allows for early mobilization of the patient as well as early knee range of motion. Placing interlocking screws proximal and distal to the fracture site is necessary in fractures with unstable butterfly fragments or severe comminution. This creates static fixation and prevents shortening and loss of rotatory alignment. Transverse fractures and those with minimal comminution may be left unlocked at one end. This creates dynamic fixation and allows interfragmentary compression with weight bearing, which in turn stimulates healing (Figures 28-5, 28-6, 28-7, 28-8, 28-9, 28-10, 28-11, 28-12).

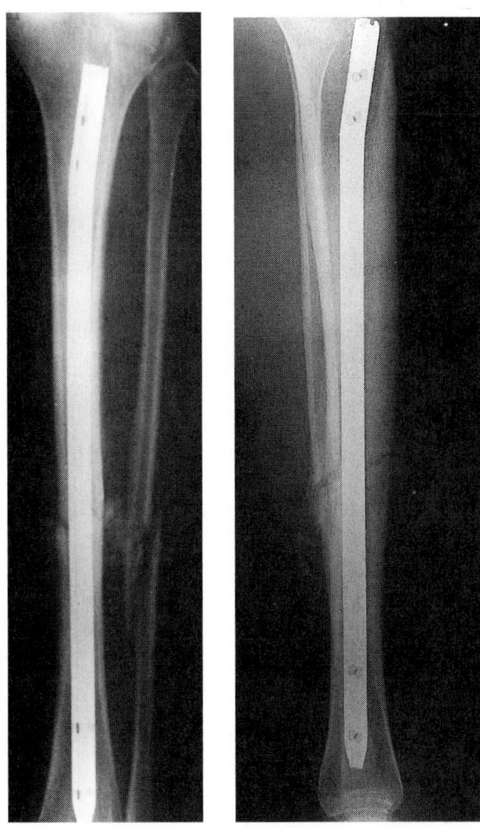

FIGURE 28-5 *(above, left)* Intramedullary rod fixation (unlocked) for a tibial shaft fracture. Note the callus formation.

FIGURE 28-6 *(above, right)* Intramedullary rod fixation of a transverse tibial fracture using a reamed unlocked nail. Note the tight fit of the rod against the tibial cortex (lateral view).

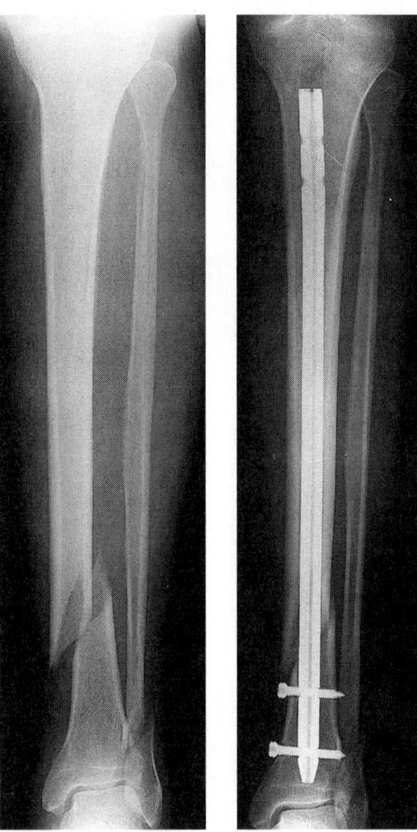

FIGURE 28-7 *(above, left)* Fracture of the distal tibial shaft and fibula.

FIGURE 28-8 *(above, right)* Fracture of the distal tibia and fibula treated with a reamed intramedullary rod and distal dynamic locking. The proximal end is well fixed by the rod, and the distal end is secured with the locking screws. This allows interfragmentary compression with weight bearing.

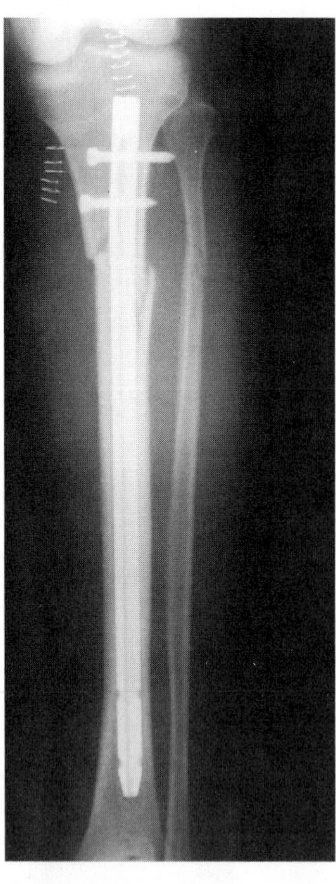

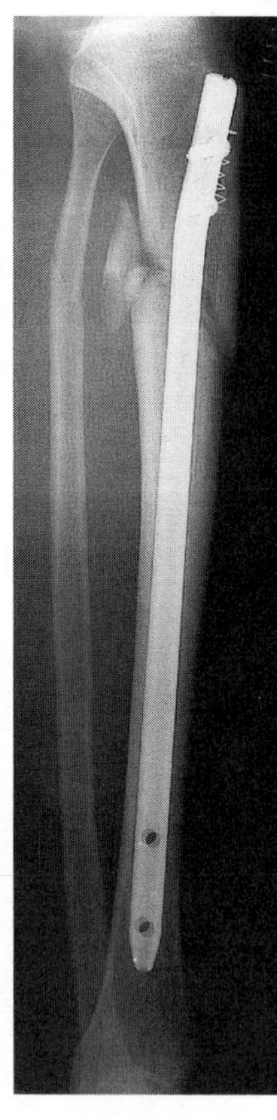

FIGURE 28-9 *(far left)* Fracture of the proximal end of the tibial shaft and fibula treated with a reamed intramedullary rod locked proximally. The distal fragment is well controlled by the tight fit of the rod against the tibial cortex.

FIGURE 28-10 *(left)* Fractured tibial shaft, proximal end, treated with a reamed intramedullary rod locked proximally (lateral view). Leaving the fracture unlocked at one end creates dynamic fixation and allows compression at the fracture site with weight bearing.

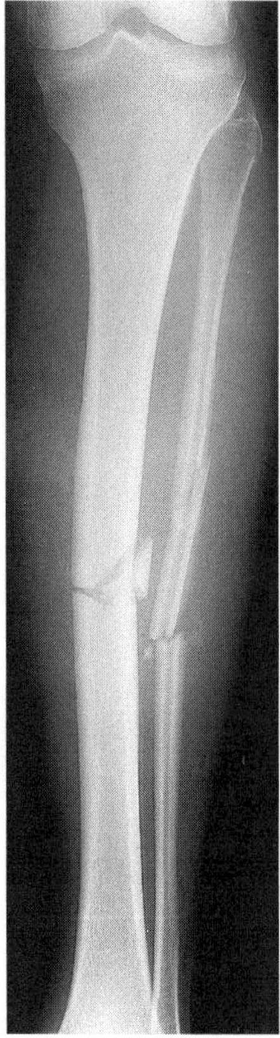

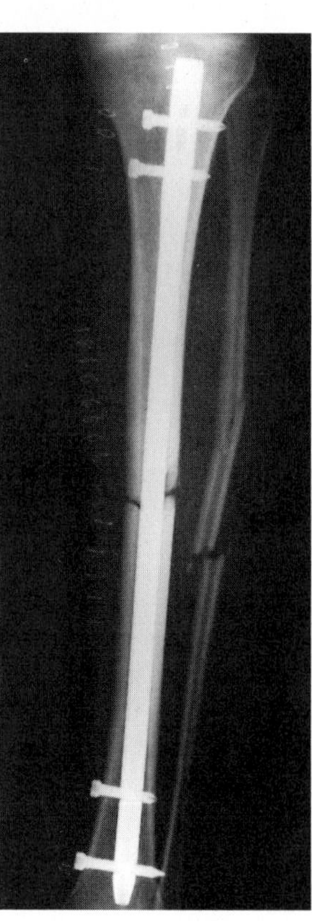

FIGURE 28-11 *(far left)* Midshaft fracture of the tibia and fibula following an automobile accident.

FIGURE 28-12 *(left)* Midshaft tibia and fibula fracture treated with an intramedullary rod fixed proximally and distally with interlocking screws. This creates static fixation and prevents shortening and loss of rotatory alignment.

External Fixator

Biomechanics: Stress-sharing device.

Mode of Bone Healing: Secondary.

Indications: This method is often used in open fractures with significant bone loss and comminution as well as contamination. In these instances, it is used in conjunction with intraoperative débridement and pulsatile irrigation. This form of treatment should be considered provisional until soft tissue coverage is achieved by skin grafting. Intramedullary rodding usually follows as the definitive form of treatment (Figures 28-13, 28-14, and 28-15).

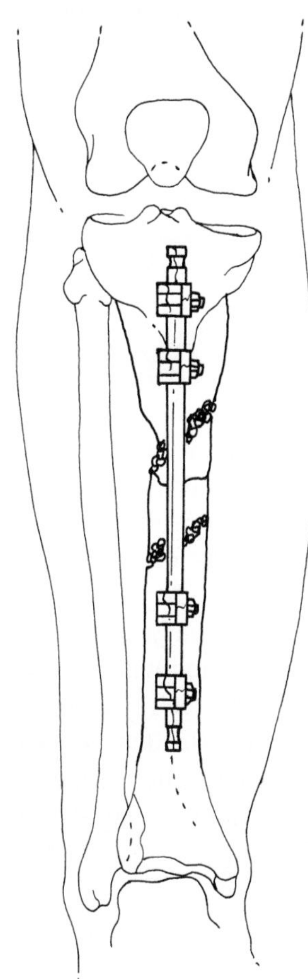

FIGURE 28-13 Segmental fracture of the tibia treated with an external fixator. This is a stress-sharing device.

Open Reduction and Internal Fixation with Plates

Biomechanics: Stress-shielding device.

Mode of Bone Healing: Primary.

Indications: This method of fixation requires violation of soft tissues for fixation as well as significant periosteal stripping. For these reasons, open reduction and internal fixation has limited application in tibial shaft fractures; it is occasionally performed for nonunion of the tibia in conjunction with bone grafting. This treatment is not discussed further in this section.

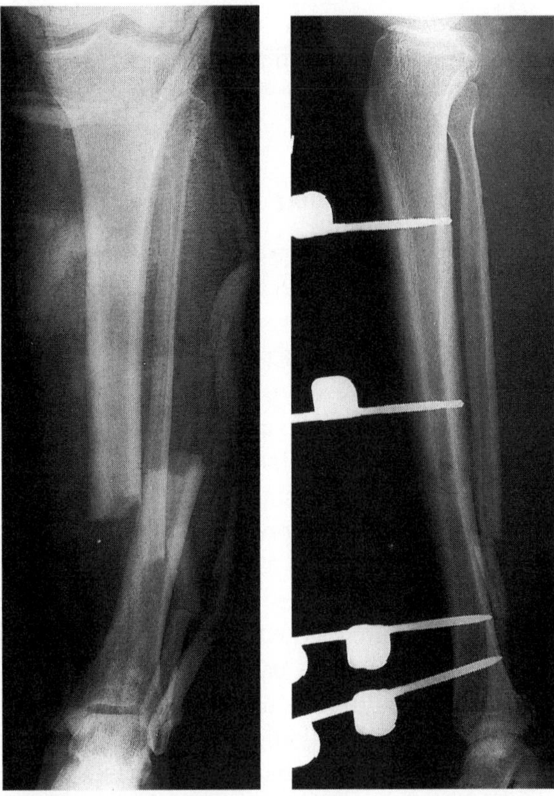

FIGURE 28-14 *(above, left)* Fracture of the shaft of the tibia and fibula with displacement, shortening, and angulation. There is associated soft tissue loss and major wound contamination.

FIGURE 28-15 *(above, right)* Fracture of the shaft of the tibia and fibula treated with an external fixator. This fixation allows maintenance of reduction and access for soft tissue coverage and wound débridement.

Special Considerations of the Fracture

The rate of bone healing in tibial fractures depends on the fracture pattern and the extent of soft tissue injuries. The major blood supply to the tibial shaft is a branch of the posterior tibial artery, which enters posterolaterally. Closed injuries with stable fracture patterns are able to bear weight and heal the most rapidly. Spiral fractures do less damage to the periosteum, which distributes the blood supply, than do higher-energy bending fractures that tear the periosteum transversely. Therefore, the spiral fracture heals much more readily. Open fractures have significantly more soft tissue damage and often require much more time for healing. In cases of nonunion or delayed union, this fracture and those with severe comminution may require bone grafting to stimulate bone healing.

Associated Injury

Compartment Syndrome

Compartment syndrome can result when soft tissue swelling and bleeding into a closed compartment lead to pressures that exceed venous and later arterial circulation. These occur most commonly in the anterior compartments where the tibia, fibula, and interosseous membrane form an unyielding space. Normal resting intracompartmental pressure is 0 to 8 millimeters of mercury. Compartmental pressure of 30 mm of pressure or greater requires immediate decompression.

Compartment syndrome is diagnosed by symptoms. (The patient is often casted, which makes a physical examination difficult.) A patient who has or in whom compartment syndrome is developing can be expected to have pain out of proportion to the injury and symptoms of increasing numbness and paresthesia, even after the cast or bandage has been removed. Exquisite pain with passive toe extension of the metatarsophalangeal joint is an important sign. If compartment syndrome is suspected, compartment pressure should be measured immediately. If the diagnosis is made, the patient should undergo a fasciotomy.

Embolism

Because of the risk of fat or pulmonary emboli, a baseline arterial blood gas measurement should be considered in every patient and definitely done in those with multiple injuries.

Fat emboli syndrome may occur in the acute phase within the first 72 hours after fracture. It causes sudden respiratory distress and hypoxia. Petechiae in the conjunctiva and axilla as well as tachypnea and tachycardia are the signs of this condition.

Pulmonary embolism may occur after 72 hours of bed rest or venous pooling. Its symptoms are similar to those of fat emboli, except there is no petechiae. Early mobilization by operative fracture fixation helps reduce the risk of this condition.

Soft Tissue Injury

Soft tissue injury associated with tibial shaft fractures is common because the anteromedial tibia is subcutaneous. The skin must be examined thoroughly for signs of contusion or compounding of the fracture. These wounds must be examined for surrounding erythema or fluctuance. They require meticulous cleaning and frequent dressing changes to prevent infection. If the fracture has been treated operatively, the operative wound should be evaluated. Edema distal to the fracture site and in the toes must also be evaluated and treated with elevation of the extremity (see Chapter 9).

Weight Bearing

The potential for weight bearing varies with the fracture pattern as well as the method of fixation. Patients with fractures with a stable pattern that are treated either by casting or with dynamically or statically locked intramedullary nails are often able to begin weight bearing early, as soon as pain permits. Unstable fractures treated with external fixators, statically locked nails, or open reduction and internal fixation usually require extended periods of non-weight bearing or toe-touch weight bearing, depending on the comminution. This limited weight bearing should continue for the first 6 to 8 weeks until a callus is seen radiographically.

Gait

Stance Phase

The stance phase is 60% of the gait cycle.

Heel Strike

The dorsiflexors, tibialis anterior, and extensor hallucis longus contract to hold the foot up in the neutral position upon heel strike (concentric contraction). Occasionally, the fracture or cast treatment may reduce range of motion of the ankle. In this case, the ankle must be stretched to attain a neutral position. The heel acts as a shock absorber because some stress from the impact is also taken in the tibia. The response to the load may be pain at the fracture site. This should decrease with healing (Figure 28-16 and *see* Figure 6-1).

Foot-Flat

The dorsiflexors go through eccentric contraction and elongate to allow smooth transition from heel strike to foot-flat and to prevent foot slap. The patient may experience pain as these muscles eccentrically contract and stretch after injury (*see* Figure 6-2).

Mid-Stance

This phase represents single-limb support because the full weight of the body is borne on the tibial shaft. This too can be painful, resulting in an antalgic gait. Patients may have an early heel rise to reduce the duration of the mid-stance phase in order to avoid pain (Figure 28-17 and *see* Figure 6-3).

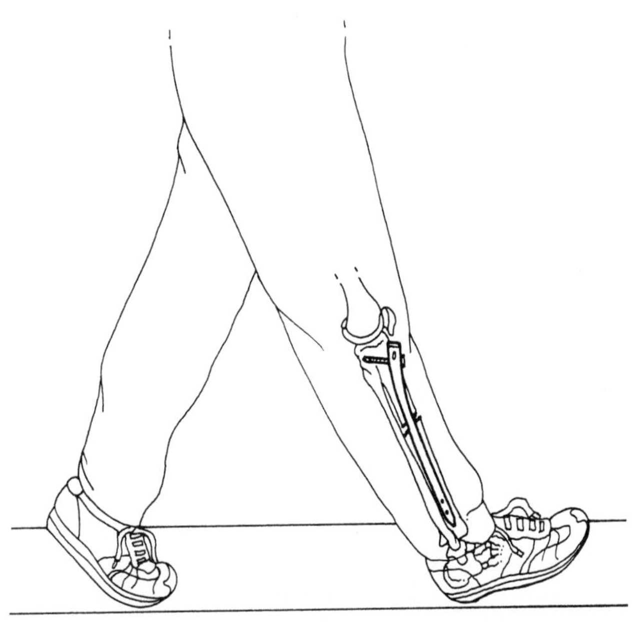

FIGURE 28-16 Transverse fracture of the tibial shaft treated with an intramedullary rod. At heel strike, the tibia absorbs the impact and the response to the load is pain at the fracture site.

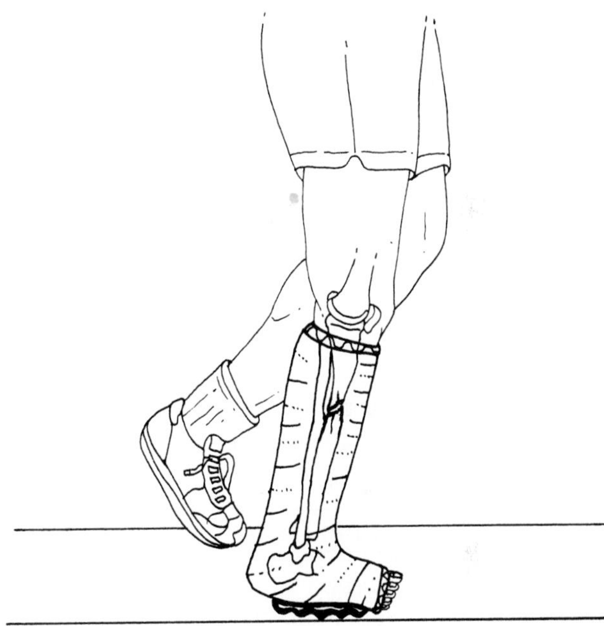

FIGURE 28-17 Transverse tibial fracture originally treated in a long leg cast, now in a short leg cast. At mid-stance, the full weight of the body is borne on the tibial shaft. This can be painful, causing an antalgic gait.

Push-Off

At this phase, the foot is getting ready to leave the ground and propel forward into the swing phase. The gastroc-soleus muscle group has to contract strongly for the forward propulsion. The patient may experience pain at the fracture site secondary to the strong contraction of the soleus (*see* Figures 6-4 and 6-5).

Swing Phase

The swing phase is 40% of the gait cycle.

Acceleration

Knee motion must be regained through stretching exercises. During the swing phase, the quadriceps must be able to extend the knee and to assist in acceleration.

Ankle dorsiflexion must be sufficient to allow the foot to clear the floor during the swing phase (*see* Figure 6-6). Hip flexion must be maintained to allow the leg to clear the ground during any form of tibial shaft fracture treatment because there may be reflex inhibition of the psoas muscle.

TREATMENT

Treatment: Early to Immediate (Day of Injury to One Week)

BONE HEALING

Stability at fracture site: None.

Stage of bone healing: Inflammatory phase. The fracture hematoma is colonized by inflammatory cells, and débridement of the fracture begins.

X-ray: No callus.

Orthopaedic and Rehabilitation Considerations

Physical Examination

Carefully evaluate for points of pressure or tightness underneath the cast or bandage. If present, reevaluate the patient for alleviation of his or her symptoms of discomfort and decreased sensation after the cast or bandage has been loosened or removed. Check for capillary refill and edema and elevate the affected limb as necessary. There should not be excessive pain with passive extension of the metatarsophalangeal joints, which is an early sign of anterior compartment syndrome. Evaluate and compare the physical examination of the affected limb with that examination done before the operative treatment or casting.

Alignment of the limb must be evaluated clinically by comparison with the normal leg. In addition, the anterior-superior iliac spine, midline of the patella, tibial tubercle, and second toe should be in the same physiologic alignment as the unaffected extremity.

Dangers

Avoid compressive neuropathy by placing generous padding at the head of the fibula where the peroneal nerve wraps around the fibular neck before casting. In addition, compartment syndrome is always a danger in tibial shaft fractures.

Radiography

Examine anteroposterior and lateral radiographs, which must include both knee and ankle joints. Radiographs should always be compared with those of the original injury and with the most recent prior films. The radiographic image should demonstrate no more than 5 degrees of varus or valgus angulation and no more than 10 degrees of anterior or posterior angulation. Rotation of up to 5 degrees is acceptable, as is a leg-length discrepancy of up to 1 cm. There should be no distraction of the fracture present on the radiograph, and cortical contact should be a minimum of 50%. In addition to evaluating the fracture alignment, look for changes in the position of any hardware used for fixation (e.g., interlocking screws, intramedullary rods, Shanz pins, or external fixators).

Weight Bearing

1. Cast. Fractures treated by closed casting methods should be of sufficient stability to allow early partial weight bearing. This may begin after soft tissue swelling subsides at the end of the first week.
2. Intramedullary Rod. If a statically locked nail has been used to treat an unstable fracture (comminution, bone loss) the patient should be allowed toe-

touch to partial weight bearing with crutches or a walker. Full weight bearing must be avoided (*see* Figure 28-12).

3. A patient with a stable fracture (good cortical contact) that was treated with a dynamically locked or statically locked nail may immediately be weight bearing as tolerated with crutches or a walker (*see* Figure 28-10).
4. External Fixator. Patients in external fixators should initially be non-weight bearing. If soft tissue swelling and wound care allow, and if there is good cortical contact, the patient may be toe-touch weight bearing with crutches or a walker and a three-point gait. This form of treatment is not designed for full weight bearing (*see* Figure 28-15).

Range of Motion

Once the initial pain subsides, the patient can actively range the knee, in flexion and extension, and range the ankle and foot, in all planes as tolerated.

Muscle Strength

Isometric exercises to the quadriceps are instructed. Initially the patient may experience pain in the whole extremity secondary to the injury. Once the pain subsides, the patient should be able to perform the exercises. Ankle isotonic exercises are prescribed to tolerance.

Functional Activities

The patient is taught to use crutches or a walker for transfer from bed to chair and vice versa. A non–weight-bearing patient should be instructed in stand/pivot transfers.

The patient dons the pants with the involved extremity first and doffs them with the uninvolved extremity first.

Gait

Depending on weight-bearing status, a two-point or three-point gait is taught with crutches or a walker. If non-weight bearing, the patient is taught stand/pivot transfers and a two-point gait, in which the crutches and affected extremity act as one unit and the unaffected extremity as the other unit. Weight is borne on the crutches (*see* Figures 6-16 and 6-17).

When ascending stairs, the patient leads with the unaffected extremity; when descending stairs, the patient leads with the affected extremity (*see* Figures 6-20, 6-21, 6-22, 6-23, 6-24, and 6-25).

Patients should be carefully supervised for ambulatory stability and safety. Stair walking may be delayed until a patient's pain level is reduced.

Methods of Treatment: Specific Aspects

Cast

Check the cast fitting, including padding and edges. Beware of skin breakdown at the margins of the cast and painful pressure points that may need windowing to check skin integrity. The cast should be examined for any softening and wear caused by weight bearing or moisture. The cast should be trimmed as necessary to ensure that the toes are exposed and the skin is protected at the cast margins. Fractures treated in casts should be radiographically examined for maintenance of the molding and tightness of the cast as soft tissue swelling subsides.

As the knee and ankle are immobilized in a long leg cast, the patient is instructed in quadriceps and ankle isometric exercises as tolerated once the pain subsides (i.e., trying to extend the knee and dorsiflex and plantar-flex the ankle inside the cast).

Intramedullary Rod

The leg should be elevated and care taken to be sure that the patient is able to range the ankle past the neutral position in dorsiflexion and plantar flexion. The knee and ankle are free, so their active range is encouraged. Full range of the ankle should be possible.

External Fixator

Examine all pin sites for discharge, erythema, purulence, exudate, or any sign of infection. Instruct the patient on appropriate pin care and signs of infection. Evaluate the stability of the fixator and tighten any loose screws or pins as necessary. Evaluate the maintenance of the fracture position with radiographs. As the knee joint and ankle joint are free, active range of motion is instituted.

Prescription

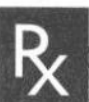

DAY ONE TO ONE WEEK

Precautions Avoid rotary motion with the foot on the floor.

Range of Motion Active range of motion to ankle and knee if not in a cast.

Strength Isometric exercises to quadriceps, tibialis anterior, and gastroc-soleus.

Functional Activities Stand/pivot transfers and non–weight-bearing ambulation with assistive devices for unstable fractures.

Weight bearing as tolerated to partial weight bearing transfers with assistive devices for stable fractures.

Weight Bearing Weight bearing as tolerated for stable fracture patterns (restoration of cortical contact, no comminution, no segmental bone loss).

No weight bearing to toe-touch for unstable fracture patterns (minimal cortical contact, comminution, segmental bone loss).

Treatment: Two Weeks

BONE HEALING

Stability at fracture site: None to minimal.

Stage of bone healing: Beginning of reparatory phase of fracture healing. Osteoprogenitor cells differentiate into osteoblasts, which lay down woven bone.

X-ray: No callus; fracture line is visible.

Orthopaedic and Rehabilitation Considerations

Physical Examination

Swelling and neurovascular function of the toes should be evaluated. Examine any areas of constant pressure or tightness underneath the cast or bandage. All wounds and surgical incisions should be examined and receive local wound care as needed. All joints that are not immobilized with an orthopaedic apparatus should be examined for active and passive range of motion. Active dorsiflexion of the ankle should be stressed to prevent an equinus deformity. Patients whose extremities demonstrate edema distal to the fracture site or in the toes should be told to keep the extremity elevated.

Dangers

Continue to watch for compressive neuropathy.

Radiography

Assess alignment and maintenance of correction and length. Any fracture treated by closed methods that demonstrates loss of alignment according to the guidelines outlined earlier should be either recasted in a well-molded cast or treated operatively.

Weight Bearing

1. Cast. Midshaft fractures of the tibia with sufficient stability for treatment in a long leg cast benefit from early partial weight bearing. Cyclical loading secondary to weight bearing has been shown to produce osteogenesis. Transverse fractures should be weight bearing as tolerated. Stable short oblique and spiral fractures may begin partial weight bearing. Weight bearing may progress as the stability at the fracture site increases with time.
2. Intramedullary Rod. Continue weight bearing as tolerated for stable fracture patterns (good cortical contact without comminution or segmental defect) treated with dynamically locked nails. Non–weight bearing to partial weight bearing is prescribed for unstable fracture patterns (comminution, poor cortical contact, segmental defects) treated with statically locked nails. Patients use crutches or a walker and a three-point gait (*see* Figure 6-17).
3. External Fixator. Continue non-weight bearing to toe-touch weight bearing using crutches or a walker and a three-point gait.

Range of Motion

The patient should not encounter any problems in actively ranging the hip. Active motion of the knee and ankle should be continued as allowed by the type of fixation. The swelling and pain should have decreased considerably at this point. The patient is instructed in writing the alphabet with the foot so that the ankle and foot are ranged in all planes.

Muscle Strength

Continue with isometric quadriceps exercises and with ankle isotonics and isometric exercises. The gastrocnemius muscle acts as a vascular pump, avoiding pooling of blood in the leg. This is important to prevent thrombophlebitis and deep vein thrombosis in the leg.

Functional Activities

Continue with stand/pivot transfers using crutches or a walker.

Gait

Continue with a two-point or three-point gait on level surfaces and stairs using assistive devices. The gait pattern depends on weight-bearing status (*see* Figure 6-16).

When ascending stairs, the patient leads with the unaffected extremity; when descending stairs, the patient leads with the affected extremity (*see* Figures 6-20, 6-21, 6-22, 6-23, 6-24, and 6-25).

Methods of Treatment: Specific Aspects

Cast

Check the cast fitting, including padding and cast margins. Beware of skin breakdown at the margins and painful areas of pressure inside the cast. Window any areas in question and examine the skin integrity. Examine the heel for softening and wear. Trim the cast to expose all toes and protect the skin. Continue with isometric strengthening exercises to the quadriceps and dorsiflexors and plantar flexors within the cast

Intramedullary Rod

Continue active motion of the hip, knee, and ankle. Continue strengthening exercises to the muscles in this region. Evaluate operative and wound sites for local care as needed. Sutures and staples may need to be removed at this time.

External Fixator

Check pin sites for discharge, purulence, or cellulitis. Check the stability of the fixator after tightening all pins and screws as necessary. Continue with full range of motion.

Prescription

TWO WEEKS

Precautions Avoid rotary movements with the foot planted.

Range of Motion Active range of motion to ankle and knee if not in a cast.

Strength Isometric exercises to quadriceps, tibialis anterior, and gastroc-soleus.

Functional Activities Stand/pivot transfers and non–weight-bearing ambulation with assistive devices for unstable fractures.

Weight bearing as tolerated or partial weight bearing with assistive devices, depending on the method of treatment.

Weight Bearing Weight bearing as tolerated for stable fracture patterns (restoration of cortical contact, no comminution, no segmental bone loss).

Non-weight bearing to toe-touch for unstable fracture patterns (comminution, bone loss, minimal cortical contact).

Treatment: Four to Six Weeks

BONE HEALING

Stability at fracture site: With advancing callus, the fracture becomes stable for axial loading but must still be protected from torsional loading.

Stage of bone healing: Reparative phase. Further organization of the callus and very early formation of lamellar bone begins. Callus is observed bridging the fracture site, and the fracture is usually stable. However, the strength of this callus, especially with torsional load, is significantly lower than that of normal bone. To avoid refracture, further protection of bone is required.

X-ray: Early callus may be visible in the posterolateral aspect of the tibia where blood supply is best. If the fracture is rigidly fixed, little callus is seen.

Orthopaedic and Rehabilitation Considerations

Physical Examination

Assess all wounds or pin sites and treat them appropriately. In those rare open fractures with severe bone loss, a significant leg-length discrepancy may be found. Leg-length inequality may also be encountered in comminuted fractures that are dynamically locked with a medullary nail. In these cases, prescribe a shoe lift to equalize the leg length, and consider bone grafting if the inequality is extensive.

Dangers

See previous section (page 372).

Radiography

Examine the anteroposterior and lateral interval radiographs to confirm fixation, rotation, and position hardware. Pay special attention to the entry point of any nail that is unlocked proximally to identify possible nail migration. In fractures being treated by closed methods, be sure the cast continues to maintain contact with the soft tissues as swelling decreases. Wedge the cast or change it to a new well-molded cast if increased angulation has occurred as a result of the cast loosening from atrophy and resolution of the soft tissue swelling.

Weight Bearing

1. Cast. Continue weight bearing as tolerated for transverse fractures. As the fracture callus becomes visible, advance short oblique fractures and spiral fractures from partial to full weight bearing.
2. Intramedullary Rod. Continue weight bearing as tolerated for dynamically locked rods and begin weight bearing as tolerated for rods that are dynamized. As weight bearing progresses, examine the unlocked end clinically for any evidence of rod migration. Non-weight bearing to partial weight bearing should be continued for rods that are statically locked. A patient with this treatment should continue to use crutches or a walker and a three-point gait (*see* Figure 6-17).
3. External Fixator. Continue non-weight bearing using crutches or a walker and a three-point gait until bony congruity has been reestablished, at which time partial weight bearing may begin.

Range of Motion

At this point, unless the patient is in a cast, he or she should have no discomfort while actively ranging the knee and ankle. Full range of motion should be maintained.

Muscle Strength

Continue isometric and isotonic exercises to the knee and ankle as appropriate.

Functional Activities

Patients who are not fully weight bearing at this stage may still need assistive devices for transfers and ambulation.

Gait

Continue with a two- or three-point gait (*see* Figures 6-16 and 6-17). Watch for structural limb shortening. If it is present, a shoe lift may be needed. Work on static balance and weight-shifting activities. Concentrate on gait training. Postural sway and the risk of falling decrease with strengthening and training. Depending on weight-bearing status, the patient may still need ambulatory assistive devices.

Methods of Treatment: Specific Aspects

Cast

Examine the cast fitting, including padding and margins. Beware of skin breakdown at the margins and any painful areas that may indicate pressure beneath the cast. Window these areas and examine skin integrity. Examine the heel for softening and wear. Trim cast margins as needed. Wedge or replace the cast as deemed necessary by interval radiographs. A long leg cast may be changed to a patella-tendon-bearing cast at this time to allow for knee range of motion. If the long leg cast is not removed, continue with isometric exercises to the quadriceps, hamstrings, gastrocnemius, and dorsiflexors of the foot. There should be no limitations on digit range of motion (Figure 28-18).

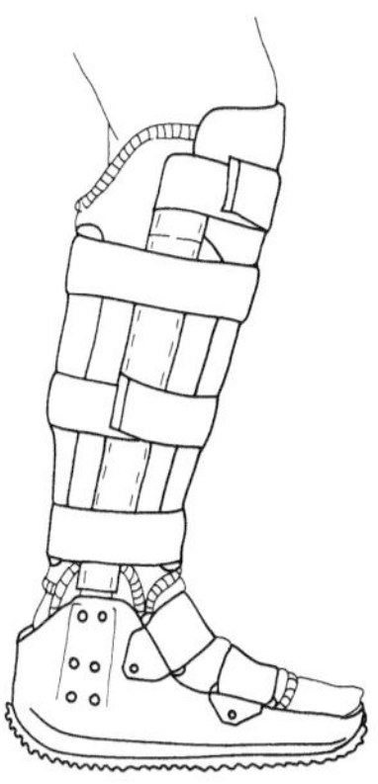

FIGURE 28-18 A long leg cast may be changed for a patellar tendon-bearing cast or patellar-tendon bearing tibia brace to allow knee range of motion.

Intramedullary Rod

Because of increased motion at the fracture site, fractures treated with rods that are not interlocked have more callus seen on radiographs than those treated with rods that are interlocked. Any fractures that are interlocked proximally and distally and still present with significant gaping at the fracture site should be considered for dynamization. Removal of an interlocking screw at either the proximal or distal end allows the fracture to collapse. This allows closer apposition of the fracture ends and promotes bone healing (*see* Figures 28-7 and 28-8).

Any open fracture that was initially treated with a narrow-diameter intramedullary rod and which exhibits instability at the fracture site should be considered for exchange nailing, with a larger diameter rod.

At this time, fractures with significant bone loss or a delayed healing process should be considered for bone grafting or bone marrow injection as an induction factor for promoting bone healing.

Continue with isotonic exercises to the knee and ankle. Eversion and inversion of the foot should also be continued, because these motions play a major role in normal gait. Drawing the alphabet with the foot is helpful for maintaining this range.

External Fixator

Examine all pin sites for discharge, erythema, or any sign of infection. Examine the frame and all pins and screws, and tighten if necessary. Pins with any evidence of infection may need to be replaced with larger pins or pins in a different site. Because the pins do not go through the joint, the patient should not have any stiffness when ranging the ankle.

Prescription

FOUR TO SIX WEEKS

Precautions Avoid rotation of the extremity on a fixed foot.

Range of Motion Active range of motion to knee and ankle if not in a cast.

Strength Isometric and isotonic exercises to knee and ankle.

Functional Activities Stand/pivot transfers and non–weight-bearing ambulation with assistive devices for unstable fractures.

Weight bearing as tolerated, to partial weight bearing, to full weight-bearing transfers and ambulation with assistive devices, depending on the method of treatment.

Weight Bearing Weight bearing as tolerated for stable fracture patterns (restoration of cortical contact, no comminution, no segmental bone loss).

Non-weight bearing to toe-touch for unstable fracture patterns (comminution, bone loss, minimal cortical contact).

Treatment: Eight to Twelve Weeks

BONE HEALING

Stability at fracture site: Fractures having minimal to no comminution are increasingly stable to completely stable. Fractures that have significant bone loss or have required bone grafting for bone loss have limited stability until the bone graft begins to consolidate and the callus is visible.

Stage of bone healing: Early remodeling phase. Woven bone is being replaced with lamellar bone. The process of remodeling takes months to years for completion.

X-ray: Bony consolidation is progressing, and the callus should be visible at the posterolateral surface of the tibia in extending around to the other surfaces. The fracture line should become cloudy and begin to disappear. If bone grafting was required, consolidation of this bone graft should begin to be seen.

Orthopaedic and Rehabilitation Considerations

Physical Examination

Assess all wounds or pin sites and treat appropriately. Compare leg lengths and prescribe a shoe lift for the rare case of significant leg-length discrepancy in excess of half an inch. Observe the gait for any functional disability and continue to measure joint motion and muscle strength.

Dangers

No change. See previous section (page 372).

Radiography

Examine the anteroposterior and lateral interval radiographs to confirm fixation, rotation, and position of hardware. Pay special attention to the entry point of any nail that is unlocked at one end for dynamization, because the nail may protrude. Examine both the tibia and fibula for healing. Radiographs that show a healed fibula fracture with a persistent un-united tibial fracture cleft must be evaluated for possible osteotomy of the fibula. This allows interfragmentary compression of the tibia and stimulation of healing.

Weight Bearing

1. Cast. Full weight bearing should be as tolerated in a patella-tendon-bearing cast or orthosis (*see* Figure 28-18).
2. Intramedullary Rod. Continue full weight bearing as tolerated. If the fracture is not united, consider cast bracing or other orthosis as an adjunct treatment to further reduce motion at the fracture site.
3. External Fixator. Partial weight bearing should be initiated once the external fixator has been removed and the leg is placed in a cast or orthosis, or if the fixator is replaced with an intramedullary rod.

Range of Motion

Continue active range of motion in all planes of the hip, knee, and ankle. If range of motion is limited, active-assisted or passive range-of-motion exercises can be instituted as the fracture becomes increasingly stable.

Muscle Strength

Depending on callus formation and the stability of the fracture site, isotonic exercises with increasing resistance are initiated to the ankle musculature. Other exercises should continue as previously stated.

Functional Activities

Depending on weight-bearing status, the patient may need to use assistive devices for transfers and ambulation.

Gait

No change.

Methods of Treatment: Specific Aspects

Cast

All casts should be removed and the limb evaluated for clinical stability. The fracture site should be palpated for tenderness and the presence of callus. The underlying skin and soft tissues should be inspected as well for areas of erythema where the cast may have been exerting too much pressure.

Fractures that exhibit clinical stability and minimal or no tenderness at the callus site may be amenable to further treatment with either a short leg weight-bearing cast or a patella-tendon-bearing cast. Use a short leg cast for patients with no tenderness and more callus. Use a patella-tendon-bearing cast for patients with some tenderness and less callus formation. In addition, a patella-tendon-bearing orthosis, if available, may be useful for patients at this stage of healing (*see* Figure 28-8).

Once the patient has been placed in a shorter cast or an orthosis, active range of motion of the knee can be initiated. Isotonic exercises to the quadriceps are encouraged. The weight of the short leg cast or orthosis may be used for some resistance in strengthening the quadriceps muscles.

Intramedullary Rod

Rods that are statically locked should be examined for any persistent cleft at the fracture site. If a fracture cleft is still present, the rod should be dynamized by removing the proximal interlocking screw. If the fibula is healed by this time and the fracture cleft is still visible, then consider performing a fibular osteotomy or ostectomy at the time of dynamization. Bone graft or injection of bone morphogenic protein may also be of benefit at this time to induce healing. Range-of-motion and strengthening exercises of the hip, knee, and ankle should continue.

External Fixator

By this time, all wounds should be closed either by primary healing and skin or flap coverage. The fixator should be removed and the limb examined for stability of the fracture and palpable callus. The leg should then be placed in a patella-tendon-bearing cast or patella-tendon-bearing orthosis. Range-of-motion and strengthening exercises should be continued. Gentle resistive exercises to the knee may be started with weights used in gradation. This should continue until a normal healing pattern is restored.

Prescription

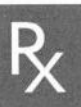

EIGHT TO TWELVE WEEKS

Range of Motion Active, active-assistive, and passive range of motion to knee and ankle.

Strength Gentle progressive resistive exercises prescribed to quadriceps, dorsiflexors, and plantar flexors.

Functional Activities If fracture site is still tender, patient may still need assistive devices for transfers and ambulation.

Weight Bearing As tolerated.

LONG-TERM CONSIDERATIONS AND PROBLEMS

Nonunion or delayed union occurs most commonly in highly comminuted or open tibia fractures. The high-energy injury that causes these fractures leads to disruption of the blood supply to the tibia, and an atrophic nonunion may occur. Hypertrophic nonunions occur when there is too much motion at the fracture site. Nonunions may be initially treated with progressive weight bearing. This often stimulates bone healing. If a tibia nonunion occurs in a leg with a healed fibula fracture, then a fibula ostectomy may be necessary to allow the tibia to transfer weight from the proximal to the distal segment across the nonunion. This may also promote healing.

A nonunion may also be treated with bone grafting and plating, intramedullary rodding, or exchange rodding to a larger reamed nail if it occurs in a tibia fracture that has initially been treated with an intramedullary nail.

IMMEDIATE TO ONE WEEK

	Cast	*Open Reduction and Internal Fixation*	*External Fixation*
Stability	None.	None.	None.
Orthopaedics	Trim cast back to the metatarsophalangeal (MTP) joints to allow dorsi and plantar flexion of the toes. Elevate the lower extremity to decrease swelling.	Perform wound care over incisions in any open wounds.	Evaluate pin sites and tendon functions as well as any open wounds that require wound management.
Rehabilitation	Isometric exercises to the quadriceps and calf musculature within the cast and active dorsi and plantar flexion of the toes.	Isometric exercises to strengthen the quadriceps and calf musculature as well as range of motion to the knee and ankle and ankle joints and the toes.	Isometric exercises to strengthen the quadriceps and calf musculature as well as range of motion to the knee joints and the toes.

TWO WEEKS			
	Cast	***Open Reduction and Internal Fixation***	***External Fixation***
Stability	None to minimal.	None to minimal.	None to minimal.
Orthopaedics	Trim cast back and continue elevation when necessary to decrease swelling.	Remove any sutures and continue wound care to any open wounds.	Evaluate pin sites and tendon functions and continue wound care.
Rehabilitation	Continue isometric exercises to the quadriceps and calf musculature within the cast and active motion of the toes.	Range of motion of the knee and the ankle as well as the digits. Isometric exercises to the quadriceps and ankle musculature.	Range of motion of the knee and the ankle as well as the digits. Isometric exercises to the quadriceps, and ankle musculature.

FOUR TO SIX WEEKS			
	Cast	***Open Reduction and Internal Fixation***	***External Fixation***
Stability	Partially stable.	Partially stable.	Partially stable.
Orthopaedics	Continue long leg cast, but this may be removed, repaired, or changed as necessary.	Consider dynamization if any fracture cleft is present.	Examine frames and all pins and screws and tighten as necessary; any pins with evidence of infection may be replaced with larger pins or pins at a different site.
Rehabilitation	Continue isometric exercises to the quadriceps and calf musculature and range of motion to the digits.	Continue active range of motion of the knee and ankle joints as well as digits. Isometric and isotonic exercises to the quadriceps and ankle musculature.	Continue active range of motion of the knee and ankle joints as well as digits. Isometric and isotonic exercises to quadriceps and ankle musculature.

EIGHT TO TWELVE WEEKS

	Cast	*Open Reduction and Internal Fixation*	*External Fixation*
Stability	Stable.	Stable.	Stable.
Orthopaedics	Remove cast.	Most fractures will be completely healed; however, those with a persistent fracture cleft must be dynamized with a fibula osteotomy or a fibula ostectomy if the fibula has healed and the tibia has a persistent fracture cleft.	Remove pins and fixator.
Rehabilitation	Begin active range of motion of the knee and ankle joints and gradually begin resistive exercises.	Continue active range of motion and resistive exercises to the knee and ankle joint.	Active range of motion should continue at the knee and ankle joints. Progressive resistive exercises to the quadriceps and ankle musculature.

BIBLIOGRAPHY

Lindsey RW, Blair SR. Closed tibial-shaft fractures: which ones benefit from surgical treatment? *J Am Acad Orthop Surg* 4:35–43, 1996.

McKibbin B. The biology of fracture healing in long bones. *J Bone Joint Surg* 60-B:150–161, 1978.

Puno RM, Vaughan JJ, Stetten ML, et al. Long-term effects of tibial angular malunion on the knees and ankle joints. *J Orthop Trauma* 5:247–254, 1991.

Puno RM, Teynor JT, Nagano J, Gustilo RB. Critical analysis of treatment of 201 tibial shaft fractures. *Clin Orthop* 212: 113–121, 1985.

Sarmiento A, Gersten LM, Sobol PA, Shankwiler JA, Vangsness CT. Tibial shaft fractures treated with functional braces. *J Bone Joint Surg* 71-B:602–609, 1989.

Trafton PG. Tibial shaft fractures In: Browner BD, Jupiter JB, Levine AM, Trafton PG, eds. *Skeletal Trauma,* Vol 2. Philadelphia: W.B. Saunders, 1992, pp. 1771–1869.

CHAPTER *Twenty-nine*

Tibial Plafond Fractures

ANNE P. MCCORMACK, MD

INTRODUCTION

Definition

Tibial plafond fractures involve the horizontal weight-bearing surface of the distal tibia—the plafond. Isolated fractures of the medial or lateral malleoli may or may not involve the plafond.

Fractures of the pilon (the supramalleolar portion of the distal tibia) are a subset of plafond fractures. These fractures extend into the plafond but may or may not have displacement, extensive comminution, or impaction. Pilon fractures are not discussed in this chapter (Figures 29-1, 29-2, 29-3, 29-4).

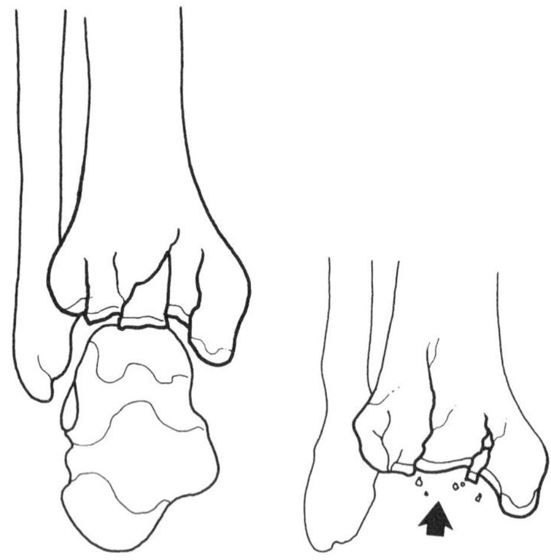

FIGURE 29-1 *(above, left)* Tibial plafond fracture with comminution. Restoration of the articular surface is essential to prevent arthritis.

FIGURE 29-2 *(above, right)* Plafond fracture with displacement of the articular surface. Reduction is necessary to prevent arthritis. Partial weight bearing is not allowed until 6 or 8 weeks in patients who have minimally displaced fractures with good callus formation. Full weight bearing is permitted at 3 to 4 months.

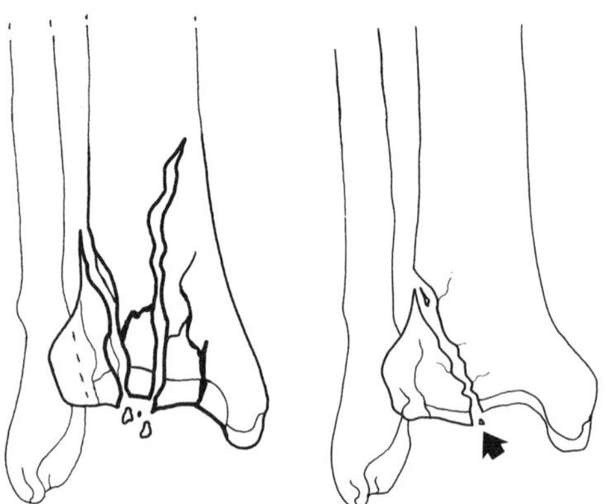

FIGURE 29-3 *(above, left)* Comminuted displaced plafond fracture with extension into the pilon (supramalleolar portion of the distal tibia). Open reduction and internal fixation is necessary to restore the articular surface.

FIGURE 29-4 *(above, right)* Oblique plafond fracture requiring open reduction and internal fixation. Rigid fixation allows for early motion of the ankle joint.

Mechanism of Injury

These fractures are caused by a high-energy impact, usually a deceleration force such as occurs in a fall from a height or a motor vehicle accident.

Treatment Goals

Orthopaedic Objectives

Alignment

Restore an intact articular surface along the tibial plafond of the ankle mortise. This is of critical importance for pain-free weight bearing across the ankle joint.

Restore the tibial and fibular length to promote healing in an anatomic position and prevent leg-length discrepancy.

Stability

Stable reconstruction of bony structures such as the lateral, medial, and posterior malleoli is important to static (weight bearing) and dynamic (walking) stability across the ankle joint.

Reconstruction of ligamentous structures, including the distal tibiofibular syndesmosis, which may have been damaged, is also important for maintaining the dynamic stability of the ankle and a normal gait.

Rehabilitation Objectives

Range of Motion

Restore the full range of motion of the ankle joint in all planes (Table 29-1).

TABLE 29-1 *Ankle Ranges of Motion*

Motion	Normal	Functional
Ankle plantar flexion	45°	20°
Ankle dorsiflexion	20°–25°	10°
Foot inversion	35°	10°
Foot eversion	25°	10°

Inadequate reduction of the fracture fragments and stabilization of the ligaments across the ankle joint can lead to significant loss of range of motion, particularly in plantar flexion and dorsiflexion. Residual loss of the range of motion of the tibiotalar joint increases stress on the subtalar articulation.

Muscle Strength

Improve the strength of the muscles that cross the ankle joint, which are affected by the fracture or by cast immobilization:

Plantar flexors of the ankle and foot:

Gastrocnemius

Soleus

Tibialis posterior (also acts as an invertor)

Flexor digitorum longus

Flexor hallucis longus

Dorsiflexors of the ankle and foot:

Tibialis anterior (also acts as an invertor)

Extensor digitorum longus

Extensor hallucis longus

Evertors of the ankle and foot

Peroneus longus

Peroneus brevis

Invertors of the ankle and foot:

Tibialis posterior (also acts as a plantar flexor)

Tibialis anterior (also acts as a dorsiflexor)

Functional Goals

Restore the ankle mortise and the congruity of the ankle in static (weight-bearing) and dynamic (walking) conditions to normalize the gait.

Restore the length of the tibia and fibula to avoid leg-length discrepancy and allow normalization of the gait.

Expected Time of Bone Healing

Six to 8 weeks.

Expected Duration of Rehabilitation

Three to 6 months.

Methods of Treatment

Open Reduction and Internal Fixation

Biomechanics: Stress-shielding device.

Mode of bone healing: Primary, without callus formation.

Indications: This method is the first choice for plafond fractures. Anatomic reduction with restoration of the articular surface and tibial length greatly improves the patient's long-term prognosis.

Bone graft is used as necessary to support defects caused by impaction of the articular surface and metaphyseal bone. Buttress plates are used in conjunction with carefully placed screws to lag (draw together) large fragments and to maintain reduction. This method provides rigid fixation and allows for early motion of the ankle joint. A protective cast or splint may be used postoperatively (Figures 29-5, 29-6, 29-7, 29-8, 29-9, and 29-10).

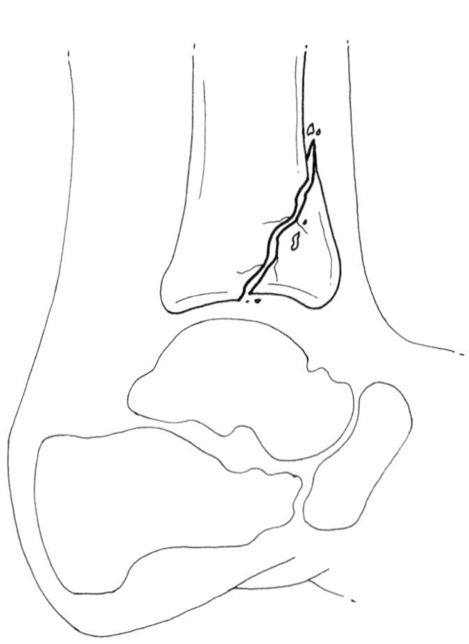

FIGURE 29-5 Plafond fracture involving the weight-bearing surface of the tibia.

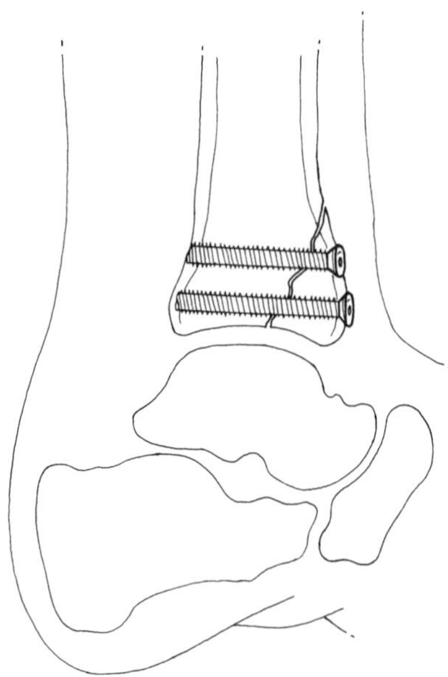

FIGURE 29-6 Anatomic reduction with restoration of the articular surface is essential. Screws are carefully placed to lag (draw together) the large fragments and to maintain reduction. Callus formation may be seen.

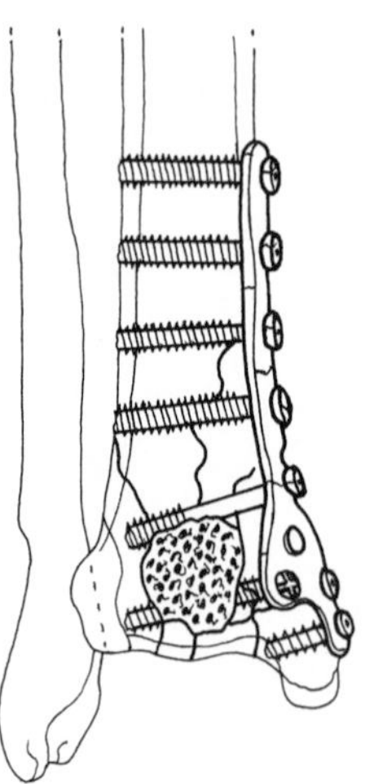

FIGURE 29-7 Anatomic reduction and restoration of the articular surface improves the patient's long-term prognosis. Bone graft is used as necessary to support defects caused by impaction of the articular surface and metaphyseal bone. A plate is used in conjunction with screws to lag large fragments and to maintain reduction. This provides rigid fixation and allows for early motion of the ankle joint. A protective cast or splint may be used postoperatively.

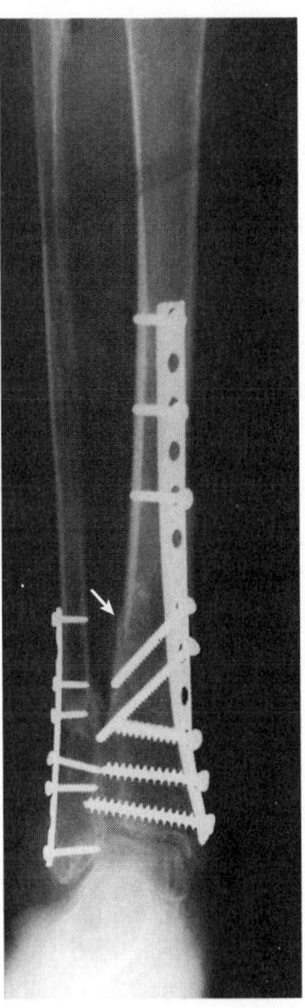

FIGURE 29-8 Healing fracture of the plafond treated with open reduction and internal screw and plate fixation. Note the callus formation indicating healing *(arrow)*. Partial weight bearing is permitted at 6 to 8 weeks when there is good callus formation.

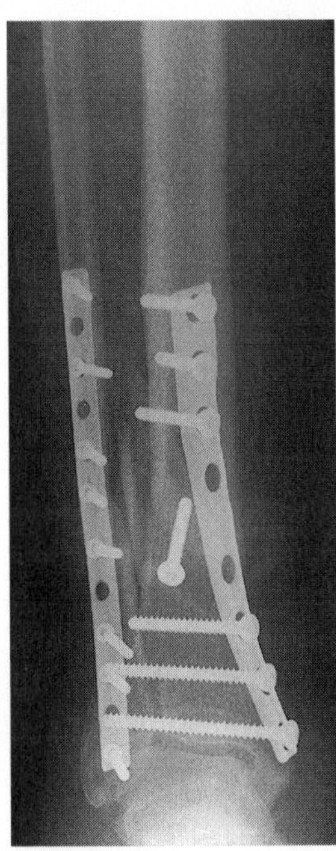

FIGURE 29-9 Plafond fracture with internal fixation with screws and plates (anteroposterior/mortise view). Note the lag screw fixation across the distal tibiofibular syndesmosis to maintain reduction. This fracture is caused by high-energy impact, usually a deceleration force, as in a fall from a height or a motor vehicle accident.

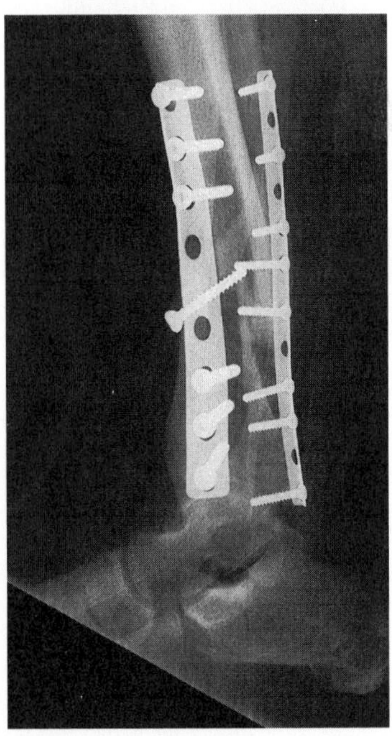

FIGURE 29-10 Lateral view of the distal tibia and ankle. The plafond fracture has been treated with plates and screws to maintain reduction. Postoperatively the patient is maintained in a cast to help control soft tissue injury. All plafond fractures are initially kept non-weight bearing.

External Fixation

Biomechanics: Stress-sharing device.

Mode of bone healing: Secondary, with callus formation.

Indications: For plafond fractures with significant soft tissue injury that are not amenable to open reduction and internal fixation, this option allows the restoration of length and possible articular congruity. It also allows for the care of soft tissue wounds that include a muscular flap or skin graft.

Cast

Biomechanics: Stress-sharing device.

Mode of bone healing: Secondary, with callus formation.

Indications: Nondisplaced or minimally displaced plafond fractures that have maintained the articular joint surface and have little or no impaction are amenable to closed reduction and long leg casting. Although this method obviates the need for a surgical incision, its drawback is that it does not allow early motion at the ankle joint (Figures 29-11 and 29-12).

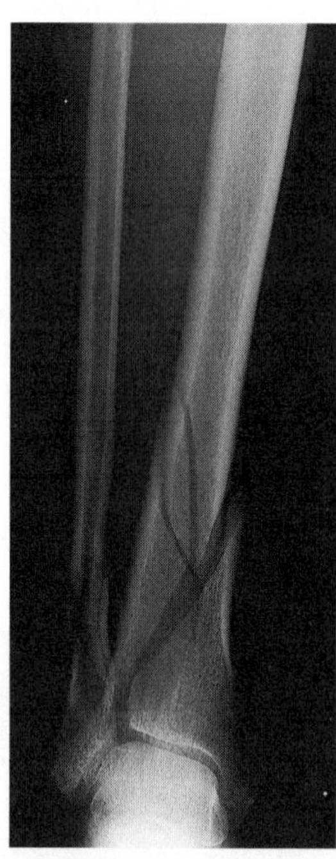

FIGURE 29-11 Radiograph of the ankle revealing a plafond fracture with minimum displacement of the articular surfaces.

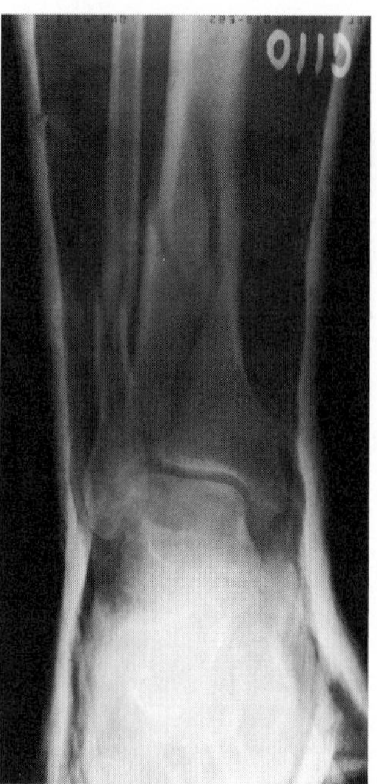

FIGURE 29-12 Newly displaced fracture of the plafond successfully treated with closed reduction and cast fixation. Although this method obviates the need for a surgical incision, it does not allow early motion at the ankle joint.

Primary Arthrodesis

Biomechanics: Stress-shielding device.

Mode of bone healing: Primary, without callus formation.

Indications: If there has been significant comminution that precludes a successful open reduction and internal fixation because of bone impaction and loss, a primary arthrodesis with bone graft gives the patient a stable pain-free ankle. This is a treatment of last resort; it is not discussed further in this chapter.

Special Considerations of the Fracture

Age

The patient's age alone does not appear to significantly affect the outcome of the healing of a tibial plafond fracture. Elderly patients may not have as high-quality bone stock to support fixation devices, however, and are at more risk for development of joint stiffness. In addition, concomitant systemic diseases, including peripheral vascular disease and diabetes, may complicate healing, because of poor blood supply.

Articular Involvement

All plafond fractures by definition involve the weight-bearing articular surface of the distal tibia. Although undisplaced or minimally displaced fractures of the plafond do well with either operative or nonoperative treatment, significant posttraumatic arthritis is possible if there has been severe comminution or displacement. These patients may later need an ankle fusion or total ankle joint replacement (Figure 29-13).

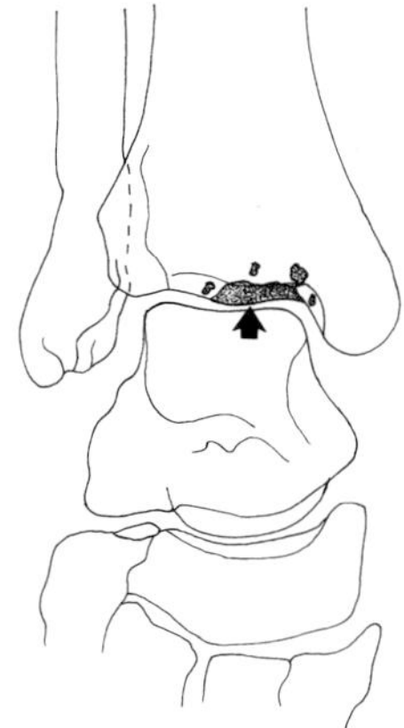

FIGURE 29-13 Undisplaced fracture of the tibial plafond. These patients may do well with either operative or nonoperative treatment; however, significant posttraumatic arthritis is possible, in which case an ankle fusion may be needed later.

Open Fractures

All open fractures should be treated aggressively with irrigation, débridement and intravenous antibiotics. Open fractures of the tibial plafond are usually associated with a significant high-energy force; therefore, severe soft tissue injury is common. There is minimal subcutaneous tissue or muscle around the ankle joint to support the skin; skin sloughing or loss is also common with open fractures. At the time of initial presentation, the patient should be carefully evaluated for any injury to the nerves or arteries around the ankle joint.

Tendinous and Ligamentous Injuries

Injuries that cause severely comminuted fractures to the tibial plafond are often associated with disruption of the ligamentous complex around the ankle joint, rendering it unstable. Repair of the tendons and ligaments may be necessary. In addition, adequate fixation, whether open reduction and internal fixation or external fixation, is important to maintain the congruity of the ankle mortise as well as the joint surface.

Associated Injury

Fractures of the tibial plafond are usually caused by a fall from a height or a high-energy deceleration injury, both of which can result in significant damage to the thin soft tissue envelope that surrounds the ankle. Although an open wound may or may not be present, the forces absorbed by the soft tissues at the moment of injury can be severe enough to cause necrosis or prevent healing of the surgical incision. If impending blisters or skin slough is suspected, the patient should be placed in either external fixation or calcaneal pin traction until the skin has become clean and free of blisters and edema.

Weight Bearing

Weight bearing is not permitted for plafond or pilon fractures until there are radiographic signs of early healing. Full weight bearing is not permitted for 3 or 4 months. Partial weight bearing is permitted at 6 to 8 weeks in patients who have minimally displaced fractures with good callus formation.

Gait

The gait cycle is profoundly affected by serious fractures of the tibial plafond. Any incongruity in the surfaces or damage to the cartilage predisposes the patient to early degenerative arthritis, which narrows the joint space and causes pain as the tibia attempts to slide over the upper surface of the talus. Posttraumatic arthritic changes may cause severe pain across the tibiotalar joint and may require subsequent fusion or joint replacement to relieve the disability and discomfort. Stresses not taken up by the tibiotalar joint are transmitted to both the subtalar joint and the medial plantar arch in an attempt to compensate for the derangement across the ankle joint. Energy expenditure for walking increases, smooth forward translation of walking is interrupted, and normal navigation of uneven surfaces is compromised.

Stance Phase

The stance phase constitutes 60% of the gait cycle.

Heel Strike

As weight is transferred through the tibial plafond onto the surface of the talus, patients who have sustained intraarticular fractures experience discomfort. Any disruption of the cartilaginous weight-bearing surface of the tibial plafond or the talus causes pain as the weight is transferred through the tibial shaft into the foot. Patients who have been immobilized in a cast may have stiffness of the joint capsule and weakness of the dorsiflexors, which prevents patients from maintaining dorsiflexion and results in an initial foot slap. This usually resolves with time (*see* Figure 6-1).

Foot-Flat

During this portion of the gait cycle, pain continues as more body weight is transferred through the tibia, over the talus, and toward the midfoot. Capsular stiffness and weak plantar flexors (resulting from immobilization) also contribute to discomfort (*see* Figure 6-2).

Mid-Stance

The single-stance phase usually is also painful. The foot is positioning itself to take the weight of the entire body as the opposite foot lifts from the floor. The increased pressure transferred through the tibial plafond into the talus causes discomfort in the ankle joint and into the fracture extending into the tibia (*see* Figure 6-3).

Push-Off

This phase may be the least painful portion of the gait cycle for patients with plafond fractures, because the hindfoot is being unloaded and weight is transferred to the opposite leg. The most difficult part is the positioning of the tibia over the talus as the foot begins to plantar flex. The weak plantar flexors have difficulty bearing load across the ankle. Pain is likely to cause inadequate push-off for the affected foot. The entire stance phase is shortened, and the patient may attempt to hop off a painful ankle to reduce pain (antalgic gait). (*See* Figures 6-4 and 6-5.)

Swing Phase

The swing phase, which constitutes 40% of the gait cycle, is also affected, but to a lesser extent. The dorsiflexors must bring the foot up, causing compressive forces across the ankle joint that extend into the plafond and pilon. This causes discomfort through the tibiotalar joint and into the distal tibia. This limits the amount of ankle dorsiflexion or plantar flexion. Occasionally, the patient may hike up the affected limb to clear the ground or bend the knee to a greater degree as a result of limited dorsiflexion (*see* Figures 6-6, 6-7, and 6-8).

TREATMENT

Treatment: Early to Immediate (Day of Injury to One Week)

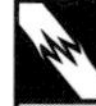

BONE HEALING

Stability at fracture site: None.

Stage of bone healing: Inflammatory phase. The fracture hematoma is colonized by inflammatory cells and débridement of the fracture begins.

X-ray: No callus. Fracture lines are visible.

Orthopaedic and Rehabilitation Considerations

Physical Examination

Pay special attention to complaints of pain, paresthesia, or cast discomfort as an indicator of a cast that is too tight or a tibial compartment syndrome. Also note whether the cast is loose; it may need replacing. Check capillary refill and sensation. Toes should be pink with brisk refill after light compression. It should be possible to reach the first web space of the toe and stroke it lightly with a blunt instrument to ensure that there is no deep peroneal nerve compression in the anterior compartment. If external fixation has been used, check the pin sites for drainage or erythema and treat appropriately.

Dangers

High-energy or crush injuries to the ankle and lower leg are at risk for tibial compartment syndrome. Compartment syndrome is a potential complication whenever a cast has been placed on a very swollen ankle and leg. The cast and padding must be cut during the early posttrauma period to prevent constriction and to allow adequate monitoring. If compartment syndrome is suspected, measure the compartment pressures in the leg and perform fasciotomies involving the compartments as necessary.

For fractures that were open or had significant fracture blisters, evaluate the skin for any erythema or drainage that may indicate infection. The patient should be advised to keep the extremity elevated above the heart level and to place ice packs over the ankle and lower leg to decrease the swelling and increase venous return.

Radiography

Obtain and check anteroposterior, lateral, and mortise radiographs of the ankle, including the distal tibia, to evaluate for any loss of correction. If internal fixation has been applied, check that all screws and plates remain in the correct position (*see* Figures 29-9 and 29-10).

Weight Bearing

All fractures of the tibial plafond should be non-weight bearing.

Range of Motion

A patient who has had stable internal fixation and is in a compressive bulky dressing may begin gentle active range of motion at the ankle as tolerated. Active range-of-motion exercises are prescribed for the metatarsophalangeal joints. A patient who has had internal fixation or is in an external fixator may also begin range of motion at the knee as tolerated.

Muscle Strength

Maintain quadriceps strength with quad sets. Patients in long leg casts as well as those in external fixators may try to engage in quadriceps strengthening.

Functional Activities

Patients are instructed in non–weight-bearing stand/pivot transfers using crutches or a walker. Patients should don pants with the affected extremity first and doff them from the unaffected extremity first. Pants may be split along a seam to facilitate their placement over the cast.

Gait

The patient uses a non–weight-bearing two-point gait in which the crutches form one unit and the unaffected extremity the other unit (*see* Figure 6-16). When ascending stairs, the patient leads with the unaffected extremity; when descending stairs, the patient leads with the affected extremity (*see* Figures 6-20, 6-21, 6-22, 6-23, 6-24, and 6-25).

Methods of Treatment: Specific Aspects

Open Reduction and Internal Fixation

The patient should be watched carefully for any evidence of skin sloughing or necrosis and should be placed in a well-padded, nonconstricting splint to ensure the ankle is maintained in a neutral position (foot at right angle to the tibia). The leg should be moderately elevated to help decrease the swelling. The surgical wound should be observed carefully; if any significant skin sloughing occurs, consider prompt coverage with a free muscle flap. Start active ankle range of motion while the patient is in a compressive dressing.

External Fixation

Evaluate the pin sites for erythema, discharge, or fluctuance. Examine the skin for evidence of demarcation or necrosis. Open fractures are often associated with an increased risk of infection and residual deformity, as well as a decreased range of motion.

Cast

Inspect the cast and trim it if necessary to allow visualization of all the toes. The patient should have free movement at the metatarsophalangeal joints. Check the cast padding and edges; evaluate for any softening and repair appropriately. If the patient has any complaints of loss of sensation or there is marked swelling of the toes and decreased temperature, consider bivalving the cast and splitting padding to release the pressure on the extremity.

Prescription

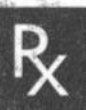

Day One to One Week

Precautions Ankle and leg are immobilized in either a cast, splint, fixator, or traction.

Range of Motion For rigidly fixed fractures, active range of motion at the metatarsophalangeal joints and the knee joint; gentle active range of motion to the ankle while in a compressive dressing.

For nonrigidly fixed fractures, range of motion at the metatarsophalangeal joints.

Strength No strengthening exercises to the ankle or foot. Quadriceps isometric exercises as tolerated.

Functional Activities Non–weight-bearing stand/pivot transfers and ambulation with assistive devices.

Weight Bearing None.

Treatment: Two Weeks

Bone Healing

Stability at fracture site: None to minimal.

Stage of bone healing: Beginning of reparative phase. Osteoprogenitor cells differentiate into osteoblasts, which lay down woven bone.

X-ray: None to very early callus.

Orthopaedic and Rehabilitation Considerations

Physical Examination

Check capillary refill and sensation of the toes, and, if possible, the first dorsal web space. Check the active and passive range of motion of all metatarsophalangeal and interphalangeal joints.

Dangers

Pay particular attention to complaints of pain, paresthesia, and cast discomfort. The patient should be made aware that any pronounced swelling could lead to skin sloughing and should be immediately brought to the physician's attention. The patient should be advised to keep the extremity elevated above the heart level to minimize swelling and improve venous return.

Radiography

Check radiographs in anteroposterior, lateral, and mortise positions with extension of these films into the tibial shaft. Evaluate the position of the fracture to assess any loss of reduction. Also assess that any hardware remains in its original position. Early callus may be evident in some patients (*see* Figure 29-8).

Weight Bearing

All patients should remain non-weight bearing.

Range of Motion

Continue active and passive range of motion at the metatarsophalangeal joints. Patients with stable internal fixation who are in a bivalved cast or posterior splint may continue active ankle range of motion. Patients who are not in a long leg cast should continue range of motion at the knee.

Muscle Strength

Maintain the strength of the quadriceps. Repetitive movements of the toes in flexion and extension strengthen the flexors and extensors across the ankle.

Functional Activities

Continue non–weight-bearing stand/pivot transfers using crutches or a walker.

Gait

Continue using a non–weight-bearing two-point gait with crutches (*see* Figure 6-16).

Methods of Treatment: Specific Aspects

Open Reduction and Internal Fixation

Evaluate the surgical incision and remove any sutures or staples. If a skin graft or muscle flap has been necessary, evaluate the viability of these grafts. The graft should be taking. If there is any evidence of infection or loss of the graft, consider reoperation. Encourage active range of motion to the ankle joint. Replace the cast or posterior splint if there is pain or tenderness.

External Fixation

Check for infection at the pin sites. Evaluate for any loosening of the bars and connectors to the pins. If the soft tissues are adequately healed, consider removing the external fixator and placing the patient in a long leg cast.

Cast

Evaluate the integrity of the cast. Repair any soft areas. Check the cast padding and cast edges and trim any sharp edges.

Prescription

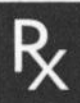

TWO WEEKS

Precautions Patients in a long leg cast or external fixator do not have stable fractures.

Range of Motion For rigidly fixed fractures, active range of motion of the metatarsophalangeal joints and knee joint; active range of motion to ankle out of splint or bivalved cast.

For nonrigidly fixed fractures, active range of motion of the metatarsophalangeal joints only.

Strength For rigidly fixed fractures, isometric exercises to dorsiflexors and plantar flexors of the ankle and toes; no resistive exercises; isometric quadriceps exercises.

For nonrigidly fixed fractures, no strengthening or resistive exercises.

Functional Activities Non–weight-bearing stand/pivot transfers; ambulation with assistive devices.

Weight Bearing None.

Treatment: Four to Six Weeks

BONE HEALING

Stability at fracture site: Usually stable. Fractures should be showing bridging callus and are stable. However, the strength of this callus, especially with torsional load, is significantly less than that of normal bone. Confirm this with physical examination and x-rays.

Stage of bone healing: Reparative phase. Further organization of the callus and formation of lamellar bone begins.

X-ray: Bridging callus is visible as a small amount of fluffy material on the periosteal surface of cortical bone. For fractures rigidly fixed with screws and plates, callus may not be visible, because there is primary bone healing. For fractures treated in a cast, expect more callus formation. There is a consolidation of the fracture and filling in of lucent lines.

Orthopaedic and Rehabilitation Considerations

Physical Examination

Remove the cast and perform the radiographic examination out of plaster. Check for stability, tenderness, and range of motion at the ankle joint. Patients whose treatment has been primarily in a long leg cast will likely be very stiff at both the knee and the ankle. Reassess all wounds and pin sites out of plaster for any evidence of infection and treat appropriately. There should be some fracture stability. Evaluate this carefully, looking for tenderness or motion at the fracture site.

Dangers

Most of the swelling from acute fractures should be resolved. Check for any trophic signs of reflex sympathetic dystrophy (RSD), characterized by vasomotor disturbances, hyperesthesias, pain, and tenderness out of proportion to the stage of fracture healing. If evidence of RSD is noted, start the patient on an aggressive physical therapy program. If the patient has had severe soft tissue injury and exhibits eschar, evaluate this carefully to ensure that there is no necrosis or infection beneath the scar tissue. Evaluate the integrity and viability of any skin or muscle grafts.

Radiography

Radiographs should be examined in the anteroposterior, lateral, and mortise positions of the ankle and distal tibia and fibula for evidence of healing and any loss of reduction, although this is uncommon at this stage. Evaluate the integrity of the hardware and check for screws that may have backed out or plates that may have fractured.

Weight Bearing

All patients should remain non-weight bearing.

Range of Motion

Continue metatarsophalangeal joint range of motion. If the patient's cast has been removed, active range of motion at the ankle may be added (dorsiflexion and plantar flexion) to tolerance. Patients who have had internal fixation may also begin gentle inversion and eversion exercises, and continue with ankle dorsiflexion and plantar flexion. This helps prevent stiffening of the ankle joint capsule.

Range of motion at the knee is also continued for any patient who is not in a long leg cast. A patient in a cast who has some evidence of healing may attempt limited dorsiflexion and plantar flexion as well as inversion and eversion within the cast, which should be loose enough to allow some limited range of motion. However, this should not be attempted as a resistive exercise.

Muscle Strength

Continue isometric exercises to the dorsiflexors and plantar flexors of the ankle. The patient should continue quadriceps strengthening exercises. A patient whose cast has been removed may also begin further strengthening of the peronei, tibialis posterior, and tibialis anterior with inversion and eversion exercises, as long as there is adequate healing evidenced by callus and decreased tenderness at the fracture site.

Functional Activities

Patients should continue non–weight-bearing stand/pivot transfers and ambulation with assistive devices.

Gait

The patient should continue to use crutches and a non–weight-bearing gait.

Methods of Treatment: Specific Aspects

Open Reduction and Internal Fixation

If a cast has been placed for safety reasons, remove it and examine the ankle. If the fracture area is nontender, without any motion, and callus has been noted on radiograph, the protective cast may be discontinued at 6 weeks. Allow the patient to begin passive and continue active range-of-motion exercises at the ankle. The posterior half of the cast may be used as a night splint to control residual pain and edema. An Unna paste boot may be applied to control the swelling.

If there is tenderness or motion at the fracture site without good radiologic evidence of healing, however, the cast should be replaced. For patients who have been allowed active range of motion before this visit, evaluate the progression and extent of the range of motion. Evaluate the skin for healing of any skin sloughing or necrosis.

External Fixation

If soft tissue healing allows, the fixator may be removed and a cast or other appropriate supportive device placed on the foot and leg while healing is completed.

Cast

Perform an examination out of plaster to check the stability, tenderness, and range of motion of the fracture. A patient who is still significantly tender should again be placed into a long leg cast for at least an additional 2 weeks. Minimally tender or nontender fractures may be placed into either a patella-tendon-bearing cast (PTB) or a short leg cast.

Prescription

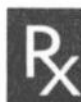

FOUR TO SIX WEEKS

Precautions Unstable fractures or those with limited fixation are still in a cast.

Range of Motion For rigidly fixed fractures, active range of motion to the ankle, metatarsophalangeal joints, and knee.

For nonrigidly fixed fractures, active range of motion to the metatarsophalangeal joints, ankle, and knee as immobilization devices allow.

Strength For rigidly fixed fractures, isometric exercises to dorsiflexors and plantar flexors of the ankle. No resistive exercises to long flexors and extensors of the toes. Quadriceps strengthening continues.

For nonrigidly fixed fractures, gentle isometric exercises to dorsiflexors and plantar flexors within a cast. No resistive exercises to the long flexors and extensors of the toes. Quadriceps strengthening continues.

Functional Activities Non–weight-bearing stand/pivot transfers and ambulation with assistive devices.

Weight Bearing None.

Treatment: Six to Eight Weeks

BONE HEALING

Stability at fracture site: With bridging callus, the fracture is usually stable. However, the strength of this callus, especially with torsional load, is significantly less than that of normal lamellar bone. Confirm with physical examination.

Stage of bone healing: Reparative phase. Further organization of the callus and formation of lamellar bone continues.

X-ray: Bridging callus is visible and indicates increasing rigidity. With rigid fixation, less callus is seen and fracture lines are less distinct. Less bridging callus is noted, and healing with endosteal bone predominates.

Orthopaedic and Rehabilitation Considerations

Physical Examination

All fractures come out of a cast for examination and radiographic study. Examine the fracture site for tenderness. If there was a wound or an operative site, evaluate it for healing and evidence of infection. Evaluate any trophic or sensory changes as an indication of RSD.

Dangers

If there has been skin or muscle grafting, evaluate the graft for viability and incorporation. Check any wounds or operative sites for evidence of infection and treat appropriately.

Radiography

Evaluate all fractures with anteroposterior, lateral, and mortise views and anteroposterior and lateral views of the tibia and fibula to assess for the loss of reduction as well as the status of healing. Evaluate the position and integrity of all hardware.

Weight Bearing

Patients with nondisplaced or minimally displaced fractures who show evidence of good callus and have a nontender physical examination may progress to partial weight bearing using crutches or a walker.

Patients with significant displacement of their fractures or those who have not had full rigid fixation must continue strict non-weight bearing using crutches or a walker. Patients who have had bone grafts may not yet be stable and should also continue non-weight bearing.

Range of Motion

The ankle will be quite stiff secondary to soft tissue trauma and immobilization. Active range-of-motion and active-assistive range-of-motion exercises in all planes are instituted. Hydrotherapy helps increase the range of motion.

Muscle Strength

Isotonic and isokinetic exercises are prescribed for the dorsiflexors, plantar flexors, evertors, and invertors of the foot. Continue quadriceps and hamstring strengthening.

Functional Activities

Patients with callus formation, minimal or no tenderness to palpation, and minimal displacement may perform transfers with partial weight bearing on the affected extremity.

Patients whose fractures are still tender to palpation and who have poor callus deposition and comminution remain non-weight bearing and continue stand/pivot transfers with crutches.

Patients who are allowed partial weight bearing should still dress the affected extremity first.

Gait

Patients who are allowed partial weight bearing use a three-point gait in which the two crutches form one point and the affected and unaffected extremities the other two points (*see* Figure 6-17). The patient climbs stairs with the unaffected extremity first, followed by the crutches and the affected extremity, and descends stairs, placing the crutches first, followed by the affected extremity and then the unaffected extremity (*see* Figures 6-20, 6-21, 6-22, 6-23, 6-24, and 6-25).

Methods of Treatment: Specific Aspects

Open Reduction and Internal Fixation

If adequate callus is visible on radiographs, any protective cast or splint may be removed and the patient may begin active and passive range-of-motion exercises at the ankle. Carefully evaluate the range of motion of patients who have been allowed previous ankle motion. Patients who have early signs of arthritis secondary to displacement or loss of articular cartilage may complain of some discomfort with range of motion.

External Fixation

The fixator may be removed if there is visible callus, even if the soft tissue wounds are not fully closed. This decreases the risk of pin track infection. Place the patient in a protective splint or, if there is full wound healing and the patient has tenderness on examination, in a cast. Continued protection of the fracture may be necessary because of inadequate healing and because focal areas of stress may develop from pin placement in the tibia.

Cast

Remove the cast to evaluate the condition of the skin and the stability of the fracture. If the fracture site is nontender and stable to palpation, the patient may be changed to a short leg or patella-tendon-bearing cast and begin partial weight bearing. Evaluate the stiffness of the ankle joint, which is generally more severe in a plafond fracture than malleoli fractures.

Prescription

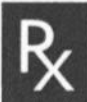

SIX TO EIGHT WEEKS

Precautions Patients undergoing conservative treatment may not yet have stable fractures.

Range of Motion For rigidly fixed fractures, begin active range of motion in all planes of the ankle and subtalar joint.

For nonrigidly fixed fractures, range the ankle and knee as the immobilization device allows. Continue active range of motion to metatarsophalangeal joints.

Strength For rigidly fixed fractures, continue isometric exercises to the dorsiflexors and plantar flexors of the ankle; no resistive exercises to the long flexors and extensors of the toes; continue quadriceps isotonic strengthening.

For nonrigidly fixed fractures, continue gentle isometric exercises to dorsiflexor and plantar flexors within a cast; no resistive exercises to the long flexors and extensors of the toes; continue quadriceps strengthening.

Functional Activities For rigidly fixed fractures, begin partial weight bearing with three-point stance. For fractures with evidence of healing, ambulation with assistive devices.

For nonrigidly fixed fractures, remain non-weight bearing.

Weight Bearing None for fractures that have not shown evidence of healing. Partial weight bearing for fractures that are nontender to palpation and appear stable on radiograph.

Treatment: Eight to Twelve Weeks

BONE HEALING

Stability at fracture site: Stable. Bridging callus is being reorganized as lamellar bone. There is increased rigidity. Ligamentous healing across the ankle joint is well established.

Stage of bone healing: Reparative phase/early remodeling phase. Lamellar bone continues to be laid down at the fracture site.

X-ray: Bridging callus is visible across the fracture. With fracture consolidation, fracture lines are less visible. Healing with endosteal callus predominates. There is evidence of incorporation of bone graft.

Orthopaedic and Rehabilitation Considerations

Physical Examination

Evaluate for tenderness at the fracture site. Evaluate the integrity of any surgical incisions for skin breakdown or infection. Check the integrity and viability of skin grafts. If fractures treated in casts are nontender, remove the cast.

Dangers

Evaluate for RSD.

Radiography

Examine anteroposterior, lateral, and mortise views of the ankle and anteroposterior and lateral views of the tibia and fibula. Use these radiographs to evaluate the integrity of the ankle joint as well as evidence of healing and the incorporation of the bone graft in the distal tibia.

Patients who have had open reduction and internal fixation should be evaluated for the integrity of their fixation devices.

Weight Bearing

Patients with minimal or nondisplaced fractures may continue partial weight bearing using crutches or a walker. Patients with more comminuted fractures or bone loss who have shown adequate healing begin toe-touch weight bearing, progressing as the graft incorporates and fracture healing is evident.

Range of Motion

Patients treated with a cast will have ankle stiffness. Begin active range of motion of the ankle in all planes as well as range of motion of the subtalar joint.

Patients who have undergone open reduction and internal fixation are likely to have better range of motion because they are allowed earlier range of motion than patients whose treatment was in a cast. Continue range-of-motion exercises, adding assistive range of motion of the ankle in all planes.

Muscle Strength

Patients whose fractures were treated with open reduction and internal fixation can continue gentle to more aggressive resistive exercises to the ankle in all planes. Patients should adjust the resistance according to their pain tolerance.

Patients whose fractures were treated conservatively and who are stable may begin gentle resistive exercises if there is no tenderness at the fracture site.

Patients should also continue with isotonic exercises to strengthen the quadriceps and hamstrings.

Functional Activities

As fracture consolidation allows, transfers are performed with toe-touch to full weight bearing on the affected extremity.

When dressing, the patient should don pants on the affected extremity first.

Gait

As the fracture consolidation increases, wean the patient from crutches or a walker to a cane as tolerated. Patients should be retrained to regain their normal gait pattern. Those who have been in a cast for an extended period tend to walk with a flat-footed gait as a result of ankle stiffness. Heel strike, foot-flat, and mid-stance as well as push-off phases should be retaught (*see* Figures 6-1, 6-2, 6-3, 6-4, and 6-5). As the ankle range of motion improves in dorsiflexion and plantar flexion, the gait pattern tends to normalize. Heavy pounding activities such as jogging, jumping, running, and twisting should be avoided until at least 12 to 16 weeks after the injury for those who are fully weight bearing at this point.

Methods of Treatment: Specific Aspects

Open Reduction and Internal Fixation

All patients should be out of a cast. The fracture site should be nontender and stable on palpation. Callus is visible on radiograph. The patient may begin partial to full weight bearing with crutches or a walker if the fracture was minimally displaced or nondisplaced. Patients with extensive comminution and injury to the articular surface should remain non-weight bearing or toe-touch weight bearing only.

External Fixation

Remove the fixator. A patient whose injury is nontender and shows good healing on radiograph may progress in weight bearing and resistive exercises. If there is not adequate healing, place the leg in a short leg cast until further healing has occurred.

Cast

Remove the cast and examine the ankle for stability and tenderness at the fracture site. If the fracture is nontender and stable to motion, remove the cast and begin range-of-motion exercises at the ankle. Patients with minimally displaced or nondisplaced plafond fractures may begin partial weight bearing with crutches or a walker if callus is visible on radiograph and the fracture is nontender to palpation.

Patients who were placed in a cast after external fixation or skeletal traction, and who may have had significant comminution, may have the cast removed if they have minimal tenderness. They should continue non-weight bearing to toe-touch weight bearing using crutches or a walker. A patient who is unlikely to comply with his or her instructions to avoid weight bearing may be placed in a patella- tendon-bearing or short leg cast for an additional 4 weeks.

Prescription

EIGHT TO TWELVE WEEKS

Precautions Avoid heavy pounding activities.

Range of Motion For rigidly fixed fractures, begin more aggressive resistive exercises in all planes of the ankle and subtalar joint.

For nonrigidly fixed fractures, begin active and active-assisted as well as passive range of motion of the ankle and subtalar joints. Patients in a cast may actively range the metatarsophalangeal joints and perform isometric exercises of the ankle and subtalar joints within their casts.

Strength For rigidly fixed fractures, begin more aggressive resistive exercises to the dorsiflexors and plantar flexors, as well as the invertors and evertors.

For nonrigidly fixed fractures, begin gentle patient-controlled resistive exercises.

Functional Activities For rigidly fixed fractures, progress from partial to full weight bearing as tolerated for transfers and ambulation using assistive devices as necessary.

For nonrigidly fixed fractures, begin partial weight bearing using assistive devices.

Weight Bearing Toe-touch to full weight bearing.

LONG-TERM CONSIDERATIONS AND PROBLEMS

Fractures of the tibial plafond involve some degree of injury to the articular cartilage of the plafond and the talar dome. This can result in long-term (chronic) disability that permanently affects the patient's ability to work and perform other activities of daily living. Early degenerative changes may progress to severe ankle arthritis pain and require a fusion of the ankle joint or total joint replacement.

Appropriately reducing both the ankle mortise and the syndesmosis and restoring the tibia and fibula to their normal length is crucial to ankle stability and normal function. Patients whose injuries have been diagnosed late or treated inadequately may have significant ankle pain as a result of the instability in the ankle joint. This disrupts gait and causes severe discomfort during weight bearing.

Ligamentous injuries at the ankle frequently have long-term sequelae. Particularly on the lateral side, persistent instability may cause repeated ankle sprains and further damage to the articular cartilage of the tibiotalar articulation. Patients who have had severe lateral ankle ligamentous injury may later need ligamentous repair to maintain the integrity of the ankle joint.

Patients who have had large amounts of bone loss secondary to fracture impaction will have a leg-length discrepancy unless the surface has been restored. Without this restoration, the talus moves up into the impacted tibial joint surface. The leg-length discrepancy alters the gait and affects the joints both above and below the ankle. Patients may need shoe lifts and other aids to give them equal leg length and near-normal gait. Leg-length discrepancy can affect the knee, the hip, and the lower back and add to the patient's overall disability.

EARLY IMMEDIATE (DAY OF INJURY TO ONE WEEK)

	Open Reduction and Internal Fixation	*External Fixation*	*Cast*
Stability	None.	None.	None.
Orthopaedics	Elevate leg to help decrease swelling.	Evaluate pin sites.	Trim to metatarsal heads. Check for adequate padding at edges.
Rehabilitation	Active range of motion at metatarsophalangeal (MTP) and knee joints.	Active range of motion at MTP and knee joints.	Range of motion at MTP joints.

TWO WEEKS

	Open Reduction and Internal Fixation	*External Fixation*	*Cast*
Stability	Minimal to none.	Minimal to none.	Minimal to none.
Orthopaedics	Remove sutures or staples. Evaluate viability of any grafts placed.	Evaluate pin sites and check for loosening of connectors or bars.	Check cast padding and edges. Repair any soft areas.
Rehabilitation	Active range of motion of the MTP and knee joints. Gentle active range of motion to the ankle joint out of bivalved cast or splint.	Active range of motion of the MTP and knee	Active range of motion of the MTP joints. joints.

FOUR TO SIX WEEKS

	Open Reduction and Internal Fixation	External Fixation	Cast
Stability	Partially stable.	Partially stable.	Partially stable.
Orthopaedics	If cast has been placed, evaluate for adequate cast padding. Trim to metatarsal heads.	May remove fixator. Replace with cast or other supportive device.	May change to patella tendon bearing (PTB) or shortleg cast if stable.
Rehabilitation	Active range of motion, to MTP joints, ankle joint, and knee.	Active range of motion to MTP joints, ankle joint, and knee.	Active range of motion to MTP joints, range ankle and knee as immobilization device allows.

SIX TO EIGHT WEEKS

	Open Reduction and Internal Fixation	External Fixation	Cast
Stability	Stable.	Stable.	Stable.
Orthopaedics	May remove cast if stable.	Remove fixator if not already done. Place in splint or other protective device if not fully stable.	If not already done, may change to short leg or PTB cast.
Rehabilitation	Begin resistive exercises of ankle and subtalar joint.	Begin resistive exercises of ankle and subtalar joint.	Continue to range ankle, knee, and MTP joints.

EIGHT TO TWELVE WEEKS

	Open Reduction and Internal Fixation	External Fixation	Cast
Stability	Stable.	Stable.	Stable.
Orthopaedics	Cast should be removed if not already done.	Remove fixator. Replace with short-leg cast if not fully stable.	May remove cast if not already done.
Rehabilitation	Continue resistive exercises of the ankle and subtalar joint.	Continue resistive exercises of the ankle and subtalar joint.	Begin active and active assistive and passive range of motion of ankle and subtalar joints. If still in cast, actively range MTP joints and perform isometrics of ankle and subtalar joint within cast.

BIBLIOGRAPHY

Bonar SK, Marsh JL. Tibial plafond fractures: changing principles of treatment. *J Am Acad Orthop Surg* 2:297–305, 1994.

Brumback RJ, McGarvey WC. Fractures of the tibial plafond: the pilon fracture. Evolving treatment concepts. *Orthop Clin North Am* 26:273–285, 1995.

Chapman M. Ankle injuries. In: Mann RA, ed. *Surgery of the Foot,* 5th ed. St. Louis: CV Mosby, 1986, pp. 572–576.

Geissler W, Tsao A. Tibial fractures. In: Rockwood CA, Green DP, eds. *Fractures in Adults,* 4th ed. Philadelphia: J.B. Lippincott, 1995, pp. 2036–2041.

Griffith GP, Thordarson DB. Tibial plafond fractures: limited internal fixation and a hybrid external fixator. *Foot Ankle* 17:8: 444–448, 1996.

Leone VJ, Reeland RT, Meinhard BP. The management of the soft tissues in pilon fractures. *Clin Orthop* 292:315–320, 1993.

Mann R. In: Chapman M, ed. *Operative Orthopaedics.* Philadelphia: J.B. Lippincott, 1993.

Manoli A II. Compartment syndromes of the foot: current concepts. *Foot Ankle* 10:340–344, 1990.

McFerran MA, Smith SW, Boulas HJ, et al. Complications encountered in the treatment of pilon fractures. *J Orthop Trauma* 6: 195–200, 1992.

Mizel M, Sobel M. In: Miller M, ed. *Review of Orthopaedics,* 2nd ed. Philadelphia: W.B. Saunders, 1996, pp. 241, 390.

Perry J. Ankle and foot gait deviations. In: Perry J, ed. *Gait Analysis.* Thorofare, NJ: SLACK, 1992, pp. 185–219.

Tile M. Fractures of the distal tibial metaphysis involving the ankle joint: the pilon fracture. In: Schatzker J, Tile M, eds. *The Rationale of Operative Fracture Care,* 2nd ed. Berlin: Springer, 1996, pp. 491–496, 605–607.

Trafton PG, Bray TJ, Simpson LA. Foot injuries. In: Browner B, Jupiter J, Levine AM, Trafton PG, eds. *Skeletal Trauma,* Vol. 2. Philadelphia: W.B. Saunders, 1992, pp. 1931–1941.

VanderGriend R, Michelson JD, Bone LB. Fractures of the ankle and distal part of the tibia. *Instructional Course Lectures* 46:311–321, 1997.

Yablon IG, Segal D. In: Evarts CM, ed. *Surgery of the Musculoskeletal System,* 2nd ed. New York: Churchill Livingstone, 1990, pp. 3849–3859.

CHAPTER *Thirty*

Ankle Fractures

ANNE P. MCCORMACK, MD

STANLEY HOPPENFELD, MD

INTRODUCTION

Definition

Ankle fractures include fractures of the medial and lateral malleoli as well as the distal articular surface of the tibia and fibula. (Fractures of the tibial plafond with extension into the pilon are discussed in Chapter 29.)

Fractures of the ankle are more specifically described as:

- Isolated lateral malleolar fractures (extraarticular; Figures 30-1 and 30-2)
- Bimalleolar fractures (intraarticular; Figures 30-3 and 30-4)
- Medial malleolar fractures (intraarticular; Figures 30-5 and 30-6)
- Bimalleolar equivalent fractures (intraarticular), in which the lateral malleolus is fractured and the medial side of the ankle mortise is widened (Figures 30-7 and 30-8)

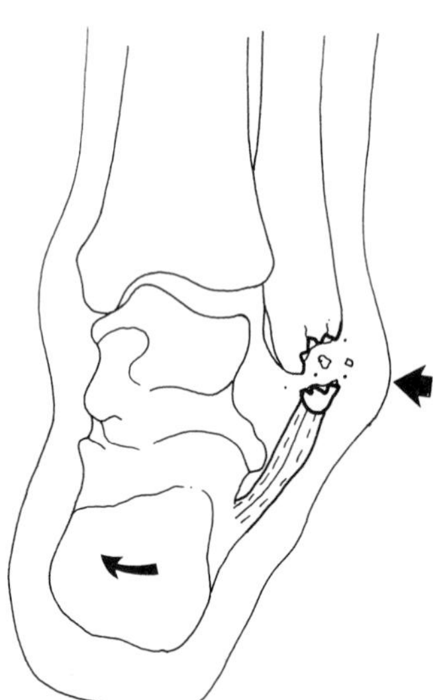

FIGURE 30-1 Lateral malleolar fracture. Avulsion of the distal portion of the lateral malleolus.

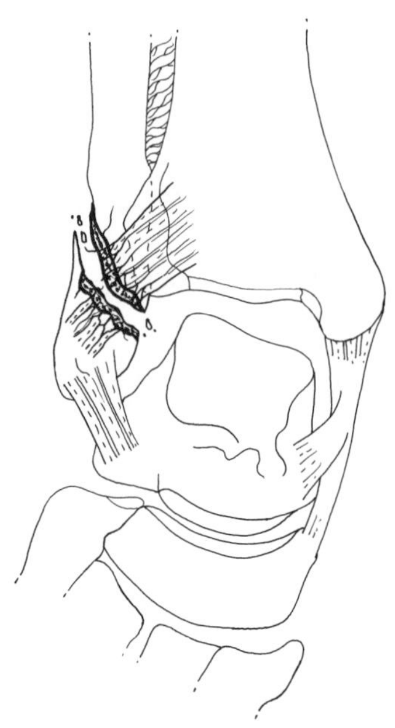

FIGURE 30-2 Isolated lateral malleolar fracture. Oblique fracture of the lateral malleolus at the level of the ankle mortise.

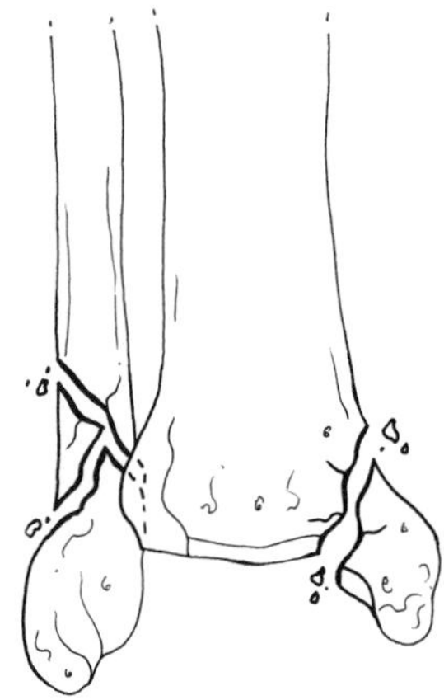

FIGURE 30-3 Bimalleolar fracture of the distal fibula with an oblique fracture of the medial malleolus.

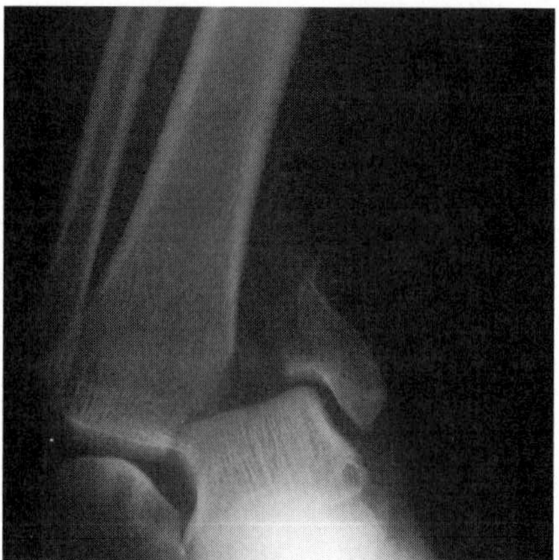

FIGURE 30-4 Bimalleolar fracture/dislocation of the ankle. Extreme example of a supination/adduction type of ankle fracture with dislocation of the talus from the tibia. Note the distal transverse fibula fracture and the vertical shear-type medial malleolar fracture.

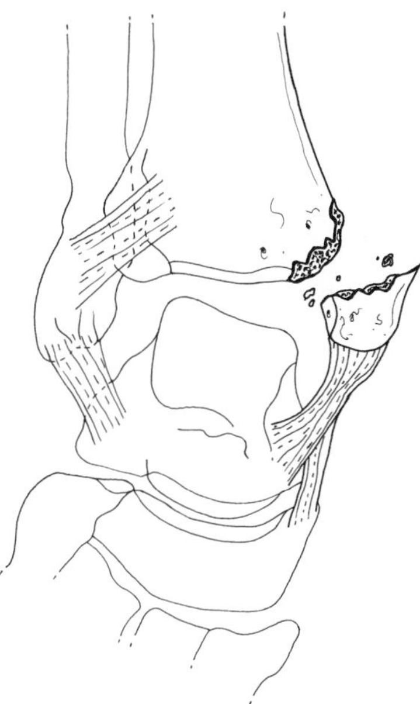

FIGURE 30-5 Medial malleolar fracture. Note that the medial malleolar fracture extends into the intraarticular surface of the tibial plafond.

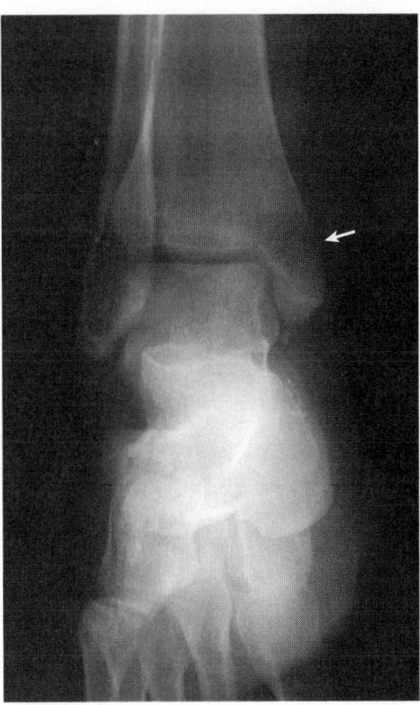

FIGURE 30-6 Minimally displaced medial malleolar fracture.

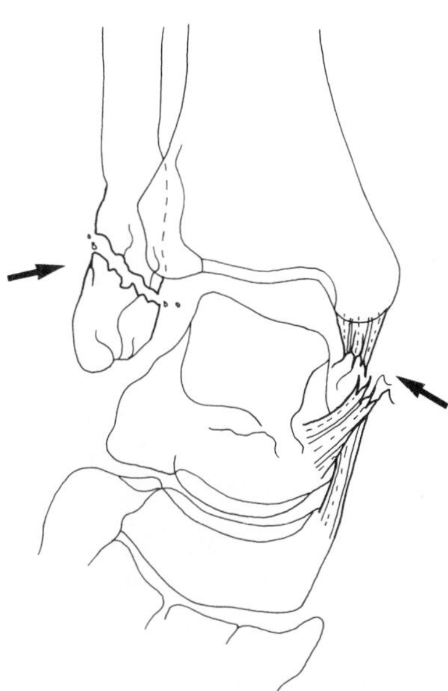

FIGURE 30-7 Bimalleolar equivalent fracture of the ankle. Note the oblique fracture of the fibula at the level of the ankle mortise and the disruption of the deltoid ligament on the medial side of the ankle. (This is equivalent to a medial malleolar fracture.) Disruption of the medial side in association with a lateral malleolar fracture often produces a lateral subluxation of the talus under the tibia.

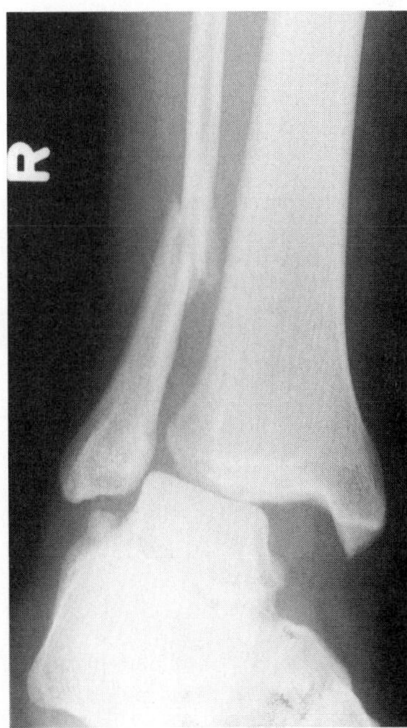

FIGURE 30-8 Bimalleolar equivalent fracture of the ankle. Note the oblique fracture of the fibula above the level of the ankle mortise and the disruption of the deltoid ligament on the medial side of the ankle, producing a subluxation of the talus laterally under the tibia. The disruption of the deltoid ligament is equivalent to a fracture of the medial malleolus.

- Trimalleolar fractures (intraarticular), involving the medial and lateral malleolus as well as the posterior aspect of the tibial plafond (posterior malleolus; Figure 30-9)

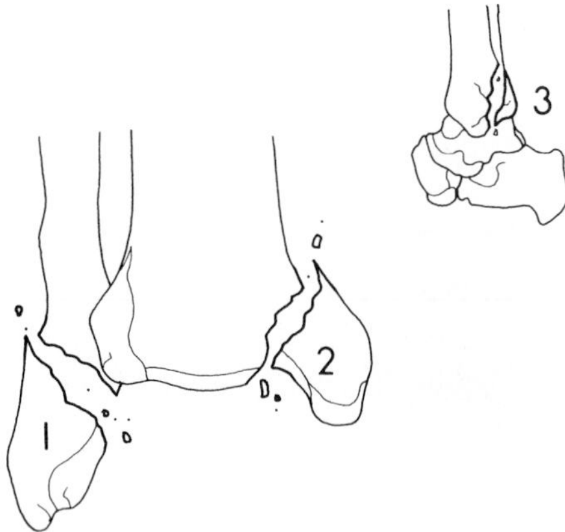

FIGURE 30-9 Trimalleolar fracture. Note the fracture of the lateral malleolus at the level of the ankle joint (1), oblique fracture of the medial malleolus (2), and fracture of the posterior malleolus (3), an avulsion fracture of the posterior tibia.

In addition, ankle fractures may disrupt the distal syndesmosis between the tibia and fibula. All ankle fractures involve some ligamentous injury.

Mechanism of Injury

Relatively low-energy forces, due to actions such as tripping on or twisting an ankle, are the most common cause of ankle fractures. Direct or indirect high-energy forces, such as those incurred in motor vehicle accidents, can also cause ankle fractures. Such fractures are often associated with significant soft-tissue injuries as well as dislocation of the ankle joint.

The pattern of ankle injury depends on the position of the foot at the time of injury, which can be in either supination or pronation. The combination of foot position and deforming force provides a characteristic pattern of ankle fracture. The four most common deforming forces (in order of frequency) are supination/external rotation, pronation/external rotation, supination/adduction, and pronation/abduction (*see* Figures 30-20, 30-21, 30-22, 30-23, 30-24, and 30-25). The body moves on a planted foot, which propagates the injury. Twisting produces external rotation. Falling to one side produces adduction or abduction injury.

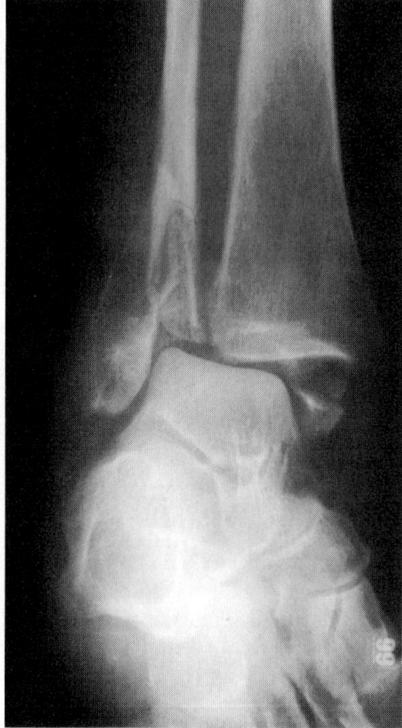

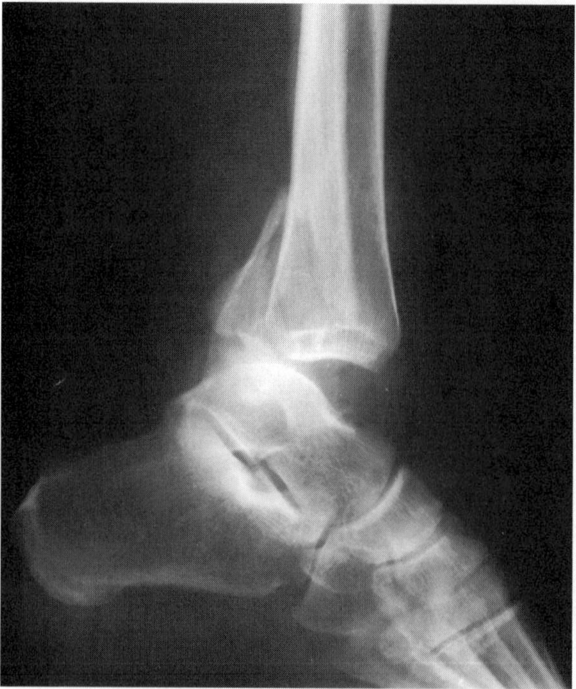

FIGURE 30-9A,B Trimalleolar fracture involving the medial malleolus, lateral malleolus, and posterior malleolus.

Treatment Goals

Orthopaedic Objectives

Alignment

The ankle mortise is the joint formed by the surfaces of the lateral malleolus, tibial plafond, and medial malleolus, which articulates with the underlying dome of the talus. Restoration of the ankle mortise is of critical importance for pain-free weight bearing across the ankle joint. Restoring the position of the talus underneath the plafond is also crucial (Figures 30-10, 30-11, and 30-12).

Loss of articular congruity by as little as 1 mm in the ankle joint may lead to posttraumatic arthritis and significant long-term disability, pain, and limp.

Stability

Reconstruction of the medial, lateral, and posterior malleoli is crucial to the static (standing still) and dynamic (walking) stability of the ankle joint.

Reconstitution or healing of ligamentous structures that may have been damaged by a fracture is also important for the dynamic stability of the ankle and proper distribution of forces during gait. This is espe-

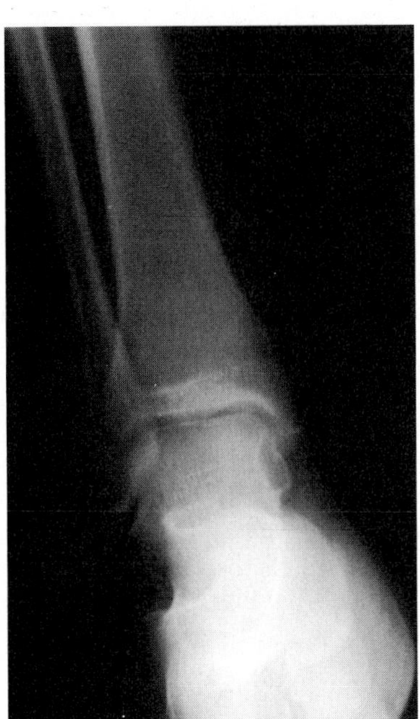

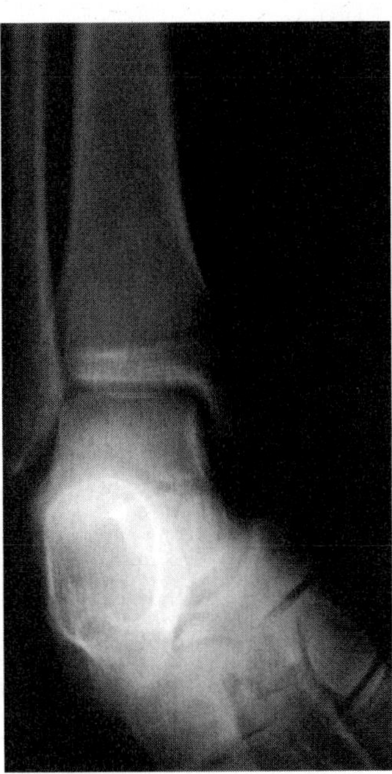

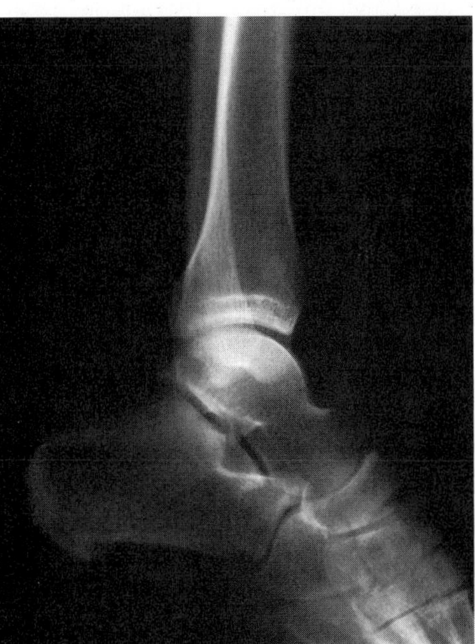

FIGURE 30-10 *(above, left)* Normal ankle (anteroposterior view). Note the talus lying beneath the distal tibia (tibial plafond).

FIGURE 30-11 *(above, middle)* Mortise view of the ankle. Anteroposterior view with the ankle in 20 degrees of internal rotation (oblique view). This view is taken to visualize the ankle mortise, which is formed by the tibial plafond lying over the talus and lateral malleolus. To confirm an intact joint, a space equivalent to that seen on the mortise view should be visualized between the medial malleolus and talus, tibial plafond and talus, and lateral malleolus and talus.

FIGURE 30-12 *(above, right)* Lateral view of the ankle. This view is used to visualize fractures of the lateral and posterior malleolus.

cially important for a patient with recurrent instability, in which the ligaments may have to be surgically reconstructed.

Rehabilitation Objectives

Range of Motion

Restore the full range of motion of the ankle joint in all planes.

Inadequate reduction or stabilization of the ankle joint can lead to significant loss of motion, specifically plantar flexion and dorsiflexion. Residual loss of range of motion of the tibiotalar joint may increase stress on the subtalar articulation and the midtarsal joints because they compensate for motion lost at the tibiotalar joint (Table 30-1).

TABLE 30-1 *Ankle Ranges of Motion*

Motion	Normal[a]	Functional
Ankle plantar flexion	45°	20°
Ankle dorsiflexion	20°[b]	10°
Foot inversion	35°	10°
Foot eversion	25°	10°

[a] These are average ranges.
[b] Range of motion most frequently lost after fracture.

Muscle Strength

Improve the strength of the muscles affected by the fracture or subsequent immobilization:

Plantar flexors of the ankle and foot:

- Gastrocnemius
- Soleus
- Tibialis posterior (also acts as an invertor)
- Flexor digitorum longus
- Flexor hallucis longus

Dorsiflexors of the ankle and foot:

- Tibialis anterior (also acts as invertor of the foot)
- Extensor digitorum longus
- Extensor hallucis longus

Evertors of the foot:

- Peroneus longus
- Peroneus brevis

Invertors of the foot:

- Tibialis posterior (also acts as a plantar flexor)
- Tibialis anterior (also acts as a dorsiflexor)

Functional Goals

Restore gait to its preinjury level.

Expected Time of Bone Healing

Extraarticular malleolar (isolated lateral malleolar) fractures: Six to 10 weeks.
Intraarticular malleolar (bimalleolar, trimalleolar, bimalleolar equivalent, and medial malleolar) fractures: Eight to 12 weeks.

Expected Duration of Rehabilitation

After cast removal:

Extraarticular malleolar fractures: Twelve to 16 weeks.
Intraarticular malleolar fractures: Sixteen to 24 weeks.

Methods of Treatment

Cast

Biomechanics: Stress-sharing device.

Mode of bone healing: Secondary, with callus formation.

Indications: Nondisplaced or minimally displaced malleolar fractures can usually be treated satisfactorily in a non–weight-bearing long leg cast with the ankle in neutral position.

Isolated fractures of the distal fibula may also be treated in this manner or, more commonly, in a short leg cast with weight bearing as tolerated if there is good pain control.

Minimally to moderately displaced fractures in patients who are not amenable to surgical intervention may be treated with closed reduction and casting if a satisfactory reduction (maintenance of the ankle mortise) is obtained and the foot can be maintained in a relatively neutral position. The patient needs frequent radiographic monitoring of the reduction until the healing is secure with good callus formation at 3 to 4 weeks. If the reduction is lost and rereduction cannot be obtained, an open reduction and internal fixation is necessary (Figures 30-13 and 30-14).

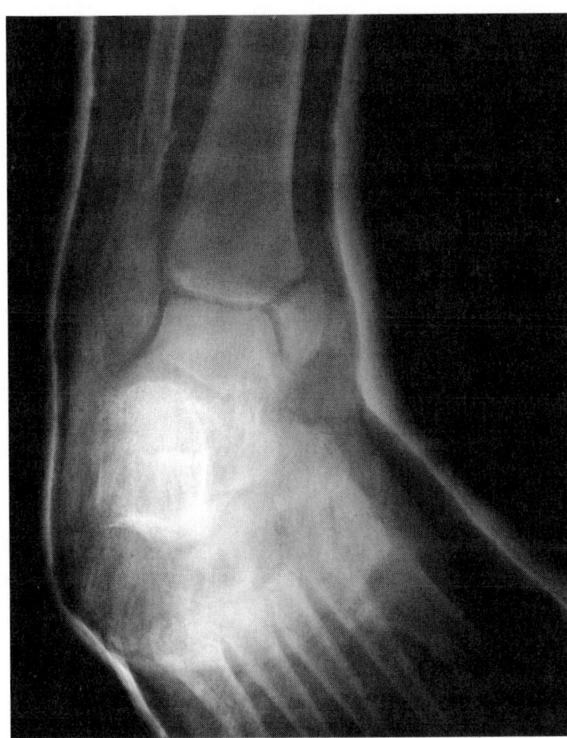

FIGURE 30-13 Bimalleolar fracture treated with cast mobilization. Note the adequate bony alignment of the fibula and inadequate alignment of the medial malleolus with a gap seen at the fracture site. Fracture reduction cannot be maintained in a cast; this patient required open reduction and internal fixation.

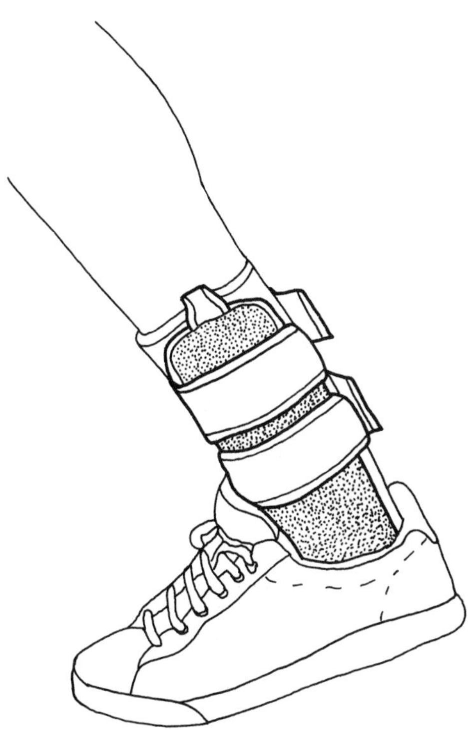

FIGURE 30-14 Stirrup air cast used for the treatment of avulsion fractures of the distal fibula to decrease postinjury pain and allow early mobilization.

Open Reduction and Internal Fixation

Biomechanics: Stress-shielding device with rigid fixation (compression); stress-sharing system without rigid fixation.

Mode of bone healing: Primary, with rigid fixation.

Indications: Displaced malleolar fractures and any syndesmotic disruptions often involve significant subluxation or dislocation of the tibiotalar joint (ankle mortise). Anatomic reduction is often difficult to maintain without placing the foot in an extreme position. Fractures that are not amenable to closed reduction or are inherently anatomically unstable require open reduction and internal fixation utilizing Kirschner wires (K-wires), screws, or plates to fix the ankle joint rigidly while the bone and soft tissues heal. This also allows the patient to be mobilized in a short leg cast, which is markedly less cumbersome and debilitating than a long leg cast. It also allows earlier weight bearing (Figures 30-14, 30-15, 30-16, 30-17, 30-18, 30-19, 30-20, 30-21, 30-22, 30-23, 30-24, 30-25, 30-26, 30-27, 30-28, and 30-29).

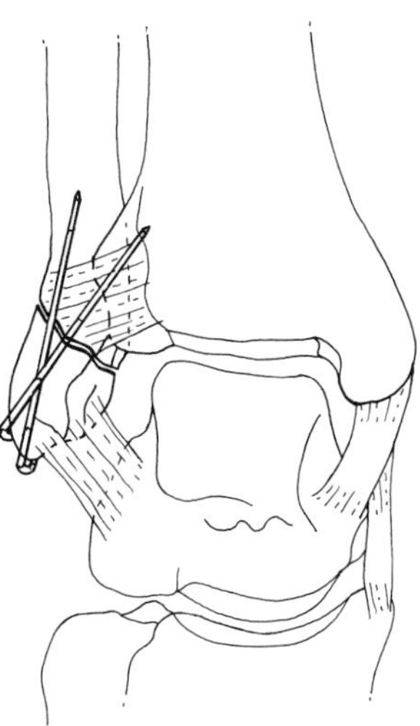

FIGURE 30-15 Lateral malleolar fractures treated with pin fixation, an alternative to plate fixation, although less secure.

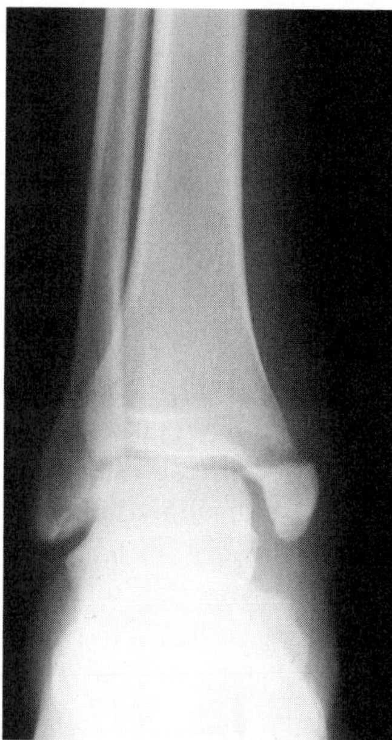

FIGURE 30-16 Medial malleolar fracture. Note the transverse fracture of the medial malleolus, with a displaced and rotated medial malleolar fragment.

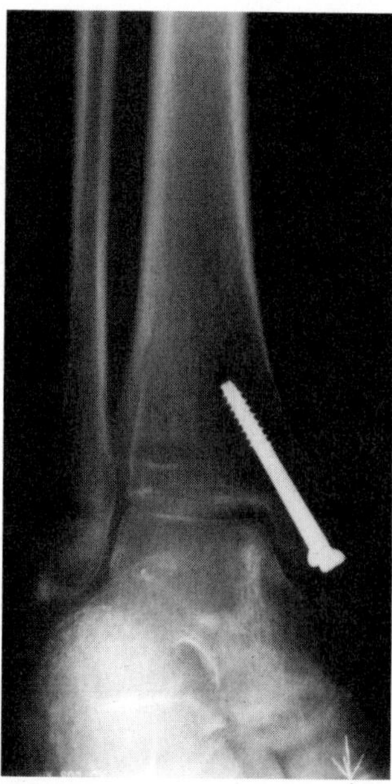

FIGURE 30-17 Medial malleolar fracture treated with parallel screw fixation. This is preferred to achieve bony compression across the fracture site. The screws achieve a lag effect, with the threads at the distal end of the screw obtaining purchase at the proximal side of the fracture.

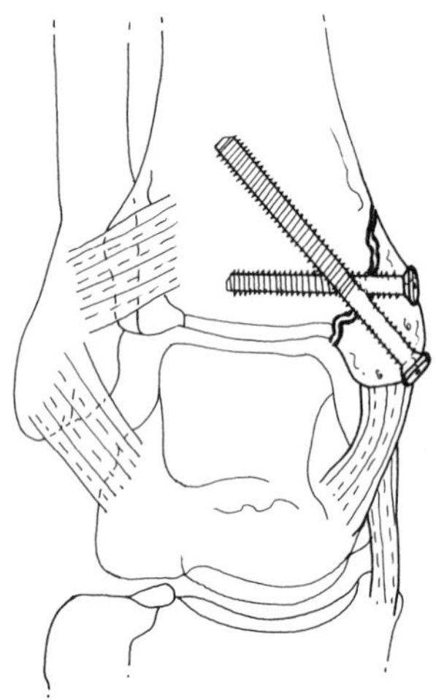

FIGURE 30-18 Oblique medial malleolar fracture treated with two screws. This fixation is better performed with parallel screws inserted in a lag fashion.

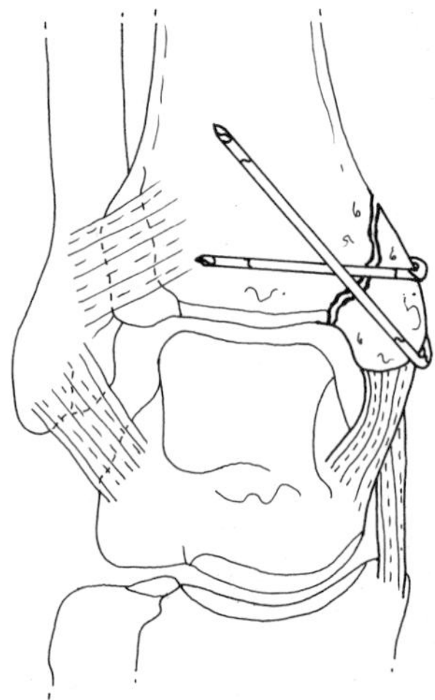

FIGURE 30-19 Oblique medial malleolar fracture treated with pin fixation. Pin fixation is inferior to screw fixation because the lag effect is not achieved across the fracture site. Early motion usually is not allowed with pin fixation.

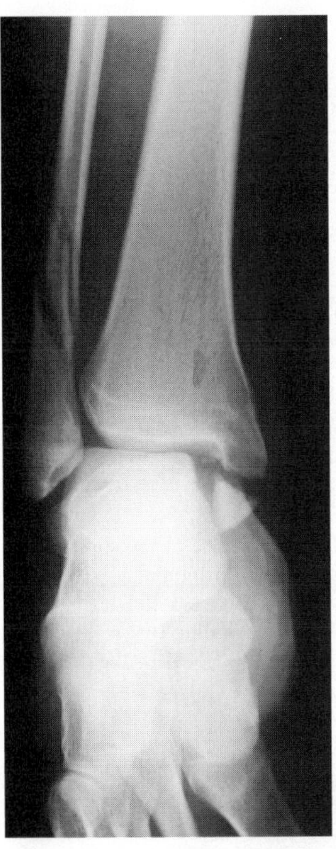

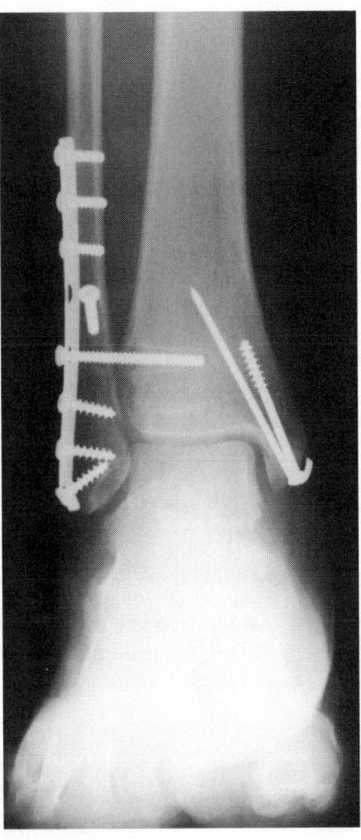

FIGURE 30-20 *(far left)* Bimalleolar fracture of the pronation/external rotation type. Note the oblique fracture of the lateral malleolus above the level of the ankle mortise and the transverse fracture of the medial malleolus. Also note the lateral subluxation of the talus under the tibia with the associated fibula fracture above the level of the ankle joint, which indicates a rupture of the inferior tibiofibular syndesmosis. This fracture requires fixation of the lateral malleolus and medial malleolus and restoration of the syndesmosis.

FIGURE 30-21 *(left)* Bimalleolar fracture of the ankle with disruption of the inferior tibiofibular syndesmosis. This is a pronation/external rotation injury. The fibular fracture is fixed with a one-third tubular plate and screws; the medial malleolus is fixed with a lag screw and pin fixation; the syndesmosis is restored with a syndesmotic screw through the fibular plate.

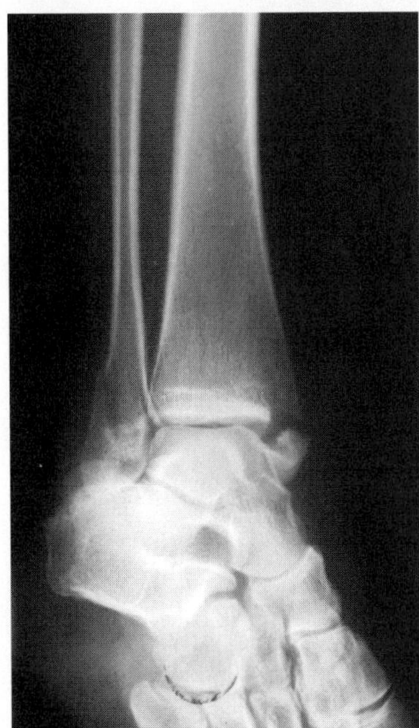

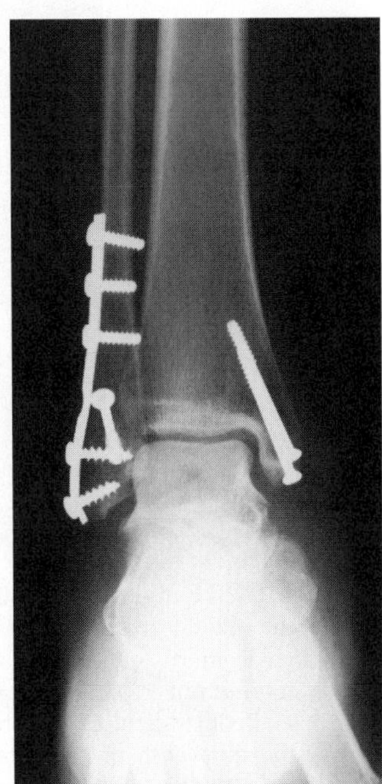

FIGURE 30-22 *(far left)* Bimalleolar fracture of the supination/external rotation type, the most common mechanism of injury. Note the oblique fibular fracture at the level of the ankle joint and the oblique medial malleolar fracture.

FIGURE 30-23 *(left)* Bimalleolar fracture, supination/external rotation type. Fibular fracture treated with a one-third tubular plate and screws with the addition of a lag screw across the fracture. The medial malleolus is fixed with two parallel lag screws.

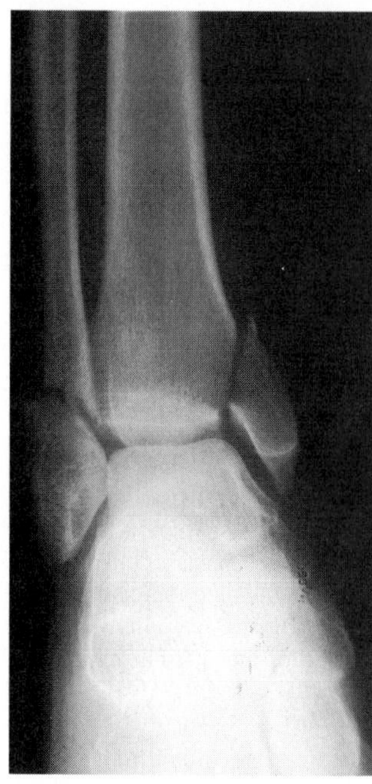

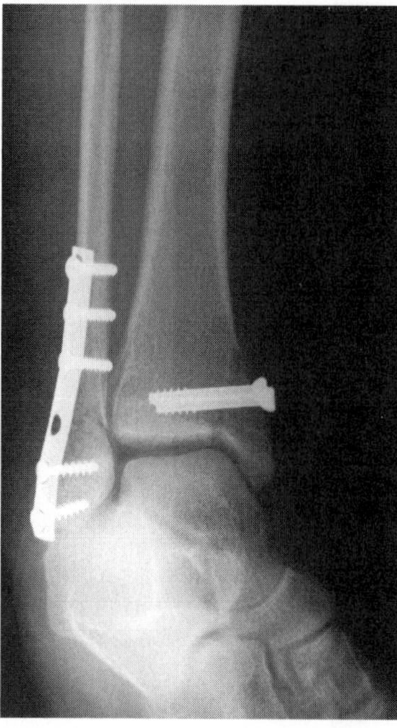

FIGURE 30-24 *(far left)* A bimalleolar fracture of the ankle, supination/adduction type. The lateral malleolar fracture is a transverse fracture at the level of the ankle joint, and the medial malleolar fracture is a vertical shear-type fracture.

FIGURE 30-25 *(left)* Bimalleolar fracture of the supination/adduction type, treated with a one-third tubular plate and screws of the lateral malleolus and two parallel lag screws across the medial malleolus, perpendicular to the fracture. Note the restoration of the ankle mortise after the fracture reduction and fixation.

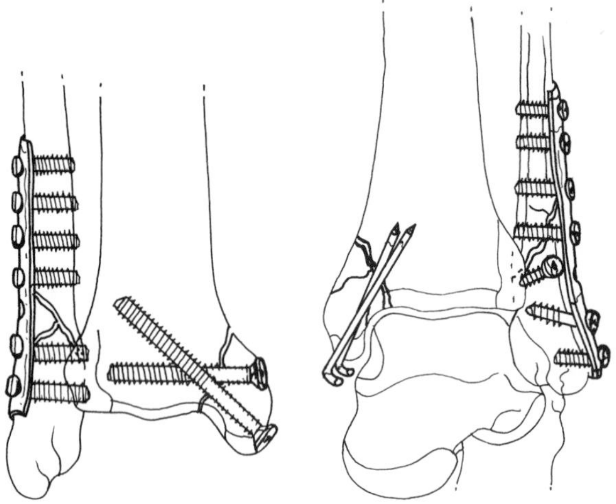

FIGURE 30-26 *(above, left)* Bimalleolar fracture, with the lateral malleolus treated with plate and screws and the medial malleolus with two lag screws. The lag screws are best positioned parallel to achieve compression across the fracture site.

FIGURE 30-27 *(above, right)* Bimalleolar fracture of the ankle treated with plate and screw fixation of the lateral malleolus and a lag screw across the lateral malleolar fracture site. The medial malleolus is fixed with parallel pins. This fixation is inferior to screw fixation, which achieves a lag effect across the fracture site to the medial malleolus.

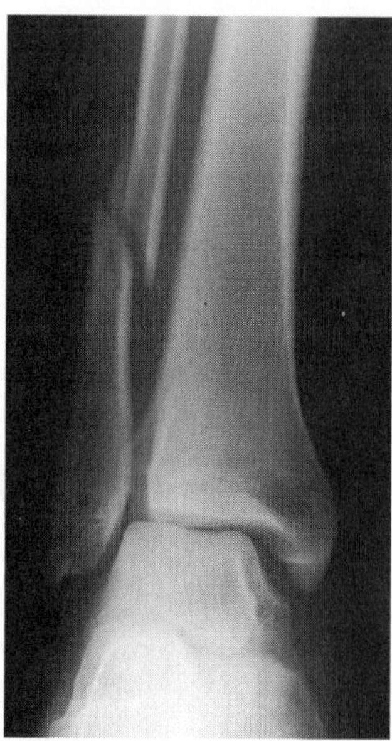

FIGURE 30-28 Bimalleolar equivalent fracture of the ankle. Note the oblique fracture of the lateral malleolus above the level of the ankle mortise and the disruption of the medial side of the ankle mortise due to a deltoid ligament tear (this is equivalent to a medial malleolus fracture). Note the lateral subluxation of the talus under the tibia with the associated high fibular fracture, indicating an inferior tibiofibular syndesmotic tear or disruption. This fracture is treated with plate fixation and reduction of the lateral malleolus and reduction of the syndesmosis with a syndesmotic screw.

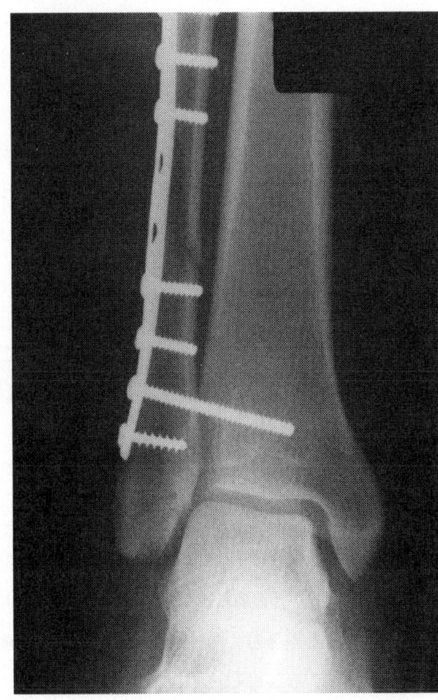

FIGURE 30-29 Bimalleolar-equivalent fracture treated with reduction and plate fixation of the lateral malleolus and a syndesmotic screw through the lateral fibular plate parallel with the ankle mortise. Note the reduction of the ankle mortise and closing of the medial clear space.

Special Considerations of the Fracture

Age

Elderly patients have an increased risk of poor healing in both skin and bone, and may exhibit osteopenia such that the screws do not hold well. Less-than-perfect anatomic alignment must be weighed carefully considering the risks of surgery versus the resultant disability in an elderly patient.

Systemic Disease

A patient with systemic disease who may not be mobile because of the energy expenditure needed for a long leg cast or who has a skin or neuropathic condition that precludes long-term immobilization in a cast requires surgical intervention. The risks and benefits of various treatments for patients with systemic disease (e.g., diabetes) must be carefully considered, such as skin not healing and infection versus early mobilization.

Articular Involvement

Fractures of the ankle, when they involve the medial or lateral malleolus as well as more than 20% to 25% of the posterior malleolus, require anatomic reduction to restore normal function of the ankle joint. If the fracture involves the plafond or pilon, rehabilitation may be complicated by pain and antalgic gait. Posttraumatic arthritis is a complication of intraarticular ankle fractures. A patient with intractable pain after fracture healing is complete may benefit from an ankle arthrodesis, or total ankle joint replacement.

Fracture Pattern

Ankle fractures usually involve the lateral or medial malleoli and other structures such as the posterior malleolus (posterior aspect of the tibial plafond); the medial, anterior, and lateral ligament complexes; and the distal tibiofibular syndesmosis.

Several classifications of ankle fractures have been described, including those by Danis-Weber and Lauge-Hansen. These classifications are based on the more common mechanisms of injury and generalized information about the orderly progression of injury to the bones and ligaments of the ankle. Ligamentous and other soft-tissue injuries that occur at the time of fracture must also be considered. An extensive network of ligaments surrounds the ankle. The deltoid ligament on the medial side, the anterior tibiofibular ligament on the lateral side, and the calcaneofibular ligament on the lateral side provide dynamic stability. A distal tibiofibular syndesmotic ligament just proximal to the ankle is also crucial for maintaining the congruity of the ankle joint. All of these must be considered in both treatment and rehabilitation.

Open Fractures

Any open fracture of the ankle must be treated initially with aggressive irrigation, débridement, and intravenous antibiotics. The fracture may be amenable only to limited internal fixation when there is much soft-tissue injury or bone fragmentation. Open reduction and internal fixation should be performed at the time of injury, if possible. Application of an external fixator is useful when soft-tissue devitalization is a main component of the injury.

Compartment Syndrome

The ankle itself usually is not involved in a tibial compartment syndrome. However, the associated injury to the foot may cause sufficient swelling to produce a compartment syndrome of the foot, particularly with a high-energy (but not a low-energy) ankle fracture.

Any suspicion of compartment syndrome, especially after a cast has been placed on a swollen foot and ankle, requires that the cast and padding be immediately split. Pressures measured in the foot or leg indicate any need for fasciotomy. The cast may need to be bivalved so that the soft-tissue swelling can be adequately accommodated during the early posttrauma period.

In a severe fracture or dislocation of the ankle, the plantar flexors or the peronei can lose strength because of injury to the tendon or tendon sheath.

Missed compartment syndromes of the leg (which are rare) or the foot can cause muscle contracture in any of the previously noted muscles, resulting in severe loss of residual muscle strength, deformity, and decreased range of motion.

Tendon and Ligamentous Injuries

Although tendon injuries are not common in ankle fractures, tendons can become trapped in a fracture site. Surgical repair must be considered for any tendon injury resulting from ankle trauma. If displaced tendons inhibit reduction, they need to be relocated at the time of surgery.

Complete rupture of the lateral collateral ligament complex may be treated conservatively; surgical repair has not been shown to improve ankle function. However, if a patient shows late instability with frequent sprain of the ankle, then reconstruction of this lateral ligament complex prevents recurrent inversion injury to the ankle joint (Figure 30-30).

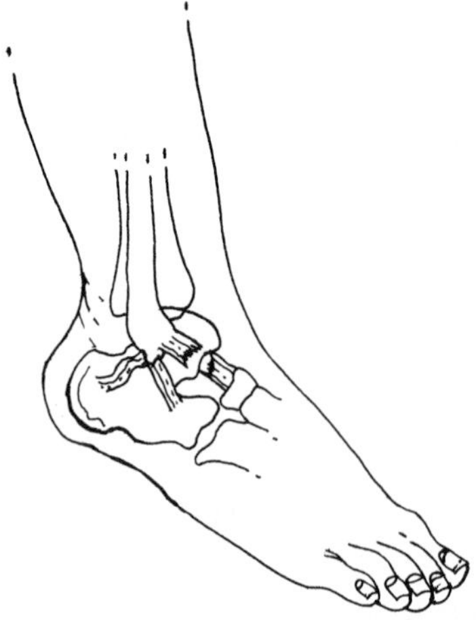

FIGURE 30-30 Lateral ligament ankle sprain. There is disruption of the anterior talofibular ligament and attenuation of the calcaneofibular and posterior talofibular ligaments. Recurrent sprains of the ankle of the inversion type may produce a chronic attenuation of the lateral ligamentous complex, leading to ankle instability.

The medial ligament complex is rarely injured as an isolated injury. On occasion, it may be torn in association with a medial malleolar fracture, but it is well restored after internal fixation of the fracture. Most commonly, it is disrupted in combination with a lateral malleolar fracture, known as a bimalleolar equivalent fracture (*see* Figures 30-28 and 30-29).

The distal tibiofibular syndesmosis may be disrupted in a fibular fracture that occurs above the ankle joint. If the syndesmosis is unstable after the associated fracture has been repaired, then surgical screw fixation of the syndesmosis is required.

Rupture of the posterior tibial tendon usually results in a symptomatic flat-foot deformity unless repaired. Lacerations or ruptures of other tendons across the foot may be less disabling if they are not repaired.

Some tendons, such as the extensor tendons of the lesser toes, are not as functionally significant and can be allowed to scar in without loss of function.

Associated Injury

Fractures of the ankle joint may occur from low- or high-energy forces. In either case, there is usually soft-tissue swelling across the ankle and often into the foot and the lower leg. The dorsalis pedis as well as posterior tibial pulses should be monitored carefully, and all soft-tissue swelling should be measured and checked every 2 hours during the first 24 hours to screen for a foot compartment syndrome. Increased pain with passive range of motion of the toes and decreased sensation are signs associated with compartment syndrome. Significant swelling of the foot or ankle can lead to necrosis and loss of soft tissue over the dorsum and particularly the dorsolateral aspect of the foot, potentially requiring soft-tissue skin grafting.

Loss of the posterior tibial nerve is particularly disabling because that nerve provides sensation to the weight-bearing (plantar) surface of the foot. Fortunately, this is a rare injury, seen only in high-energy accidents with major joint disruption. If it cannot be repaired, the patient runs a high risk for development of plantar breakdown, pressure ulcers, and associated complications.

Injuries to other nerves that cross the ankle are also rare and seen only in high-energy injuries. These can result in painful neuromas embedded in scar tissue. This can be prevented by transecting injured nerves and burying them deep in the soft tissues or bone away from scar and moving or weight-bearing structures.

Weight Bearing

Initially, no weight bearing is permitted with either open reduction and internal fixation or casting, except for isolated nondisplaced fibular fractures. After stable internal fixation, the patient is non-weight bearing for 6 weeks and then begins progressive weight bearing when there has been sufficient healing.

Gait

Stance Phase

The stance phase comprises 60% of the gait cycle.

Heel Strike

As weight is transferred through the tibial plafond onto the surface of the talus, there may be pain for patients who have sustained intraarticular fractures. A patient who has been immobilized for a long period and has weakness in the dorsiflexors (which are attempting to dorsiflex or decelerate the foot to prevent slap) experiences muscular pain and may have an initial foot slap. Any disruption of the cartilaginous surface of the tibial plafond or the talus causes discomfort because weight is applied to a smaller area of remaining intact articular cartilage. As weight is transferred through the tibial shaft into the foot, nerve endings receive increased pressure, thereby increasing pain. Rapid degeneration of the remaining cartilage may occur because of this increased load over a smaller area (*see* Figure 6-1).

Foot-Flat

Pain continues as the tibia rotates over the talus, transferring weight toward the midfoot. At this point, the plantar flexors contract and there may be muscular soreness and tension in the back of the calf. The anterior muscle group (mainly the extensor hallucis longus and tibialis anterior) is weak and undergoes eccentric elongation to allow the sole of the foot to reach the floor; this may be painful. In addition, the joint capsule is tight, and stretching during weight bearing causes pain (*see* Figure 6-2).

Mid-Stance

Single stance begins and is usually the most painful portion of the gait cycle. The foot is positioned to take the weight of the entire body as the opposite foot lifts. The increased pressure transferred through the tibia into the talus causes discomfort in the ankle joint. The patient attempts to shorten this phase, hopping off the affected leg as soon as possible (antalgic gait; *see* Figure 6-3).

Push-off

This may be the least painful portion of the gait cycle. The patient starts to unload the hind foot and transfer weight onto the opposite leg. Impaired push-off for the affected foot is likely because the plantar flexors are weak and the joint capsule is tight. In general, the patient takes smaller steps and spends less time on the affected foot (*see* Figure 6-4).

Swing Phase

The swing phase comprises 40% of the gait cycle.

In the swing phase, the dorsiflexors must bring the toes up. This generates forces across the ankle joint that may cause discomfort. Because push-off is inadequate and patients tend to try to limit the amount of dorsiflexion or plantar flexion, they may compensate by knee flexion to have the foot clear the ground (*see* Figures 6-6, 6-7, and 6-8).

Any incongruity in the joint surfaces or damage to the cartilage predisposes the patient to early degenerative arthritis. This narrows the joint space and causes rough transitioning of the tibia as it attempts to slide over the upper surface of the talus. With joint surface disruption, posttraumatic arthritic changes may cause severe pain across the tibiotalar joint. Fusion relieves the discomfort, but is rarely needed.

Stresses not absorbed by the tibiotalar joint are transmitted to the subtalar joint and the medial plantar arch in an attempt to compensate for the derangement in the ankle joint. This increases energy expenditure, interrupts smooth translation or forward progression of walking, and compromises the normal navigation of uneven ground surfaces.

TREATMENT

Treatment: Early to Immediate (Day of Injury to One Week)

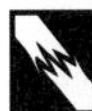

Bone Healing

Stability at fracture site: None

Stage of bone healing: Inflammatory phase. The fracture hematoma is colonized by inflammatory cells, and débridement of the fracture begins.

X-ray: No callus.

Orthopaedic and Rehabilitation Considerations

Physical Examination

Note if the patient feels that the cast is loose. Check for toe capillary refill and sensation. The toes should be pink, with brisk refill after light compression. Evaluate passive plantar flexion and dorsiflexion for increased pain. It should be possible to reach the first web space of the toe through the cast and stroke it lightly with a blunt instrument to ensure that there is no deep peroneal nerve compression in the lower ankle and foot. This is not a common injury.

If external fixators have been used, check the pin sites for evidence of drainage or erythema and treat appropriately. In cases of crush injury, evaluate the dorsum of the foot for any evidence of skin sloughing.

Dangers

Evaluate for any evidence of a dorsal foot compartment syndrome as well as tibial compartment syndrome. Pay special attention to complaints of pain, paresthesia, and cast discomfort. For fractures that were open or had significant fracture blisters, evaluate the skin for any evidence of erythema or drainage, which may indicate infection. The patient should be advised to keep the extremity elevated above the heart level and place ice packs over the ankle and foot to decrease the swelling.

Radiography

Obtain and check anteroposterior, lateral, and mortise (15-degree internal rotation) radiographs of the ankle to evaluate for any loss of correction. If internal fixation has been applied, ensure that all screws, plates, and K-wires are still in the correct position. Oblique views should be obtained if the fracture cannot be adequately assessed with the aforementioned radiographs.

Weight Bearing

All fractures of the ankle should be non-weight bearing. The single exception is an isolated distal fibula fracture without any further ligamentous or bony disruption. This injury may be weight bearing as tolerated in a short leg cast.

Range of Motion

Patients in a long leg cast may begin active range-of-motion exercises for the metatarsophalangeal joints.

Patients who have had internal fixation may still be in a postoperative short leg splint and may begin range of motion of the knee and the metatarsophalangeal joints. If stable fixation is achieved and there is good bone stock, the patient may begin early range of motion at the ankle.

Muscle Strength

Maintain the strength of the quadriceps with quadriceps sets. Patients in long leg casts may attempt isometric quadriceps exercises by trying to extend the knee within the cast and by attempting to lift the heel of the cast off the bed. Patients in external fixators may engage in quadriceps strengthening as well. No strengthening of the dorsiflexors, plantar flexors, invertors, or evertors of the ankle should be prescribed.

Functional Activities

Patients are instructed in stand/pivot transfers using assistive devices such as crutches, with no weight bearing on the affected extremity. Patients should don pants on the affected extremity first and doff them from the unaffected extremity.

Gait

The patient is instructed in a non–weight-bearing, two-point gait in which the crutches are one unit and the unaffected extremity the other unit (*see* Figure 6-16). The patient climbs stairs one step at a time by placing the good foot first, then hopping up to the step with the crutches and the affected extremity. The patient descends stairs placing the crutches first, followed by the unaffected extremity, one step at a time (*see* Figures 6-20, 6-21, 6-22, 6-23, 6-24, and 6-25).

Methods of Treatment: Specific Aspects

Cast

Evaluate the condition of the long leg cast. Check the cast margins and make sure they are adequately padded. The cast must reach the metatarsal heads but should allow free movement of the metatarsophalangeal joints. Evaluate the skin at the edges of the cast to make sure that swelling has not caused skin breakdown and that there is no evidence of cyanosis or compartment syndrome. If the cast has softened under the foot, reinforce and repair it. Continue with metatarsophalangeal joint range of motion. Patients in a short leg cast should continue knee range-of-motion exercise.

Open Reduction and Internal Fixation

If the patient is in a short leg cast, check the cast margins to make sure they are well padded. Again, the metatarsophalangeal joints should have free movement. Also ensure that there is no irritation at the knee in the popliteal area or fibular neck from a cast that is placed too high or has inadequate padding. Look for any breakdown of the skin at the cast edges and trim appropriately. Repair any breakdown or softening of the cast.

If the patient is not yet in a cast, examine the padding to make sure there is no irritation or constriction from the splint. Evaluate any surgical incisions for evidence of infection. Continue range of motion of the metatarsophalangeal joints as well as range of motion of the knee and strengthening of the quadriceps.

Prescription

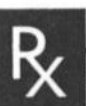

DAY ONE TO ONE WEEK

Range of Motion

For rigidly fixed fractures, active range of motion at metatarsophalangeal joints and knee joint. No ankle range of motion.

For nonrigidly fixed fractures, range of motion at metatarsophalangeal joint. No range of motion at ankle or knee.

Muscle Strength No strengthening exercises to ankle or foot. Quadriceps isometric exercises as tolerated.

Functional Activities Non–weight-bearing stand/pivot transfers and ambulation with assistive devices.

Weight Bearing None, except weight bearing as tolerated for nondisplaced distal fibula fractures.

Treatment: Two Weeks

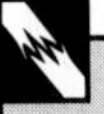

BONE HEALING

Stability at fracture site: None to minimal.

Stage of bone healing: Beginning of reparative phase. Osteoprogenitor cells differentiate into osteoblasts that lay down woven bone.

X-ray: No changes noted. Fracture lines are visible; no callus present.

Orthopaedic and Rehabilitation Considerations

Physical Examination

Check for capillary refill of the toes and sensation of the toes and, if possible, the first dorsal web space. Check the active and passive range of motion of all metatarsophalangeal and interphalangeal joints.

Dangers

Pay particular attention to complaints of pain, paresthesia, and cast discomfort, which may be caused by pressure points at the medial or lateral malleoli or over other exposed bony surfaces such as the anterior tibia and the knee. These areas may have not been adequately padded.

The patient should be made aware that any pronounced swelling could lead to skin sloughing, and should be immediately brought to the physician's attention. The patient should be advised to keep the extremity elevated above the level of the heart to control swelling.

Radiography

Check radiographs in anteroposterior, lateral, and mortise views to assess any loss of reduction and to determine that implanted hardware is still in its original position (*see* Figures 30-10, 30-11, and 30-12). Look for evidence of early callus. Oblique views may be obtained if the fracture pattern cannot be well delineated on the aforementioned radiographs.

Weight Bearing

All fractures remain non-weight bearing except nondisplaced distal fibula fractures. Toe-touch weight bearing is allowed for rigidly fixed fractures.

Range of Motion

Patients should continue active and passive range of motion at the metatarsophalangeal joints. Patients who have had internal fixation and are not in a long leg cast should continue active range of motion at the knee.

Muscle Strength

Once the patient's pain has subsided, begin active range of motion with flexion and extension of the toes. Repetitive movement of the toes strengthens the flexors and extensors across the ankle.

Patients with rigidly fixed fractures can perform isometric dorsiflexion and plantar flexion exercises within the cast.

Maintain the strength of the quadriceps.

Functional Activities

Continue with stand/pivot transfers using crutches or a walker.

Gait

Continue a non–weight-bearing gait with crutches. If weight bearing is allowed, as for nondisplaced fibula fractures, the patient may bear weight to tolerance using a two- or three-point gait (*see* Figures 6-16 and 6-17).

Methods of Treatment: Specific Aspects

Cast

Trim the cast to allow visualization of the toes to the metatarsophalangeal joints. The cast usually is not changed at this visit unless there has been a loss of reduction. Reinforce any cast that has broken down at the foot or at the metatarsophalangeal joints. The cast probably is not loose because there usually is residual swelling. Continue with metatarsophalangeal joint range of motion. Patients in a short leg cast should continue range of motion at the knee.

Open Reduction and Internal Fixation

All patients are in a cast except for those who had significant open fractures that required external fixation. They should continue range of motion of the metatarsophalangeal joints as well as range of motion of the knee and strengthening of the quadriceps.

Prescription

TWO WEEKS

Precautions Patients treated in long leg cast or external fixator do not have stable fractures.

Range of Motion

For rigidly fixed fractures, active range of motion of the metatarsophalangeal joints and knee joint. No range of motion to ankle.

For nonrigidly fixed fractures, active range of motion of the metatarsophalangeal joints. No range of motion of the ankle or knee.

Muscle Strength

For rigidly fixed fractures, isometric exercises of dorsiflexors and plantar flexors of the toes and ankle. No resistive exercises.

For nonrigidly fixed fractures, no strengthening exercises.

Functional Activities Non–weight-bearing stand/pivot transfers. Ambulation with assistive devices.

Weight Bearing None, except for stable fractures of the distal fibula. Toe-touch weight bearing for rigidly fixed fractures.

Treatment: Four to Six Weeks

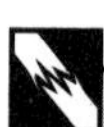

BONE HEALING

Stability at fracture site: Acute fractures should be showing bridging callus, and the fracture is usually stable. However, the strength of this callus, especially with torsional load, is significantly lower than that of normal bone.

Stage of bone healing: Reparative phase. Further organization of the callus and formation of lamellar bone begins.

X-ray: Bridging callus is visible as a fluffy material on the periosteal surface of cortical bone. For fractures rigidly fixed with screws and plates, callus may not be visible and there is a consolidation of the fracture and filling in of lucent lines. Amount of callus deposition is less than that at a midshaft fracture.

Orthopaedic and Rehabilitation Considerations

Physical Examination

The cast is removed for radiographic examination out of plaster. Check for stability, tenderness, and range of motion at the ankle joint. Patients who have been treated primarily in a long leg cast will likely be very stiff at both the ankle and the knee.

Dangers

Most of the swelling from acute fractures should be relieved. Check for any trophic signs of reflex sympathetic dystrophy: redness, swelling, vasomotor disturbances, hyperesthesias, pain, and tenderness out of proportion to the stage of fracture healing. If evidence of reflex sympathetic dystrophy is noted, the patient should begin a more aggressive physical therapy program.

Patients who have had severe soft-tissue injury and continue to have eschar should have this evaluated carefully to ensure that there is no evidence of necrosis or infection beneath scar tissue. Check the integrity of any skin grafts.

Radiography

Examine radiographs of the anteroposterior, lateral, and mortise views of the ankle for evidence of healing and any loss of reduction. Also evaluate the integrity of the hardware. Check for screws that may have backed out or plates that may have fractured.

Weight Bearing

Patients who have had internal fixation and are now showing adequate consolidation may begin toe-touch weight bearing on the affected extremity.

If there is adequate evidence of callus, a long leg cast may be converted to a short leg cast, a patellar tendon-bearing (PTB) cast, or a cam walker. However, weight bearing may not begin for at least another 2 weeks.

Patients who have had massive soft-tissue damage and were treated with an external fixator should have the fixator removed; if the skin allows, they may be placed in either a protective splint or a cast and remain non-weight bearing.

Patients with nontender nondisplaced distal fibula fractures may have their casts removed and begin weight bearing as tolerated.

Range of Motion

Continue with metatarsophalangeal joint and knee range of motion. If the patient has had internal fixation and is now out of a cast, active dorsiflexion and plantar flexion to tolerance, as well as gentle inversion and eversion at the ankle may be added. This helps to prevent stiffening of the ankle joint capsule. Hydrotherapy is helpful to decrease stiffness of the ankle during range of motion.

If the patient is in a cast, attempt dorsiflexion and plantar flexion, as well as inversion and eversion within the cast. The cast should now be loose enough to allow some limited range of motion. Continue with active range of motion of the knee.

Muscle Strength

Continue isometric exercise to the ankle dorsiflexors and plantar flexors. The patient should continue quadriceps strengthening exercises. If the cast has been removed, begin strengthening of the peronei, tibialis posterior, and tibialis anterior with inversion and eversion exercises. No resistive exercises in inversion and eversion should be prescribed.

Functional Activities

Patients allowed toe-touch weight bearing may use the affected extremity during transfers, using crutches for balance and support.

If weight bearing is still not allowed, non–weight-bearing pivot transfers using crutches should continue.

Gait

Non–weight-bearing patients continue ambulation with crutches.

Patients who are allowed to begin weight bearing use a three-point gait in which two crutches constitute one point and the affected and unaffected extremities the other two points (*see* Figure 6-17). The patient may climb stairs placing the unaffected extremity first, followed by the crutches and then the affected extremity, and descends stairs placing the crutches first, followed by the affected extremity and then the unaffected extremity (*see* Figures 6-20, 6-21, 6-22, 6-23, 6-24, and 6-25).

Methods of Treatment: Specific Aspects

Cast

Evaluate the patient for range of motion at the ankle joint. The joint is likely to be stiff after immobilization. Be careful not to confuse discomfort due to stiffness with pain at an unstable fracture site. If the radiographs have shown deposition of callus and the patient is minimally to nontender at the fracture site, the patient may be placed in a PTB cast or a short leg cast and begin partial weight bearing. A patient who is still tender at the fracture site or shows no evidence of adequate callus must again be placed in a long leg cast and remain non-weight bearing. Continue range of motion of the metatarsophalangeal joints and knee.

Open Reduction and Internal Fixation

Remove the cast and examine the ankle joint. Evaluate the surgical sites for any evidence of infection or skin breakdown. If the patient is nontender and radiographs show deposition of callus or adequate consolidation of the fracture lines, the short leg cast may be removed and partial weight bearing begun using crutches. Active range of motion is also now prescribed to the knee and ankle.

Patients who do not show adequate evidence of healing and have had a painful examination are placed back in a short leg cast and must remain non-weight bearing using crutches or a walker and a two-point gait (*see* Figure 6-16).

For the rare patient who has had internal fixation augmented with an external fixator, the fixator may be removed if there is adequate evidence of healing and the condition of the soft tissues allows for the patient to be placed in a cast or a brace. If the soft tissues are not yet sufficiently healed, the patient must be placed in another apparatus such as a cam walker that allows access to the wound while keeping the ankle joint stable.

Prescription

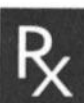

FOUR TO SIX WEEKS

Precautions Keep unstable fractures or those with limited fixation in a cast or cam walker. Stable fractures are out of a cast.

Range of Motion

For rigidly fixed fractures, active range of motion to metatarsophalangeal joints, ankle, and knee.

For nonrigidly fixed fractures, active range of motion to metatarsophalangeal joints. Range the ankle and knee as immobilization device allows.

Muscle Strength

For rigidly fixed fractures, isometric and isotonic exercises to dorsiflexors and plantar flexors of the ankle, evertors and invertors of the ankle and foot. No resistive exercises prescribed. Quadriceps strengthening continued.

For nonrigidly fixed fractures, gentle isometric exercises to dorsiflexors and plantar flexors within the cast. No resistive exercises prescribed. Quadriceps strengthening continued.

Functional Activities Non–weight-bearing stand/pivot transfers and ambulation with assistive devices for fractures with little evidence of healing. Toe-touch to partial weight bearing with assistive devices for fractures showing evidence of healing.

Weight Bearing None for fractures showing little evidence of healing. Partial weight bearing for fractures that are nontender to palpation and appear stable on radiography. Weight bearing as tolerated for nondisplaced distal fibula fractures.

Treatment: Six to Eight Weeks

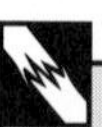

BONE HEALING

Stability at fracture site: With bridging callus, the fracture is usually stable. The strength of this callus, especially with torsional load, is significantly lower than that of normal bone. Confirm with physical examination.

Stage of bone healing: Reparative phase. Further organization of the callus and formation of lamellar bone continues. This requires further protection to avoid refracture.

X-ray: Bridging callus is visible and indicates increased rigidity. With rigid fixation, less callus is seen and fracture lines are less distinct. Healing with endosteal bone predominates.

Orthopaedic and Rehabilitation Considerations

Physical Examination

All fractures come out of a cast for examination and radiography. Examine the fracture site for tenderness. Evaluate any wound or operative site for healing or evidence of infection. Evaluate for trophic or sensory changes as indications of reflex sympathetic dystrophy. Evaluate any skin graft.

Radiography

Evaluate all fractures with anteroposterior, lateral, and mortise views to assess for loss of reduction as well as the healing status. Evaluate the position and integrity of hardware.

Weight Bearing

All fractures treated with internal fixation, as well as nondisplaced distal fibula fractures, may begin progressive partial weight bearing if there is evidence of fracture consolidation and the fracture site is nontender to palpation.

Fractures treated in a cast may begin partial weight bearing if the fracture is nontender on examination.

Open fractures that still have tenuous soft tissues may begin toe-touch to partial weight bearing as the healing of the fracture and soft tissues allows.

Patients whose fractures still need protection may use a cam walker that allows mobilization while protecting the fracture. It can be removed for range of motion and used as a splint when the leg is at rest.

Range of Motion

The ankle is quite stiff secondary to immobilization. Active range-of-motion, active-assisted range-of-motion, and gentle passive range-of-motion exercises in all planes are instituted. Hydrotherapy (to increase the range of motion and decrease the discomfort) is prescribed if necessary. Patients are instructed in drawing the alphabet with the foot to improve range of motion.

Muscle Strength

Gentle resistive exercises can be started. The patient uses his or her unaffected foot to offer resistance. Strengthening exercises such as isotonic exercises are prescribed to the dorsiflexors, plantar flexors, evertors, and invertors of the foot. Continue with quadriceps strengthening.

Functional Activities

Transfers are performed with partial to full weight bearing on the affected extremity. Patients whose fractures remain non-weight bearing should continue stand/pivot transfers using crutches. The patient dresses the affected extremity first.

Gait

Patients should be gradually weaned from crutches and walkers to a cane and retrained in a normal gait pattern. Heel strike, foot-flat, mid-stance, heel-off, and push-off phases should be emphasized and retaught. Patients tend to walk with a foot-flat gait because they have been wearing a cast for a long time. As dorsiflexion and plantar flexion improve, the gait pattern also improves. Heavy pounding activities such as jogging, jumping, running, and twisting should be avoided until at least 12 to 16 weeks.

Methods of Treatment: Specific Aspects

Cast

Evaluate the patient out of a cast. The joint is stiff after immobilization. Patients who are partially weight bearing in a PTB or short leg cast may increase weight bearing as tolerated. Patients being changed to PTB or short leg casts begin partial weight bearing. By now, it is the rare patient who needs to remain in a long leg cast because of fracture site tenderness or lack of callus. Continue to range the metatarsophalangeal joints.

Open Reduction and Internal Fixation

Remove the cast, if not already done, and examine the ankle. If the fracture site is nontender and there is adequate healing by radiography, the patient may remain out of a cast and begin partial weight bearing. Active range-of-motion exercises are continued for those patients previously out of a cast or begun for those just removed from a cast.

Patients who need to remain in a short leg cast may begin partial weight bearing.

For the rare patient who has had internal fixation augmented with an external fixator, the fixator may be removed if not already done. The patient then needs alternate support such as a short leg cast or removable split so that soft-tissue injuries can be managed.

Prescription

SIX TO EIGHT WEEKS

Precautions Keep unstable fractures or those with limited fixation in a cast or cam walker. Stable fractures are out of a cast.

Range of Motion

For rigidly fixed fractures, active, active-assistive, and passive range of motion in all planes to the ankle and subtalar joint.

For nonrigidly fixed fractures, begin active and active-assistive range of motion to the ankle and subtalar joints. Patients still in a cast may actively range the metatarsophalangeal joints and try to actively range the ankle in their casts.

Muscle Strength For rigidly and nonrigidly fixed fractures, begin resistive exercises to the dorsiflexors and plantar flexors as well as invertors and evertors of the ankle.

Functional Activities

For rigidly fixed fractures, partial to full weight bearing with assistive devices for fractures showing evidence of healing. Use assistive devices as necessary.

For nonrigidly fixed fractures, toe-touch to partial weight bearing using assistive devices for transfers and ambulation.

Weight Bearing Partial to full weight bearing.

Treatment: Eight to Twelve Weeks

BONE HEALING

Stability at fracture site: Stable, except for the most comminuted fractures.

Stage of bone healing: Remodeling phase. Woven bone is replaced with lamellar bone. The process of remodeling takes months to years for completion.

X-ray: Rigidly fixed bones should show a disappearance of the fracture line. Fractures treated in a cast show a small amount of fluffy callus at the medial malleolus and along the shaft of the distal fibula.

Orthopaedic and Rehabilitation Considerations

Physical Examination

Evaluate for residual tenderness at the fracture site. If there was a surgical procedure, evaluate the integrity of the surgical incisions.

Evaluate range of motion. Patients who have been in a cast for a prolonged period are quite stiff. If a patient treated in a cast is nontender, remove the cast and begin active range of motion as well as partial weight bearing.

Dangers

Evaluate all wounds and incisions for any evidence of erythema or infection, and treat appropriately. Evaluate for reflex sympathetic dystrophy. Evaluate fractures for tenderness. Weight bearing should be limited if the patient is tender to palpation over the fracture site.

Radiography

Anteroposterior, lateral, and mortise views of the ankle are taken to evaluate the alignment of the ankle joint as well as fracture healing. Evaluate the integrity of any hardware.

Weight Bearing

All fractures treated with open reduction and internal fixation should now be stable and patients may begin progressive weight bearing on the affected extremity.

Patients treated in a cast who show adequate evidence of callus and are no longer tender at the fracture site may also begin to progress from partial to full weight bearing.

Range of Motion

Patients treated in a cast are quite stiff secondary to fibrosis and tightness of the joint capsule. They must begin active-assistive and passive range of motion of the ankle and subtalar joint in all planes.

Patients treated with open reduction and internal fixation are likely to have better range of motion. Active-assistive and passive range-of-motion exercises are prescribed to improve the range of motion of the ankle. Using a towel to stretch the foot and ankle can assist the patient in dorsiflexion and plantar flexion of the ankle.

Muscle Strength

Patients treated with open reduction and internal fixation continue progressive resistive exercises in all planes of the ankle. Patients should control these exercises to adjust resistance to their tolerance. Start with 2-pound weights attached to the feet and gradually increase to 5 to 10 pounds.

Patients who have been treated in a cast may begin gentle resistive exercises if the fracture site is stable and nontender.

Patients should also continue with quadriceps exercises.

Functional Activities

Transfers are performed with partial to full weight bearing on the affected extremity. The patient may now dress with the affected extremity first.

Gait

Patients should be weaned from crutches or a walker to a cane as tolerated and retrained in a normal gait pattern. Heel strike, foot-flat, mid-stance, and push-off phases should be taught again. Patients who have been in a cast for an extended period tend to walk with a foot-flat gait. When the ankle range of motion improves in dorsiflexion and plantar flexion, the gait pattern tends to normalize. Heavy pounding activities such as jogging, jumping, running, and twisting should be avoided until at least 12 to 16 weeks.

Methods of Treatment: Specific Aspects

Cast

Most patients are out of a cast. Patients who are tender over the fracture site on examination may remain in a PTB or short leg cast as necessary. They may begin partial weight bearing to provide some stress to the bone and accelerate bony healing. Patients who are out of a cast work on active and active-assistive range of motion to the ankle.

Open Reduction and Internal Fixation

Patients who have undergone this method of treatment should be well healed. They may begin more aggressive range-of-motion exercises and continue partial to full weight bearing. Patients should still avoid heavy pounding activities such as jogging, jumping, and running because the fracture cannot yet withstand these forces.

Prescription

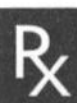

EIGHT TO TWELVE WEEKS

Precautions Essentially none.

Range of Motion

For rigidly fixed fractures, active, active-assistive, and passive range of motion in all planes to the ankle and subtalar joints.

For nonrigidly fixed fractures, begin active and active-assistive range of motion of the ankle and subtalar joints. Any patient still in a cast may actively range the metatarsophalangeal joints and try to actively range the ankle within the cast.

Muscle Strength

For rigidly fixed fractures, begin progressive resistive exercises to the dorsiflexors and plantar flexors, as well as invertors and evertors.

For nonrigidly fixed fractures, continue gentle resistive exercises.

Functional Activities

For rigidly fixed fractures, progress from partial to full weight bearing as tolerated for transfers and ambulation, using assistive devices as necessary.

For nonrigidly fixed fractures, begin partial weight bearing. Assistive devices required for transfers and ambulation.

Weight Bearing Partial to full weight bearing.

LONG-TERM CONSIDERATIONS AND PROBLEMS

Patients who have not had rigid fixation may still have limited ankle range of motion. Active-assistive and passive range of motion should be instituted. Progressive resistive exercises should be added to strengthen the ankle musculature.

Pliometric exercises such as jumping and hopping are not necessary for functional ambulation or activities of daily living. For athletes who want to improve their strength and performance, pliometric and high-performance exercises are prescribed at a later stage of rehabilitation.

Fractures of the ankle usually involve some amount of injury to the articular cartilage of the tibial plafond and the talar dome. This can result in traumatic arthritis, producing long-term chronic disability that may permanently affect the patient's ability to work and perform other activities of daily living. Early degenerative changes that progress to significant ankle pain may eventually require fusion or total joint replacement if the discomfort is great.

Appropriate reduction of both the ankle mortise and the distal tibiofibular syndesmosis is crucial for a patient to have normal function at the tibiotalar joint. Patients whose disruption is not recognized until after bony consolidation has begun and reduction is not possible, or if reduction and stabilization are inadequate, may have significant ankle pain because of the instability at the ankle joint. This affects the gait and causes ankle discomfort when the patient bears weight on that extremity because of the additional strains placed on the soft tissues, tendons, and articular surfaces.

Severe ligamentous injuries to the ankle can also have long-term sequelae. Particularly on the lateral side, recurrent instability of the lateral collateral ligament complex (which includes the anterior talofibular, calcaneofibular, and posterior talofibular ligaments) and turning of the ankle may cause repeated ankle sprains and damage to the articular cartilage of the tibiotalar articulation. Patients with lateral ankle ligamentous injury may need secondary repair to maintain the integrity of their ankle joint (*see* Figure 30-30).

Proprioception training must be instituted for all patients, especially athletes. Ankle taping, high-top shoes, and mastering balance on one leg are important to aid in reestablishing the reflex response necessary to avoid further injury in high-performance sports.

IMMEDIATE TO ONE WEEK

	Cast	*Open Reduction and Internal Fixation*
Stability	None.	None.
Orthopaedics	Check cast margins for adequate padding. Trim to the metatarsal heads. Reinforce and repair as necessary.	If a short leg cast has been placed, check cast margins for adequate padding and trim foot of cast to metatarsal heads.
Rehabilitation	Range of motion at metatarsophalangeal joint.	Range of motion at metatarsophalangeal and knee joints.

TWO WEEKS

	Cast	*Open Reduction and Internal Fixation*
Stability	None to minimal.	None to minimal.
Orthopaedics	Trim cast to metatarsal heads. Evaluate padding. Reinforce and repair as necessary	Trim cast to metatarsal heads. Evaluate padding. Reinforce and repair as necessary.
Rehabilitation	Active range of motion at metatarsophalangeal joints. Isometric quadriceps strengthening within cast.	Active range of motion at metatarsophalangeal and knee joints. Isometric quadriceps strengthening.

FOUR TO SIX WEEKS

	Cast	Open Reduction and Internal Fixation
Stability	Partially stable.	Partially stable.
Orthopaedics	If stable, may change to patella tendon-bearing or short leg weight-bearing cast. Otherwise, continue long leg cast.	May consider removing cast if stable.
Rehabilitation	Continue range of motion to metatarsophalangeal joints. Begin range of motion to ankle and knee as immobilization device allows. Isometric quadriceps and ankle dorsiflexor and plantar flexor strengthening.	Active range of motion to metatarsophalangeal joints, ankle joints, and knee joint. Isometric quadriceps and ankle dorsiflexor and plantar flexor strengthening.

SIX TO EIGHT WEEKS

	Cast	Open Reduction and Internal Fixation
Stability	Stable.	Stable.
Orthopaedics	May remove cast if stable.	May remove cast if not already done.
Rehabilitation	Continue active to active-assistive range of motion of the metatarsophalangeal, ankle, subtalar, and knee joints.	Continue active to active-assistive range of motion of the metatarsophalangeal, ankle, subtalar, and knee joints.
	Isotonic and isokinetic exercises to the ankle.	Isotonic and isokinetic exercises to the ankle.

EIGHT TO TWELVE WEEKS

	Cast	Open Reduction and Internal Fixation
Stability	Stable.	Stable.
Orthopaedics	Remove patella tendon-bearing or short leg cast if not already done.	
Rehabilitation	Begin active, active-assistive, and passive range of motion of the ankle and subtalar joints. Continue range of motion of the metatarsophalangeal joints if still in cast. Progressive resistive exercises to all muscle groups of the ankle.	Active and active-assistive and passive range of motion to ankle and subtalar joints. Progressive resistive exercises to all muscle groups of the ankle.

BIBLIOGRAPHY

Amendola A. Controversies in diagnosis and management of syndesmosis injuries of the ankle. *Foot and Ankle*, 13:44–50, 1992.

Chapman M. Ankle injuries. In: Mann RA, ed. *Surgery of the Foot*. St. Louis: C.V. Mosby, 1986, pp. 568–586.

Geissler W, Tsao A. Foot and ankle fractures. In: Rockwood CA Jr, Green DP, eds. *Fractures in Adults*, 4th ed. Philadelphia: J.B. Lippincott, 1995, pp. 2212–2235.

Manoli A II. Compartment syndromes of the foot: current concepts. *Foot and Ankle*, 10:340–344, 1990.

Mann R. Lower extremeties. In: Chapman M, ed. *Operative Orthopaedics*. Philadelphia: J.B. Lippincott, 1993, pp. 2143–2178.

Michelson JD. Fractures about the ankle. *J Bone Joint Surg Am*, 77:142–152, 1995.

Mizel M, Sobel M. Trauma—Section 1. In: Miller M, ed. *Review of Orthopaedics*, 2nd ed. Philadelphia: W.B. Saunders, 1996, pp. 390–391.

Perry J. Ankle and foot gait deviations. In: Perry J, ed. *Gait Analysis*. Thorofare, NJ: Slack, 1992, pp. 185–219.

Segal D, Wiss DA, Whitelaw GP. Functional bracing and rehabilitation of ankle fractures. *Clin Orthop*, 199:39–45, 1985.

Tile M. Fractures of the ankle. In: Schatzker J, Tile M, eds. *The Rationale of Operative Fracture Care*, 2nd ed. Berlin, Springer-Verlag, 1996, pp. 523–530.

Trafton PG, Bray TJ, Simpson LA. Fractures and soft tissue injuries of the ankle. In: Browner B, Jupiter J, Levine AM, Trafton PG, eds. *Skeletal Trauma*, Vol 2. Philadelphia: W.B. Saunders, 1992, pp. 1887–1931.

VanderGriend R, Michelson JD, Bone LB. Fractures of the ankle and distal part of the tibia. *Instr Course Lect*, 46:311–321, 1997.

Yablon IG, Segal D. Foot and ankle injuries. In: Evarts CM, ed. *Surgery of the Musculoskeletal System*, 2nd ed. New York: Churchill Livingstone, 1990, pp. 3827–3849.

CHAPTER *Thirty-one*

Talar Fractures

ANNE P. MCCORMACK, MD

INTRODUCTION

Definition

Fractures of the hindfoot are those involving the calcaneus (os calcis) and the talus.

Fractures of the talus include fractures of the talar neck, the talar body, or the talar head, as well as osteochondral fractures and fractures of the lateral process (Figure 31-1; *see* Figures 31-2, 31-4, and 31-7).

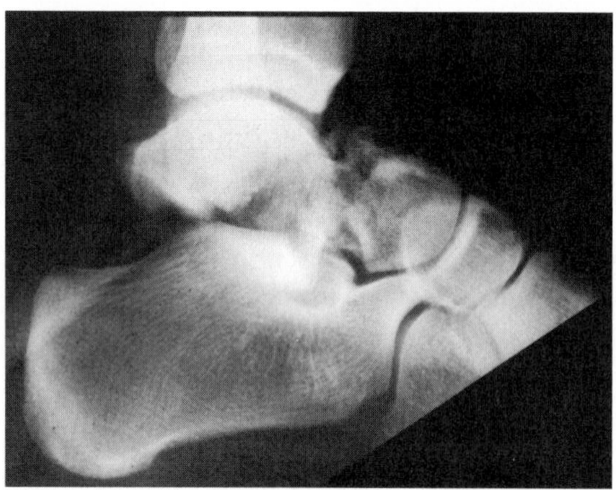

FIGURE 31-1 Fracture of the talar neck due to a high-energy injury in a motor vehicle accident. Closed reduction and casting was attempted and failed; open reduction and internal fixation was necessary.

Mechanism of Injury

Fractures of the body and neck of the talus usually result from high-energy injuries such as motor vehicle accidents. Fractures of the head and posterior aspects of the talus usually result from axial load. Osteochondral fractures and lateral process fractures are often seen with ankle or subtalar sprains and fracture/dislocations of the subtalar joint.

Treatment Goals

Orthopaedic Objectives

Alignment

Anatomic realignment is more critical for the articular surfaces of the talus than for any other bone in the foot. This is because of the high risk of avascular necrosis due to a poor blood supply (*see* Figures 31-11 and 31-12).

Stability

Stable fixation of talar neck fractures is crucial to reduce the risk of avascular necrosis of the talar head. Fractures of the talar body must be stably fixed to restore subtalar joint congruity. Fractures of the talar head must be stably maintained to allow for load transfer across the talonavicular joint.

Rehabilitation Objectives

Range of Motion

Restore the range of motion of the ankle and foot in all planes.

Restore the full range of motion of the subtalar joint (Table 31-1).

TABLE 31-1 *Ankle Ranges of Motion*

Motion	Normal	Functional
Ankle plantar flexion	45°	20°
Ankle dorsiflexion	20°	10°
Foot inversion	35°	10°
Foot eversion	25°	10°

Intraarticular fractures of the talar body involving the subtalar joint may have residual loss of range of motion. This causes increased stress on the subtalar articulation and leads to further degeneration and arthritic changes.

Muscle Strength

Strengthen the muscles of the foot.

Invertors of the foot:

Tibialis posterior (inverts and plantar flexes the foot and supports the medial talonavicular articulation)

Evertors of the foot:

Peroneus brevis

Peroneus longus

Dorsiflexors of the foot:

Tibialis anterior (acts as a dorsiflexor and invertor of the foot)

Extensor hallucis longus

Plantar flexors of the ankle and foot:

Gastrocnemius

Soleus

Flexor digitorum brevis (originates on the calcaneal tuberosity and does not cross the ankle joint)

Functional Goals

Normalize the gait pattern.

Expected Time of Bone Healing

Six to 10 weeks.

Expected Duration of Rehabilitation:

Twelve to 16 weeks. Patients in whom avascular necrosis develops usually need further surgery and extensive rehabilitation for up to 12 months.

Methods of Treatment

Open Reduction and Internal Fixation (Multiple Screws)

Biomechanics: Stress-shielding device with rigid fixation.

Mode of bone healing: Primary, without callus formation.

Indications: Displaced fractures of the talus. Over 60% of the talar surface is articular. Normal gait mechanics are not possible unless all of the joints articulating with the talus have nearly full range of motion. Because no tendons or muscles attach to the talus, there is a very limited blood supply and the talus is prone to avascular necrosis, particularly after the talar body has been subluxed or dislocated (*see* Figures 31-11 and 31-12). Open reduction and internal fixation may lessen the chance of avascular necrosis in fractures of the talar body and the talar neck. Fractures of the talar head, although they are less common, should also have large fracture fragments reduced to limit potential devascularization. The postoperative patient is initially treated with a bulky compressive dressing. An internally fixed fracture is placed in a cast after the edema subsides. Talar fractures tend to have less swelling than calcaneal fractures (Figures 31-2, 31-3, 31-4, 31-5, 31-6, 31-7, 31-8, 31-9, and 31-10).

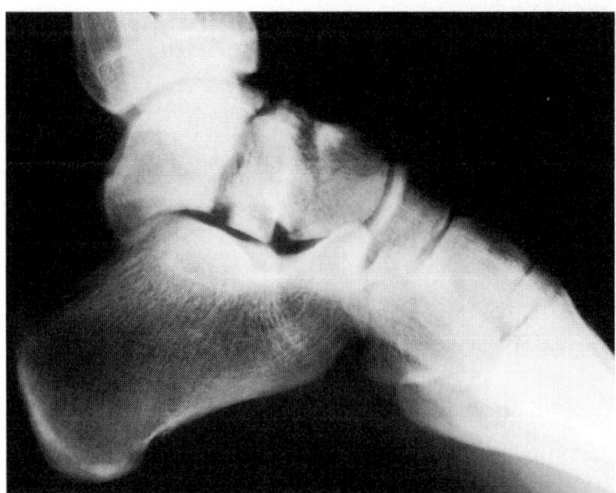

FIGURE 31-2 Fracture of the talar neck. A failed attempt at closed reduction.

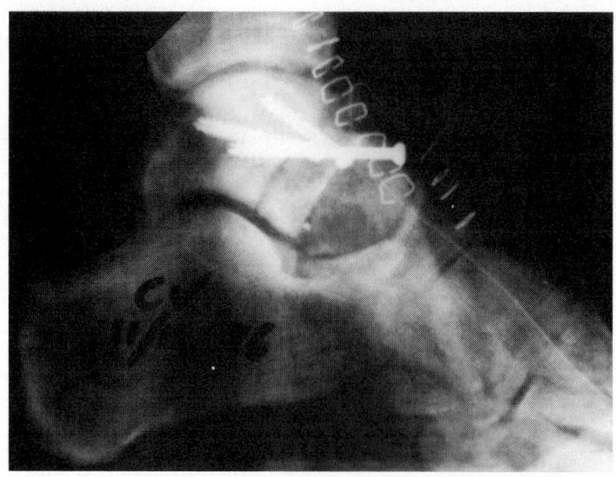

FIGURE 31-3 Fracture of the talar neck treated with open reduction and internal fixation. After surgery, the patient initially had a bulky compressive dressing. The fracture was placed in a cast after the edema subsided. Talar fractures tend to have less swelling than calcaneal fractures.

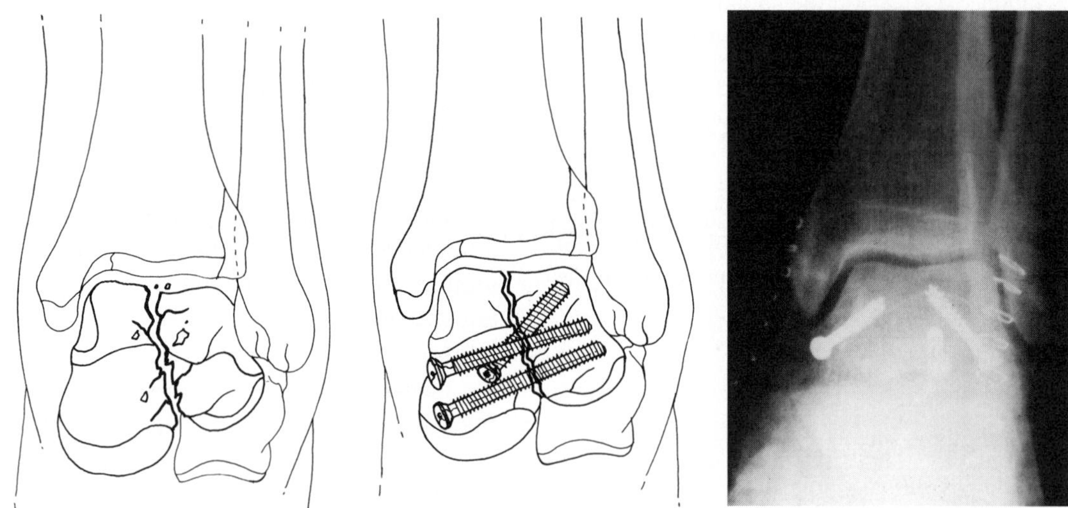

FIGURE 31-4 *(above, left)* Fracture of talar body. Because over 60% of the talar surface is articular, as close to anatomic reduction as possible is necessary.

FIGURE 31-5 *(above, middle)* Open reduction and internal screw fixation of the talus. Intraarticular fractures of the talar body involving the subtalar joint may have residual loss of range of motion. Note that no tendons or muscles attach to the talus.

FIGURE 31-6 *(above, right)* Internal fixation of talar fracture with lag screws. It is important to regain anatomic alignment and maintain it throughout healing to minimize further degenerative changes in the subtalar joint and to restore a pain-free gait.

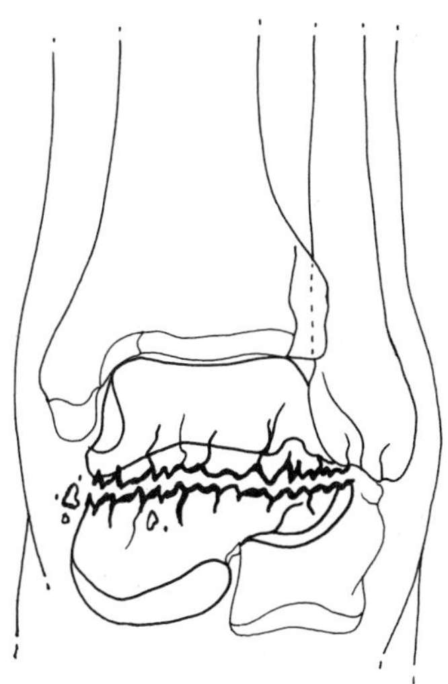

FIGURE 31-7 Fracture of the talar body.

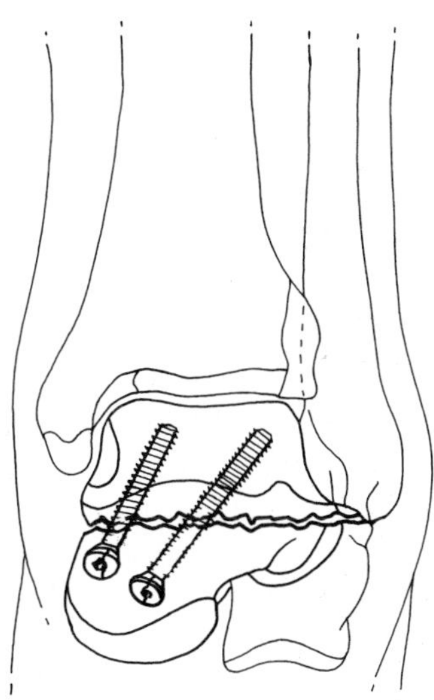

FIGURE 31-8 Internal fixation with lag screws across the talar body fracture to produce anatomic reduction.

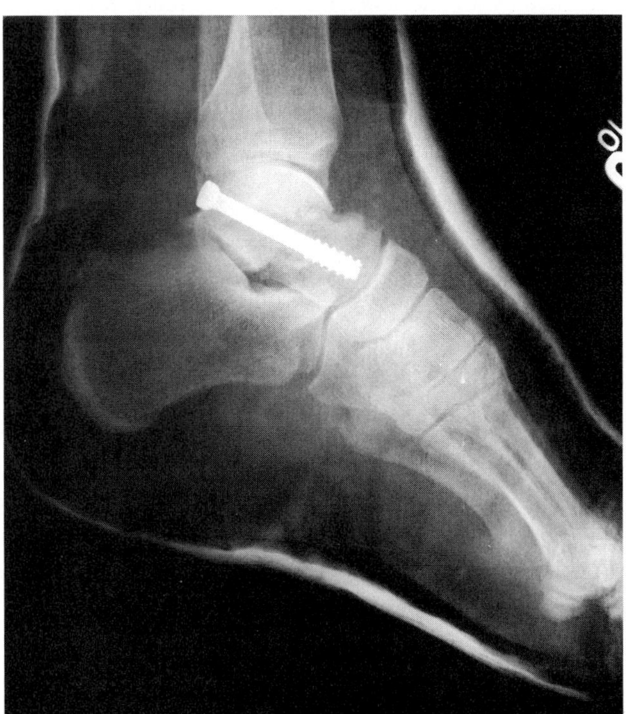

FIGURE 31-9 Fracture of the talar neck treated with internal reduction and screw fixation. The fracture was treated in a cast in the immediate postoperative period because there was very little swelling.

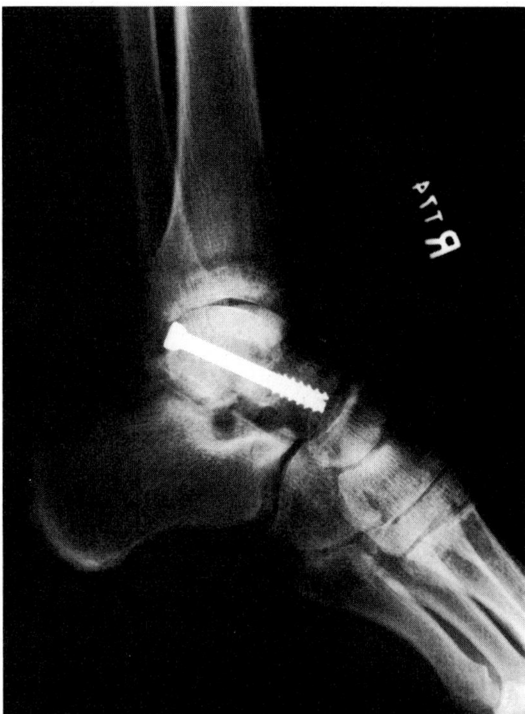

FIGURE 31-10 Postoperative internal fixation of the talar neck. There is healing. Active range of motion of the ankle and subtalar joint has begun.

Cast

Biomechanics: Stress-sharing device.

Mode of bone healing: Secondary, with callus formation. This mainly cancellous bone shows only a small amount of callus because the cortex is quite thin and there is minimal periosteum.

Indications: A nondisplaced or minimally displaced fracture of the talar neck may be anatomically reduced with a closed technique and then placed in a cast. A problem with this method is that maintaining the patient in a cast precludes the early motion important for successful rehabilitation of the tibiotalar and subtalar joints. In general, casting as a primary form of treatment should be considered a temporary and not an acceptable final method of treatment.

Special Considerations of the Fracture

Age

Elderly patients are at greater risk for development of joint stiffness after fractures of the talus. Patients of all ages are prone to avascular necrosis; however, elderly patients with compromised circulation may be even more susceptible. Rehabilitation may be more prolonged and may never be complete for elderly patients who have preexisting arthritic changes in the tibiotalar or the subtalar joint.

Articular Involvement

Because the talus is approximately 60% articular surface, almost all talar fractures are intraarticular, and therefore anatomic reduction is of critical importance. It is important to regain anatomic alignment and maintain it throughout healing both to minimize further degenerative changes within the subtalar joint and restore a pain-free gait.

Location

No muscles insert or originate on the talus. Residual weakness of muscle groups related to fractures of the talus is caused by disuse during immobilization and healing. Serious subtalar dislocations can cause additional injury to the peroneal tendons only on the lateral side and the posterior tibial tendon on the medial side.

Fractures of the talus, particularly those that result in avascular necrosis, significantly impair the patient's ability to transfer weight from the tibia to the foot and then from the hindfoot to the midfoot. The resultant pain and alteration of gait can be quite disabling.

Open Fractures

Any open fracture of the talus must be treated aggressively with irrigation, débridement, and intravenous antibiotics. The likelihood of infection also increases after the placement of hardware. Open fractures with talar subluxation or dislocation must be carefully monitored because this significant trauma may disrupt the tenuous vascular supply of the talus.

Tendon and Ligamentous Injuries

Severe fractures and dislocations of the talus may have associated peroneal tendon injury if the talus has been dislocated laterally. The posterior tibial tendon may be injured by medial talus displacement. The function of these muscles should be evaluated when the patient is able to tolerate testing.

Associated Injury

Because of the large-magnitude force involved with most of these fractures, there can be significant soft-tissue damage secondary to swelling. Even with open fractures, isolated compartments may still swell and need to be observed. The patient must be watched carefully for the development of foot compartment syndrome.

Weight Bearing

Fractures of the talus are initially placed in a bulky compressive dressing or cast with the foot elevated for 2 to 5 days. When a walking cast is applied, the patient may be allowed weight bearing (weight of leg) if the fixation can tolerate it. It is very important with talar fractures for the patient to keep the foot elevated as much as possible in the first 3 weeks to optimize circulation to the talus, in the hope of preventing avascular necrosis (Figures 31-11 and 31-12). In the depen-

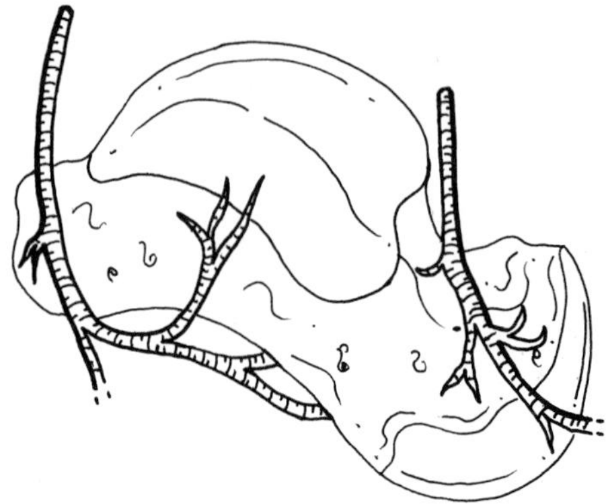

FIGURE 31-11 The limited blood supply to the talus makes it prone to avascular necrosis, particularly after the talar body has been subluxed or dislocated.

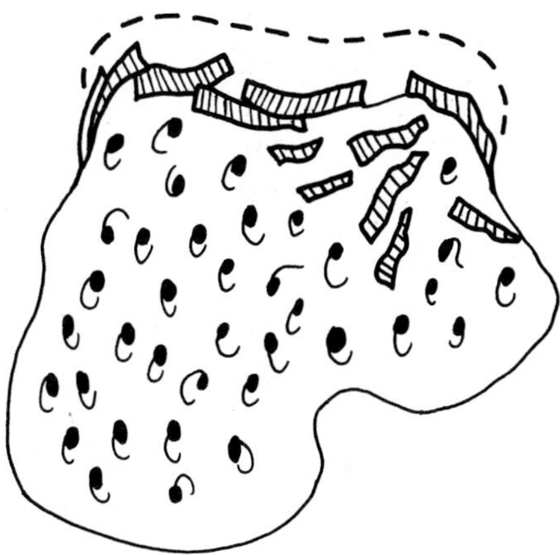

FIGURE 31-12 Avascular necrosis of the talus. Note the collapse of the subtalar bone of the dome of the talus.

dent position, there is inadequate venous return secondary to the vascular congestion caused by the swelling. Early motion is extremely important for a satisfactory final outcome, and the patient with rigid internal screw fixation frequently is put in a bivalve cast or removable cam walker (a rigid, padded, supportive splint with a rocker bottom) 2 weeks after surgery to expedite exercise of the joints. The patient should ideally remain partial weight bearing for up to 3 months and then progress with weight bearing as tolerance and radiographic evidence of healing suggest.

Gait

Stance Phase

The stance phase constitutes 60% of the gait cycle.

Heel Strike

The initial impact causes significant discomfort as the body's weight is transferred onto the posterior facet of the subtalar joint. This pain continues as the weight is transferred from the hindfoot to the midfoot and the anterior and medial facets are engaged.

Fractures of the talus are also painful during the heel strike as the posterior facet of the os calcis engages the undersurface of the talus. At this point, the talus is caught between the calcaneus and the undersurface of the tibial articular surface, causing compression at both surfaces.

During the initial healing phase of talar fractures, the patient abbreviates the time spent on the affected leg because the talus is involved with bearing weight throughout stance phases. The patient attempts a shallow angle of attack in heel strike and maintains plantar flexion to minimize the extremes of load placed across the talus (*see* Figure 6-1).

Foot Flat

This portion of the gait cycle is also painful because the weight is now being transferred from the posterior facet to the anterior and medial facets and the talonavicular joint. This places significant force across both the os calcis facets and the talar body and neck (*see* Figure 6-2).

Mid-Stance

The single-stance phase is also usually painful because the talus is being compressed and fully engaged into the talonavicular joint (*see* Figure 6-3).

Push-off

Fractures of the talus are painful at this point because the talar head is pushed into the navicular and weight is transferred across the midfoot into the forefoot. The patient may try to limit the amount of ankle plantar flexion to limit this transmission of force. Thus, there is inadequate push-off with the affected foot, and this portion of the gait cycle is limited. The entire weight-bearing phase is painful, producing an antalgic gait that reduces the overall time spent in the stance phase (*see* Figures 6-4 and 6-5).

Swing Phase

The swing phase constitutes 40% of the gait cycle. It usually is not affected by fractures of the talus.

The gait cycle may be profoundly affected by serious fractures of the talus, including dislocations and subluxations that affect peroneal or the posterior tibial tendons. Significant pain from irregular articular surfaces of the talus may necessitate fusion to relieve pain and improve function of the foot (*see* Figures 6-6, 6-7 and 6-8).

TREATMENT

Treatment: Early to Immediate (Day of Injury to One Week)

BONE HEALING

Stability at fracture site: None.

Stage of bone healing: Inflammatory phase. The fracture hematoma is colonized by inflammatory cells, and débridement of the fracture begins.

X-ray: No callus; visible fracture lines.

Orthopaedic and Rehabilitation Considerations

Physical Examination

Pay special attention to complaints of pain, paresthesia, and cast discomfort as indicators of a compartment syndrome. Check the fit of any compressive dressing or cast. Check for capillary refill and sensation. The toes should be pink, with brisk refill after light compression. It should be possible to reach the first web space of the foot and stroke it lightly with a blunt instrument to ensure that there is no peroneal nerve compression in the lower ankle and foot. Evaluate fractures of the talus for evidence of significant edema or fracture blisters.

Dangers

Patients with significant soft-tissue swelling in the foot are at increased risk for compartment syndrome. Symptoms that should raise suspicions include significant swelling, tightness of the skin, and the presence of fracture blisters. Pay special attention to complaints of severe pain, paresthesia, and cast or compressive dressing discomfort. For patients with fracture blisters, evaluate the skin for erythema or drainage that might indicate the presence of infection. The patient should be advised to keep the extremity elevated above heart level and to place ice packs over the ankle and foot to decrease the swelling.

Radiography

Obtain and check anteroposterior and lateral radiographs of the foot for any loss of correction.

Weight Bearing

All fractures of the talus should be non-weight bearing. For most of the initial week, the patient should be at bed rest with the foot elevated above heart level to control swelling.

Range of Motion

Once the initial pain subsides, start active range-of-motion exercises to the ankle in dorsiflexion, plantar flexion, eversion, and inversion as tolerated while awaiting casting, if the fracture has been rigidly fixed. Range of motion is avoided if the fracture has not been internally fixed. The patient should perform active range of motion of the knee and the metatarsophalangeal joints.

Muscle Strength

Quadriceps sets are prescribed to maintain quadriceps strength.

Functional Activities

The patient is taught to don pants on the involved extremity first and doff them from the uninvolved extremity first.

The patient is taught non–weight-bearing stand/pivot transfers from the bed to a chair, and vice versa. The patient needs assistive devices such as crutches or a walker for transfers and ambulation.

Gait

The patient is taught a two-point gait using crutches or a walker, with no weight bearing on the affected extremity. To climb stairs, the patient places the good foot first on the step above and then hops to the step with the affected extremity and the crutches; to descend stairs, the patient places the crutches first, followed by the unaffected extremity (*see* Figures 6-20, 6-21, 6-22, 6-23, 6-24, and 6-25).

Methods of Treatment: Specific Aspects

Open Reduction and Internal Fixation

A cast may be placed during the first 2 to 5 days if swelling and resolution of fracture blisters allow. While awaiting casting, start range-of-motion and isometric exercises to the ankle and foot muscles to help reduce swelling. Check the cast margins to make sure they are well padded. Again, note that the metatarsophalangeal joints have free movement. Look for any breakdown of the skin at the edges of the cast and trim appropriately. If there is any breakdown or softening of the cast, repair it as necessary.

Cast

Evaluate the condition of the cast. The cast margins should be adequately padded. There should be free movement of the metatarsophalangeal joints and full extension and flexion at the knee. Evaluate the skin at the cast edges to make sure that swelling has not caused skin breakdown and that there is no evidence of cyanosis or compartment syndrome. If the cast has softened under the foot, this is an appropriate time to reinforce and repair it.

Prescription

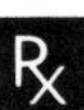

Day One to One Week

Precautions Fixation is not rigid unless the patient has had open reduction and internal fixation. Avoid passive range of motion.

Range of Motion Active range of motion of the toes and metatarsophalangeal joints as well as the knee. Before casting, do not move the ankle and subtalar joint unless rigidly fixed.

Muscle Strength No strengthening exercises to the ankle and foot.

Functional Activities Non–weight-bearing stand/pivot transfers and ambulation with assistive devices.

Weight Bearing None.

Treatment: Two Weeks

Bone Healing

Stability at fracture site: None to minimal.

Stage of bone healing: Beginning of reparative phase. Osteoprogenitor cells differentiate into osteoblasts that lay down woven bone.

X-ray: No changes noted. Fracture lines are visible. No callus formation.

Orthopaedic and Rehabilitation Considerations

Physical Examination

Check for capillary refill and sensation of the toes and, if possible, the first dorsal web space. Check the active and passive range of motion of all metatarsophalangeal and interphalangeal joints. Change the cast. Examine the skin of the ankle and heel for any evidence of infection or skin breakdown secondary to associated swelling. Remove sutures.

Dangers

Pay particular attention to complaints of pain, paresthesia, and cast discomfort. The patient should be made aware that any pronounced amount of swelling could lead to skin sloughing and should be immediately brought to the physician's attention. The patient should be advised to continue to keep the extremity elevated above the heart level as much as possible to reduce swelling and improve circulation.

Radiography

Check radiographs taken in anteroposterior and lateral positions. Check for any loss of reduction, movement of hardware, or extrusion of bone graft. At this point, it is too early to assess whether there will be avascular necrosis in the talus.

Weight Bearing

Patients with talar fractures that have been rigidly fixed may begin toe-touch weight bearing as tolerated by the fixation device and the patient's pain. Any weight bearing requires the use of assistive devices.

Range of Motion

Patients with talar fractures treated with internal fixation should be placed in a bivalved short leg cast or a cam walker so that they can range the tibiotalar and the subtalar joints out of the apparatus.

Muscle Strength

Maintain the strength of the quadriceps. As pain allows, the patient may attempt to strengthen the toe muscles by repetitive flexion and extension exercises.

Functional Activities

Patients with talar fractures may have toe-touch weight bearing transfers using crutches or a walker.

Gait

Patients with talar fractures continue a non–weight-bearing gait using crutches.

Patients who have rigidly fixed talar fractures progress to toe-touch weight bearing as tolerated, using assistive devices.

Methods of Treatment: Specific Aspects

Open Reduction and Internal Fixation

Trim the cast to allow visualization of the toes and the metatarsophalangeal joints, if this has not already been done. Reinforce any portion of the cast that has broken down at the foot or the metatarsophalangeal joints. These patients should continue with range of motion at the metatarsophalangeal joints. Begin baseline exercises of the gastrocnemius-soleus group and the anterior tibialis by having the patient attempt to plantar flex and dorsiflex in the cast. If there has been stable internal fixation of the fracture, begin gentle isometric exercises of the peroneal group by gentle eversion out of the cast. Try to invert the foot to strengthen the tibialis posterior, as well as create some subtalar motion.

Cast

Trim the cast to allow visualization of the toes to the metatarsophalangeal joint, if this has not already been done. Reinforce the cast if it has broken down at the foot or at the metatarsophalangeal joints. Continue metatarsophalangeal joint range of motion. If casting is the primary method of treatment, the patient should not begin any exercises across the ankle or subtalar joints.

Prescription

Two Weeks

Precautions Fixation is not rigid unless the patient has had open reduction and internal fixation. Avoid passive range of motion.

Range of Motion Rigidly fixed fractures of the talus may begin active ankle and subtalar range of motion. Continue metatarsophalangeal joint exercises. Patients who have not had internal fixation may range the metatarsophalangeal joints only.

Muscle Strength Rigidly fixed talar fractures may begin isometric exercises in dorsiflexion and plantar flexion as well as inversion and eversion out of the bivalved cast or cam walker.

Functional Activities Toe-touch weight-bearing transfers with assistive devices for rigidly fixed talar fractures.

Weight Bearing Talar fractures that have been rigidly fixed may begin toe-touch weight bearing.

Treatment: Four to Six Weeks

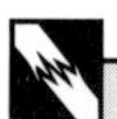

Bone Healing

Stability at fracture site: Some stability at fracture site. There is some callus formation, but the strength of this callus, especially with torsional load, is significantly lower than that of normal bone. The foot requires further protection to avoid refractures. Confirm with physical examination and radiography.

Stage of bone healing: Reparative phase. Further organization of the callus and formation of lamellar bone begins.

X-ray: The tarsal bones, which are mainly cancellous in composition, with minimal periosteum, begin to show consolidation of the fracture and filling in of lucent lines. With increased rigidity, lucency disappears, and healing with endosteal callus predominates because there is little periosteum.

Orthopaedic and Rehabilitation Considerations

Physical Examination

Remove the cast and perform radiographic examination out of plaster.

Check for stability, tenderness, and range of motion.

Dangers

Most of the swelling from acute fractures should now be resolved. Check for any trophic signs of reflex sympathetic dystrophy (RSD), characterized by vasomotor disturbances, hyperesthesias, and pain and tenderness disproportionate to the stage of fracture healing. If evidence of RSD is noted, the patient should begin an aggressive physical therapy program, including hydrotherapy.

Radiography

Examine radiographs taken in the anteroposterior and lateral positions for evidence of healing or any loss of reduction. In fractures of the talus, the patient should be evaluated radiographically for evidence of avascular necrosis.

Fractures of the talus should now exhibit Hawkins sign (presence of a lucent zone at the talar neck beneath the subchondral plate of the talus; this is seen on the anteroposterior radiograph of the ankle). The presence of this sign is a good indicator of the revascularization of the talus and a decreased likelihood of avascular necrosis. If a Hawkins' sign is not present, some amount of avascular necrosis is likely to become apparent on future radiographs.

Patients who have undergone bone grafting for talar fractures should be carefully assessed for incorporation of their bone graft.

Evaluate all hardware for any evidence of loosening by looking for lucency around the pins. Check for the maintenance of alignment to ensure there has been no change since the last examination.

Weight Bearing

A patient with a rigidly fixed talar fracture may continue partial weight bearing as the fixation and the patient's pain tolerance allow. Patients who were treated with closed reduction should remain non-weight bearing.

Range of Motion

Talar fractures that have been rigidly fixed may continue active range of motion of the ankle and the subtalar joints out of the cast or cam walker, as previously prescribed. Patients who have had closed reduction for talar fractures may continue only with metatarsophalangeal joint range of motion because the fracture is not yet stable enough to tolerate ankle or subtalar motion out of the cast without risking displacement. The cast is loose enough to allow for the patient a small amount of ankle and subtalar motion.

Muscle Strength

Repeated range-of-motion exercises gradually increase the strength of the affected muscles. Continue quadriceps strengthening. Begin ankle isometric exercises to improve the strength of the gastrocnemius-soleus group and the tibialis anterior in the cast.

Functional Activities

Rigidly fixed talar fractures may continue partial weight-bearing transfers, and ambulation. Patients still need to use crutches or a walker during transfers.

Fractures of the talus with closed treatment should remain non-weight bearing for transfers and ambulation.

Gait

Patients who are non-weight bearing continue to use crutches or a walker for ambulation. Patients who have begun weight bearing may use a three-point gait in which the crutches form one point and the affected and unaffected extremities the other two points. The patient climbs stairs with the unaffected extremity first, followed by the crutches and then the affected extremity. The patient descends stairs by placing the crutches first, followed by the affected extremity and then the unaffected extremity.

All weight bearing at this point is in either a cast, a splint, or a cam walker. Attempts to normalize the gait cycle have not yet begun.

Methods of Treatment: Specific Aspects

Open Reduction and Internal Fixation

Fractures that have been rigidly fixed are in a removable cast or cam walker. Evaluate and encourage range of motion at the tibiotalar joint, subtalar joint, and metatarsophalangeal joints.

Cast

Talar fractures that are not rigidly fixed should not have range of motion to the tibiotalar or subtalar joints.

Prescription

FOUR TO SIX WEEKS

Precautions Rigidly fixed talar fractures are in a bivalved cast or cam walker.

Range of Motion

For rigidly fixed fractures, continue active range of motion as the metatarsophalangeal joints, tibiotalar joints, and subtalar joints. Remove bivalved cast or cam walker to perform range of motion.

For nonrigidly fixed fractures, continue active range of motion at the metatarsophalangeal joints only. The patient is still in a cast. The patient may attempt a small amount of ankle and subtalar motion within the cast.

Muscle Strength

For rigidly fixed fractures, begin isometric exercises to the dorsiflexors and plantar flexors of the ankle and the invertors and evertors in the cast.

For nonrigidly fixed fractures, no strengthening exercises.

Functional Activities For rigidly fixed fractures, continue partial weight-bearing stand/pivot transfers and a three-point gait.

Weight Bearing

For rigidly fixed fractures, continue toe-touch to partial weight bearing.

Nonrigidly fixed fractures are non-weight bearing in a short leg cast.

Treatment: Six to Eight Weeks

BONE HEALING

Stability at fracture site: Increasing stability. There is callus formation, but the strength of this callus, especially with torsional load, is significantly lower than that of normal lamellar bone. The foot requires further protection to avoid refracture. Confirm with physical examination and radiography.

Stage of bone healing: Reparative phase. Further organization of callus and formation of lamellar bone begins. Small amounts of callus are observed.

X-ray: The fracture line is less distinct. In the tarsal bones, which are mainly cancellous, no appreciable amount of callus is visible because the periosteum is thin.

Orthopaedic and Rehabilitation Considerations

Physical Examination

All fractures treated by open reduction and internal fixation should be out of a cast. Fractures being treated conservatively should be examined out of plaster, after which the non–weight-bearing short leg cast is replaced. Examine the fracture site for tenderness. If there was a wound or an operative site, evaluate it for healing and evidence of infection, and treat appropriately. Evaluate any trophic or sensory changes as possible evidence of RSD.

Radiography

Fractures of the talus should be evaluated with anteroposterior and lateral radiographs. If avascular necrosis is suspected, evaluate radiographs critically for Hawkins' sign. If there is evidence of vascularization (as would be noted by the lucent line seen on radiographs) and this is incomplete, the patient should remain partially weight bearing to limit the risk of collapsing the talar head (*see* Figure 31-12). This continues until there are obvious signs of either healing with increased vascularity or collapse of the talar head. Obvious signs of talar head collapse will most likely not be evident now even if avascular necrosis is present.

Weight Bearing

It is important to stress to the patient that weight bearing should only be partial, particularly if there is tenderness at the fracture site.

Talar fractures treated with internal fixation may now begin progressive partial weight bearing as the fixation and the patient's pain allow.

Talar fractures that have been treated conservatively must remain non-weight bearing in a short leg cast.

Range of Motion

Patients who remain in a cast because they have had conservative management of talar fractures should continue metatarsophalangeal joint range of motion.

Patients with internal fixation of the talus should attempt active range of motion in all planes out of the bivalved cast or cam walker.

Muscle Strength

Patients with rigid fixation of talar fractures begin resistive exercises in dorsiflexion, plantar flexion, inversion, and eversion out of the cast. Increase the resistive exercises as pain allows and continued healing at the fracture site demonstrates stability.

Patients treated conservatively may begin isometric exercises within the cast for dorsiflexion and plantar flexion as well as inversion and eversion as pain allows and as is permitted by room in the cast.

Functional Activities

Patients with talar fractures treated by internal fixation begin partial weight bearing using crutches and a three-point gait. Patients whose fractures were treated conservatively should remain non-weight bearing and continue to use assistive devices for transfers and gait.

Gait

Patients treated conservatively for talar fractures should remain fully non-weight bearing and use a two-point gait. Patients who are allowed to begin partial weight bearing with crutches use a three-point gait, placing the crutches first, followed by the unaffected extremity and then the affected extremity. To climb stairs, the patient places the unaffected extremity first, followed by the crutches and then the affected extremity, and descends stairs placing the crutches first, followed by the affected extremity and then the unaffected extremity. Patients who are allowed to toe-touch still have an antalgic gait because the fracture is not fully healed. However, it is too soon to attempt to normalize their gait because they are only partial weight bearing on their toes.

Methods of Treatment: Specific Aspects

Open Reduction and Internal Fixation

Any protective casts should have been removed by now. The patient may begin active and active-assistive range of motion as noted earlier, particularly of the tibiotalar and subtalar joints. There may be residual pain secondary to stiffness, which may be improved with hydrotherapy.

Cast

Patients being treated conservatively for talar fractures should remain fully non-weight bearing and in a short leg cast because the fracture may not yet be totally stable. They may continue range of motion at the knee as well as the metatarsophalangeal joints and begin isometric exercises of the plantar flexors and dorsiflexors and the invertors and evertors of the ankle within their casts.

Prescription

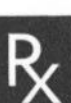

SIX TO EIGHT WEEKS

Precautions No passive range of motion.

Range of Motion

Rigidly fixed fractures may begin active-assistive range of motion in dorsiflexion and plantar flexion as well as inversion and eversion at the ankle and subtalar joint, out of the cast.

Nonrigidly fixed fractures may actively range the metatarsophalangeal joints as well as ankle and subtalar joints within or without a cast.

Muscle Strength

Rigidly fixed fractures may begin isometric exercises out of the cast.

Nonrigidly fixed fractures continue isometric exercises at the ankle and subtalar joint in the cast. Continue quadriceps strengthening.

Functional Activities

Rigidly fixed fractures continue partial weight bearing for transfers and ambulation with assistive devices.

Nonrigidly fixed fractures continue non–weight-bearing transfers and mobilization.

Weight Bearing

Rigidly fixed fractures may begin partial weight bearing as tolerated in a cast.

Nonrigidly fixed fractures must remain non-weight bearing.

Treatment: Eight to Twelve Weeks

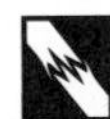

BONE HEALING

Stability at fracture site: Fractures treated with internal fixation are stable. Talar neck fractures that are not rigidly fixed may not be stable.

Stage of bone healing: Reparative/early remodeling phase. Woven bone is replaced with lamellar bone. The process of remodeling takes months to years for completion.

X-ray: Tarsal bones show that fracture lines are disappearing. This is more obvious with fractures that have had internal fixation. The amount of callus formation is significantly less than in midshaft long bone fractures because the periosteum is quite thin in this region.

Orthopaedic and Rehabilitation Considerations

Physical Examination

Evaluate for tenderness at the fracture site. Evaluate any wounds or operative sites for evidence of skin breakdown or infection. Blister healing should be complete. Evaluate all wounds and incisions for erythema or infection and treat appropriately. Evaluate for possible RSD. Restrict weight bearing for patients who are tender to palpation.

Radiography

For all fractures of the talus, anteroposterior and lateral views are crucial to determine if revascularization has occurred. Evaluate for evidence of Hawkins' sign. If there is avascular necrosis, there may be early evidence of partial or complete talar head collapse. This is seen by the flattening of the normally rounded talar head articulation or possibly by crescentic lucency at the talar head.

Weight Bearing

Talar fractures that have been treated with internal fixation may progress to full weight bearing if radiographs show evidence of adequate healing and they are nontender on weight bearing and palpation.

Talar fractures that have been treated conservatively remain non-weight bearing unless they are fully nontender and have shown reconsolidation of their fracture as evidenced by the loss of distinct fracture lines. These fractures are progressed to partial weight bearing.

Range of Motion

Patients whose fractures have been treated with internal fixation should continue with full active and passive range of motion at the ankle and subtalar joint in all planes.

All fractures that were treated conservatively should be able to come out of a cast and begin active and gentle passive range of motion of the ankle at the tibiotalar and subtalar joints.

Muscle Strength

For all fractures treated with internal fixation, patients continue gentle to more aggressive resistive exercises in dorsiflexion and plantar flexion and inversion and eversion. These all should be controlled by the patient to allow him or her to alter resistance according to pain tolerance. Patients should also continue quadriceps resistive exercises. Patients who have been treated conservatively should not engage in resistive exercises because inadequate healing may cause displacement of the fracture. This is particularly important in the talus because most of its surface is articular and displacement of fracture fragments could precipitate avascular necrosis and posttraumatic arthritis; the exception to this is the quadriceps, where isometric and isotonic exercises continue as before.

Functional Activities

All fractures treated by internal fixation may progress to full weight bearing as tolerated. Even if radiographs show adequate fracture healing, the patient may still need to use a crutch or cane for support and stability during transfers and ambulation.

Patients with conservatively treated talar fractures still need to use crutches but may be able to progress to some partial weight bearing using a three-point gait for transfers and ambulation.

Gait

Patients with talar fractures have tenderness from heel strike through single stance and into early push-off because the talar articular surfaces are involved in weight transfer through all these stages of the stance phase.

Particularly if there has been avascular necrosis of the talar head, the patient tries to avoid a steep-angle of push-off because this forces the talar head into the articular surface of the navicular.

Patients with inadequately healed fractures of the talar body have more discomfort in mid-stance and try to spend a little more time either on the heel or on the toe, depending on what portion of the body of the talus was affected. Patients with fractures of the talar neck tend to spend a little more time on their heel; those with more posterior body fractures tend to spend more time on their toes.

Methods of Treatment: Specific Aspects

Open Reduction and Internal Fixation

Casts should have been removed from all fractures by now. Patients should be undergoing active and resistive strengthening and range-of-motion exercises at the ankle, subtalar joint, and metatarsophalangeal joints. If they are pain free, they may progress at their own tolerance from partial to full weight bearing. The goal is to normalize gait.

Cast

Patients being treated conservatively in a cast remain non-weight bearing unless there has been adequate evidence of fracture consolidation, which allows them to begin partial weight bearing. They may continue active range of motion of the metatarsophalangeal joints as well as isometric exercises, plantar flexion and dorsiflexion, and inversion and eversion in the cast. With adequate evidence of healing, range of motion is done out of the cast. They should avoid resistive exercises.

Prescription

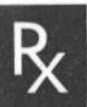

Eight to Twelve Weeks

Precautions Nonrigidly fixed fractures may need to limit the amount of weight bearing and the performance of resistive exercises.

Range of Motion

Rigidly fixed fractures may do active, active-assistive, and passive range of motion at the ankle and subtalar joints.

Nonrigidly fixed fractures allow active range of motion at the metatarsophalangeal joints and isometric exercises of the ankle and subtalar joints out of the casts.

Muscle Strength

Rigidly fixed fractures may begin gentle resistive exercises to the dorsiflexors and plantar flexors, evertors and invertors, and flexors and extensors of the toes.

For nonrigidly fixed fractures, no resistive exercises.

Functional Activities

Rigidly fixed fractures may progress to full weight bearing as tolerated for transfers and ambulation, using assistive devices as necessary.

Nonrigidly fixed fractures are either non-weight bearing or partial weight bearing. They require the use of assistive devices for transfers and ambulation.

Weight Bearing

Rigidly fixed fractures are partial to full weight bearing.

Nonrigidly fixed fractures are non-weight bearing to partial weight bearing.

Treatment: Twelve to Sixteen Weeks

Orthopaedic and Rehabilitation Considerations

Patients with rigidly fixed fractures are usually doing well if they have anatomic reduction of their fracture. They are out of their casts or immobilization devices. Progress patients to full weight bearing and normalize their gait. Avoid high-impact activities for 6 months.

Patients with nonrigidly fixed fractures are variable in the need to continue wearing the cast. Talar fractures are usually consolidated at this point and the cast is removed. Progress to full weight bearing and normalize their gait. Check radiographs for development of avascular necrosis, especially of the talar head. This precludes weight bearing.

LONG-TERM CONSIDERATIONS AND PROBLEMS

Fractures of the talus that lead to avascular necrosis can cause significant disability because the main articular surface that allows smooth weight transfer from the hindfoot to the midfoot through the talonavicular joint may be completely disrupted. Normal gait mechanics for these patients are virtually impossible because the talonavicular joint is affected. Additional surgery may be required to fuse the midfoot and hindfoot. This permanently precludes a normal gait in the affected extremity. Before surgery, the patient may need special stiff-soled shoes for ambulation.

Fractures of the talus, particularly those of the talar body, that do not regain anatomic alignment lead to serious impairment of tibiotalar and subtalar joint function secondary to arthritis. Disruption of these articular surfaces causes significant pain, and normal gait mechanics are not possible. In addition, significant posttraumatic arthritis develops in both joints in these patients, most likely requiring a fusion, or a total ankle joint replacement.

The extended immobilization that is often required for conservatively managed hindfoot fractures may lead to significant shortening of the posterior joint capsule. This limits full ankle motion (particularly dorsiflexion) and leads to tightening of the Achilles tendon. This in turn increases the load across the hindfoot/midfoot junction. Such changes further impede attempts to normalize the gait by overstressing these joints and possibly accelerating degenerative changes.

IMMEDIATE TO ONE WEEK

	Open Reduction and Internal Fixation	*Cast*
Stability	None.	None.
Orthopaedics	Trim cast to metatarsal heads to allow full range of motion at the knee.	Trim cast to metatarsal heads to allow full range of motion at the knee.
Rehabilitation	Range of motion of the metatarsophalangeal (MTP), interphalangeal (IP), and ankle joints while in compressive dressing awaiting casting.	Range of motion of the MTP and IP joints.

TWO WEEKS

	Open Reduction and Internal Fixation	*Cast*
Stability	None to minimal.	None to minimal.
Orthopaedics	Trim cast to metatarsal heads or change bivalved cast to cam walker.	Trim cast to metatarsal heads.
Rehabilitation	Range of motion of metatarsophalangeal (MTP), interphalangeal (IP), and knee joints. Also range the ankle and subtalar joints out of the cast or cam walker.	Range of motion of MTP, IP, and knee joints.

FOUR TO SIX WEEKS

	Open Reduction and Internal Fixation	*Cast*
Stability	Stable.	Stable.
Orthopaedics	Evaluate cast for breakdown and repair as necessary. Trim and pad cast as necessary.	Evaluate cast for breakdown and repair as necessary. Trim and pad cast as necessary.
Rehabilitation	Continue range of motion of the ankle and subtalar joints out of the cast.	Range of motion at the metatarsophalangeal, interphalangeal, and knee joints. Attempt small amount of subtalar and ankle motion within the cast.

SIX TO EIGHT WEEKS

	Open Reduction and Internal Fixation	Cast
Stability	Stable.	Stable.
Orthopaedics	Remove cast if not already done.	Continue short leg non–weight-bearing cast.
Rehabilitation	Continue active range of motion and dorsiflexion and plantar flexion, and inversion and eversion of ankle and subtalar joint out of the cast.	Actively range metatarsophalangeal and ankle joints within or out of a cast.

EIGHT TO TWELVE WEEKS

	Open Reduction and Internal Fixation	Cast
Stability	Stable.	Stable.
Orthopaedics	Remove cast.	Remove the cast. Occasionally may need cast for immobilization for weight bearing.
Rehabilitation	Active, active-assistive, and passive range of motion of ankle and subtalar joints.	Active range of motion of the metatarsophalangeal joints and isometric exercises to the ankle and subtalar joints out of a cast.

BIBLIOGRAPHY

Adelaar RS. Complex fractures of the talus. *Instr Course Lect*, 46:323–338, 1997.

Canale ST, Kelly FB. Fractures of the neck of the talus. *J Bone Joint Surg Am*, 60:143–156, 1978.

DeLee J. Talus and MTP injuries. In: Mann RA, ed. *Surgery of the Foot*, 5th ed. St. Louis: C.V. Mosby, 1986, pp. 656–711.

Geissler W, Tsao A. Foot and ankle fractures. In: Rockwood CA Jr, Green DP, eds. *Fractures in Adults*, 4th ed. Philadelphia: J.B. Lippincott, 1995, pp. 2212–2235.

Hansen ST Jr. Foot injuries. In: Browner B, Jupiter J, Levine AM, Trafton PG, eds. *Skeletal Trauma*, Vol 2. Philadelphia: W.B. Saunders, 1992, pp. 1960–1972.

Inokuchi S, Ogawa K, Usami N. Classification of fracture of the talus: clear differentiation between neck and body fractures. *Foot and Ankle*, 17:748–750, 1996.

Jahss MH. *Disorders of the Foot and Ankle: Medical and Surgical Management*. Philadelphia: W.B. Saunders, 1990.

Mann R. Lower extremity. In: Chapman M, ed. *Operative Orthopaedics*. Philadelphia: J.B. Lippincott, 1993, pp. 2143–2178.

Mann RA, Coughlin MJ. *Surgery of the Foot and Ankle,* 7th ed. St. Louis: Mosby, 1999.

Manoli A II. Compartment syndromes of the foot: current concepts. *Foot and Ankle*, 10:340–344, 1990.

Mizel M, Sobel M. Trauma—Section 1. In: Miller M, ed. *Review of Orthopaedics*, 2nd ed. Philadelphia: W.B. Saunders, 1996, pp. 390–391.

Perry J. Ankle and foot gait deviations. In: Perry J, ed. *Gait Analysis*. Thorofare, NJ, Slack, 1992, pp. 185–219.

Tile M. Fractures of the talus. In: Schatzker J, Tile M, eds. *The Rationale of Operative Fracture Care*, 2nd ed. Berlin, Springer-Verlag, 1996, pp. 563–569.

Yablon IG, Segal D. Foot and ankle injuries. In: Evarts CM, ed. *Surgery of the Musculoskeletal System*, 2nd ed. New York: Churchill Livingstone, 1990, pp. 4257–4267.

CHAPTER *Thirty-two*

Calcaneal Fractures

ANNE P. MCCORMACK, MD

INTRODUCTION

Definition

Fractures of the hindfoot are those involving the calcaneus (os calcis) and the talus or any of its processes.

Fractures of the calcaneus are often intraarticular, involving the subtalar and sometimes the calcaneocuboid joint (*see* Figure 32-10). Nonarticular fractures of the calcaneus usually involve the so-called posterior beak (the posterior aspect of the calcaneus including the bony insertion of the Achilles tendon; *see* Figure 32-10) and may or may not involve injury to the Achilles tendon (Figures 32-1, 32-2, 32-3, and 32-4).

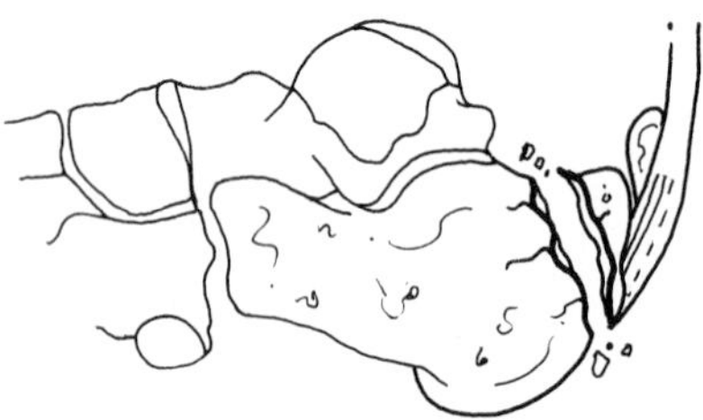

FIGURE 32-1 A posterior beak fracture of the calcaneus (os calcis). The posterior aspect of the calcaneus is involved, including the bony insertion of the Achilles tendon.

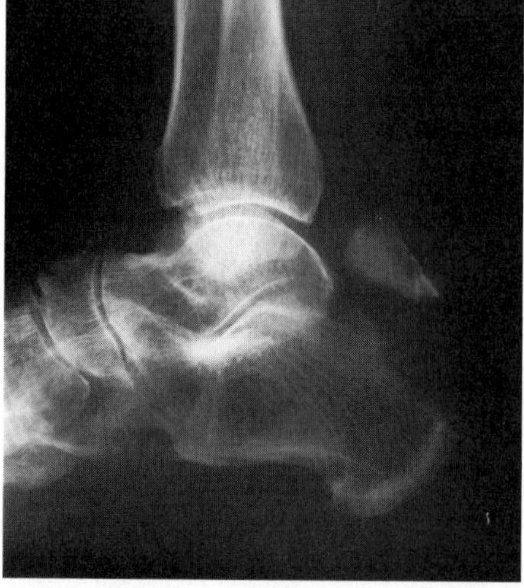

FIGURE 32-2 Lateral radiograph of the calcaneus revealing a posterior beak fracture. This is a nonarticular fracture. (Courtesy of Dr. Jerry Sallis, Albert Einstein College of Medicine, Bronx, NY.)

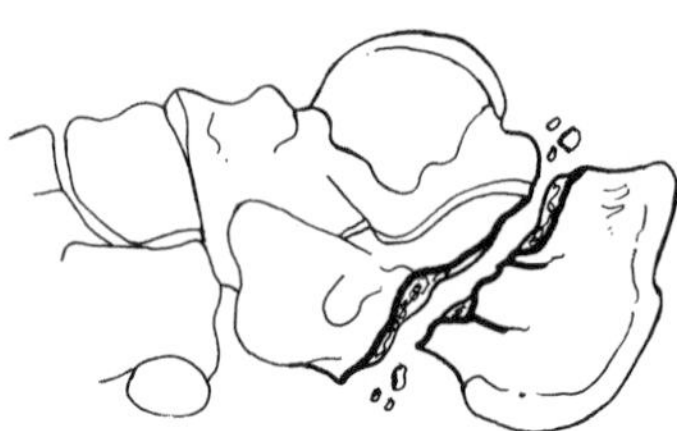

FIGURE 32-3 Extraarticular calcaneal fracture involving the posterior aspect. This fracture is often caused by a sudden, high-velocity impact on the heel such as in a motor vehicle accident or a fall of 3 feet of more directly onto the heel.

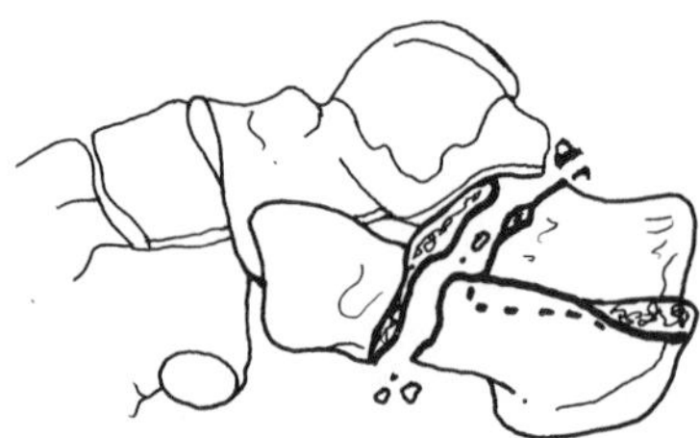

FIGURE 32-4 Intraarticular calcaneal fracture involving the subtalar joint. It is important to reestablish the length and normal width of the calcaneus and restore the calcaneal surface of the subtalar joint.

Mechanism of Injury

Calcaneus (os calcis) fractures are often caused by a sudden, high-velocity impact on the heel, such as in a motor vehicle accident or landing from a fall of 3 feet or more directly onto the heel.

Treatment Goals

Orthopaedic Objectives

Alignment

Reestablish the length and normal width of the calcaneus and restore the calcaneal surface of the subtalar joint (*see* Figures 32-12 and 32-13).

Stability

Stable fixation of the calcaneus is crucial to allow restoration and maintenance of Böhler's angle (a radiographic measurement seen on the lateral view; it is the angle formed by the intersection of a line drawn along the upper surface of the calcaneus with a line connecting the highest points of the anterior and posterior facets; Figures 32-5 and 32-6). This is also important to restore the normal anatomy of the subtalar joint at the posterior, anterior, and medial facets (Figure 32-7).

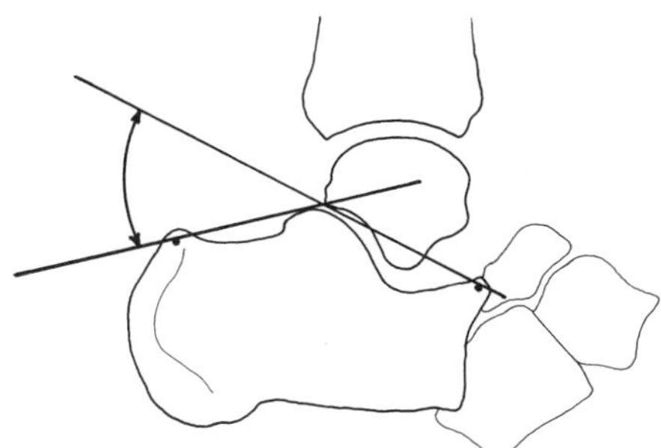

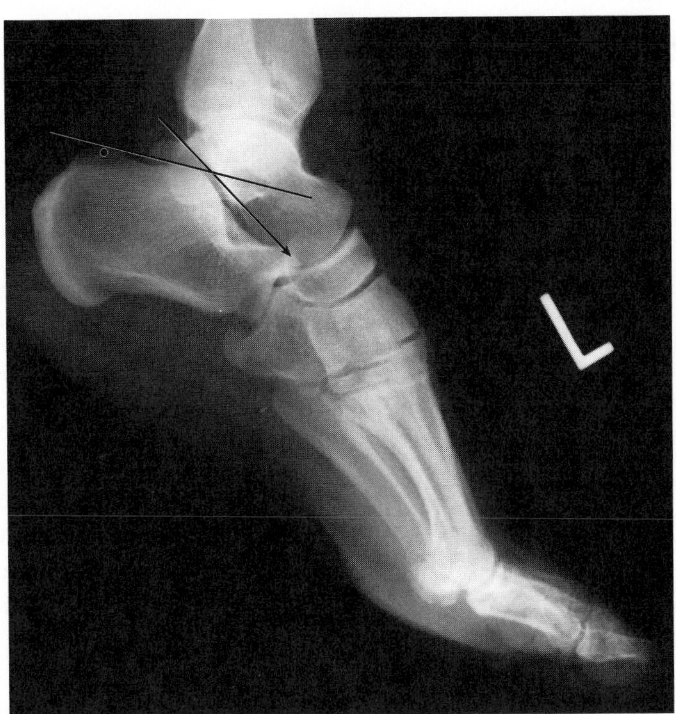

FIGURE 32-5 *(above)* Lateral view of Böhler's angle radiographic measurement, the angle formed by the intersection of a line drawn from the upper surface of the calcaneus with a line connecting the highest point of the anterior and posterior facets.

FIGURE 32-6 *(right)* Böhler's angle as seen on a lateral radiograph of the foot and ankle. Loss of this angle implies loss of the appropriate articulation of the subtalar joint at the posterior, anterior, and middle facets.

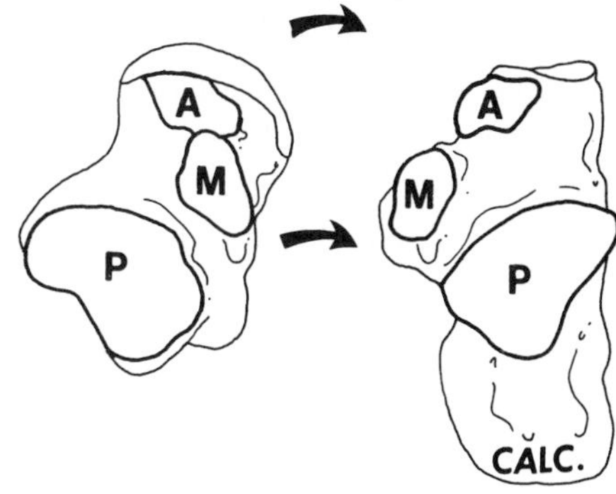

FIGURE 32-7 Subtalar joint. The talus and calcaneus are opened like a clam. To the right, the dorsal surface of the calcaneus is noted, revealing the anterior, middle, and posterior facets. To the left is the ventral surface (undersurface) of the talus, revealing the anatomy of the subtalar joint at the posterior, anterior, and middle facets. It is critical to restore normal articulation of these joints after an intraarticular calcaneal fracture.

Rehabilitation Objectives

Range of Motion

Restore the range of motion of the ankle and foot in all planes.

Restore the full range of motion of the subtalar joint, which is likely to be affected by intraarticular calcaneus (os calcis) fractures (Table 32-1).

TABLE 32-1 *Ankle Ranges of Motion*

Motion	Normal	Functional
Ankle plantar flexion	45°	20°
Ankle dorsiflexion	20°	10°
Foot inversion	35°	10°
Foot eversion	25°	10°

Intraarticular fractures of the calcaneus that are not anatomically reduced may result in loss of range of motion. This causes increased stress on the subtalar articulation and leads to degeneration and arthritic changes (*see* Figure 32-7).

Muscle Strength

Improve the strength of the muscles that cross the ankle joint, which are affected by the fracture or by cast immobilization:

Plantar flexors of the ankle and foot:

- Gastrocnemius
- Soleus
- Tibialis posterior (also acts as an invertor)
- Flexor digitorum longus
- Flexor hallucis longus

Dorsiflexors of the ankle and foot:

- Tibialis anterior (also acts as an invertor)
- Extensor digitorum longus
- Extensor hallucis longus

Evertors of the ankle and foot:

- Peroneus longus
- Peroneus brevis

Invertors of the ankle and foot:

- Tibialis posterior (also acts as a plantar flexor)
- Tibialis anterior (also acts as a dorsiflexor)

Functional Goals

Normalize the gait pattern. If a calcaneal fracture has left the patient with a shortened or widened calcaneus, shoe inserts and custom footwear help to restore a normal and pain-free gait.

Expected Time of Bone Healing

Eight to 12 weeks.

Expected Duration of Rehabilitation

Twelve to 16 weeks. Patients treated nonoperatively may take as long as 12 to 18 months.

Methods of Treatment

Open Reduction and Internal Fixation (Screw and Plate Fixation)

Biomechanics: Stress-shielding device.

Mode of bone healing: Primary, with rigid fixation.

Indications: A large percentage of calcaneus fractures are intraarticular, involving the facets of the subtalar joint (*see* Figures 32-4 and 32-7). Restoration of the normal anatomy is the key to minimizing the possibility of subtalar arthritis as well as to allow for a normal and pain-free gait. Open reduction may also be indicated for large nonarticular calcaneal fractures that involve the Achilles tendon (Figures 32-8 and 32-9). The return of function directly corresponds to how accurately the talocalcaneal joint is restored and to what degree the normal height, width, and alignment of the heel are reestablished. Screws, plates, and bone grafting are the usual methods of fixation (Figures 32-10, 32-11, 32-12, and 32-13). Factors that preclude

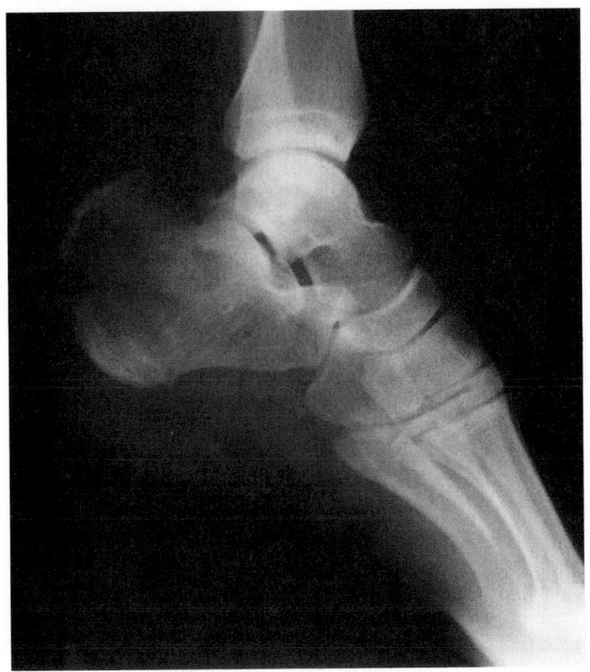

FIGURE 32-8 A large nonarticular calcaneal fracture involving the Achilles tendon.

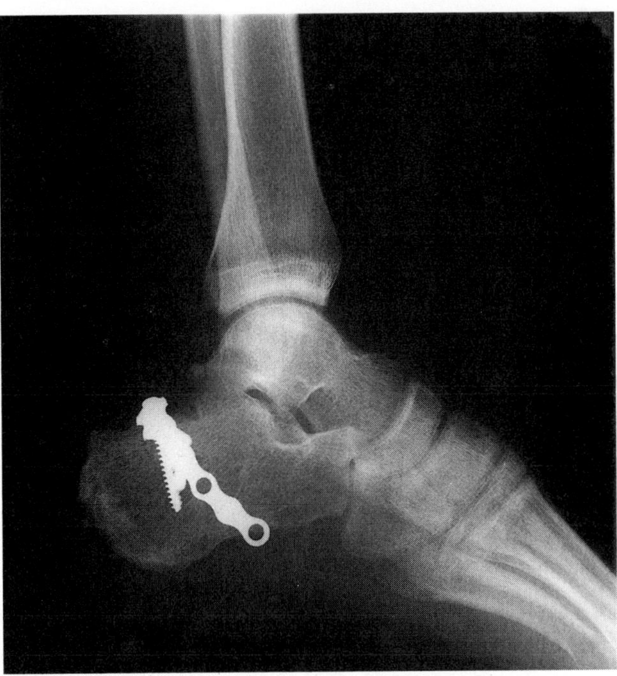

FIGURE 32-9 Open reduction and internal fixation of a nonarticular calcaneal fracture with screws and plates.

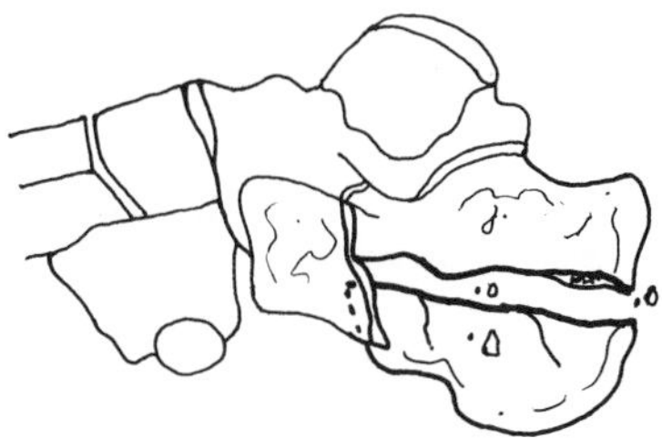

FIGURE 32-10 Intraarticular calcaneal fracture. The calcaneocuboid joint is involved.

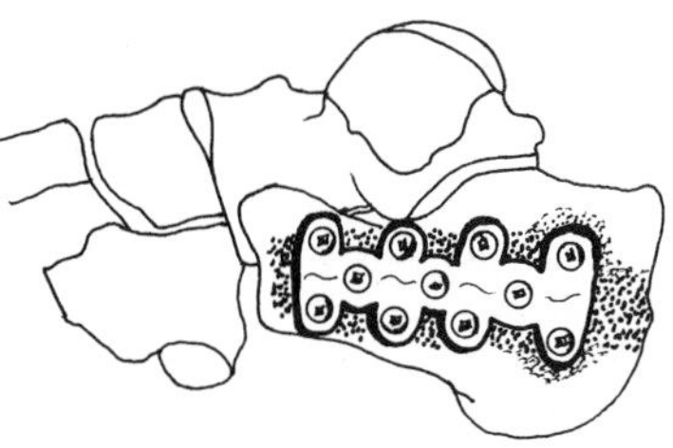

FIGURE 32-11 Internal fixation of a calcaneal fracture with a plate. This restores articular congruity.

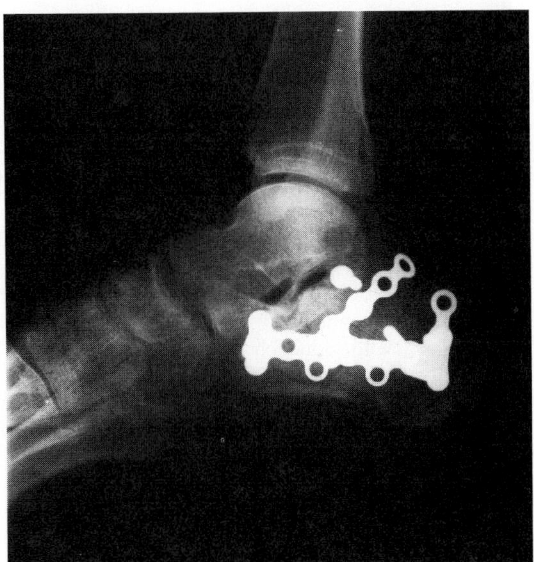

FIGURE 32-12 Intraarticular calcaneal fracture that occurred when the patient jumped from a first-story window. The height and length of the calcaneus have been restored as well as the calcaneal surface of the subtalar joint.

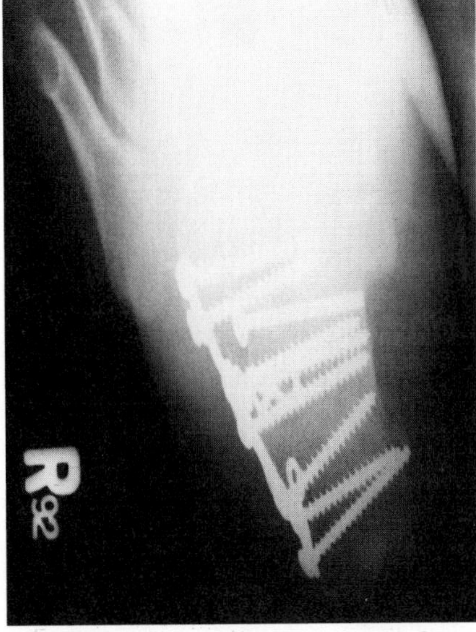

FIGURE 32-13 Width and alignment of the heel have been reestablished with the use of screws and plates. The return to function directly corresponds to how accurately the talocalcaneal joint is restored and to what degree the normal height, width, and alignment of the heel are reestablished.

surgery include excessive swelling of the soft tissues of the foot. Surgery must be postponed if skin (fracture) blisters develop. Primary reduction is still possible after 3 to 4 weeks but becomes more difficult because of consolidation of the fracture. If surgery cannot be performed by 4 weeks, the preferred treatment is to allow the fracture to consolidate for 3 to 12 months and then reconstruct the os calcis with an osteotomy and subtalar joint fusion.

Patients treated with open reduction and internal fixation are placed in a cast after edema subsides. They can expect to remain in a cast for 8 weeks. Calcaneal fractures tend to have more swelling than talar fractures (Figures 32-14, 32-15, 32-16, and 32-17).

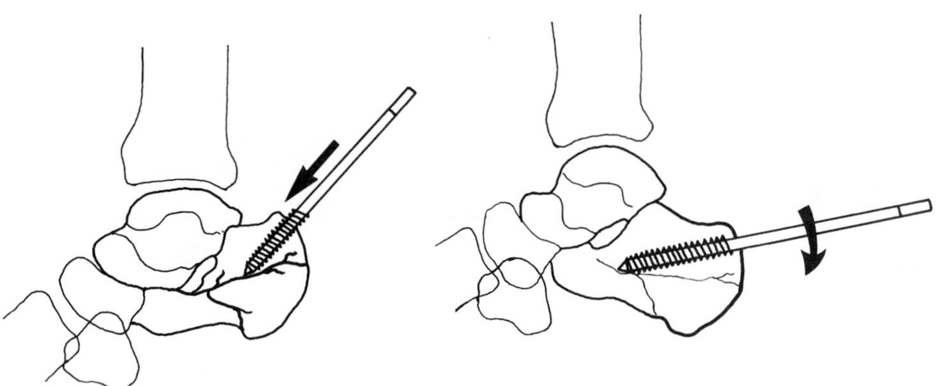

FIGURE 32-14 *(above)* Essex-Lopresti method of treating a calcaneal fracture. A pin is placed into the calcaneus and reduction is attempted by levering the pin toward the plantar surface of the foot in order to restore the subtalar joint, Böhler's angle, and the height of the calcaneus.

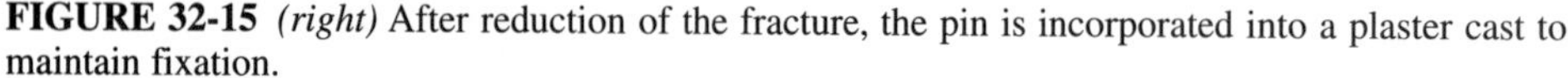

FIGURE 32-15 *(right)* After reduction of the fracture, the pin is incorporated into a plaster cast to maintain fixation.

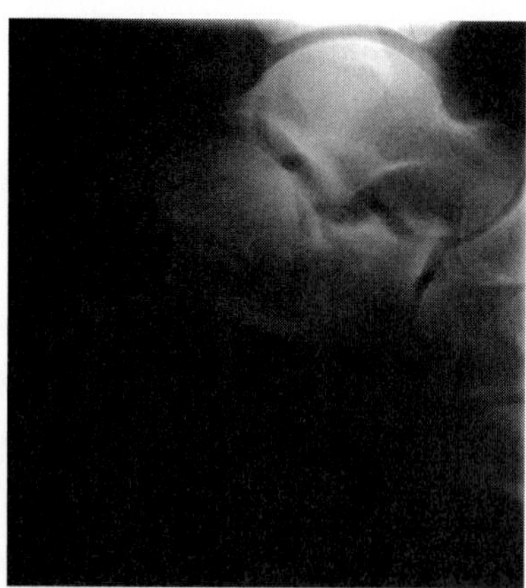

FIGURE 32-16 Calcaneal fracture with loss of height and reduction of Böhler's angle.

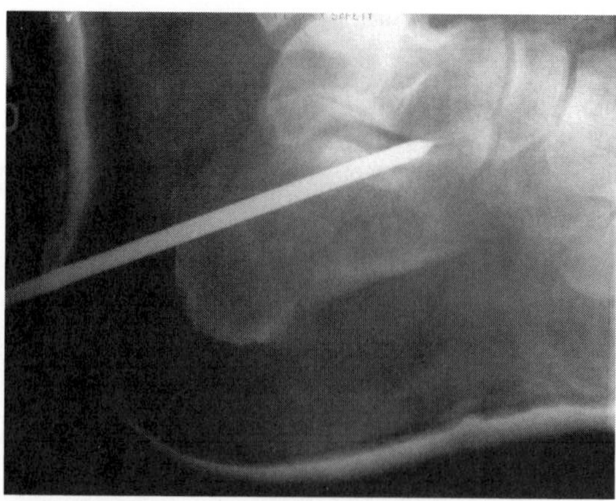

FIGURE 32-17 Treatment of the calcaneal fracture, Essex-Lopresti method, with reduction of the fracture restoring height and Böhler's angle. The fracture and pin are then maintained in the corrected position in a cast. The pin had to be reinserted because of its involvement with the subtalar joint. This method of treatment is used less frequently than open reduction and plate fixation.

Cast

Biomechanics: Stress-sharing device.

Mode of bone healing: Secondary, with callus formation, although little callus is formed in this mainly cancellous bone with a relatively thin cortex.

Indications: Any minimally displaced nonarticular calcaneal fractures may be treated nonoperatively. These fractures are often considered posterior beak fractures. If the Achilles tendon is involved, surgery should be performed.

Closed reduction does not restore normal anatomy, leaving the patient with significant functional disabilities, especially in the area of gait. Most of these fractures take 8 to 12 weeks to heal, with a tolerable level of residual pain. Rehabilitation may take as long as 12 to 18 months. However, the patient rarely returns to a normal activity level or a normal gait. Many of these patients may require fusion at a later date. Patients treated conservatively can expect to be in a cast for 12 to 16 weeks, depending on their healing and pain tolerance. Patients are first treated in a bulky compressive dressing to control swelling. Initial casting may be delayed 1 week to 10 days if there is marked swelling or skin (fracture) blisters.

Special Considerations of the Fracture

Age

Elderly patients are at greater risk for development of joint stiffness. Patients of all ages are prone to avascular necrosis, although elderly patients with compromised circulation may be even more susceptible. Rehabilitation may be prolonged and never be complete for elderly patients with preexisting arthritic changes in the subtalar joint.

Articular Involvement

Fractures of the calcaneus may interrupt the articular facets of the subtalar joint. It is important to regain anatomic alignment and maintain it until full healing to minimize further degenerative changes in the subtalar joint, as well as to restore a pain-free gait (*see* Figures 32-12 and 32-13).

Location

Fractures of the calcaneus that are treated closed and do not attain anatomic realignment have a prolonged course of healing and rehabilitation. In many cases, the patient may never regain a pain-free, normal gait.

Open Fractures

Any open fracture of the calcaneus must be treated aggressively with irrigation, débridement, and intravenous antibiotics. The likelihood of infection increases after the placement of hardware.

Tendon and Ligamentous Injuries

Nonarticular fractures of the calcaneus that involve the Achilles tendon must be surgically addressed. The gastrocnemius-soleus complex converges to become the Achilles tendon at the posterior aspect of the calcaneus. Loss of Achilles tendon function disables the gastrocnemius-soleus complex, and the patient is unable to plantar flex the ankle or foot. There can be a residual loss of strength from disuse as well as from any avulsion of the Achilles tendon from the calcaneus.

Associated Injury

There is a risk of a foot compartment syndrome secondary to a calcaneus fracture. The relatively closed and small compartment that surrounds the calcaneus is prone to massive soft-tissue swelling. Significant soft-tissue edema or the presence of skin (fracture) blisters precludes any surgical intervention until these can be addressed.

Because of the force involved with most of these fractures, there may be significant soft-tissue damage. Even with open fractures, isolated compartments may still swell and need to be observed. The patient must be watched carefully for the possibility of a foot compartment syndrome.

Weight Bearing

In the immediate postoperative period, patients with calcaneus fractures should be at bed rest for 2 to 5 days with the leg elevated. Once swelling is reduced, the patient is placed in a short leg cast and allowed out of bed. The patient may use toe-touch weight bearing for balance only. At approximately 2 to 3 weeks after surgery, the patient may begin partial (weight-of-leg) weight bearing for an additional 3 weeks. The patient then increases weight bearing in a cast until 8 weeks after surgery. If healing is satisfactory, weight bearing after 8 weeks may be out of a cast. Full weight bearing is initiated approximately 3 months after surgery as pain tolerance and healing allow.

Gait

Stance Phase

The stance phase constitutes 60% of the gait cycle.

Heel Strike

The initial impact causes significant discomfort as the body's weight is transferred onto the posterior facet of the subtalar joint. This pain continues as the weight is transferred from the hindfoot to the midfoot and the anterior and medial facets are engaged.

During the initial healing phase of calcaneal fractures, the patient tries to limit the time spent on the heel and midfoot and to decrease the angle of attack at heel strike to minimize axial loading across the calcaneus (Figure 32-18). Patients tend to toe walk to avoid

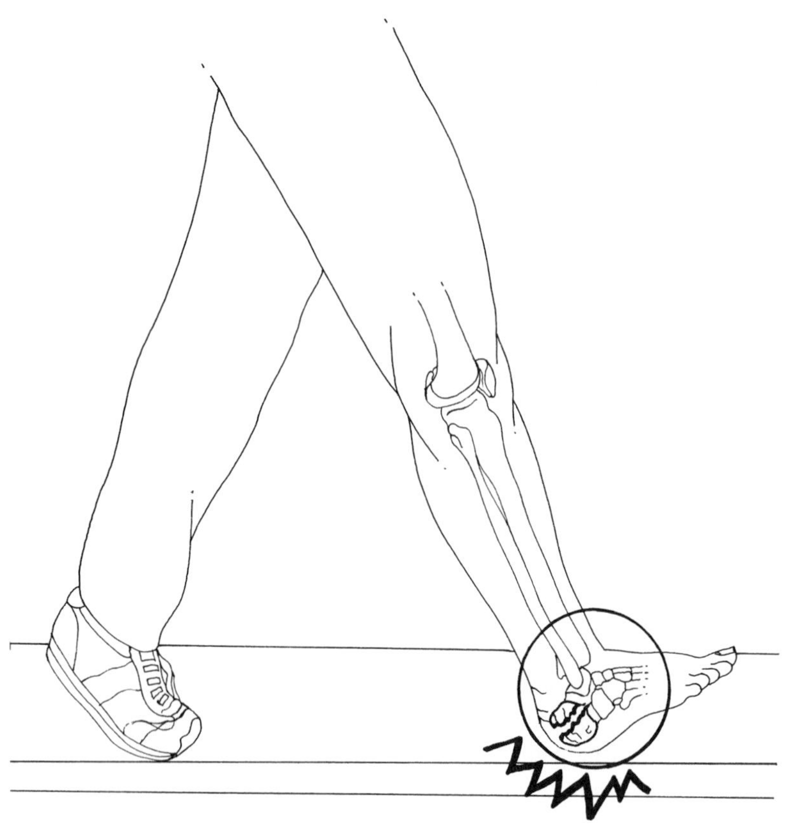

FIGURE 32-18 The initial impact of heel strike may cause significant discomfort as the body weight is transferred onto the previously fractured calcaneus and posterior facet of the subtalar joint. The patient spends as little time at heel strike as possible, frequently hopping off the foot (antalgic gait), and may tend to toe walk to avoid placing weight directly on the calcaneus.

placing weight directly on the calcaneus. Exceptions to this would be posterior beak fractures, in which stress across the Achilles tendon increases the discomfort. These patients may try to spend more time on their heel and keep the gastrocnemius-soleus complex from firing (*see* Figure 6-1).

Foot Flat

This portion of the gait cycle is also painful as weight is transferred from the posterior facet to the anterior and medial facets and the talonavicular joint. This places significant force across both the calcaneus facets and the talar body and neck (*see* Figure 6-2).

Fractures of the calcaneus involving the anterior and medial facet are also somewhat painful because weight is transferred as the foot transitions from inversion to eversion.

Mid-Stance

Because the weight is borne on one foot, mid-stance is quite painful (*see* Figure 6-3).

Push-off

Most of the load has been removed from the calcaneus at this point, and except for fractures of the posterior beak that involve the Achilles tendon, push-off is relatively pain free (*see* Figures 6-4 and 6-5).

Swing Phase

The swing phase constitutes 40% of the gait cycle.

The swing phase usually is not affected by fractures of the calcaneus except those in which there has been a posterior beak fracture involving the Achilles tendon. In this case, the patient may limit the force of ankle dorsiflexion and adopt a steppage-type gait to avoid discomfort (*see* Figures 6-6, 6-7, and 6-8).

TREATMENT

Treatment: Early to Immediate (Day of Injury to One Week)

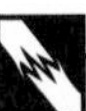

BONE HEALING

Stability at fracture site: None

Stage of bone healing: Inflammatory phase. The fracture hematoma is colonized by inflammatory cells, and débridement of the fracture begins.

X-ray: No callus; visible fracture lines.

Orthopaedic and Rehabilitation Considerations

Physical Examination

Pay special attention to complaints of pain, paresthesia, and cast discomfort as indicators of a compartment syndrome. Check the looseness of any compressive dressing or cast. Check for capillary refill and sensation. The toes should be pink, with brisk refill after light compression. It should be possible to reach the first web space of the foot and stroke it lightly with a blunt instrument to ensure that there is no peroneal nerve compression. Evaluate fractures of the calcaneus for evidence of edema or skin (fracture) blisters.

Dangers

Patients with significant soft-tissue swelling in the foot are at increased risk for compartment syndrome. Suspect symptoms include significant swelling, tightness of the skin, and the presence of fracture blisters. Pay particular attention to complaints of severe pain, paresthesia, and cast or compressive dressing discomfort. For patients with fracture blisters, evaluate the skin for erythema or drainage that might indicate the presence of infection. The patient should be advised to keep the extremity elevated above heart level and to place ice packs over the ankle and foot to decrease the swelling.

Radiography

Obtain and check anteroposterior and lateral radiographs of the foot as well as Harris views (posterior tangential views of the calcaneus in which the x-ray beam is angled 45 degrees to the heel) for any loss of intraoperative correction.

Weight Bearing

All fractures of the calcaneus should be non-weight bearing. For most of the initial week, the patient should be at bed rest with the foot elevated above heart level to control swelling.

Range of Motion

Once the initial pain subsides, start active range-of-motion exercises in dorsiflexion, plantar flexion, eversion, and inversion as tolerated while awaiting casting, providing the fracture has been rigidly fixed. Range of motion is avoided if the fracture has not been internally fixed. The patient should be able to perform active range of motion of the knee in flexion and extension. The metatarsophalangeal joints should also be actively ranged.

Muscle Strength

Quadriceps sets are prescribed to maintain quadriceps strength.

Functional Activities

The patient is taught to don pants on the involved extremity first and doff them from the uninvolved extremity first.

The patient is taught non–weight-bearing stand/pivot transfers from the bed to a chair, and vice versa. The patient needs assistive devices such as crutches or a walker for transfers and ambulation.

Gait

The patient is taught a two-point gait using crutches or a walker, with no weight bearing on the affected extremity (*see* Figure 6-16). To climb stairs, the patient places the crutches first and then hops to the step with the unaffected extremity; to descend stairs, the patient places the crutches first, followed by the unaffected extremity (*see* Figures 6-21, 6-22, 6-23, 6-24, and 6-25).

Methods of Treatment: Specific Aspects

Open Reduction and Internal Fixation

A cast may be placed during the first 2 to 5 days if swelling and the resolution of fracture blisters allow. While awaiting casting, begin range-of-motion and isometric exercises to the muscles of the ankle and foot for edema reduction. Check the cast margins to make sure they are well padded. Again, note that the metatarsophalangeal joints have free movement. Look for any breakdown of the skin at the edges of the cast and trim the cast appropriately. If there is any breakdown or softening of the cast, repair it as necessary.

Cast

Evaluate the condition of the cast. The cast margins should be adequately padded. There should be free movement of the metatarsophalangeal joints and full extension and flexion at the knee. Evaluate the skin at the edges of the cast to ensure that any swelling has not caused skin breakdown and there is no evidence of cyanosis or compartment syndrome. If the cast has softened under the foot, this is an appropriate time to reinforce and repair it.

Prescription

DAY ONE TO ONE WEEK

Precautions Fixation is not rigid unless the patient has had open reduction and internal fixation. Avoid passive range of motion.

Range of Motion Active range of motion of the toes, metatarsophalangeal joints, and knee. Before casting, do not move the ankle and subtalar joint unless rigidly fixed.

Muscle Strength No strengthening exercises to the ankle or foot.

Functional Activities Non–weight-bearing stand/pivot transfers and ambulation with assistive devices.

Weight Bearing None.

Treatment: Two Weeks

BONE HEALING

Stability at fracture site: None to minimal.

Stage of bone healing: Beginning of reparative phase. Osteoprogenitor cells differentiate into osteoblasts that lay down woven bone.

X-ray: No changes noted. Fracture lines are visible. No callus formation.

Orthopaedic and Rehabilitation Considerations

Physical Examination

Check for capillary refill and sensation of the toes. If possible, check the first dorsal web space. Check the active and passive range of motion of all metatarsophalangeal and interphalangeal joints. Change the cast. Examine the skin of the ankle and heel for any evidence of infection or skin breakdown. Remove any sutures.

Dangers

Pay particular attention to complaints of pain, paresthesia, and cast discomfort. The patient should be made aware that any pronounced amount of swelling could lead to skin sloughing and should be immediately brought to the physician's attention. The patient should be advised to continue extremity elevation above the heart level as much as possible to reduce swelling and improve circulation.

Radiography

Check anteroposterior, lateral, and Harris view radiographs. Assess any loss of reduction or movement of hardware as well as extrusion of bone graft.

Weight Bearing

All patients with calcaneal fractures should still be non-weight bearing.

Range of Motion

Patients with calcaneal fractures should continue range of motion to the metatarsophalangeal and knee joints while in the cast.

Patients with rigidly fixed fractures of the calcaneus should be placed back in a short leg cast for a total of 6 weeks' immobilization. Nonrigidly fixed calcaneal fractures should be placed back in a short leg cast for a total of 8 to 12 weeks.

Muscle Strength

Maintain quadriceps strength. As pain allows, the patient may attempt to strengthen the toe flexors and extensors by repetitive flexion and extension exercises.

Functional Activities

Patients with calcaneus fractures remain non-weight bearing and continue stand/pivot transfers.

Gait

Patients with calcaneal fractures continue a non–weight-bearing gait using crutches (*see* Figure 6-16).

Methods of Treatment: Specific Aspects

Open Reduction and Internal Fixation

Trim the cast to allow visualization of the toes and the metatarsophalangeal joints, if this has not already been done. Reinforce any cast breakdown at the foot or the metatarsophalangeal joints. Patients should continue with range of motion at the metatarsophalangeal joints. Begin exercises of the gastrocnemius-soleus group, the tibialis anterior, and toe extensors by having the patient attempt to plantar flex and dorsiflex within the cast. If there has been stable internal fixation of the fracture, begin gentle isometric exercises of the peronei group by gentle eversion within the cast. Try to invert the foot to strengthen the tibialis posterior as well as provide subtalar motion.

Cast

Trim the cast to allow visualization of the toes to the metatarsophalangeal joint, if this has not already been done. Reinforce the cast if it has broken down. Continue metatarsophalangeal joint range of motion. If casting is the primary method of treatment, the patient should not begin any exercises across the ankle or subtalar joints.

Prescription

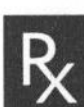

TWO WEEKS

Precautions Fixation is not rigid, unless the patient has had open reduction and internal fixation. Avoid passive range of motion.

Range of Motion Rigidly fixed and nonrigidly fixed fractures may range the metatarsophalangeal joints only.

Muscle Strength Rigidly fixed calcaneal fractures may begin isometric exercises in dorsiflexion and plantar flexion as well as inversion and eversion in the cast only.

Functional Activities Non–weight-bearing stand/pivot transfers for calcaneus fractures.

Weight Bearing Calcaneus fractures are non-weight bearing.

Treatment: Four to Six Weeks

BONE HEALING

Stability at fracture site: Some stability at fracture site. There is some callus formation, but the strength of this callus, especially with torsional load, is significantly lower than that of normal bone. The foot requires further protection to avoid refractures. Confirm with physical examination and radiography.

Stage of bone healing: Reparative phase. Further organization of the callus and formation of lamellar bone begins.

X-ray: The tarsal bones, which are mainly cancellous in composition, with minimal periosteum, begin to show consolidation of the fracture and filling in of lucent lines. With increased rigidity, lucency disappears, and healing with endosteal callus predominates because there is little periosteum.

Orthopaedic and Rehabilitation Considerations

Physical Examination

Remove the cast and perform the radiographic examination out of plaster.

Check for stability, tenderness, and range of motion.

Dangers

Most of the swelling from acute fractures should be relieved. Check for any trophic signs of reflex sympathetic dystrophy (RSD), characterized by vasomotor disturbances, hyperesthesias, and pain and tenderness out of proportion to the stage of fracture healing. If evidence of RSD is noted, the patient should begin a more aggressive physical therapy program, including hydrotherapy.

Radiography

Examine radiographs for evidence of healing and any loss of reduction. These are taken in the anteroposterior and lateral positions. Include a Harris view.

Patients who have undergone bone grafting for calcaneus fractures should be carefully assessed for incorporation of their bone graft.

Evaluate all hardware for any evidence of loosening by looking for lucency around the pins. Check the alignment to ensure there has been no change in the interval between examinations.

Weight Bearing

A patient with a calcaneus fracture treated with open reduction and internal fixation may gradually begin toe-touch weight bearing and slowly progress to partial weight bearing until 8 weeks after surgery. The amount of weight bearing is determined by the patient's pain. Patients who were treated with closed reduction should remain non-weight bearing.

Range of Motion

Patients with rigidly fixed or closed-reduced calcaneal fractures may continue with metatarsophalangeal joint range of motion. Patients with rigidly fixed fractures may also begin to range the ankle joint in the cast. Note that the cast will have had some compression of the padding and should be loose enough to allow the patient to move the ankle slightly.

Muscle Strength

Repeated range-of-motion exercises gradually increase the strength of the involved muscles. Continue quadriceps strengthening. Begin isometric ankle exercises to improve the strength of the gastrocnemius-soleus group and the tibialis anterior. Posterior beak fractures of the calcaneus that involve the Achilles tendon should not undergo gastrocnemius-soleus strengthening exercises.

Functional Activities

Rigidly fixed calcaneus fractures may continue with partial weight-bearing transfers and ambulation. Patients still need to use crutches or a walker during transfers.

Fractures of the calcaneus that have been treated closed should remain non-weight bearing for transfers and ambulation.

Gait

Patients who are non-weight bearing continue to use crutches or a walker for ambulation. Patients who have begun weight bearing may use a three-point gait in which the crutches form one point and the affected and unaffected extremities the other two points (*see* Figure 6-17). The patient climbs stairs with the unaffected extremity first, followed by the crutches and then the affected extremity, and descends stairs by placing the crutches first, followed by the affected extremity and then the unaffected extremity (*see* Figures 6-20, 6-21, 6-22, 6-23, 6-24, and 6-25).

All weight bearing is in either a cast, splint, or cam walker. Attempts to normalize the gait cycle do not begin yet.

Methods of Treatment: Specific Aspects

Open Reduction and Internal Fixation

Rigidly fixed fractures of the calcaneus are still in a short leg cast. The cast should be evaluated for adequate padding and any evidence of breakdown. Evaluate range of motion at the metatarsophalangeal joints and encourage range of motion of the tibiotalar and subtalar joints in the cast.

Cast

Patients who have been treated with closed reduction and casting are non-weight bearing and should have the cast removed only for examination and radiography out of plaster. A non–weight-bearing short leg cast should be replaced. Evaluate the range of motion at the metatarsophalangeal joints. As before, isometric exercises may be done in the cast.

Prescription

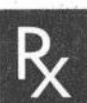

FOUR TO SIX WEEKS

Precautions All calcaneus fractures are still in a non–weight-bearing short leg cast.

Range of Motion

Rigidly fixed fractures are still casted. Continue active range of motion to the metatarsophalangeal joints as well as isometric exercises of the ankle, plantar flexion and dorsiflexion, and inversion and eversion in the cast.

Nonrigidly fixed fractures continue active range of motion at the metatarsophalangeal joints only. The patient is still in a cast.

Muscle Strength

Rigidly fixed fractures begin isometric exercises to the dorsiflexors and plantar flexors of the ankle and the invertors and evertors in the cast.

For nonrigidly fixed fractures, no strengthening exercises.

Functional Activities Rigidly fixed fractures of the calcaneus and talus may continue partial weight-bearing stand/pivot transfers and a three-point gait.

Weight Bearing

Rigidly fixed fractures may continue toe-touch to partial weight bearing.

Nonrigidly fixed fractures are non-weight bearing in a short leg cast.

Treatment: Six to Eight Weeks

BONE HEALING

Stability at fracture site: Increasing stability. There is callus formation, but the strength of this callus, especially with torsional load, is significantly lower than that of normal lamellar bone. The foot requires further protection to avoid refracture. Confirm with physical examination and radiography.

Stage of bone healing: Reparative phase. Further organization of callus begins and formation of lamellar bone begins. Small amounts of callus are observed.

X-ray: The fracture line is less distinct. In the tarsal bones, which are mainly cancellous, no appreciable amount of callus is visible because the periosteum is thin.

Orthopaedic and Rehabilitation Considerations

Physical Examination

All fractures treated with open reduction and internal fixation should be out of a cast. Fractures treated conservatively should be examined out of plaster, after which the non–weight-bearing short leg cast is replaced. Examine the fracture for tenderness. If there was a wound or an operative site, evaluate it for healing and any evidence of infection, and treat appropriately. Evaluate any trophic or sensory changes as possible signs of RSD.

Radiography

Evaluate all fractures of the calcaneus with anteroposterior, lateral, and Harris views to assess the status of healing and any loss of reduction, particularly for patients who are being treated without internal fixation and who may have inadvertently increased their weight bearing.

Weight Bearing

It is important to stress to the patient that weight bearing should be partial only, particularly if there is any tenderness at the fracture site.

Patients with calcaneus fractures treated by internal fixation remain out of a cast so that they may begin active range of motion and partial weight bearing. Patients with calcaneus fractures treated by closed reduction without internal fixation should remain non-weight bearing or toe-touch weight bearing in a short leg cast for a total of 8 to 12 weeks. Otherwise, they risk displacing the fracture by beginning full weight bearing.

Range of Motion

Begin active range of motion for calcaneus fractures treated with internal fixation. This is most important to attempt to regain the full range of motion at the tibiotalar and subtalar joints.

Patients with calcaneus fractures treated conservatively should continue metatarsophalangeal joint range of motion. They may begin isometric exercises in the cast in dorsiflexion and plantar flexion as well as inversion and eversion, as pain allows.

Muscle Strength

Patients with calcaneus fractures treated by rigid fixation begin exercises in plantar flexion, dorsiflexion, inversion, and eversion. Initially these should be nonresistive and then progress to resistive exercises as stability is demonstrated and pain allows. Subtalar exercises (particularly inversion and eversion) should also be initiated. Active but nonresistive eversion and inversion should be started. Once the patient has adequate pain tolerance, resistive exercises for inversion and eversion may begin. The same follows for strengthening the ankle plantar and dorsiflexors. A patient who is still in a cast may begin these exercises as permitted by the room in the cast.

Functional Activities

Patients with calcaneus fractures treated with internal fixation begin partial weight bearing using crutches and a three-point gait. Patients whose fractures were treated conservatively should remain non-weight bearing and continue to use assistive devices for transfers and gait.

Gait

Patients treated conservatively for calcaneus fractures should remain fully non-weight bearing and use a two-point gait (*see* Figure 6-16). Patients who are allowed to begin partial weight bearing with crutches use a three-point gait, placing the crutches first, followed by the unaffected extremity and then the affected extremity (*see* Figure 6-17). To climb stairs, the patient places the unaffected extremity first, followed by the crutches and then the affected extremity, and descends stairs placing the crutches first, followed by the affected extremity and then the unaffected extremity (*see* Figures 6-21, 6-22, 6-23, 6-24, and 6-25). Patients who are allowed to toe-touch still have an abnormal gait due to pain because the fracture is not fully healed. However, it is too soon to attempt to normalize their gait because they are only partial weight bearing on the toes.

Methods of Treatment: Specific Aspects

Open Reduction and Internal Fixation

Any protective casts should have been removed. The patient may begin active and active-assistive range of motion as noted previously, particularly of the tibiotalar and subtalar joints. There may be residual pain secondary to stiffness, which can be improved with hydrotherapy.

Cast

Patients treated conservatively should remain non-weight bearing in a short leg cast because the fracture may not be totally stable. They continue range of motion at the knee and metatarsophalangeal joints and begin isometric exercises of the plantar flexors and dorsiflexors and the invertors and evertors in their casts.

Prescription

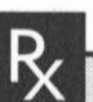

Six to Eight Weeks

Precautions No passive range of motion.

Range of Motion

Rigidly fixed fractures may begin active range of motion in dorsiflexion and plantar flexion as well as inversion and eversion to the ankle and subtalar joint, out of the cast.

Nonrigidly fixed fractures may actively range the metatarsophalangeal joints as well as ankle and subtalar joints in or out of a cast.

Muscle Strength

Rigidly fixed fractures begin isometric exercises out of the cast.

Nonrigidly fixed fractures continue isometric exercises to the ankle and subtalar joint in the cast. Continue quadriceps strengthening.

Functional Activities

Rigidly fixed fractures continue partial weight bearing for transfers and ambulation with assistive devices.

Nonrigidly fixed fractures continue non–weight-bearing transfers.

Weight Bearing

Rigidly fixed fractures may begin partial weight bearing as tolerated in a cast.

Nonrigidly fixed fractures must remain non-weight bearing.

Treatment: Eight to Twelve Weeks

Bone Healing

Stability at fracture site: Fractures treated with internal fixation are stable.

Stage of bone healing: Remodeling phase. Woven bone is replaced with lamellar bone. The process of remodeling takes months to years for completion.

X-ray: Tarsal bones show fracture lines disappearing. This is more obvious with fractures that have had internal fixation. Amount of callus formation is significantly less than in midshaft long bone fractures because the periosteum is quite thin in this region.

Orthopaedic and Rehabilitation Considerations

Physical Examination

Evaluate for tenderness at the fracture site. Evaluate any wounds or operative sites for evidence of skin breakdown or infection. Blister healing should be complete. Evaluate all wounds and incisions for erythema or evidence of infection, and treat appropriately. Evaluate for RSD. Evaluate the fracture for any evidence of tenderness. Restrict weight bearing for patients who are tender to palpation.

Radiography

Anteroposterior and lateral radiographs as well as Harris views should be taken out of plaster both for patients who have been treated conservatively and for those with internal fixation. Fractures treated conservatively may have lost some correction if there was early full weight bearing. Loss of correction is unusual for internally fixed fractures.

Weight Bearing

Calcaneus fractures that have been treated with internal fixation may progress to full weight bearing if radiographs show adequate healing and the fracture is nontender on weight bearing and palpation.

Calcaneus fractures that have been treated conservatively remain non-weight bearing unless they are fully nontender and have shown reconsolidation, as evidenced by the loss of distinct fracture lines.

Range of Motion

Patients whose fractures have been treated with internal fixation should continue with full active range of motion and resistive strengthening of the ankle and subtalar joint in all planes.

Fractures that were treated conservatively should be able to come out of the cast and begin active and gentle passive range of motion at the tibiotalar and subtalar joints. Resistive exercises should not be undertaken if the fracture is inadequately healed because they may cause displacement of the fracture.

Muscle Strength

For all fractures treated with internal fixation, the patient can continue gentle to more aggressive resistive exercises in dorsiflexion, plantar flexion, inversion, and eversion at the subtalar joint. These are controlled by the patient to allow resistance appropriate for his or her pain and tolerance. Patients should also continue quadriceps resistive exercises. Patients who have been treated conservatively should not engage in resistive exercises, except for the quadriceps. Isometric and isotonic exercises should continue.

Functional Activities

All fractures treated with internal fixation may progress to full weight bearing as tolerated. Even if radiographs show adequate fracture healing, the patient may still need to use a crutch or cane for support and stability during transfers and ambulation.

Patients with conservatively treated calcaneus fractures still need to use crutches but may be able to progress to partial weight bearing, using a three-point gait for transfers and ambulation (*see* Figure 6-17).

Gait

Calcaneus fractures are still likely to have tenderness on heel strike. Because the weight transfers forward from the hindfoot to the midfoot and forefoot, the patient has less discomfort and thus attempts to do more toe walking rather than planting fully on the heel and rolling through (*see* Figure 32-18).

Methods of Treatment: Specific Aspects

Open Reduction and Internal Fixation

Casts should have been removed from all fractures by now. Patients should be undergoing active and resistive range-of-motion exercises (and isotonic strengthening) of the ankle and subtalar and metatarsophalangeal joints. If they are pain free, they may progress as tolerated from partial to full weight bearing. The goal now is to normalize the gait.

Cast

Patients being treated conservatively in a cast should continue non-weight bearing unless there has been adequate evidence of fracture consolidation, which allows them to begin partial weight bearing. They continue active range of motion of the metatarsophalangeal joints as well as isometric exercises, plantar flexion and dorsiflexion, and inversion and eversion in the cast. They should avoid resistive exercises.

When the calcaneus fracture has healed enough so that the cast can be removed, the patient may begin partial weight bearing with assistive devices, and advance weight bearing as dictated by fracture healing and pain tolerance.

Prescription

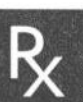

Eight to Twelve Weeks

Precautions Nonrigidly fixed fractures may need to limit the amount of weight bearing and the ability to perform resistive exercises.

Range of Motion

Rigidly fixed fractures may have active and active-assistive as well as passive range of motion of the ankle and subtalar joints.

Nonrigidly fixed fractures may actively range the metatarsophalangeal joints and perform isometric exercises of the ankle and subtalar joints within their casts.

Muscle Strength

Rigidly fixed fractures may begin gentle resistive exercises to the dorsiflexors and plantar flexors, evertors and invertors, and flexors and extensors of the toes.

For nonrigidly fixed fractures, no resistive exercises.

Functional Activities

Rigidly fixed fractures may progress to full weight bearing as tolerated for transfers and ambulation, using assistive devices as necessary.

Nonrigidly fixed fractures are either non-weight bearing or partially weight bearing and require the use of assistive devices for transfers and ambulation.

Weight Bearing

Rigidly fixed fractures are partially to fully weight bearing.

Nonrigidly fixed fractures are non-weight bearing to partially weight bearing.

Treatment: Twelve to Sixteen Weeks

Orthopaedic and Rehabilitation Considerations

Patients with rigidly fixed fractures are usually doing well if they have anatomic reduction of their fracture. They are out of their casts or immobilization devices. Progress the patients to full weight bearing and normalize their gait. Avoid high-impact activities for 6 months.

Patients with nonrigidly fixed fractures are variable in their need to remain in a cast. Most calcaneal fractures do not have anatomic reduction and have more pain and less consolidation of the fracture than rigidly fixed fractures. Many of these patients need continued protective weight bearing in a cast for an additional 4 to 6 weeks. At that time, begin progressive weight bearing as tolerated out of the cast, and normalize the gait.

LONG-TERM CONSIDERATIONS AND PROBLEMS

Fractures of the calcaneus are often work related and may result in long-term disability. This may permanently affect the patient's ability to work and perform activities of daily living. If there has been significant comminution and intraarticular involvement, post-traumatic subtalar arthritis is likely to develop. This initially causes significant discomfort and ultimately requires fusion of the hindfoot.

Patients who have not had anatomic reduction or internal fixation may experience more significant disability from calcaneus fractures because they have intraarticular malalignment of their articular surfaces (the anterior, middle, and posterior facets) with the talus (*see* Figure 32-7). They may also have a widened and possibly shortened heel, making shoes uncomfortable. Finding properly fitting shoes can be extremely difficult and costly. Depending on the position of the calcaneal fracture fragments, shards of bone penetrating into the heel pad can cause excruciating pain at heel strike (*see* Figure 32-18).

Nonarticular fractures of the calcaneus that involve the Achilles tendon (posterior beak) and have not been appropriately reduced may cause posttraumatic bursitis as a shoe rubs over the area. Weakness in the gastrocnemius-soleus complex may result from shortening of the Achilles tendon (*see* Figure 32-1).

The extended immobilization that is often required for conservatively managed hindfoot fractures may lead to significant stiffening of the posterior joint capsule. This limits full ankle motion (particularly dorsiflexion) and may lead to tightening of the Achilles tendon, with a subsequent increased load across the hindfoot/midfoot junction. These changes further aggravate and destabilize the gait by overstressing these joints and possibly accelerating degenerative changes.

IMMEDIATE TO ONE WEEK		
	Open Reduction and Internal Fixation	*Cast*
Stability	None.	None.
Orthopaedics	Trim cast to metatarsal heads to allow full range of motion at the knee.	Trim cast to metatarsal heads to allow full range of motion at the knee.
Rehabilitation	Range of motion of the metatarsophalangeal (MTP), interphalangeal (IP), and ankle joints while in compressive dressing awaiting casting.	Range of motion of the MTP, IP, and ankle joints.

TWO WEEKS		
	Open Reduction and Internal Fixation	*Cast*
Stability	None to minimal.	None to minimal.
Orthopaedics	Trim cast to metatarsal heads.	Trim cast to metatarsal heads.
Rehabilitation	Range of motion of metatarsophalangeal (MTP), interphalangeal (IP), and knee joints.	Range of motion of MTP, IP, and knee joints.

FOUR TO SIX WEEKS		
	Open Reduction and Internal Fixation	*Cast*
Stability	Stable.	Stable.
Orthopaedics	Evaluate cast for breakdown and repair as necessary. Trim and pad cast as necessary.	Evaluate cast for breakdown and repair as necessary. Trim and pad cast as necessary.
Rehabilitation	Continue range of motion of the metatarsophalangeal (MTP), interphalangeal (IP), and knee joints. Start range of motion of the ankle and subtalar joint in the cast.	Range of motion at the MTP, IP, and knee joints.

SIX TO EIGHT WEEKS		
	Open Reduction and Internal Fixation	*Cast*
Stability	Stable.	Stable.
Orthopaedics	Remove cast if not already done.	Continue short leg non–weight-bearing cast.
Rehabilitation	Begin active range of motion and dorsiflexion and plantar flexion, and inversion and eversion of ankle and subtalar joint out of the cast.	Actively range metatarsophalangeal and ankle joints within or out of a cast.

EIGHT TO TWELVE WEEKS

	Open Reduction and Internal Fixation	*Cast*
Stability	Stable.	Stable.
Orthopaedics	Remove cast.	May remove cast or continue with protective immobilization as necessary.
Rehabilitation	Active, active-assistive, and passive range of motion of ankle and subtalar joints.	Active range of motion of the metatarsophalangeal joints and isometric exercises to the ankle and subtalar joints in or out of a cast.

BIBLIOGRAPHY

DeLee J. Talus and MTP injuries. In: Mann RA, ed. *Surgery of the Foot*, 5th ed. St. Louis: C.V. Mosby, 1986, pp. 656–711.

Geissler W, Tsao A. Foot and ankle fractures. In: Rockwood CA Jr, Green DP, eds. *Fractures in Adults*, 4th ed. Philadelphia: J.B. Lippincott, 1995, pp. 2291–2353.

Giachino AA, Unthoff HK. Current concepts review: intraarticular fractures of the calcaneus. *J Bone Joint Surg Am*, 71:784–787, 1989.

Hansen ST Jr. Foot injuries. In: Browner B, Jupiter J, Levine AM, Trafton PG, eds. *Skeletal Trauma*, Vol 2. Philadelphia: W.B. Saunders, 1992, pp. 1960–1972.

Jahss MH. *Disorders of the Foot and Ankle: Medical and Surgical Management*. Philadelphia: W.B. Saunders, 1990.

Macey LR, Benirschke SK, Sangeorzan BJ, Hansen ST. Acute calcaneal fractures: treatment, options, and results. *Journal of the American Academy of Orthopedic Surgeons*, 2:36–43, 1994.

Mann R. Lower extremity. In: Chapman M, ed. *Operative Orthopaedics*. Philadelphia: J.B. Lippincott, 1993, pp. 2143–2178.

Mann RA, Coughlin MJ. *Surgery of the Foot and Ankle,* 7th ed. St. Louis: Mosby, 1999.

Manoli A II. Compartment syndromes of the foot: current concepts. *Foot and Ankle*, 10:340–344, 1990.

Mizel M, Sobel M. In: Miller M, ed. *Review of Orthopaedics*, 2nd ed. Philadelphia: W.B. Saunders, 1996, pp. 241, 390–391.

Myerson M, Manoli A. Compartment syndromes of the foot after calcaneal fractures. *Clin Orthop*, 290:142–150, 1993.

Perry J. Ankle and foot gait deviations. In: Perry J, ed. *Gait Analysis*. Thorofare, NJ, Slack, 1992, pp. 185–219.

Sangeorzan BJ, Benirschke SK, Carr JB. Surgical management of fractures of the os calcis. *Instr Course Lect*, 44:359–370, 1995.

Yablon IG, Segal D. Foot and ankle injuries. In: Evarts CM, ed. *Surgery of the Musculoskeletal System*, 2nd ed. New York: Churchill Livingstone, 1990, pp. 4257–4267.

CHAPTER Thirty-three

Midfoot Fractures

ANNE P. MCCORMACK, MD

INTRODUCTION

Definition

Fractures of the midfoot involve the tarsometatarsal (or Lisfranc) joint, the cuneiforms, the tarsal navicular (or scaphoid) bone, and the cuboid bone (Figures 33-1, 33-2, and 33-3). Injuries of the tarsometatarsal joint may or may not include fractures of the metatarsal bases and can be further described as homolateral (involving all metatarsals subluxed in the same direction), isolated (with one or two metatarsals displaced), or divergent (displacement in both coronal and sagittal planes; Figures 33-4, 33-5, and 33-6; *see* Figures 33-12 and 33-15).

The various fractures of the tarsal navicular (or scaphoid) bone include cortical avulsion, fractures of the tuberosity (which may involve the posterior tibial tendon), body fractures, and stress fractures (Figures 33-7, 33-8, and 33-9; *see* Figure 33-12).

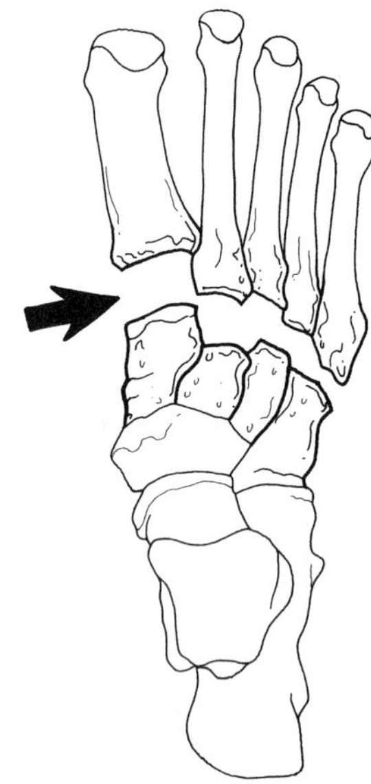

FIGURE 33-1 Lisfranc joint, between the tarsal and metatarsal bones of the midfoot. This joint (the first and second metatarsal articulations with the medial cuneiform) is the keystone of the foot, of critical importance to normal weight bearing and load distribution. It supplies stability between the midfoot and the forefoot during gait.

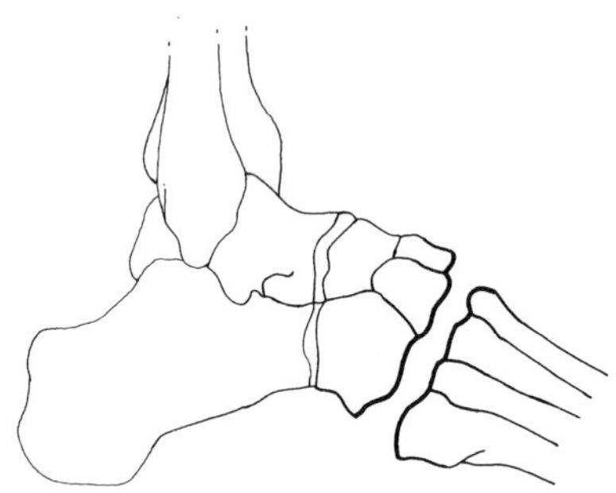

FIGURE 33-2 Lisfranc joint (lateral view).

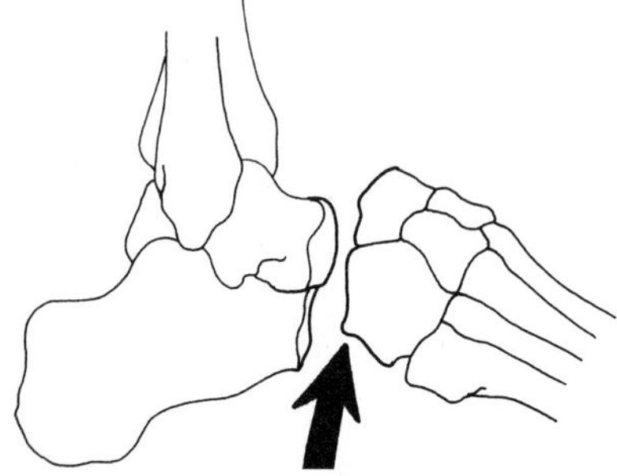

FIGURE 33-3 Chopart's joint involves the midtarsal joints. The talocuboid and calcaneonavicular joints are involved.

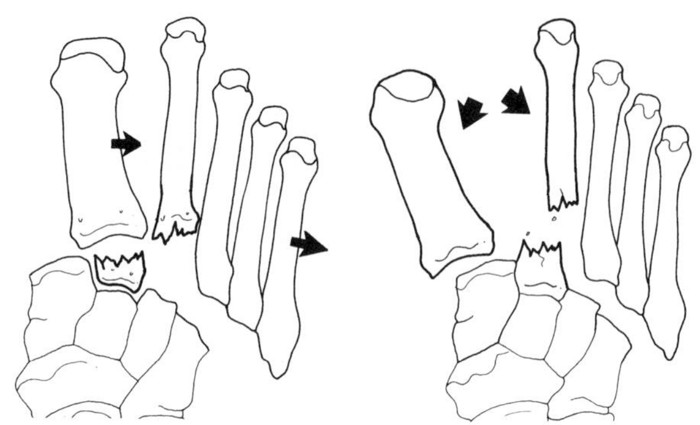

FIGURE 33-4 *(above, left)* Fracture/dislocation of the Lisfranc joint. All of the metatarsals are dislocated or subluxed homolaterally (in the same direction).

FIGURE 33-5 *(above, right)* Fractures of the Lisfranc joint, divergent type. The metatarsals are being subluxed in different directions. With fracture/dislocations of the Lisfranc joint complex, weight bearing may not begin for at least 6 weeks or until the patient is pain free.

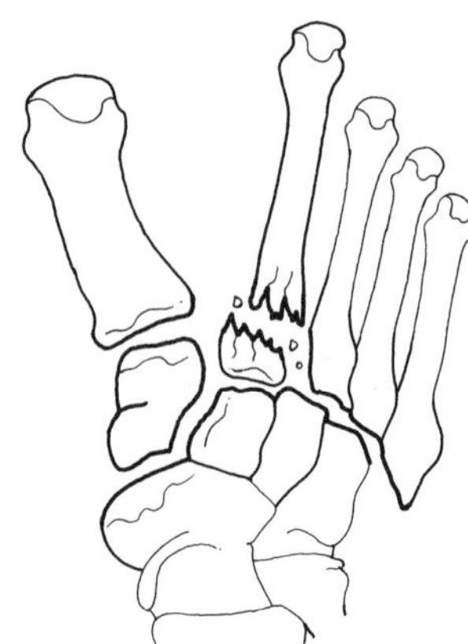

FIGURE 33-6 Fracture through the Lisfranc joint, divergent type, in both the coronal and sagittal planes. Note that the subluxation extends through the cuneiform bones.

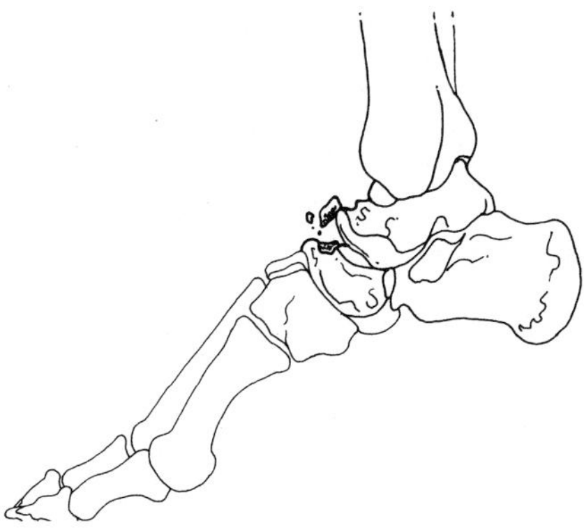

FIGURE 33-7 Cortical avulsion fracture of the dorsum of the dorsal navicular tuberosity. Cortical avulsion fractures (dorsal lip) may bear weight as tolerated.

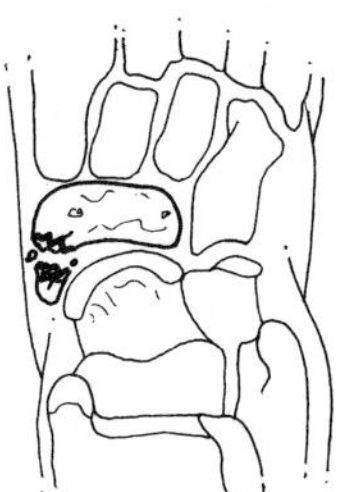

FIGURE 33-8 Fracture of the navicular tuberosity. The posterior tibial tendon inserts into the tuberosity, causing pain and separation of the fracture fragments. Tarsal navicular tuberosity fractures that fail to unite may be very painful and may require subsequent surgery to reattach the avulsed fragment and the posterior tendon to the bone.

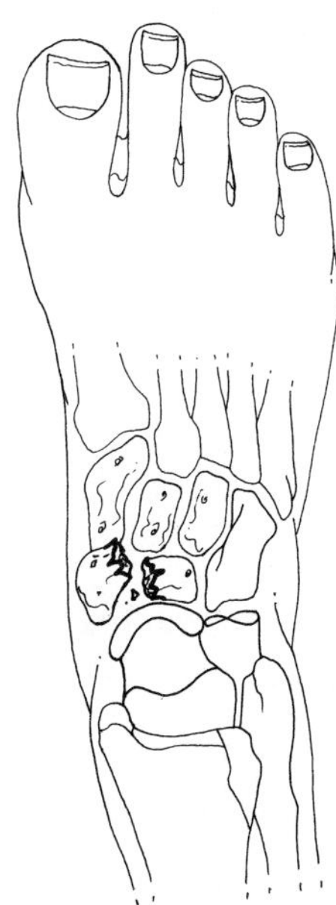

FIGURE 33-9 Fracture of the body of the navicular (scaphoid). This fracture is intraarticular by definition. These patients frequently have posttraumatic arthritis and discomfort in all phases of gait. Fractures of the tarsal navicular body may require immobilization in a non–weight-bearing short leg cast for 7 to 10 weeks. Limited weight bearing then gradually progresses over the next 6 to 12 weeks, depending on the degree of fracture comminution.

Fractures of the cuboid are usually related to calcaneal fractures and often metatarsal fractures. They are known as nutcracker fractures. The cuboid is cracked like a nut between the fifth metatarsal and the calcaneus as the forefoot is forced into abduction (Figures 33-10 and 33-11).

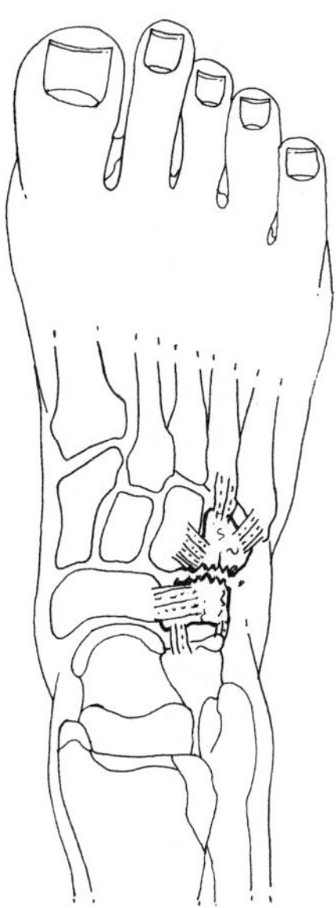

FIGURE 33-10 Cuboid fracture, frequently called a nutcracker fracture. The cuboid is cracked like a nut between the fifth metatarsal and the calcaneus as the forefoot is forced into abduction. Cuboid fractures are usually associated with calcaneal fractures and often with metatarsal fractures.

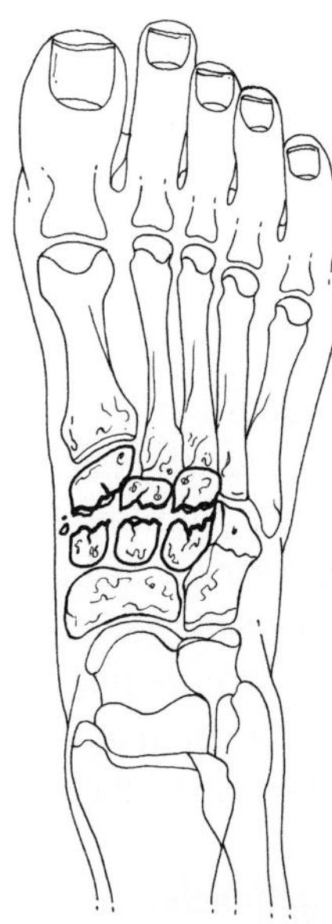

FIGURE 33-11 Cuneiform fractures. Isolated cuneiform fractures are uncommon and usually occur in association with high-energy injuries. Open reduction and internal fixation is recommended if there is displacement; it is followed by 6 weeks of non-weight bearing.

Mechanism of Injury

The three most common causes of midfoot fractures are injury due to twisting of the forefoot, axial loading of a fixed foot, and crushing. Twisting injuries often occur during motor vehicle accidents when the foot is forcefully abducted, or when the forefoot is fixed and the midfoot and hindfoot twist around it, as when a foot is caught in the rung of a ladder. Axial loading of the fixed foot can occur in one of two ways: extrinsic axial compression applied to the heel, as in a fall on an extremely dorsiflexed foot, or an extreme ankle equinus with axial loading from the body weight, as when stepping off a curb. Direct crushing blows to the dorsum of the foot usually occur in industrial accidents. The clinician must be extremely cautious in such injuries and evaluate the foot for compartment syndrome and injury to the dorsalis pedis artery.

Treatment Goals

Orthopaedic Objectives

Alignment

Restoring the alignment of the metatarsals with the cuneiforms, thus restoring the keystone of the midfoot (the first and second metatarsal articulations with the medial cuneiform), is of critical importance to normal weight bearing and load distribution of the foot. This keystone provides stability between the midfoot and forefoot during gait.

Restoring the length and alignment of the cuneiforms, cuboid, and navicular is crucial to maintaining the medial arch of the foot. This is important because the longitudinal and transverse arches of the foot control direct distribution of weight of the body on the foot during gait.

Stability

A stable reconstruction of the Lisfranc joint complex is critically important to maintaining the medial arch of the foot as well as to a pain-free and secure gait.

Stable fixation of the navicular and cuboid is critical to maintaining the transverse tarsal joint (calcaneocuboid and talonavicular joints) position. This allows effective transfer of weight from the hindfoot as well as facilitating inversion and eversion of the subtalar joint.

Rehabilitation Objective

Range of Motion

Restore the full range of motion to the transverse tarsal and tarsometatarsal joints in inversion and eversion.

Restore the full range of motion to the ankle in all planes (Table 33-1).

TABLE 33-1 *Range of Motion of the Ankle*

Motion	Normal	Functional
Ankle plantar flexion	45°	20°
Ankle dorsiflexion	20–25°	10°
Foot inversion	35°	10°
Foot eversion	25°	10°

Only a small amount of motion occurs at the naviculo-cuneiform and cuneiform metatarsal joints because these joints primarily serve as stabilizers. Any loss of range of motion there is insignificant.

Restore or maintain range of motion at the fourth and fifth metatarsal cuboid joints. A greater arc of dorsiflexion and plantar flexion as well as pronation and supination occurs at the fourth and fifth metatarsocuboid joints than the first three tarsometatarsal joints. This motion, although small, is helpful to allow the foot to adapt to uneven surfaces. Residual loss of this range of motion may cause increased stress on the subtalar articulation.

Muscle Strength

Restore normal strength to the muscles of the foot and ankle.

Invertors of the foot and ankle:

Tibialis posterior (also acts as a plantar flexor; this muscle provides the primary support of the midtarsal joints)

Tibialis anterior (also acts as a dorsiflexor)

Evertors of the foot and ankle:

Peroneus longus

Peroneus brevis

Dorsiflexors of the foot and ankle:

Tibialis anterior (also acts as an invertor)

Toe extensors

Plantar flexors of the foot and ankle:

Gastrocnemius

Soleus

Tibialis posterior (also acts as an invertor)

Peroneus longus weakness can result from a severe dislocation at the Lisfranc joint complex because this muscle inserts on the first metatarsal and first cuneiform.

Functional Goals

Maintain the longitudinal and transverse arches of the foot for proper distribution of body weight during gait.

Restore the gait pattern to the preinjury level.

Expected Time of Bone Healing

Tarsometatarsal or Lisfranc Fracture/Dislocations

Eight to 10 weeks.

Tarsal Navicular or Scaphoid Fractures

Six to 10 weeks.

Cuboid and Cuneiform Fracture/Dislocations

Six to 10 weeks.

Expected Duration of Rehabilitation

Tarsometatarsal or Lisfranc Fracture/Dislocations

Eight weeks to 4 months.

Tarsal Navicular or Scaphoid Fractures

For acute fractures, 6 weeks to 4 months.

For delayed union, nonunion, or stress fractures, 6 weeks to 4 months, or longer if surgical repair is necessary.

Cuboid and Cuneiform Fracture/Dislocations

Six weeks to 4 months.

Methods of Treatment

Tarsometatarsal or Lisfranc Fracture/Dislocations

Cast

Biomechanics: Stress-sharing device.

Mode of bone healing: Secondary, with callus formation.

Indications: Fractures or dislocations of the Lisfranc joint that are identified on radiographs but have preserved anatomic reduction may be treated with short leg cast immobilization for 6 weeks. Patients may bear weight when they are pain free.

Open Reduction and Internal Fixation

Biomechanics: Stress-shielding device with screw fixation.

Mode of bone healing: Primary, with rigid fixation.

Indications: Most displaced Lisfranc fracture/dislocations should be managed with open reduction and internal fixation to ensure anatomic reduction and rigid stabilization. After surgery, the patient is placed in a non–weight-bearing cast for 6 weeks. Unprotected weight bearing is not recommended until the screws are removed, at least 10 to 12 weeks after surgery (Figures 33-12, 33-13, and 33-14).

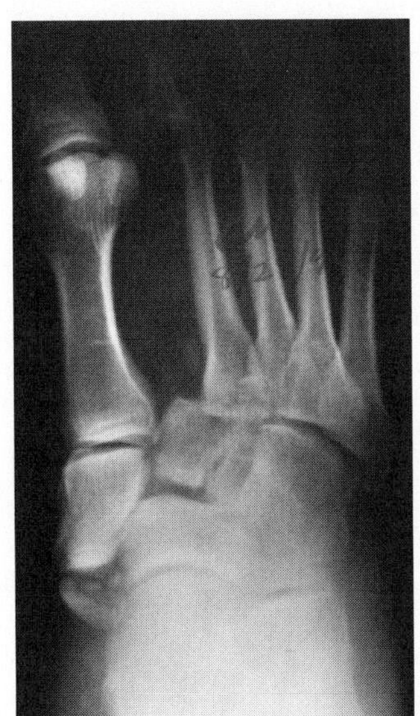

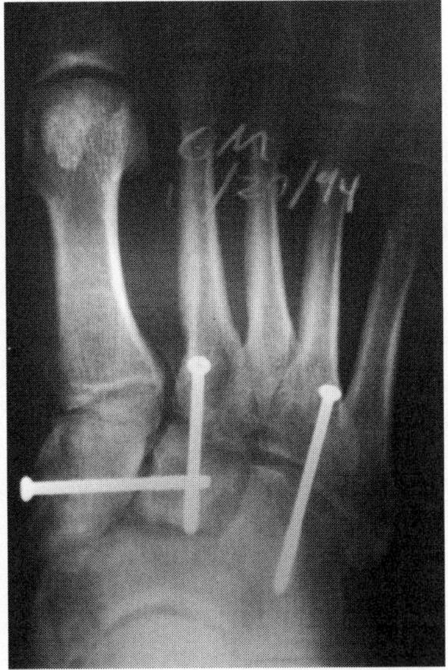

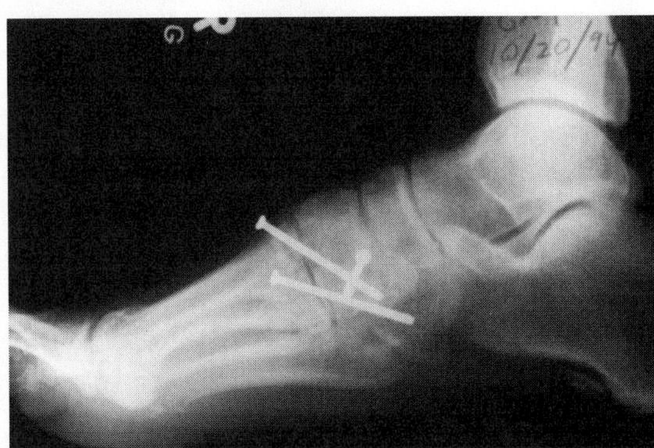

FIGURE 33-12 *(above, left)* Lisfranc fracture/dislocation, divergent type, extending through the first and second metatarsals and cuneiforms and between the first and second cuneiforms. Note avulsion of the navicular tuberosity.

FIGURE 33-13 *(above, middle)* Lisfranc fracture/dislocation, divergent type, treated with open reduction and internal screw fixation. This ensures anatomic reduction and rigid stabilization. After surgery, the patient is placed in a non–weight-bearing cast for 6 weeks. Note reduction of the navicular tuberosity.

FIGURE 33-14 *(above, right)* Open reduction and internal screw fixation of a Lisfranc fracture/dislocation (lateral view). Unprotected weight bearing is not recommended until the screws are removed at least 10 to 12 weeks after surgery.

Closed Reduction and Percutaneous Pinning

Biomechanics: Stress-sharing device with pin fixation.

Mode of bone healing: Secondary, with callus formation.

Indications: Kirschner-wire fixation is adequate when the injuries are mainly bony in nature because less time is required for healing and fixation. The patient is placed in a non–weight-bearing short leg cast after fixation. The wires are removed at approximately 6 weeks, followed by protected weight bearing (Figures 33-15 and 33-16).

Tarsal Navicular or Scaphoid Fractures

Cast

Biomechanics: Stress-sharing device.

Mode of bone healing: Secondary, with callus formation.

Indications: Cortical avulsion (dorsal lip) fractures, tuberosity fractures, and stress fractures of the navicular usually can be treated closed by placement in a short leg cast.

Cortical avulsion fractures may be treated in a short leg walking cast and managed for 4 to 6 weeks (*see* Figure 33-7).

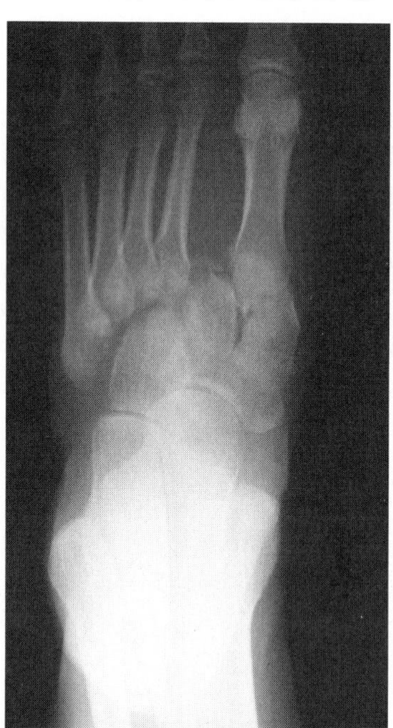

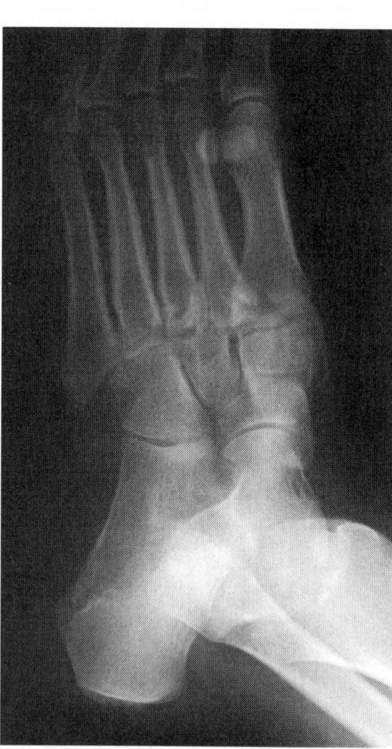

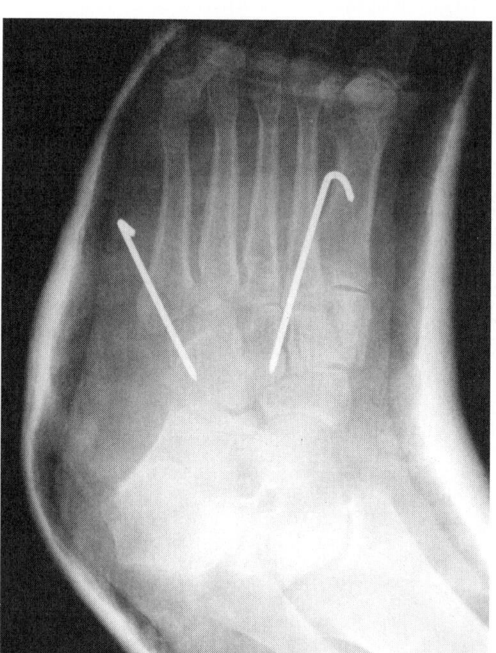

FIGURE 33-15A,B *(above, left and middle)* Lisfranc fracture dislocation with minimum bone injury.

FIGURE 33-16 *(above, right)* Closed reduction and percutaneous pinning of a Lisfranc fracture/dislocation. The patient is placed in a non–weight-bearing short leg cast after fixation. The wires are removed at approximately 6 weeks, followed by protected weight bearing.

Tuberosity fractures are also amenable to treatment with a short leg walking cast, which is maintained for 4 to 6 weeks. The cast must be well molded in the arch and maintain a neutral to slightly supinated foot posture (*see* Figure 33-8).

Nonunion of a tuberosity fracture may require subsequent surgery, often open reduction and internal fixation.

Stress fractures that are nondisplaced are often treated with a non–weight-bearing cast. Displaced fractures require open reduction and internal fixation.

Open Reduction and Internal Fixation

Biomechanics: Stress-shielding device with rigid fixation.

Mode of bone healing: Primary, without callus formation.

Indications: Fractures of the body of the navicular involve both the talonavicular and naviculocuneiform joints. To avoid severe deformity and traumatic arthritis of the midfoot, these must be treated with anatomic reduction and rigid fixation. If a fracture is comminuted, it may require temporary placement of an external fixator as well as an interpositional bone graft to restore a neutral alignment to the forefoot.

Stress fractures that have not responded to cast treatment or that are displaced may require rigid fixation as well as an inlay bone graft.

A painful nonunion or a problematic medial prominence of the navicular tuberosity (causing shoe problems) may require reattachment of the posterior tibial tendon and removal of the avulsed fragment of bone.

Cuboid and Cuneiform Fracture/Dislocations

Cast

Biomechanics: Stress-sharing device.

Mode of bone healing: Secondary, with minimum callus formation.

Indications: Most cuboid injuries are minimally displaced or nondisplaced avulsion fractures. They are often seen on radiographs as flecks of bone lying along the lateral aspect of the calcaneocuboid joint. These fractures can be treated closed in a weight-bearing cast.

Nondisplaced fractures of the cuneiforms may also be treated in a short leg cast but require prolonged immobilization for healing because there is usually significant ligamentous damage (*see* Figures 33-10 and 33-11).

Open Reduction Internal Fixation

Biomechanics: Stress-shielding device.

Mode of bone healing: Primary, with rigid fixation.

Indications: A compression injury or nutcracker fracture usually results from a high-energy force. Any displacement requires open reduction and internal fixation. If there is significant comminution or bone loss, a short-term external fixator as well as an autogenous bone graft may be required to restore the lateral column length. This prevents abduction and pronation deformity of the forefoot, which may be painful and alter gait.

Most fractures and dislocations of the cuneiforms occur in association with other high-energy injuries. Open reduction and internal fixation is recommended for any amount of displacement and should be followed by a 6-week period of non-weight bearing.

Isolated cuneiform fractures are uncommon but amenable to screw fixation. After surgery, all of these fractures and fracture dislocations should be further immobilized in a non–weight-bearing short leg cast.

Special Considerations of the Fracture

Age

Elderly patients are at greater risk for development of joint stiffness, particularly with navicular fractures. Younger, active patients who have sustained navicular fractures with loss of anatomic alignment are also prone to joint stiffness in the hindfoot.

Articular Involvement

Almost all fractures of the midfoot are intraarticular because of the anatomy of these bones. Fortunately, there is normally little motion at the Lisfranc and cuboid cuneiform joints. However, improper alignment of these bones can result in pain at the plantar arch or the dorsal surface of the foot because of shoe pressure. The tarsal navicular (scaphoid) is the keystone of the medial arch of the foot; in concert with the cuboid, it forms the transverse tarsal joint (that articulates with the hindfoot) and is critical for both inversion and eversion of the hindfoot as it adapts to uneven and sloped surfaces. Intraarticular fractures of the cuboid or the navicular can lead to significant posttraumatic arthritis and a fusion may eventually be indicated. This can result in hindfoot stiffness and a lack of normal eversion and inversion at the subtalar joint.

There may also be limited pronation and supination of the ankle because of residual stiffness.

Location

Unidentified or inadequately treated Lisfranc fractures can severely impair midfoot function. As noted, any intraarticular involvement of the navicular or cuboid can result in significant long-term disability.

Tuberosity fractures of the navicular (scaphoid) bone can cause weak inversion and compromise the medial longitudinal arch because of tibialis posterior incompetence (*see* Figures 33-8 and 33-12).

Open Fractures

Any midfoot fracture associated with loss of soft tissue is usually accompanied by damage to the dorsalis pedis artery. This should be carefully evaluated at the time of initial examination. Collateral circulation to the forefoot is usually adequate; however, in rare cases the forefoot has to be amputated because of these injuries.

Most midfoot injuries that cause an open fracture involve high energy, and there should be a low threshold of suspicion for compartment syndrome. All open fractures must be treated aggressively with irrigation, débridement, and intravenous antibiotics.

Tendon and Ligament Injuries

Disruption of the Lisfranc joint complex usually is associated with disruption of the intermetatarsal and tarsal ligaments. This can be repaired during surgery, although not always.

With any open fracture, the extensor tendons of the foot should be carefully inspected for possible damage.

Laceration of tendons such as the tibialis anterior and those extending the first ray (extensor hallucis longus) should be repaired primarily.

Laceration of the lesser toe extensor tendons may be repaired primarily, but they are less important to foot function and may be allowed to scar in.

Associated Injury

Fractures of the Lisfranc joint complex may be the result of either a high-energy injury such as forceful impact on the heel of a fixed foot, or a trivial injury such as stepping off a curb in a twisted position. In either case, there is usually significant soft-tissue swelling of the dorsum of the foot. The dorsalis pedis pulse should be monitored carefully, and all soft-tissue swelling should be watched during the first 24 hours to rule out any possibility of a foot compartment syndrome. Fractures of the cuboid and cuneiforms are usually associated with Lisfranc injuries, and the same precautions hold for these fractures. Stress fractures of the tarsal navicular (scaphoid) are usually not associated with significant soft-tissue swelling, unlike avulsion fractures or other acute fractures. As noted, open fractures should be carefully evaluated for laceration of any major extensor tendons and for direct injury to the dorsalis pedis artery. Significant swelling of the foot can lead to necrosis and loss of soft tissue over the dorsum of the foot, potentially requiring skin grafting.

An untreated compartment syndrome that occurs with a crush injury may injure the evertors and invertors across the midfoot as well as the major dorsiflexors across the ankle. This causes an appreciable loss of strength.

Weight Bearing

Initially, weight bearing is not permitted for fracture/dislocations of the Lisfranc joint complex, stress fractures and body fractures of the navicular, any fracture of the cuneiform, or nutcracker fractures of the cuboid.

Cortical avulsion fractures (dorsal lip), tuberosity fractures of the navicular, and avulsion fractures of the cuboid may bear weight as tolerated.

With fracture/dislocations of the Lisfranc joint complex, weight bearing may not begin for at least 6 weeks or until the patient is pain free.

Nondisplaced stress fractures of the tarsal navicular (scaphoid) may begin weight bearing at 6 weeks. Displaced fractures that have required open reduction and internal fixation may also begin protected weight bearing at 6 weeks.

Fractures of the tarsal navicular body may require immobilization in a non–weight-bearing short leg cast for 7 to 10 weeks. Limited weight bearing then gradually progresses over the next 6 to 12 weeks, depending on the degree of fracture comminution.

Nondisplaced fractures of the cuneiforms and cuboid may begin protected weight bearing at 4 to 6 weeks. If they have been adequately stabilized with open reduction and internal fixation, grossly displaced fractures of these bones may allow partial weight bearing at 6 weeks, progressing as the patient becomes symptom free and radiographs indicate consolidation of the fragments (Table 33-2).

TABLE 33-2 *Earliest Partial Weight Bearing*

Lisfranc (tarsometatarsal) fracture/dislocation	Six to 8 weeks
Navicular fractures	
Cortical avulsion	Immediate—as tolerated
Tuberosity	Immediate—as tolerated
Stress—nondisplaced/displaced	Six weeks
Displaced intraarticular fracture with open reduction	Six to 8 weeks
Body	Seven to 10 weeks
Cuboid fractures	
Avulsion	Immediate—as tolerated
Nondisplaced	Four to 6 weeks
Displaced nutcracker with open reduction and internal fixation	Six weeks
Cuneiform fractures	
Nondisplaced	Four to 6 weeks
Grossly displaced with open reduction and internal fixation	Six weeks

Gait

Stance Phase

The stance phase constitutes 60% of the gait cycle.

During the healing phase of fractures of the midfoot, the patient initially tries to limit the time spent on the affected limb and decreases the angle of push-off to minimize axial loading across the fractured bones.

Heel Strike

Initial impact may not cause discomfort. As weight is transferred from the hindfoot to the midfoot, a patient who has sustained a fracture of the navicular and cuboid experiences an increase in pain as the foot begins to go from inversion to eversion (*see* Figure 6-1).

Foot-Flat

This portion of the gait cycle is painful because of injured bones of the medial arch, which is transferring weight from the hindfoot to the forefoot (*see* Figure 6-2).

Mid-Stance

The single-stance phase begins. This phase also is usually painful. The foot is transitioning from neutral to eversion and the roll-out of the foot over the tarsals and into the Lisfranc joints can cause pain (*see* Figure 6-3).

Push-off

At this point, most of the body's weight is over the first and second metatarsal heads. The patient may try to limit the amount of ankle plantar flexion to minimize force transmission along the metatarsal shafts, particularly in Lisfranc joint complex injuries. Thus, there is inadequate push-off with the affected foot to avoid pain, and this portion of the gait cycle is shortened (*see* Figures 6-4 and 6-5).

Swing Phase

The swing phase constitutes 40% of the gait cycle. It is not affected by any of these fractures because the foot is not in contact with the ground (*see* Figures 6-6, 6-7, and 6-8).

TREATMENT

Treatment: Early to Immediate (Day of Injury to One Week)

BONE HEALING

Stability at fracture site: None, except stress fracture of the navicular.

Stage of bone healing: Inflammatory phase. The fracture hematoma is colonized by inflammatory cells, and débridement of the fracture begins. Stress fractures have already débrided and formed a fibrous mass.

X-ray: No callus.

Orthopaedic and Rehabilitation Considerations

Physical Examination

Pay special attention to complaints of pain, paresthesia, and cast discomfort as indicators that the cast is too tight or as possible indicators of foot compartment syndrome. Also note if the patient feels that the cast is loose. Check for capillary refill and sensation. The toes should be pink, with brisk refill after light compression to blanch them. It should be possible to reach the first web space and stroke it lightly with a blunt instrument to ensure that there is no peroneal nerve compression affecting the lower ankle and foot.

If external fixators have been used as an adjunct to internal fixation, check the pin sites for drainage or erythema and treat appropriately. In cases of crushing injury, evaluate the dorsum of the foot for any evidence of skin sloughing.

Dangers

Evaluate for any evidence of a dorsal foot compartment syndrome as noted previously, paying special attention to complaints of pain, paresthesia, and cast discomfort. For fractures that were open or had significant skin (fracture) blisters, evaluate the skin for any evidence of erythema or drainage that may indicate the presence of infection. The patient should be advised to keep the extremity elevated above heart level and to place ice packs over the ankle and foot to decrease swelling and improve venous return.

Radiography

Obtain and check anteroposterior and lateral radiographs of the foot for any loss of correction (redislocation at the Lisfranc joint, displacement of bone graft, angulation, or shortening).

Weight Bearing

All fractures and dislocations of the Lisfranc joint complex should be non-weight bearing.

Patients with cortical avulsion (dorsal lip) or tuberosity fractures of the navicular can be weight bearing as tolerated in a short walking cast.

Minimally or nondisplaced avulsion fractures of the cuboid may be weight bearing in a cast as tolerated.

More serious or nutcracker fractures of the cuboid are non-weight bearing (Table 33-3).

Range of Motion

The patient is instructed in active range-of-motion exercises at the metatarsophalangeal joints. This may be painful because the long extensors and flexors cross over the tarsal joint. Active range-of-motion exercises are prescribed for the knee.

Muscle Strength

Maintain the strength of the quadriceps with isometric exercises (quadriceps sets).

Functional Activities

The patients is instructed in stand/pivot transfers using assistive devices such as crutches, with no weight bearing on the affected extremity. The patient is taught to don pants on the affected extremity first and doff them from the unaffected extremity first.

Gait

The patient uses a non–weight-bearing two-point gait, with the crutches as one unit and the unaffected extremity as the other unit (*see* Figure 6-16). The patient climbs stairs with the unaffected extremity first and brings the fractured limb either simultaneously with the crutches, or the crutches are kept on the step below until both feet are on the step above (*see* Figures 6-20, 6-21, and 6-22). The patient descends stairs by placing the crutches and the affected extremity first, followed by the unaffected extremity (*see* Figures 6-23, 6-24, and 6-25). Patients with navicular and cuboid fractures who can bear weight partially (*see* Table 33-3) are instructed in using the affected extremity during transfers and ambulation.

Methods of Treatment: Specific Aspects

Cast

Evaluate the condition of the cast. Check the cast margins and ensure they are adequately padded. There

TABLE 33-3 ***Immediate to One Week Weight Bearing***

	Partial weight bearing	Non-weight bearing
Lisfranc (tarsometatarsal) **fracture/dislocation**	None	All
Navicular fractures	Cortical avulsion Tuberosity	Stress nondisplaced/displaced Body Displaced intraarticular
Cuneiform fractures	None	All
Cuboid fractures	Avulsion Nondisplaced	Nutcracker

should be free movement of the metatarsophalangeal joints and full extension and flexion at the knee. Evaluate the skin at the edges of the cast to ensure that swelling has not caused skin breakdown and there is no evidence of compartment syndrome. If the cast has softened under the foot, reinforce it.

Open Reduction and Internal Fixation

Usually a cast has been placed by the end of the first week. Check the cast margins to make sure they are well padded. Note that the metatarsophalangeal joints have free movement. Look for any breakdown of skin at the edges and trim appropriately. Repair any breakdown or softening of the cast as necessary.

Closed Reduction and Percutaneous Pinning

Check the pin sites for discharge, erythema, or any tenting of the skin; surgically release any tenting of the skin. If the foot or pin sites have any purulence, erythema, or streaking, the patient should be admitted for intravenous antibiotics and possible pin removal. Most patients are placed in a short leg cast during the first week.

A patient who has not been placed in a cast should range the metatarsophalangeal joints cautiously. This fixation is not as rigid as internal fixation and aggressive active ranging could loosen the pins and lead to loss of reduction at the Lisfranc joint complex.

Prescription

Day One to One Week

Precautions Fixation is not rigid unless the patient has had open reduction and internal fixation. No range of motion to the midfoot.

Range of Motion Active range of motion to the toes and metatarsophalangeal joints.

Muscle Strength No strengthening exercises to the ankle and foot.

Functional Activities

Non–weight-bearing stand/pivot transfers and ambulation with assistive devices.

Partial weight bearing transfers and ambulation with assistive devices for some fractures of the navicular and cuboid (*see* Table 33-3).

Weight Bearing Partial weight bearing for cortical avulsion and tuberosity fractures of navicular, as well as avulsion or nondisplaced fractures of cuboid. Remainder are non-weight bearing (*see* Table 33-3).

Treatment: Two Weeks

Bone Healing

Stability at fracture site: None to minimal.

Stage of bone healing: Beginning of reparative phase. Osteoprogenitor cells differentiate into osteoblasts that lay down woven bone. An exception to this is nonunion of the tarsal navicular or scaphoid, in which a fibrous union may be slowly creating a reparation; however, it may not be of bony nature.

X-ray: No changes to early callus noted in the periosteal aspects of the bone.

Orthopaedic and Rehabilitation Considerations

Physical Examination

Check for capillary refill and sensation of the toes and, if possible, the first dorsal web space. Check the active and passive range of motion of the metatarsophalangeal and interphalangeal joints.

Dangers

Pay particular attention to complaints of pain, paresthesia, and cast discomfort. The patient should be made aware that any pronounced swelling could lead to skin sloughing, and that this should be brought to the physician's immediate attention. The patient should be advised to continue elevating the extremity above heart level as much as possible.

Radiography

Check anteroposterior and lateral radiographs to assess any loss of reduction of the Lisfranc joint complex, migration of any bone graft placed, or loss of length. Assess callus deposition for fractures involving cortical bone such as the metatarsal shafts.

Weight Bearing

Patients with cortical avulsion fractures and tuberosity fractures of the navicular, or nondisplaced avulsion fractures of the cuboid, may be partial weight bearing or weight bearing as tolerated.

All other fractures of the Lisfranc joint complex, tarsal navicular avulsions, displaced cuboid and cuneiform fractures, and stress fractures are still non-weight bearing (Table 33-4).

TABLE 33-4 *Two Weeks Weight Bearing*

	Partial weight bearing	Non-weight bearing
Lisfranc (tarsometatarsal) fracture/dislocation	None	All
Navicular fractures	Cortical avulsion Tuberosity	Stress nondisplaced/displaced Body Displaced intraarticular
Cuneiform fractures	None	All
Cuboid fractures	Avulsion Nondisplaced	Nutcracker

Range of Motion

Patients should continue active and passive range of motion at the metatarsophalangeal joints as well as range of motion at the knee.

Muscle Strength

Maintain the strength of the quadriceps. Repeated movements of the toes strengthen the long flexors, intrinsics, and the extensors.

Functional Activities

The patient should continue with stand/pivot transfers and a non–weight-bearing gait using crutches or a walker, depending on the type of fracture. For fractures where partial weight bearing is allowed, the affected extremity bears some weight during transfers.

Gait

The patient continues with a non–weight-bearing gait using crutches (*see* Figure 6-16).

If weight bearing is allowed, as for the previously noted stable fractures, the patient may bear weight partially or as tolerated using a three-point gait (*see* Figure 6-17). If the cast fits well, there should be no discomfort in any portion of the gait cycle.

Methods of Treatment: Specific Aspects

Cast

Trim the cast to allow visualization of the toes at the metatarsophalangeal joints. Reinforce any cast that has broken down. Continue metatarsophalangeal joint range of motion. Start exercises of the gastrocnemius-soleus group, the tibialis anterior, and the extensors by trying to plantar flex and dorsiflex in the cast. If there has been stable fixation of the fracture, begin gentle peronei group isometric exercises with gentle eversion and gentle dorsiflexion for the tibialis anterior in the cast. Try to invert the foot to strengthen the tibialis posterior.

Open Reduction and Internal Fixation

All patients are in a cast after open reduction and internal fixation and can begin to follow the exercise and range-of-motion protocol prescribed previously.

Closed Reduction and Percutaneous Pinning

Check the pin sites for discharge, erythema, or skin tenting and treat any problems appropriately. Admit the patient for antibiotics if the pin sites are infected.

Because the patient is in a cast, check the padding and cast edges for signs of wear. The padding at the edges of the cast should be adequate to prevent skin breakdown. Also check for cast softening and repair appropriately.

The patient in a cast may engage in the exercises described previously.

Occasionally, a patient is not in a cast because of extensive soft-tissue injury. In this case, continue gentle flexion and extension only at the metatarsophalangeal joints because further ankle plantar flexion and dorsiflexion or inversion and eversion could cause a loss of reduction.

Prescriptions

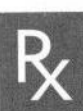

Two Weeks

Precautions Fixation is rigid and stable only for patients treated with open reduction and internal fixation.

Range of Motion Active ankle range of motion to the toes and metatarsophalangeal joints.

Muscle Strength No resistive exercises to the long flexors and extensors of the toes and metatarsophalangeal joints. Isometric exercises to the dorsiflexors and plantar flexors and invertors and evertors of the ankle are performed in the cast.

Functional Activities

Non–weight-bearing stand/pivot transfers and ambulation with assistive devices, depending on type of fracture.

Partial weight bearing to weight bearing as tolerated with assistive devices for stable fractures of the navicular and cuboid (*see* Table 33-4).

Weight Bearing None except for stable fractures of the tarsal navicular and cuboid (*see* Table 33-4).

Treatment: Four to Six Weeks

Bone Healing

Stability at fracture site: Usually stable. Acute fractures should show bridging callus. Confirm with physical examination and radiography. With ligamentous injuries that occur in Lisfranc fracture/dislocations and tarsal bone avulsions, the reconstruction may not yet be stable secondary to the slower healing of ligaments.

Stage of bone healing: Reparative phase. Further organization of the callus and formation of lamellar bone begins. If callus is observed on radiographs and there is bridging at the fracture site, the fracture is usually stable. However, the strength of this callus, especially with torsional load, is significantly lower than that of normal bone.

X-ray: Bridging callus is visible as a fluffy material on the periosteal surface of cortical bone. The tarsal bones, which are mainly cancellous in composition, begin to show consolidation and filling in of lucent fracture lines. With increased rigidity, less bridging callus and lucency are noticed, and healing with endosteal callus predominates. In stress fractures and nonunions of the tarsal navicular, a fibrous nonunion with a smooth fracture edge may be observed.

Orthopaedic and Rehabilitation Considerations

Physical Examination

Remove the cast and perform radiographic examination. Check for stability, tenderness, and range of motion.

Dangers

Most of the swelling from acute fractures should now be resolved. If the patient has noticed vasomotor disturbances, hyperesthesias, pain, and tenderness out of proportion to the stage of fracture healing, it is important to check for any trophic signs of reflex sympathetic dystrophy (RSD). If evidence of RSD is noted, the patient should begin transcutaneous epidural neurostimulation and fluidotherapy in addition to an aggressive physical therapy program.

Radiography

Examine radiographs in the anteroposterior, lateral, and oblique positions of the foot for evidence of healing or any loss of reduction. For Lisfranc fracture/dislocations treated solely in a cast, it is important to assess that reduction has been maintained.

For stress fractures of the tarsal navicular, it is important to evaluate if the fracture line has disappeared.

Patients who have undergone bone grafting to treat avulsions of the tarsal navicular or the cuboid should be carefully assessed for incorporation of the graft. In cases of tarsal navicular or cuboid avulsion, evaluate foot alignment to ensure that the medial or lateral arch is maintained.

Weight Bearing

Lisfranc fracture/dislocations may begin weight bearing as tolerated if they are nontender. The patient should not walk barefoot or on uneven ground, and should keep the foot protected by a rigid shoe for several more weeks.

If percutaneous pins have been placed, they should be removed and the patient may begin partial weight bearing as tolerated.

Patients treated with open reduction and internal fixation should remain non-weight bearing.

Patients with cortical avulsion fractures, tuberosity fractures, and consolidating stress fractures of the tarsal navicular may begin partial weight bearing as

TABLE 33-5 *Four to Six Weeks Weight Bearing*

	Partial weight bearing	Non-weight bearing
Lisfranc (tarsometatarsal) **fracture/dislocation**	Closed reduction—percutaneous pinning (at 6 weeks with stiff-soled shoes) Cast	Open reduction with internal fixation
Navicular fractures	Cortical avulsion Tuberosity Stress fracture nondisplaced (stiff-soled shoe)	Body Stress displaced Displaced intraarticular
Cuneiform fractures	Nondisplaced	Displaced with screw fixation
Cuboid fractures	Nondisplaced Avulsion	Nutcracker—displaced

tolerated out of a cast. Those who have had displaced stress fractures or avulsion of the body of the navicular as well as intraarticular fractures remain non-weight bearing.

Nondisplaced avulsion fractures of the cuboid may now begin weight bearing as tolerated. Nutcracker fractures of the cuboid and displaced or crush fractures of the cuneiforms treated with screw fixation should remain non-weight bearing in a cast. Nondisplaced fractures of the cuneiforms should remain non-weight bearing (Table 33-5).

Range of Motion

Continue with metatarsophalangeal joint range of motion. If the patient is not in a cast, active range of motion of the ankle may be added as dorsiflexion and plantar flexion to tolerance. Gentle active inversion and eversion exercises may also begin. This is helpful to prevent stiffening of the ankle joint capsule. A patient in a cast should continue metatarsophalangeal range-of-motion exercises and perform isometric strengthening by attempting dorsiflexion and plantar flexion and inversion and eversion in the cast. Knee active range of motion should also continue.

Muscle Strength

Continue with isometric exercises of the ankle dorsiflexors and plantar flexors. The patient should continue with quadriceps strengthening exercises. If the cast has been removed, the patient may begin strengthening of the peronei and the tibialis anterior with inversion and eversion exercises. The patient may also work the ankle in dorsiflexion to strengthen the tibialis anterior and plantar flexion for the gastrocnemius-soleus complex.

Functional Activities

If weight bearing is still not allowed, non–weight-bearing pivot transfers using crutches should continue. If weight bearing is allowed, the patient can use the affected extremity during transfers, although crutches may still be needed for balance and support.

Gait

Patients who are non-weight bearing continue ambulation with crutches (*see* Figure 6-16). Patients beginning to weight bear may use a three-point gait in which two crutches act as one point and the affected and the unaffected extremities the other two points (*see* Figure 6-17). The patient may climb stairs with the unaffected extremity first, followed by the affected extremity and then the crutches (*see* Figure 6-20, 6-21, and 6-22). When descending stairs, the patient places the affected extremity first, followed by the crutches and then the unaffected extremity (*see* Figures 6-23, 6-24, and 6-25).

Patients who had Lisfranc fracture/dislocations treated in a cast may find that they are still significantly tender as they move from heel strike into midstance and the foot goes from eversion to inversion. They may try to prolong the heel strike portion of the gait cycle and will probably attempt to shift their weight to the lateral aspect of the foot to keep pressure off the Lisfranc joint complex. Toe-off is shortened and incomplete to minimize motion across the midfoot as the body weight shifts (*see* Figures 6-4 and 6-5).

Cortical avulsion fractures, tuberosity fractures, and well healed stress fractures of the navicular should be pain free at this time and cause no aberrations in gait.

Nondisplaced avulsion fractures of the cuboid, if they are well healed, should also be pain free during the gait.

Cuneiform fractures usually involve ligamentous disruption and are still tender as the patient goes from heel strike to early and mid-stance across the midfoot. The patient may attempt to shift more of the lateral weight of the foot onto the fifth metatarsal. He or she may minimize stance and toe-off so that the cuneiforms spend the least amount of time in torsion and loading.

Methods of Treatment: Specific Aspects

Cast

The cast should be removed at this visit to evaluate for stability and tenderness at the fracture site. Fracture/dislocations of the Lisfranc joint complex that have not had operative intervention may now come out of plaster, and the patient placed in a bunion shoe with protective weight bearing or non-weight bearing.

Cortical avulsion fractures, tuberosity fractures, and nondisplaced or incomplete stress fractures of the tarsal navicular may come out of plaster and begin weight bearing as tolerated in a stiff-soled shoe. Stress fractures that are still tender should again be placed in a non–weight-bearing short leg cast.

Nondisplaced avulsion fractures of the cuboid as well as nondisplaced fractures of the cuneiforms may be removed from plaster and begin partial weight bearing if they are nontender. If there is tenderness over the region of the cuneiforms, a short leg cast should be replaced because these injuries may require prolonged immobilization to allow for healing of the ligamentous injuries.

Open Reduction and Internal Fixation

The cast may be removed and the stability of the fracture, tenderness, and range of motion all evaluated out of plaster.

Fractures of the Lisfranc joint complex are still not stable despite rigid internal fixation, and they should remain non-weight bearing for at least another 4 to 6 weeks or until the screws are ready to be removed.

Fractures of the body of the tarsal navicular involve both the talonavicular and naviculocuneiform joints. If the patient has a significant amount of tenderness at the fracture site, a non–weight-bearing short leg cast should be placed. If nontender, the patient may remain out of plaster but must remain strictly non-weight bearing.

Compression injuries, or nutcracker fractures, of the cuboid usually involve significant comminution or bone loss. If an external fixator has been placed, as well as an autogenous bone graft to restore the lateral column length, remove the fixator if it is thought, based on radiographic and physical examination, that this construct is stable. If the patient is still significantly tender or not thought to be stable, the patient should be placed in a non–weight-bearing short leg cast.

Multiple cuneiform fractures that have had screw fixation should continue to be immobilized in a non–weight-bearing short leg cast.

Closed Reduction and Percutaneous Pinning

Check the pin sites for discharge, erythema, or any evidence of tenting. Release tenting of the skin as necessary. If the foot or pin sites have any purulence and there is erythema or streaking, the patient should be admitted for intravenous antibiotics and the pin removal.

After radiographic examination, if it appears the fracture is adequately stable, the pins may be removed. If the fracture/dislocation across the Lisfranc joint appears adequately stable, the patient may be placed in a stiff-soled shoe and begin partial protected weight bearing.

Prescription

FOUR TO SIX WEEKS

Precautions The fracture/dislocation is not fully stable unless the rigid fixation device is in place. However, the fracture is still not fully healed and cannot bear weight.

Range of Motion Active range of motion to toes and metatarsophalangeal joints. If out of cast, gentle active range of motion to the ankle and subtalar joint.

Muscle Strength Isometric exercises to the dorsiflexors and plantar flexors of the ankle. No resistive exercises to the long flexors or extensors of the toes.

Functional Activities Partial or non–weight-bearing stand/pivot transfers and ambulation with assistive devices, depending on type of fracture.

Weight Bearing None for patients with open reduction and internal fixation, or multiple cuneiform fractures and displaced stress fractures of the tarsal navicular. Partial weight bearing as tolerated for all other fractures, including percutaneous pinning after hardware removal (*see* Table 33-5).

Treatment: Six to Eight Weeks

BONE HEALING

Stability at fracture site: With bridging callus, the fracture is usually stable. Confirm with physical examination.

Stage of bone healing: Reparative phase. Further organization of callus and formation of lamellar bone begins. Once the bridging callus is observed, the fracture is usually stable. This requires further protection to avoid refracture because the strength of this callus, especially with torsional load, is significantly lower than that of normal lamellar bone.

X-ray: Bridging callus is visible in cortical bone, indicating increased rigidity. Healing with endosteal bone predominates. In the region of the tarsal bones, which are mainly cancellous, an appreciable amount of callus is not seen because the cortex is quite thin, but the fracture line is less distinct.

Orthopaedic and Rehabilitation Considerations

Physical Examination

All fractures should be out of a cast. Examine the fracture for tenderness. If there was a wound or an operative site, evaluate it for healing and evidence of infection. Evaluate any trophic or sensory changes as indications of RSD. Evaluate wounds or operative sites for any evidence of infection, and treat appropriately.

Radiography

Evaluate fractures that are tender with anteroposterior, lateral, and oblique views. Assess maintenance of reduction as well as the status of healing.

Weight Bearing

Patients with Lisfranc fractures who were treated with a cast or closed reduction and percutaneous pinning and have previously begun partial weight bearing may continue to increase their weight bearing as tolerated at this time. Fracture/dislocations that have required open reduction and internal fixation should remain non-weight bearing unless it is decided that the screws will be removed.

Patients with cortical avulsion fractures, tuberosity fractures, and healed stress fractures of the tarsal navicular continue partial weight bearing and progress as tolerated. Fractures of the body of the tarsal navicular that required open reduction and internal fixation, as well as displaced stress fractures, should not be weight bearing.

Nondisplaced avulsion fractures of the cuboid may continue to bear weight progressively as tolerated. Nutcracker fractures of the cuboid that required open reduction and internal fixation should continue non-weight bearing. Nondisplaced fractures of the cuneiform, if they are nontender on examination, may begin toe-touch to partial weight bearing (Table 33-6).

TABLE 33-6 *Six To Eight Weeks Weight Bearing*

	Partial weight bearing	Non-weight bearing
Lisfranc (tarsometatarsal) **fracture/dislocation**	Closed reduction—percutaneous pinning Cast	Open reduction with internal fixation
Navicular fractures	Cortical avulsion Tuberosity Stress nondisplaced healed	Body (with open reduction and internal fixation) Stress displaced
Cuneiform fractures	Nondisplaced	Displaced
Cuboid fractures	Nondisplaced Avulsion	Nutcracker (with open reduction and internal fixation)

Range of Motion

Active and active-assistive range-of-motion exercises are performed at the metatarsophalangeal joints, interphalangeal joints, and ankle in all planes. If the ankle is particularly stiff from immobilization, begin gentle passive range-of-motion exercises. The patient can be instructed in passively flexing and extending the toes; the same can be done with the ankle if the ankle joint is stiff. These exercises are all done to patient tolerance. Caution the patient not to be overly aggressive with ranging in inversion and eversion because this places particular stress across the midfoot.

Muscle Strength

Once the patient actively extends and flexes the toes fully in a repeated fashion, the muscles are being strengthened isotonically. When the fracture site is stable, gentle resistance can be applied to the toes during ranging. The patient can use one hand to apply and control the force over the toes. To strengthen the dorsiflexors and plantar flexors of the ankle, the patient can apply resistance against the foot while ranging the ankle. Resistive exercises should not be performed for fracture/dislocations of the Lisfranc joint complex.

Functional Activities

Lisfranc joint fracture/dislocations that required open reduction and internal fixation, tarsal navicular body fractures, nonunited stress fractures, and nutcracker fractures of the cuboid remain non-weight bearing. All other midfoot fractures may now be partially to fully weight bearing. Patients may still need crutches to support their weight if the fracture is not yet pain free and stable.

Gait

As noted, patients who are non-weight bearing or partially weight bearing on the affected extremity may still need to use crutches. Those who are weight bearing now use a protective shoe. Patients who are still using crutches may use a two- or a three-point gait (*see* Figures 6-16 and 6-17). Patients who are out of casts and no longer using crutches may still note tenderness when attempting to bear full weight in the stance phase of gait, and may try to prolong heel strike. They might also tend to avoid the torsional motion of the foot coming from eversion to inversion as the foot moves from heel strike to mid-stance. This is accomplished by shifting their weight to the lateral aspect of the foot through the mid-stance phase and into the push-off phase. The push-off phase may be abbreviated and without full loading to avoid discomfort as the body's weight shifts from the midfoot to the forefoot.

Methods of Treatment: Specific Aspects

Cast

With the possible exception of unhealed stress fractures of the tarsal navicular, casts should be removed. For all fractures remaining in plaster, remove the cast and perform an examination out of plaster. A patient who is still tender should be given a stiff-soled bunion shoe or a cam walker–type device for ambulation. Active and assisted range-of-motion exercises are either begun for those just coming out of a cast or continued for those whose casts were already removed. For those coming out of a cast, the ankle may be quite stiff. Gentle subtalar motion, eversion, and inversion are instituted. These motions can be quite painful initially. Patients can be instructed to perform these exercises under water or with hydrotherapy to ease the discomfort.

Open Reduction and Internal Fixation

Casts should have been removed by now. The patient may begin active and active assistive range of motion for the ankle joint as well as the metatarsophalangeal joints, if this was not previously instituted. All fractures that required open reduction and internal fixation should remain non-weight bearing.

Closed Reduction and Percutaneous Pinning

Any casts or retained pins should be removed. Depending on the stage of fracture healing, the patient now may begin to bear weight as tolerated on the affected extremity. If the patient is unable to bear weight because of pain at the fracture site, active and active-assistive range of motion at the metatarsophalangeal, subtalar, and ankle joints should continue.

Prescription

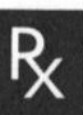

Six to Eight Weeks

Precautions Avoid passive range of motion to the midfoot. Stability of fracture/dislocations not full unless rigid fixation devices in place.

Range of Motion Gentle active to active-assistive to gentle passive range of motion, as tolerated, to the ankle and subtalar joint if not in a cast.

Muscle Strength Isometric exercises and isotonic exercises to the ankle and subtalar joint if not in a cast.

Functional Activities Partial weight bearing is permitted during transfers except in fractures treated with open reduction and internal fixation (*see* Table 33-6).

Weight Bearing Depending on tenderness at fracture site and callus formation, weight bearing is partial or full, with the exception of any fracture with open reduction and internal fixation.

Treatment: Eight to Twelve Weeks

Bone Healing

Stability at fracture site: Stable.

Stage of bone healing: Remodeling phase. Woven bone is replaced with lamellar bone. The process of remodeling takes months to years for completion.

X-ray: Callus is seen in all fractures in cortical regions of bone. Tarsal bones show fracture lines beginning to disappear. Trabeculae reform and strengthen over time.

Orthopaedic and Rehabilitation Considerations

Physical Examination

Evaluate for tenderness at the fracture site. Evaluate any wounds, pin sites, or incisions for evidence of infections and treat appropriately. Evaluate for RSD.

Radiography

If the patient is nontender and hardware has not been placed, radiographs are not necessary. If there is tenderness, presence of internal fixation devices, or a suspected nonunion, radiographs in the anteroposterior, lateral, and oblique positions should be taken and evaluated for fracture healing and bony alignment.

Weight Bearing

All fractures, with the possible exception of navicular stress fractures that have not united, may begin toe-touch to partial weight bearing. Fractures that were already weight bearing may progress to full weight bearing. Lisfranc fracture/dislocations that have undergone open reduction and internal fixation may now have their hardware removed and begin slowly progressive weight bearing. The patient should not engage in any repetitive pounding or jumping activities because these may cause a loss of reduction or damage to any retained hardware (Table 33-7).

TABLE 33-7 ***Eight to Twelve Weeks Weight Bearing***

	Full weight bearing	Partial weight bearing
Lisfranc (tarsometatarsal) **fracture/dislocation**	Closed reduction—percutaneous pinning Cast	Open reduction with internal fixation
Navicular fractures[a]	Cortical avulsion Tuberosity Stress nondisplaced healed	Body (with open reduction and internal fixation)
Cuneiform fractures	Nondisplaced	Displaced
Cuboid fractures	Nondisplaced Avulsion	Nutcracker (with open reduction and internal fixation)

[a]Nonunited stress fractures of the navicular are non-weight bearing.

Range of Motion

Continue with full active and passive range of motion of the metatarsophalangeal and ankle joints. Patients should now be regaining almost full range of motion of these joints if they have been out of a cast for at least 2 weeks. Fractures of the body of the navicular and nutcracker fractures of the cuboid may still have some residual stiffness with restricted inversion and eversion. Depending on the complexity of the fracture and the extent of intraarticular involvement, there may eventually be permanent arthritic changes that compromise these motions of inversion and eversion.

Muscle Strength

Depending on the stability of the fracture, the patient is instructed in gentle resistive exercises. The patient dorsiflexes the foot against resistance provided by the other foot and holds to a count of five. The patient can alter the resistance depending on pain and tolerance. This is repeated in all planes. Continue with quadriceps isotonic exercises.

Functional Activities

The patient is now either partially or fully weight bearing. The patient still may need to use crutches or a cane for balance and stability during transfers and ambulation.

Gait

The ankle and metatarsophalangeal joints may still have some residual stiffness from prolonged immobilization. This affects the gait during push-off and heel strike. Residual tenderness in the midfoot may cause the patient to increase his or her heel strike weight-bearing time to delay transfer of weight to the midfoot during stance. To avoid pressure across the Lisfranc joint complex, the patient may try to roll his or her weight across the lateral aspect of the foot; if the fracture/dislocation has involved all of the metatarsals, the patient may try to avoid the stance phase altogether because of tenderness. Push-off is also painful because this loads the metatarsal heads, stressing the Lisfranc joint complex. Another way for the patient to avoid torsion across the Lisfranc complex is to skip the heel-strike portion of the gait cycle and place the foot in a brief mid-stance position to spread the weight equally across the foot. In this situation, the patient spends most of the time on the unaffected leg, using the affected foot only for brief push-off to make forward progress.

Cortical avulsion fractures, tuberosity fractures, and stress fractures of the tarsal navicular, as well as nondisplaced avulsion fractures of the cuboid, should now have a normal gait pattern. Nonunited stress fractures of the tarsal navicular are still painful and need to undergo open reduction and internal fixation.

Fractures of the navicular body are by definition intraarticular. Patients experience significant discomfort when moving from heel strike into the early stance and mid-stance phases because of talar head loading across the talonavicular joint. Patients are likely to try to shift their weight to the lateral aspect of the foot to unload the talonavicular joint as it moves through stance. This lateral weight shift continues into toe-off again to unload the talonavicular joint. Crush or nutcracker fractures of the cuboid are painful as the weight shifts from heel strike to early stance and mid-stance. In this case, patients shift weight toward the medial aspect of the foot to unload the calcaneocuboid joint. As they continue through stance, they bear more of their weight on the first ray of the foot, preparing for push-off. With both of these fractures, the patient may never be able fully to normalize the gait because of posttraumatic articular changes. Severe pain may eventually require consideration of fusion.

Methods of Treatment: Specific Aspects

Cast

Casts should have been removed from all fractures. Patients should continue active, active-assistive, and passive range of motion. They continue weight bearing as tolerated.

Open Reduction and Internal Fixation

Casts should have been removed from all fractures. Patients should be performing active and active-assistive range of motion at the ankle and metatarsophalangeal joints. For patients who have had open reduction and internal fixation of the Lisfranc joint complex, internal fixation devices should be removed if there is adequate evidence of healing. If there is solid incorporation of a bone graft in navicular body or cuboid fractures, consider removing all hardware. However, until there is solid consolidation and adequate assurance that the medial and lateral columns will remain stable, hardware should remain in place. The medial column is formed by the medial cuneiform, navicular, and talar bones, the lateral column by the cuboid and calcaneus. All fractures may now begin weight bearing to tolerance.

Closed Reduction and Percutaneous Pinning

See section on Open Reduction and Internal Fixation.

Prescription

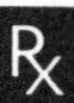

EIGHT TO TWELVE WEEKS

Precautions A rigid shoe or cam walker can be used as necessary.

Range of Motion Active, active-assistive, and passive range of motion to the ankle and subtalar joints.

Muscle Strength Gentle resistive exercises to the dorsiflexors and plantar flexors, evertors, invertors, long flexors, and extensors of the toes.

Functional Activities Partially to fully weight-bearing transfers and ambulation with assistive devices or independently, as healing dictates.

Weight Bearing Partial to full weight bearing (*see* Table 33-7).

LONG-TERM CONSIDERATIONS AND PROBLEMS

Patients with fractures and dislocations of the Lisfranc joint complex who have regained anatomic reduction should have few long-term problems at the midfoot. Increased stiffness and possible interarticular involvement may cause some discomfort in mid- to late stance when weight transfers from the midfoot to the forefoot. However, because these joints in general do not have much movement, this is not usually problematic.

Fractures of the tarsal navicular body and cuboid nutcracker fractures have the most significant long-term consequences. These fractures are intraarticular by definition. If they have not been anatomically reduced or if there has been significant articular damage, the patient may have severe posttraumatic arthritis and discomfort in all phases of the gait cycle.

Tarsal navicular tuberosity fractures that fail to unite may be very painful and require subsequent surgery to reattach the avulsed fragment as well as the posterior tibial tendon to the bone.

Inadequately treated Lisfranc fracture/dislocations may remain unstable and cause significant midfoot pain and disability during the gait cycle. Pain is particularly noticeable as the patient transfers weight across the Lisfranc joint complex during heel strike and midstance. Persistent instability causes significant midfoot pain with any torsional motion across the foot as it moves from eversion to inversion. This may ultimately need to be treated with open reduction and internal fixation.

Residual stiffness in the Lisfranc, intercuneiforms, and cuneiform-cuboid joints is usually of little consequence in the gait cycle because normally these joints have very little motion.

The gait cycle may be profoundly affected by serious fractures of the tarsal navicular or the cuboid because these bones are both part of the transverse tarsal (calcaneocuboid and talonavicular) or Chopart's joint (*see* Figure 33-3). This joint is important for transfer of load from the hindfoot to the midfoot. It also stabilizes the foot throughout the gait cycle. Posttraumatic arthritic changes may cause profound pain across these joints and require subsequent fusion to relieve disability and discomfort.

IMMEDIATE TO ONE WEEK

	Cast	*Open Reduction and Internal Fixation*	*Closed Reduction and Percutaneous Pinning*
Stability	None.	None.	None.
Orthopaedics	Trim cast to metatarsal heads and allow free range of motion of the knee.	Trim cast to metatarsal heads and allow free range of motion of the knee.	Trim cast to metatarsal heads and allow free range of motion of the knee.
Rehabilitation	Range of motion of the metatarsophalangeal (MTP) and interphalangeal (IP) joints as well as knee.	Range of motion of the MTP and IP joints as well as knee.	Range of motion of the MTP and IP as well as knee.

TWO WEEKS

	Cast	*Open Reduction and Internal Fixation*	*Closed Reduction and Percutaneous Pinning*
Stability	None to minimal.	None to minimal.	None to minimal.
Orthopaedics	Trim cast to metatarsal heads and at knee to allow full range of motion.	Trim cast to metatarsal heads and at knee to allow full range of motion.	Evaluate point sites. Trim cast to metatarsal heads and at knee to allow full range of motion.
Rehabilitation	Range of motion to the metatarsophalangeal and interphalangeal (IP) joints and the knee joint.	Range of motion to the MTP and IP joints and the knee joint.	Range of motion to the MTP and IP joints and the knee joint.

FOUR TO SIX WEEKS

	Cast	*Open Reduction and Internal Fixation*	*Closed Reduction and Percutaneous Pinning*
Stability	Stable.	Moderate to stable.	Stable.
Orthopaedics	Remove cast and replace with a stiff-soled or bunion shoe.	May remove or continue with weight bearing cast.	May remove points. Remove cast and place in stiff-soled or bunion shoe.
Rehabilitation	Continue metatarsophalangeal (MTP), interphalangeal (IP), and knee joint range of motion. Begin plantar flexion and dorsiflexion, inversion and eversion ankle and subtalar range of motion.	Continue MTP, IP, and knee joint range of motion. Begin plantar flexion and dorsiflexion, inversion and eversion ankle and subtalar range of motion.	Continue MTP, IP, and knee joint range of motion. Begin plantar flexion and dorsiflexion, inversion and eversion ankle and subtalar range of motion.

SIX TO EIGHT WEEKS

	Cast	Open Reduction and Internal Fixation	Closed Reduction and Percutaneous Pinning
Stability	Stable.	Stable.	Stable.
Orthopaedics	Remove cast if not already done.	Remove cast if not already done.	Remove pins and cast if not already done.
Rehabilitation	Continue range of motion of metatarsophalangeal (MTP), interphalangeal (IP), ankle and knee joints. Begin plantar flexion and dorsiflexion, inversion and eversion ankle and subtalar range of motion.	Continue range of motion of MTP, IP, ankle and knee joint. Begin plantar flexion and dorsiflexion inversion and eversion ankle and subtalar range of motion.	Continue range of motion of MTP, IP, ankle and knee joints. Begin plantar flexion and dorsiflexion, inversion and eversion ankle and subtalar range of motion.

EIGHT TO TWELVE WEEKS

	Cast	Open Reduction and Internal Fixation	Closed Reduction and Percutaneous Pinning
Stability	Stable.	Stable.	Stable.
Orthopaedics		May consider removing internal fixation devices.	
Rehabilitation	Continue metatarsophalangeal (MTP), interphalangeal (IP), and knee joint range of motion. Begin gentle resistive exercises except for Lisfranc injuries.	Continue MTP, IP, and knee joint range of motion. Begin gentle resistive exercises except for Lisfranc injuries.	Continue MTP, IP, and knee joint range of motion. Begin gentle resistive exercises except for Lisfranc injuries.

BIBLIOGRAPHY

Chapman M. Tarsal and metatarsal injuries. In: Mann RA, ed. *Surgery of the Foot*. St. Louis: C.V. Mosby, 1986, pp. 714–729.

Geissler W, Tsao A. Foot and ankle fractures. In: Rockwood CA Jr, Green DP, eds. *Fractures in Adults*, 4th ed. Philadelphia: J.B. Lippincott, 1995, pp. 2354–2372.

Hansen ST Jr. Foot injuries. In: Browner B, Jupiter J, Levine AM, Trafton PG, eds. *Skeletal Trauma*, Vol 2. Philadelphia: W.B. Saunders, 1992, pp. 1960–1972.

Mann R. Lower extremity. In: Chapman M, ed. *Operative Orthopaedics*. Philadelphia: J.B. Lippincott, 1993, pp. 2179–2190.

Manoli A II. Compartment syndromes of the foot: current concepts. *Foot and Ankle*, 10:340–344, 1990.

Mizel M, Sobel M. Trauma—Section 1. In: Miller M, ed. *Review of Orthopaedics*, 2nd ed. Philadelphia: W.B. Saunders, 1996, pp. 241–242, 391.

Perry J. Ankle and foot gait deviations. In: Perry J, ed. *Gait Analysis*. Thorofare, NJ, Slack, 1992, pp. 185–219.

Schenck RC Jr, Heckman JD. Fractures and dislocations of the forefoot: Operative and nonoperative treatment. *Journal of the American Academy of Orthopedic Surgeons*, 3:70–78, 1995.

Sondergaard L, Konradson L, Holmer P, et al. Acute midtarsal sprains: frequency and course of recovery. *Foot and Ankle*, 17: 195–199, 1996.

Stephen DJG. Injuries to the midfoot and forefoot. In: Schatzer J, Tile M, eds. *The Rationale of Operative Fracture Care*, 2nd ed. Berlin: Springer-Verlag, 1996, pp. 605–619.

Yablon IG, Segal D. Foot and ankle injuries. In: Evarts CM, ed. *Surgery of the Musculoskeletal System*, 2nd ed. New York: Churchill Livingstone, 1990, pp. 4269–4277.

CHAPTER Thirty-four

Forefoot Fractures

ANNE P. MCCORMACK, MD

STANLEY HOPPENFELD, MD

INTRODUCTION

Definition

Fractures of the forefoot are those involving the great toe or any of the lesser toes (phalanges), the metatarsals, or the sesamoid bones (Figure 34-1 and *see* Figures 34-4, 34-13 and 34-15).

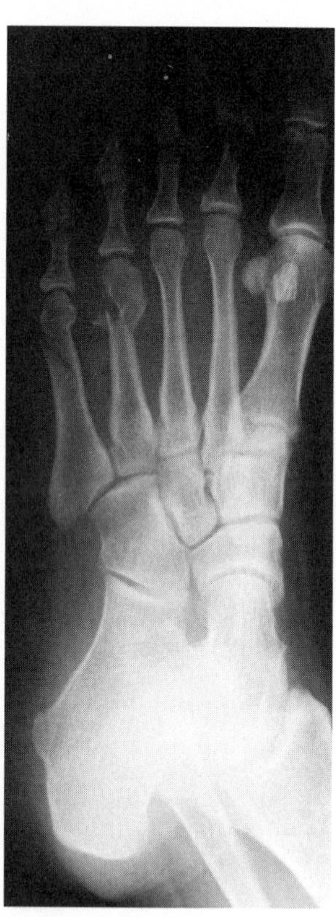

FIGURE 34-1 Fractures of the fourth and fifth metatarsals. They are extraarticular and stable.

Fractures involving the phalanges and metatarsals can be intraarticular or extraarticular. Phalangeal or metatarsal fractures can involve the neck, shaft, or base of the bone. Fractures involving the Lisfranc joints (tarsometatarsal joints) are discussed in the chapter on the midfoot (*see* Figures 33-1 and 33-2).

Metatarsal fractures are further classified as stable or unstable. Unstable configurations usually involve multiple metatarsals that are comminuted or displaced or else involve the first metatarsal (Figure 34-2). These

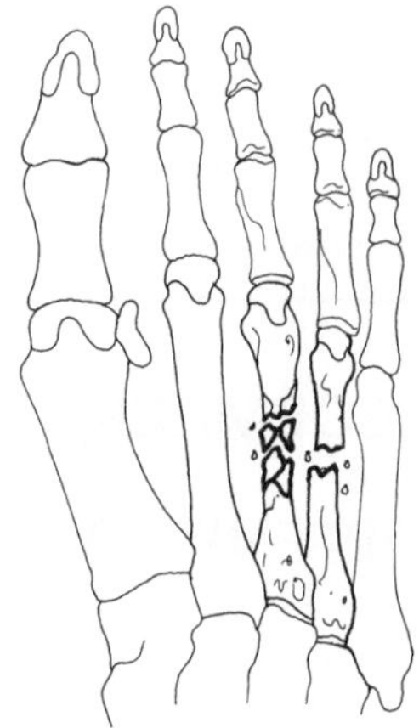

FIGURE 34-2 Fracture of the shaft of the third metatarsal; it is comminuted, unstable, and extraarticular. There is a transverse fracture of the shaft of the fourth metatarsal.

fractures can occasionally be complicated further by a compartment syndrome of the foot or skin slough.

Fractures of the proximal fifth metatarsal shaft carry the eponym of Jones fracture (Figure 34-3 and *see* Figures 34-11 and 34-12).

These are often confused with apophyseal fractures of the base of the fifth metatarsal (Figure 34-3A, *see* Figures 34-9 and 34-10).

Sesamoid fractures involve splitting or fragmentation of one or both of the two small bones contained within the tendon of the flexor hallucis longus. They are important because of their role in forefoot weight distribution (Figures 34-4 and *see* Figure 34-17).

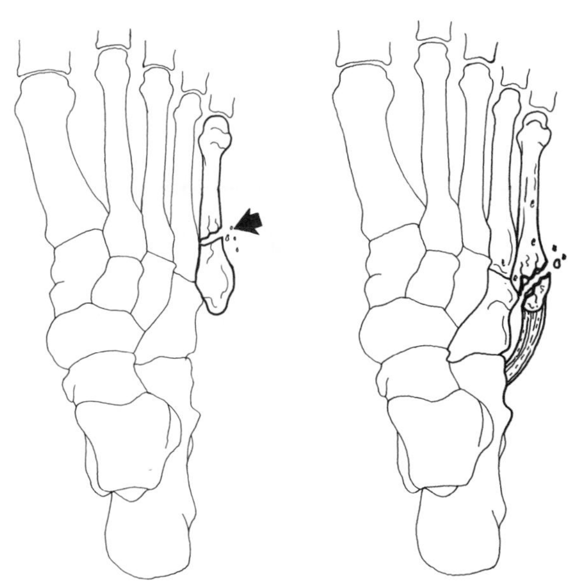

FIGURE 34-3 *(above, left)* Jones fracture of the proximal fifth metatarsal shaft. These are often confused with epiphyseal fractures of the base of the fifth metatarsal.

FIGURE 34-3A *(above, right)* Epiphyseal or avulsion fracture of the base of the fifth metatarsal. These are often confused with Jones fractures. The peroneus brevis tendon attaches to the styloid process of the fifth metatarsal and with weight bearing avulses the proximal fragment.

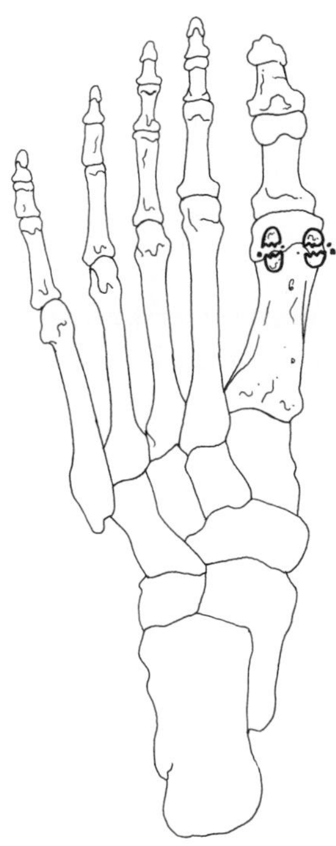

FIGURE 34-4 Sesamoid fractures involving a splitting or fragmentation of one or both of the two small bones contained within the tendon of the flexor hallucis longus. They are important because of their role in weight-bearing distribution. These fractures are often caused by the foot hitting a hard surface while the toes are dorsiflexed.

Mechanism of Injury

Phalangeal Fractures

Fractures of the first proximal phalanx result from direct trauma or an avulsion mechanism, such as when the great toe is caught on a table or chair leg (*see* Figure 34-13). Fractures of the lesser phalanges are usually the result of direct trauma.

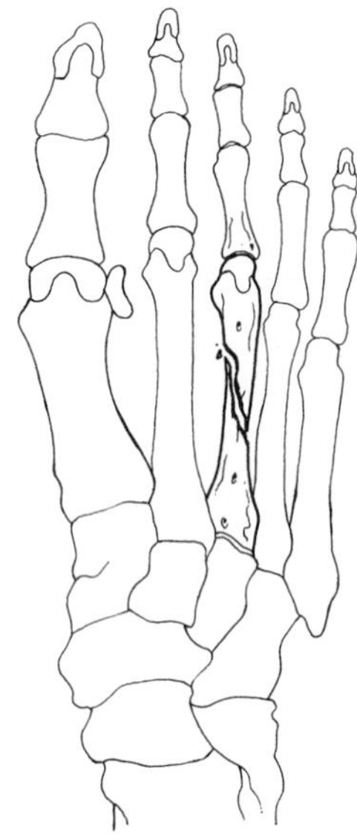

FIGURE 34-5 Oblique fracture to the shaft of the third metatarsal. This frequently occurs as the result of a twisting injury.

Metatarsal Fractures

Fractures of the first through fourth metatarsals usually result from direct trauma (*see* Figures 34-17 and 34-20). Fractures of the second through fifth metatarsals may also occur as a result of a twisting injury (Figure 34-5 and *see* Figure 33-15).

Diaphyseal stress fractures are common in the second through fourth metatarsals and commonly result from repeated trauma (Figure 34-6 and *see* Figure 34-8).

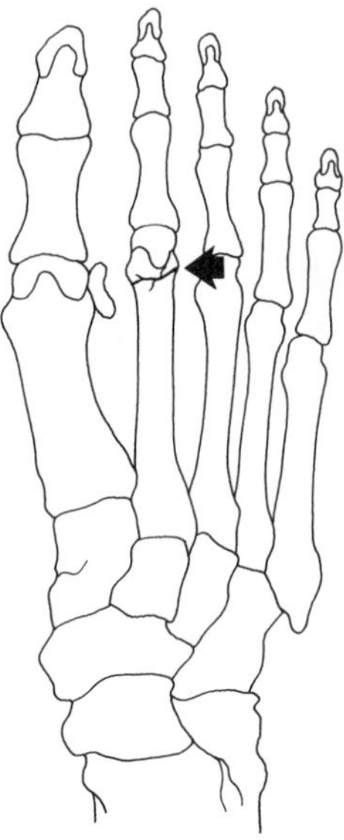

FIGURE 34-6 Stress fracture of the neck of the second metatarsal. This frequently results from a long march or after long ballet exercise and is sometimes referred to as a "march fracture."

Avulsion fractures of the proximal apophysis and proximal shaft of the fifth metatarsal may follow an inversion injury on a plantar-flexed ankle (*see* Figures 34-9 and 34-9A).

Sesamoid Fractures

Sesamoid fractures are often secondary to the impact of the foot on a hard surface while the toes are dorsiflexed. Stress fractures are not uncommon as a result of repeated impact and tension (as seen in dancers and runners).

Treatment Goals

Orthopaedic Objectives

Alignment

Restoration of great toe, phalanx, metatarsal, and sesamoid alignment is of critical importance to weight bearing and load distribution on the foot. Restoration of perfect anatomic alignment is less critical in phalanges two through five. Metatarsals two through five should be aligned as anatomically as possible to minimize problems with gait and painful fitting of shoes.

Stability

A stable union of all the forefoot bones is particularly important to maintain a pain-free, stable gait.

Rehabilitation Objectives

Range of Motion

Restore and maintain the range of motion of the metatarsophalangeal joints and the phalangeal joints; maintain the range of motion of the ankle and foot (Table 34-1).

TABLE 34-1 *Forefoot Range of Motion*

Motion	Normal
Great toe (hallux) extension or dorsiflexion metatarsophalangeal joint	75°
Great toe (hallux) flexion or plantar flexion metatarsophalangeal joint	45°
Great toe (hallux) extension interphalangeal joint	0°
Great toe (hallux) flexion interphalangeal joint	90°
Lesser toes flexion metatarsophalangeal joint	40°
Lesser toes extension metatarsophalangeal joint	70°
Lesser toes flexion distal interphalangeal joint	60°
Lesser toes flexion proximal interphalangeal joint	75°

In severe fractures of the first metatarsal and first phalanx, a patient may lose up to 75% of the normal range of motion. The residual range of motion may be painful when weight bearing, particularly in the push-off phase of gait (*see* Figures 34-18 and 34-19).

Residual loss of range of motion secondary to fractures of the first metatarsal and first phalanx are usually related to interarticular fractures.

Muscle Strength

Improve and restore the strength of the following muscles:

Long extensors of the toes:

- Extensor hallucis longus
- Extensor digitorum longus and brevis

Long flexors of the toes:

- Flexor hallucis longus
- Flexor digitorum longus

Evertors of the foot:

- Peroneus longus and brevis (insert into the first and fifth metatarsal bones, respectively)

Invertors of the foot:

- Tibialis posterior, (as expansion inserts into the base of the second and fourth metatarsals)
- Tibialis anterior, (as it inserts into the base of the first metatarsal along with the insertion into the cuneiform)

The muscle that is most likely to lose strength as a result of a sesamoid fracture is the flexor hallucis brevis, because the sesamoid bones are contained within the tendon. Fractures of the first metatarsal may cause residual weakness in the extensor hallucis longus as well as the flexor hallucis longus. Fractures of the lesser four metatarsals may weaken the extensor digitorum longus and brevis. Unless there is an untreated compartment syndrome of the foot, evertors and invertors as well as the major dorsiflexors across the ankle should not have any residual strength loss as a result of forefoot fractures.

Functional Goals

Normalize gait to its preinjury pattern.

Expected Time of Bone Healing

1. Lesser phalanx fracture: 4 to 6 weeks.
2. Second, third, and fourth metatarsal fracture: 4 to 6 weeks.
3. Fifth metatarsal fracture: 6 to 8 weeks.

4. Great (first) toe phalanx fracture: 4 to 6 weeks.
5. First metatarsal fracture: 6 to 8 weeks.
6. Sesamoid fracture: generally, 4 to 8 weeks.

Expected Duration of Rehabilitation

1. Lesser phalanx fracture: 2 to 6 weeks.
2. Second, third, and fourth metatarsal fracture: 4 to 6 weeks.
3. Fifth metatarsal fracture:
   For acute fracture, 4 to 6 weeks
   For delayed union, nonunion, or stress fracture, 6 to 10 weeks.
4. Great (first) toe phalanx fracture: 4 to 6 weeks.
5. First metatarsal fracture: 4 to 6 weeks.
6. Sesamoid fracture: For acute fracture, 8 to 12 weeks, possibly longer after sesamoidectomy.

METHODS OF TREATMENT

Lesser Phalanx Fractures

Splints or Buddy Taping

Biomechanics: Stress-sharing device.

Mode of bone healing: Secondary, with callus formation.

Indications: Diaphyseal fractures of the proximal and middle phalanges are generally closed injuries and treated with a simple splint. The injured toe is taped lightly to an adjacent uninjured toe after a piece of gauze or cast padding is placed between them to prevent skin maceration (Figure 34-7).

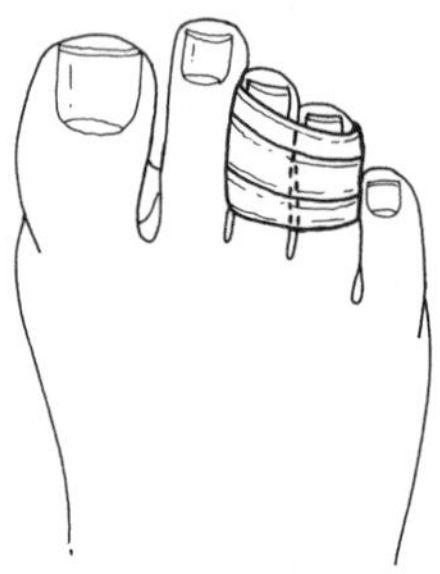

FIGURE 34-7 Buddy taping of the third and fourth toes to treat diaphyseal fractures of the proximal and middle phalanges. The injured toe is taped lightly to an adjacent uninjured toe after a piece of gauze or cast padding is placed between them to prevent maceration.

Open Reduction and Percutaneous Pinning

Biomechanics: Stress-sharing device for pin fixation.

Mode of bone healing: Secondary, with callus formation.

Indications: Open fractures, or those that cannot be aligned anatomically via closed means, require open reduction and Kirschner wire (K-wire) fixation of the fragments. A short leg cast that extends to the toes is placed postoperatively for 2 to 3 weeks, until the pins are pulled.

Second, Third, and Fourth Metatarsal Fractures

Cast

Biomechanics: Stress-sharing device.

Mode of bone healing: Secondary, with callus formation.

Indications: Undisplaced or minimally displaced fractures (including stress fractures) of the metatarsal shaft are generally closed and amenable to closed reduction and placement of a short leg walking cast (Figure 34-8 and *see* Figure 34-6).

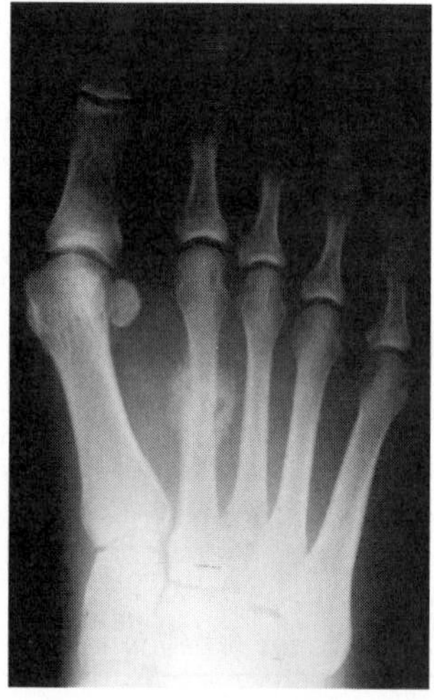

FIGURE 34-8 A healed stress fracture of the shaft of the second metatarsal. This was initially treated in a short walking cast.

Closed Reduction and Percutaneous Pinning

Biomechanics: Stress-sharing device for pin fixation.

Mode of bone healing: Secondary, with callus formation.

Indications: Intramedullary K-wire fixation is used for closed, displaced, or angulated metatarsal shaft fractures. Postoperatively the foot is immobilized in a non–weight-bearing short leg cast for 2 to 3 weeks until the pins are removed.

Open Reduction and Internal Fixation

Biomechanics: Stress-sharing device for pin fixation.

Mode of bone healing: Secondary, with callus formation.

Indications: Open displaced fractures require the best anatomic reduction possible. Intramedullary K-wire fixation maintains this reduction. Postoperatively, the foot is immobilized in a non–weight-bearing short leg cast for 2 to 3 weeks until the pins are removed.

Fifth Metatarsal Fractures

Cast/Splint

Biomechanics: Stress-sharing device.

Mode of bone healing: Secondary, with callus formation.

Indications: Acute avulsion injuries of the apophysis are usually treated in a short leg walking cast or, if displacement is less than 2 mm, with strapping and a walking boot (Figures 34-9, 34-9A, 34-10, and 34-10A). Jones fractures of the proximal end of the fifth metatarsal shaft are treated in a non–weight-bearing short leg cast (Figures 34-11 and 34-12). Stress fractures can be treated with a cast, but this is often unsuccessful.

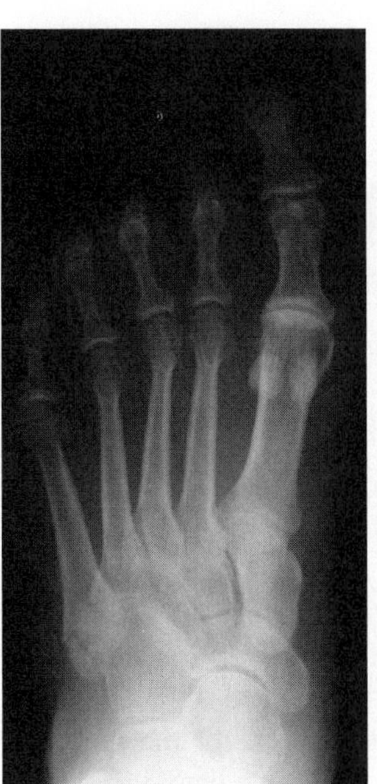

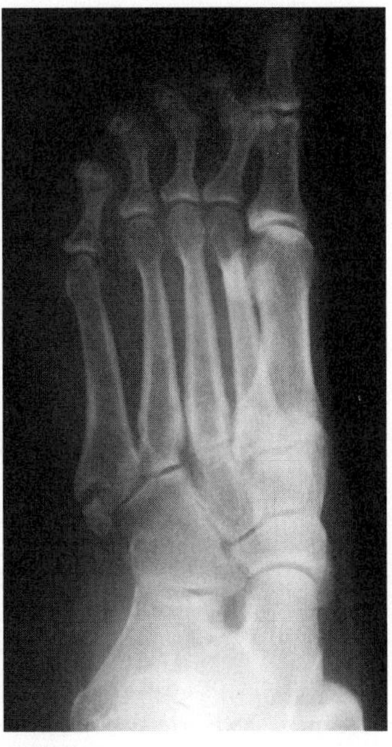

FIGURE 34-9 *(above, left)* Avulsion fracture of the styloid process of the base of the fifth metatarsal, non-weight bearing. The fracture fragments appear approximated.

FIGURE 34-9A *(above, right)* Epiphyseal fracture of the styloid process of the fifth metatarsal, weight bearing. The fracture fragments are no longer approximated because of the pull of the peroneus brevis tendon, which causes significant pain. These injuries are best treated in a short leg cast.

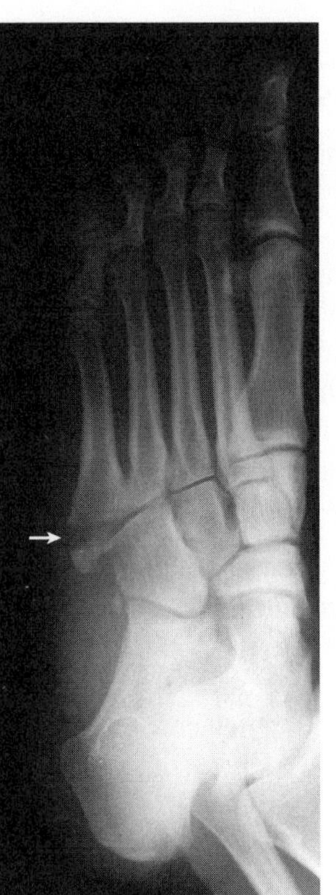

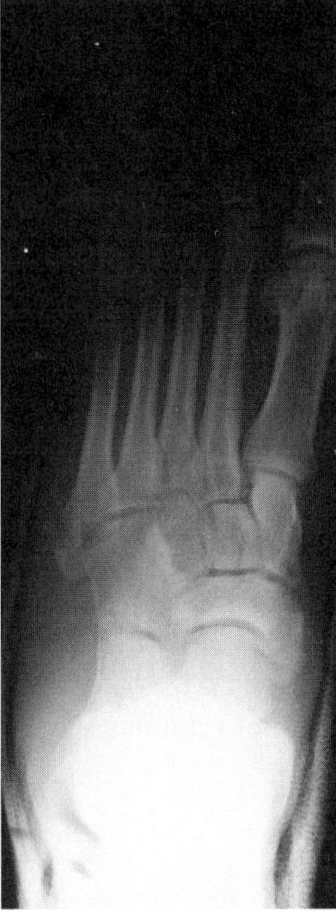

FIGURE 34-10 *(above, left)* Avulsion fracture of the styloid process of the fifth metatarsal. Note the marked separation of the fracture segments caused by the pull of the peroneus brevis tendon.

FIGURE 34-10A *(above, right)* Styloid fracture treated in a short leg cast.

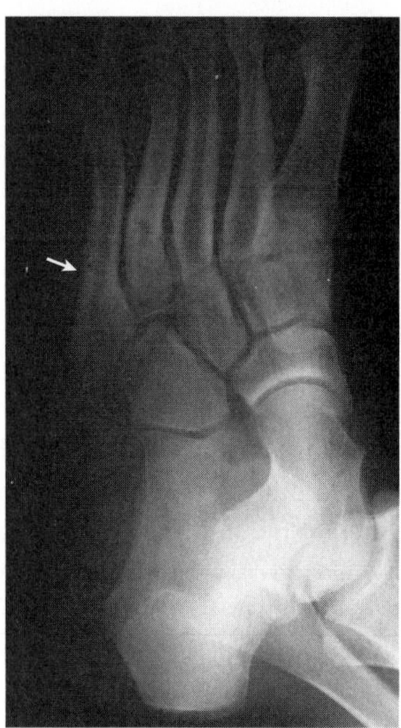

FIGURE 34-11 Acute Jones fracture of the proximal end of the fifth metatarsal requiring cast immobilization.

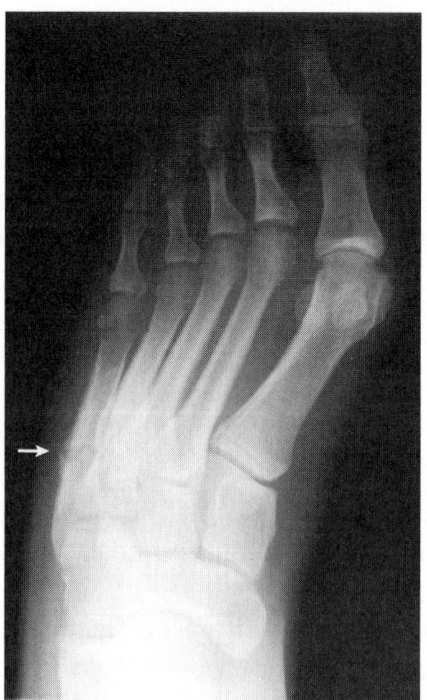

FIGURE 34-12 Healed Jones fracture. Note the callus formation.

Open Reduction and Internal Fixation

Biomechanics: Stress-shielding for screw fixation.

Mode of bone healing: Primary, no callus formation.

Indications: Avulsion fractures with greater than 2 mm displacement are treated by open reduction and internal fixation with a small tension-band wire or lag screw. Delayed unions or nonunions require bone graft and intramedullary screw fixation. Postoperatively, a non–weight-bearing short leg cast is applied for approximately 6 weeks.

Great (First) Toe Phalanx Fractures (Hallux)

Cast

Biomechanics: Stress-sharing device.

Mode of bone healing: Secondary, with callus formation.

Indications: Nondisplaced, extraarticular fractures can be buddy taped to the adjacent toe and placed in a non–weight-bearing short leg cast that extends to the end of the toes.

Closed Reduction and Percutaneous Pinning

Biomechanics: Stress-sharing device.

Mode of bone healing: Secondary, with callus formation.

Indications: Displaced or intraarticular fractures must be anatomically reduced and held in place with K-wires. A short leg cast is then placed with the toe in a neutral position for 2 to 3 weeks until the pins are removed (Figures 34-13, 34-14, 34-15, and 34-16).

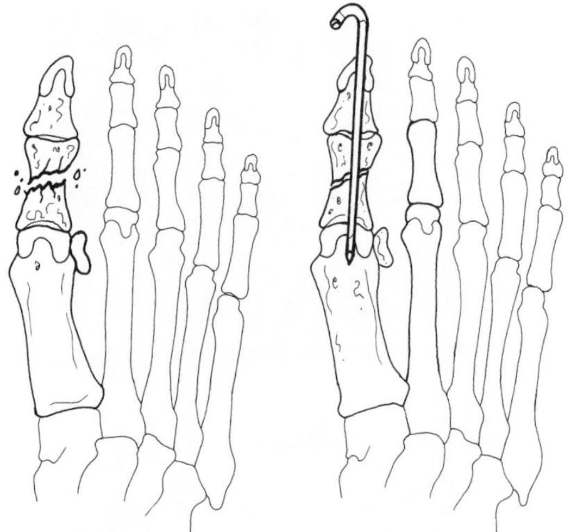

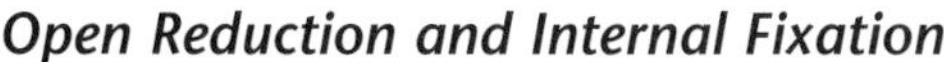

FIGURE 34-13 *(above, left)* Fracture of the shaft of the proximal phalanx of the great toe.

FIGURE 34-14 *(above, right)* Fracture of the shaft of the proximal phalanx of the great toe treated with Kirschner wire fixation. A short leg cast is then placed with the toe in a neutral position for 2 to 3 weeks until the pins are removed.

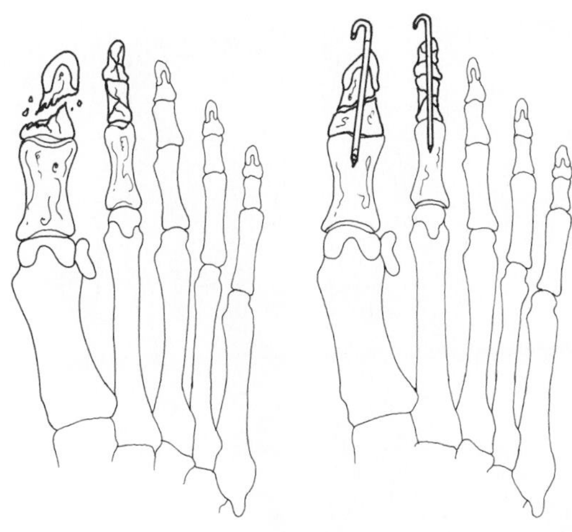

FIGURE 34-15 *(above, left)* Fracture of the distal phalanx of the great toe. This usually occurs from direct trauma or twisting. Note the associated fractures of the distal and middle phalanx of the second toe.

FIGURE 34-16 *(above, right)* Phalangeal fractures of the great and second toe treated with Kirschner wire fixation. These pins may be removed in 2 to 3 weeks.

Open Reduction and Internal Fixation

Biomechanics: Stress-shielding device when rigid fixation is obtained.

Mode of bone healing: Primary when solid fixation is achieved; no callus formation.

Indications: This technique is used when a displaced or intraarticular fracture cannot be satisfactorily reduced by closed means. Small osteochondral fragments are excised, and reduction is maintained with small compression screws or double-threaded Herbert screws. A cast is placed postoperatively with the toe in a neutral position, and it remains in place for 2 to 3 weeks. The screws are generally not removed.

First Metatarsal Fractures

Cast

Biomechanics: Stress-sharing device.

Mode of bone healing: Secondary, with callus formation.

Indications: Nondisplaced fractures can be placed in a non–weight-bearing short leg cast that extends to the end of the toes (Figures 34-17, 34-18, and 34-19).

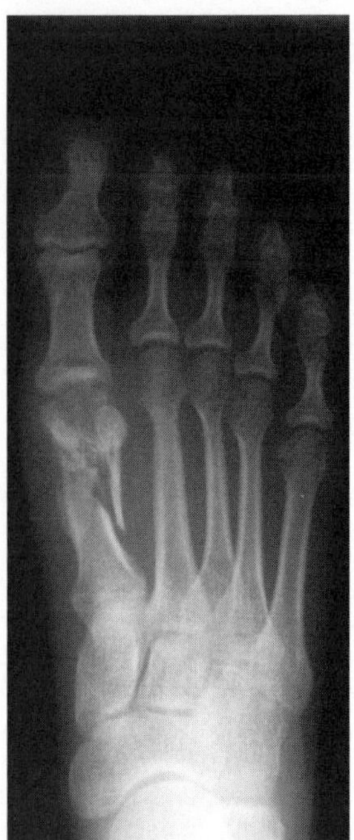

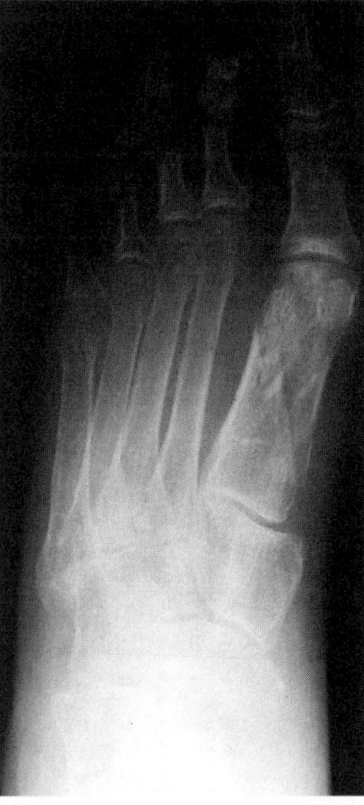

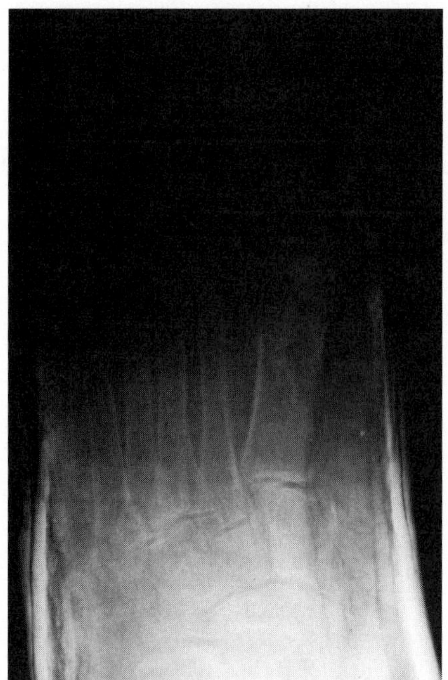

FIGURE 34-17 *(above, left)* Fracture of the shaft of the first metatarsal, which resulted from direct trauma. Note the fracture of the medial sesamoid bone. This was treated in a non–weight-bearing short leg cast that extended to the toes.

FIGURE 34-18 *(above, right)* Crush fracture of the shaft of the first metatarsal.

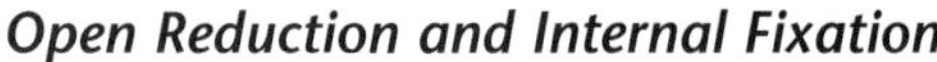

FIGURE 34-19 Crush fracture of the first metatarsal treated in a non–weight-bearing short leg cast. The cast should be trimmed dorsally so that the toes are visible. Fractures of the first phalanx affect gait, particularly at push-off, because the first metatarsal bears one third of the load distributed to the forefoot.

Open Reduction and Internal Fixation

Biomechanics: Stress-shielding device for plate fixation.

Mode of bone healing: Primary, for rigid fixation; no callus formation.

Indications: Displaced, intraarticular, or open fractures must be anatomically reduced and rigidly fixed. A one-third tubular plate or small dynamic compression plate with appropriately sized cortical screws provides the best fixation. A short leg cast is applied postoperatively (Figures 34-20 and 34-21).

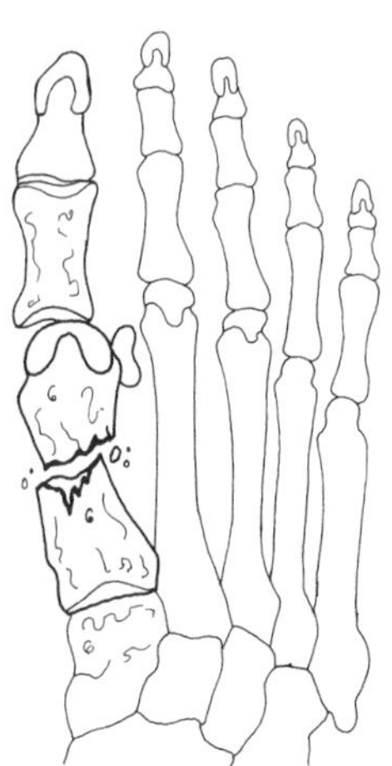

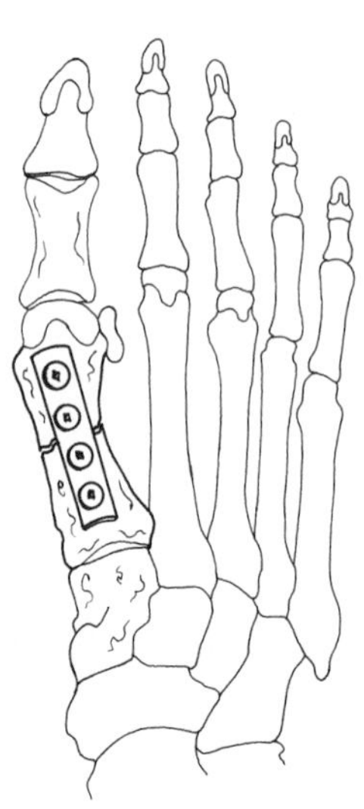

FIGURE 34-20 *(far left)* Transverse fracture of the shaft of the first metatarsal. The maintenance of reduction is critical, because one third of the body weight passes through the first ray.

FIGURE 34-21 *(left)* Open reduction and internal fixation using a plate to maintain anatomic reduction. A short leg cast is applied postoperatively to prevent additional stress at the fracture site.

Sesamoid Fractures

Cast/Splint

Biomechanics: Stress-sharing device.

Mode of bone healing: Primary membranous bone; no callus formation.

Indications: Acute fractures or suspected stress fractures are treated by placing soft padding under the arch and first metatarsal head, and strapping the metatarsophalangeal joint into a neutral or slightly plantar flexed position. The foot is then placed in a short leg cast that extends to the ends of the toes. Alternatively, a postoperative bunion shoe may be used (*see* Figure 34-4).

Sesamoidectomy

Biomechanics: Not applicable.

Mode of bone healing: Not applicable.

Indications: Surgery must be performed if casting has not been successful and there is no evidence of healing (which is common), or if pain persists. This is an extremely delicate procedure in which the bone is shelled out of the flexor hallucis brevis tendon, leaving the tendon intact. The toe is then splinted in a protected position for 4 to 6 weeks.

Special Considerations of the Fracture

Age

In all forefoot fractures, the elderly are at higher risk for development of joint stiffness secondary to immobilization of adjacent joints. This is especially true for the first metatarsophalangeal joint. The elderly also have greater risk for delayed healing or nonunion, particularly following fifth metatarsal fractures.

Articular Involvement

Fractures involving any articular surface in the forefoot require anatomic reduction. This is particularly important in the great toe and first metatarsal, because these constitute the major weight-bearing complex of the forefoot. Fractures of the fifth metatarsal that articulate with the cuboid must also be anatomically reduced to prevent painful foot plant.

Location

Unless there is severe angulation that may result in soft corns by causing pressure on adjacent toes, a small amount of angulation of the lesser phalanges is acceptable. Because they are of lesser importance in forefoot load transfer, joint stiffness is also generally not problematic.

Metatarsal shaft fractures generally heal well, and problems occur only months later when metatarsalgia or intractable plantar keratoses develop under the metatarsal heads. This can occur with as little as 2 to 4 mm of head elevation or shortening of the injured metatarsal. This displacement can cause overload of the unaffected metatarsals with subsequent pain and antalgic gait.

Stress fracture, delayed union, and nonunion of the proximal fifth metatarsal shaft can cause significant pain and disability, particularly in dancers and running athletes. Rarely there may be entrapment of the sural nerve, which runs along the lateral border of the ankle and foot. If this occurs, a Tinel sign can be elicited. (Tapping the nerve at the point of entrapment causes pain along its distal portion.) Appropriate fragment excision or bone grafting and intramedullary fixation usually resolves the problem.

In great toe and first metatarsal fractures, it is crucial to obtain as close to anatomic reduction as possible, because this ray of the foot carries one third of the load applied in foot plant. Angulation of the metatarsal head in any direction can seriously impair forefoot mechanics (*see* Figures 34-20 and 34-21).

Sesamoid fractures are usually transverse (unless associated with a metatarsophalangeal dislocation, in which case they are longitudinal) and give a bipartite appearance. Because they are enclosed within a tendon, they do not usually angulate or significantly displace. However, poor alignment can lead to great toe drift toward the opposite side (medially), which may then require surgical correction (*see* Figure 34-4).

Open Fractures

All open fractures must be treated aggressively with irrigation, débridement, and intravenous antibiotics. Trauma significant enough to cause an open fracture at the first metatarsal must also raise suspicion of serious vascular and skin compromise.

Associated Injury

An avulsion-type fracture, the typical "stubbed toe," causes only moderate swelling and is generally not a cause of soft tissue loss unless the fracture is open. However, many metatarsal fractures that follow crush injuries or direct blows have a large amount of swelling and may lead to tissue loss. Any degloving injury requires the use of special coverage techniques.

Swelling over the dorsum of the foot can lead to significant soft tissue necrosis and possible extensor mechanism damage. The possibility of dorsal foot compartment syndrome must be considered when there has been significant trauma.

Decompression may be necessary to save the neurovascular complex of the forefoot and midfoot as it crosses the ankle into the foot (between the extensor hallucis longus and extensor digitorum longus).

All open fractures should be carefully inspected for any associated tendon damage. Lacerations of lesser toe extensor tendons may be either repaired or left alone; they are not crucial to forefoot function and normal gait. Lacerations of the extensors of the great toe and foot must be repaired either primarily or at a later date.

Weight Bearing

Initially, weight bearing is not permitted at any time for sesamoid, first phalanx, or metatarsal fractures; however, patients with phalangeal fractures may be able to bear some weight as their pain allows. Patients with sesamoid, first phalanx, and metatarsal fractures may begin a progressive weight-bearing program at approximately 4 weeks, if adequate healing is evidenced on radiograph.

Gait

Stance Phase

The stance phase constitutes 60% of the gait cycle.

Heel Strike

Heel strike causes no pain. The patient may actually increase the duration of heel strike or only "heel walk" (*see* Figure 6-1).

Foot-Flat

There is usually no pain at this stage. Most of the weight is still borne on the hindfoot (*see* Figure 6-2).

Mid-Stance

The single stance phase begins. This phase is usually painful, as the foot begins to go from inversion to eversion and rolls out across the metatarsal heads, causing pain. The patient may try to further evert or invert the forefoot to reduce pressure on the healing fracture site. Pain may cause shortening of this stage (*see* Figure 6-3).

Push-Off

Most of the weight bearing is on the first and second metatarsal heads; therefore, push-off may be painful. This stage may be shortened because of the pain (antalgic gait) or totally avoided (Figures 34-22 and 34-23, and *see* Figure 6-4).

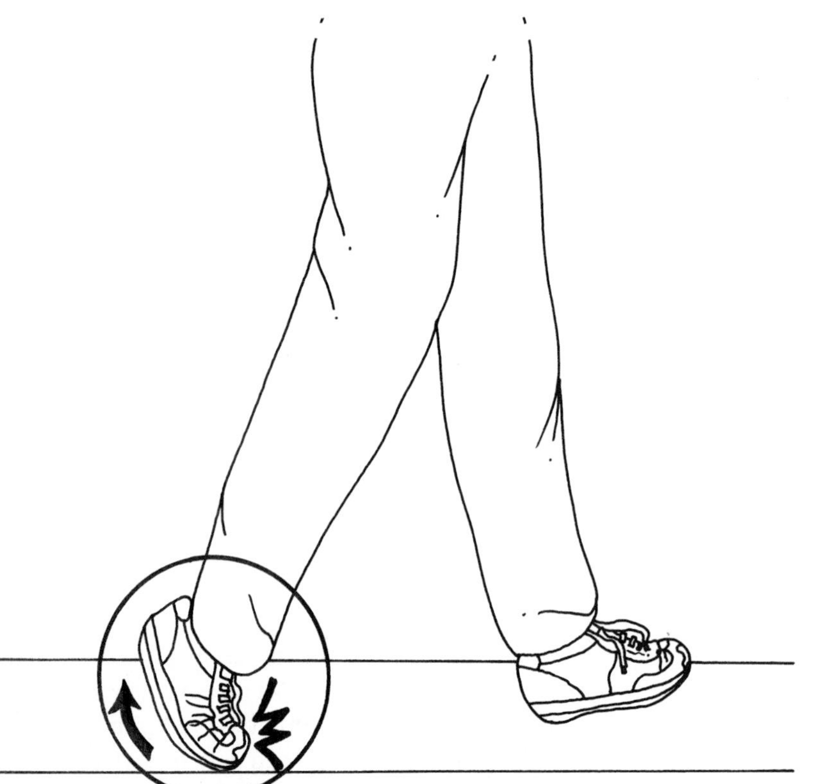

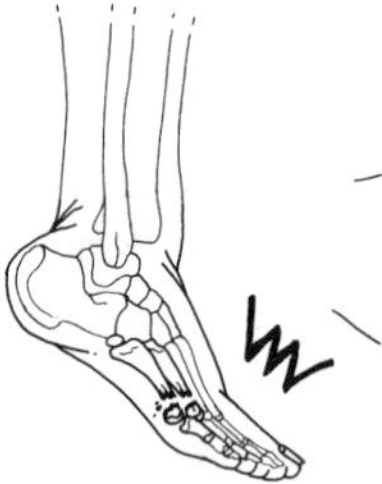

FIGURE 34-22 *(left)* Metatarsal fractures frequently result in pain during the push-off phase of gait. The patient may shorten this phase secondary to the pain (antalgic gait) or may totally avoid it.

FIGURE 34-23 *(above)* Push-off phase of gait is frequently painful particularly with fractures of the first metatarsal. A firm-bottom shoe may help temporarily relieve pain during push-off.

Swing Phase

The swing phase constitutes 40% of the gait cycle. There are no problems in this phase of gait (*see* Figures 6-6, 6-7, and 6-8).

Gait During Healing

The patient favors heel strike and early stance phase to protect the toes during the healing of uncomplicated lesser phalangeal fractures. Because these fractures usually heal quickly, permanent alterations in gait are unusual.

Fractures of the lesser metatarsals may cause pain in stance at push-off secondary to shortening, angulation, or rotation. The patient tends to spend a longer portion of the gait cycle on the heel and the lateral side of the foot to avoid pain and pressure under the metatarsal heads.

Fractures of the apophysis or proximal metaphysis of the fifth metatarsal are often tender in late stance at toe-off as the foot begins to evert. Patients with nonunions and malunions find it difficult to bear weight on the lateral aspect of the foot and shift their weight medially, which can cause painful overload in the first and second metatarsals.

Fractures of the first phalanx, first metatarsal, and sesamoids affect gait at push-off. The first ray bears one third of the load distribution of the forefoot (*see* Figure 34-23). Painful malunions or nonunions cause a shift of weight toward the lateral side of the foot. This places an increased load on the remaining metatarsals and may result in painful metatarsalgia.

TREATMENT

Treatment: Early to Immediate (Day of Injury to One Week)

Bone Healing

Stability at fracture site: None

Stage of bone healing: Inflammatory phase. The fracture hematoma is colonized by inflammatory cells, and débridement of the fracture begins. Exceptions to this are stress fractures, which have already débrided and formed a fibrous mass by the time they are noted.

X-ray: No callus.

Orthopaedic and Rehabilitation Considerations

Physical Examination

Check for capillary refill and sensation. The toes should be pink, with brisk refill after light compression of the digits. It should be possible to reach the first web space of the toe; stroke it lightly with a blunt instrument to ensure that there is no peroneal nerve compression in the lower ankle and foot. Pay special attention to complaints of pain, paresthesia, and cast discomfort as indicators of compartment syndrome or constriction of the cast. Also note whether the patient feels that the cast is loose.

For fractures of the phalanges and sesamoids, check the rotational position of the toes and make sure that there has been no deformity since application of the device. For sesamoid fractures, it is important that the toe and the metatarsophalangeal joint remain in a neutral to slightly plantar flexed position.

Dangers

Evaluate for any evidence of a dorsal foot compartment syndrome. Pay special attention to complaints of pain, paresthesia, and cast discomfort. For fractures that were open or had significant fracture blisters, evaluate the skin for erythema or drainage, which may indicate the presence of infection. The patient should be advised to keep the extremity elevated above heart level and to place ice packs over the ankle and foot to help decrease swelling.

Radiography

Obtain and check anteroposterior and lateral radiographs of the foot for any loss of correction (i.e., rotational changes, angulation, or shortening, particularly in a metatarsal fracture). If there is depression of the metatarsal head, re-reduction of the fracture is necessary.

Weight Bearing

The patient is generally on crutches at this time and is non-weight bearing. The exception to this is with a phalangeal fracture, in which case the patient may bear weight as tolerated.

Range of Motion

Phalangeal fractures usually are stable and may be moved within their buddy taping splint as patient comfort permits. Metatarsal fractures are well immobilized within a cast but it is important to encourage the patient to move the metatarsophalangeal joints (except first metatarsal fractures). This decreases any swelling of the digits and foot and inhibits any stiffness of the metatarsophalangeal joints, particularly the first metatarsophalangeal joint. At this point in the healing process, sesamoid fractures should remain immobile, and there should be no motion at the metatarsophalangeal joint. Active range-of-motion exercises are prescribed to the knee and ankle. If in a cast, the patient should try to dorsiflex and plantar flex his ankle within the cast.

Muscle Strength

No strengthening exercises to the long flexors and extensors of the toes are recommended for patients with fractures of the forefoot because this fracture is unstable. Isometric quadriceps strengthening exercises are prescribed to maintain strength. Ankle dorsiflexion and plantar flexion strengthening exercises are also prescribed to maintain ankle strength and to reduce venous pooling.

Functional Activities

Patients are instructed in stand/pivot transfers with non-weight bearing on the affected extremity, using assistive devices such as crutches. Patients are instructed to don pants on the affected extremity first and doff them from the unaffected extremity first.

Gait

The patient uses a non–weight-bearing two-point gait in which the crutches form one unit and the unaffected extremity the other unit (*see* Figures 6-16A and 6-16B). When ascending stairs, the patient leads with the unaffected extremity; when descending stairs, the patient leads with the affected extremity (*see* Figures 6-20, 6-21, 6-22, 6-23, 6-24, and 6-25).

Methods of Treatment: Specific Aspects

Cast

Evaluate the condition of the cast. For fractures of the sesamoid and first metatarsal, the cast must extend to the tips of the toes and not allow movement of the first metatarsophalangeal joint. For fractures of the second, third, fourth, and fifth metatarsals, the metatarsophalangeal joint should be allowed early range of motion. If a cast is too long, it may be trimmed back and additional padding added for comfort. It is important to evaluate the skin at the cast edges to make sure that any swelling has not caused skin breakdown and that there is no evidence of cyanosis or compartment syndrome. If the cast has softened under the foot, it should be reinforced and repaired. Isometric dorsiflexion and plantar flexion exercises are prescribed within the cast to maintain ankle strength. This also helps to decrease venous pooling.

Closed Reduction and Percutaneous Pinning

Check all pin sites for discharge or erythema and release any tenting of the skin. If the foot or the pin sites have any purulence or there is erythema or streaking, the patient should be admitted for intravenous antibiotics and possible pin removal.

If the patient is not placed in a splint or cast, the metatarsophalangeal joints should be actively moved, except for the first metatarsophalangeal joint. The patient can begin exercises for maintaining quadriceps strength and knee flexibility.

Open Reduction and Internal Fixation

For fractures of the first phalanx, first metatarsal, and sesamoids, if a cast has been placed, trim it to allow visualization of the tips of the toes. Fractures of the second through fifth metatarsals should have casts that extend to the metatarsophalangeal joint but do not impede range of motion. Evaluate for adequate padding on the cast edges, look for any skin breakdown at the edges, and trim appropriately. Repair any breakdown or softening of the cast.

All metatarsophalangeal joints can be actively ranged with the exception of the first metatarsophalangeal joint postoperatively.

Prescription

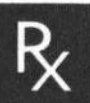

DAY ONE TO ONE WEEK

Precautions No passive range of motion.

Range of Motion

For stable phalangeal fractures, active range of motion to metatarsophalangeal joints.

For fractures of the sesamoids, first phalanx, and first metatarsal, no range of motion.

Strength No strengthening exercises.

Functional Activities

Non-weight bearing stand/pivot transfers and ambulation with assistive devices for fractures of sesamoid, first phalanx, and first and fifth metatarsals.

Weight bearing as tolerated, transfers, and ambulation for stable fractures of the metatarsals, lesser phalanges, and lesser metatarsals.

Weight Bearing

Weight bearing to tolerance for stable fractures of phalanges and lesser metatarsals.

Non-weight bearing for fractures of the sesamoid, first phalanx, and first and fifth metatarsals.

Treatment: Two Weeks

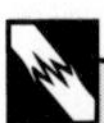

BONE HEALING

Stability at fracture site: None to minimal.

Stage of bone healing: Beginning of reparative phase. Osteoprogenitor cells differentiate into osteoblasts, which lay down woven bone. An exception to this would be nonunions of the sesamoids or the fifth metatarsal shaft, in which a fibrous union may be slowly creating a reparation; however, it may not be of a bony nature.

X-ray: No changes to early callus noted in the periosteal aspects of the bone.

Orthopaedic and Rehabilitation Considerations

Physical Examination

Check for capillary refill of the toes, sensation of the toes, and, if possible, the first dorsal web space. For phalangeal and metatarsal fractures, check the active and passive range of motion of the unaffected digits. In phalangeal fractures, any rotation deformity may be noted at this time. Palpation of the digit can give a gross impression of healing based on the presence or absence of pain.

Dangers

Pay particular attention to complaints of pain, paresthesia, and cast discomfort, which may signal a compartment syndrome. The patient should be made aware that any pronounced swelling could lead to skin sloughing and should be immediately brought to the physician's attention. The patient should be advised to continue extremity elevation above heart level as much as possible.

Radiography

Check radiographs in an anteroposterior and lateral position to assess any loss of metatarsal alignment and to assess callus deposition for all fractures.

Weight Bearing

Patients with phalangeal fractures and undisplaced second through fourth metatarsal fractures may begin or continue weight bearing as tolerated. Fractures of the sesamoids, first phalanx, and first metatarsal, as well as those of the proximal diaphyseal shaft of the fifth metatarsal (Jones fracture) and apophyseal fractures of the fifth metatarsal, should remain non-weight bearing.

Range of Motion

If the patient is not in a cast, active ankle range of motion may be added to tolerance. This helps prevent stiffening of the ankle joint capsule. A patient who is in a cast should continue active metatarsophalangeal range-of-motion exercises (with the exception of the first and fifth joints) and knee range of motion. Patients can try to actively dorsiflex and plantar flex within the cast.

Muscle Strength

The patient should continue with knee strengthening exercises and ankle isometric strengthening exercises within the cast.

Functional Activities

The patient should continue with non–weight-bearing stand/pivot transfers using crutches. If weight-bearing is allowed and the patient uses the affected extremity during transfers, crutches may still be useful for balance and support.

Gait

Continue a non-weight bearing gait using crutches. If weight bearing is allowed, the patient should use a three-point gait in which the two crutches form one point and the affected and unaffected extremities form the other two points (*see* Figure 6-17). If weight bearing is allowed, the patient may climb stairs with the unaffected extremity first, followed by the crutches and then the affected extremity (*see* Figures 6-20, 6-21, and 6-22). The patient descends stairs by placing the crutches first, followed by the affected extremity and then the unaffected extremity (*see* Figures 6-23, 6-24, and 6-25).

Patients with lesser phalangeal fractures may experience mild to moderate discomfort at push-off when the toes are loaded during roll-off over the metatarsal heads.

Patients with stable, nondisplaced lesser metatarsal fractures feel pain on weight bearing in mid-stance and push-off as weight is transferred from the hindfoot to the forefoot (*see* Figures 34-22 and 34-23). To compensate for this discomfort, the patient may prolong the duration of heel strike or walk solely on the heel.

Methods of Treatment: Specific Aspects

Cast

If it was not done previously, the cast should be trimmed to allow visualization from the tips of the toes to the metatarsophalangeal joints in metatarsal fractures. Buddy-taped splinting may be changed, and the color and swelling of the involved digits assessed. Reinforce any cast that has broken down at the foot or at the metatarsophalangeal joints.

Continue with metatarsophalangeal joint range of motion as tolerated (except for sesamoid and first metatarsal fractures. Start isometric exercises of the gastrocsoleus group, trying to plantar flex within the cast. If the fracture is of the phalanges and the metatarsals are free, start gentle isometric exercises of the peronei group by gentle eversion within the cast. Begin gentle dorsiflexion by the tibialis anterior within the cast. Do not dorsiflex the great toe if the first phalanx is involved. Try to invert the foot to strengthen the tibialis posterior.

Closed Reduction and Percutaneous Pinning

Check pin sites for discharge, erythema, or skin tenting and treat as necessary. Admit the patient if the pin sites are infected.

The pins may be removed now if the healing is satisfactory. Patients are to continue active range of motion of the metatarsophalangeal joints. Gentle isometric exercises within the cast can be performed to the patient's tolerance.

Open Reduction and Internal Fixation

For fractures of the first phalanx, trim the cast to allow visualization of the tip of the injured digit but do not allow free movement at the metatarsophalangeal joint. For all metatarsal fractures, the metatarsophalangeal joint should be free so that active and passive range of motion can be carried out. Check the cast padding and cast edges; there should be adequate padding at the edges of the cast so that skin breakdown does not occur. Also check the cast for any softening and repair appropriately.

A patient who is not in a cast may begin active range of motion of the ankle in all planes to tolerance. If the patient is in a cast, the earlier protocol should continue.

Prescription

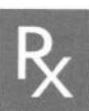

TWO WEEKS

Precautions No passive range of motion.

Range of Motion

For stable phalangeal fractures, active range of motion to the metatarsal phalangeal joints.

For fractures of the first metatarsal and Jones fracture, no range of motion.

For sesamoids and first phalanx, immobilized; no range of motion.

For fractures of the second, third, fourth, and fifth metatarsal, active range of motion to the metatarsal and interphalangeal joints.

Strength

For stable phalangeal fractures, no strengthening exercises to the long flexors and extensors of the toes.

For metatarsal fractures, no exercises; however, isometric strengthening exercises to all the ankle musculature.

Functional Activities

Non-weight bearing stand/pivot transfers and ambulation with assistive devices for fractures of the first phalanx, sesamoids, first and fifth metatarsals.

Weight bearing as tolerated transfers and ambulation for single lesser phalangeal fractures.

Weight Bearing

For lesser phalangeal and stable metatarsal fractures, weight bearing as tolerated.

For sesamoid, first, and fifth metatarsal fractures, non-weight bearing.

Treatment: Four to Six Weeks

BONE HEALING

Stability at fracture site: Acute fractures should be showing bridging callus, and the fracture is usually stable. This is confirmed by physical examination and radiography. However, the strength of this callus, especially with torsional load, is significantly lower than that of normal bone.

Stage of bone healing: Reparative phase. Further organization of the callus and formation of lamellar bone begins.

X-ray: Bridging callus is visible as a fluffy material on the periosteal surface of the bone. With increased rigidity, less bridging callus is noted, and healing with endosteal callus predominates. For stress fractures and nonunions of the sesamoids and fifth metatarsals, a fibrous nonunion with smooth fracture edges may be observed.

Orthopaedic and Rehabilitation Considerations

Physical Examination

Discontinue the cast. Radiographic study and examination are performed out of plaster. Check for stability, tenderness, and range of motion.

Dangers

Most of the swelling from acute fractures should be resolved at this point. Assess the patient for any trophic signs of reflex sympathetic dystrophy: vasomotor disturbances, hyperparesthesias, and pain and tenderness out of proportion to the stage of fracture healing. If evidence of reflex sympathetic dystrophy is noted, the patient should begin an aggressive physical therapy program in addition to hydrotherapy.

Radiography

Radiographs are examined for evidence of healing and any loss of correction. These are obtained in the anteroposterior and lateral positions. For stress fractures of the sesamoid and fifth metatarsal, it is important to evaluate whether the fracture line is disappearing.

Weight Bearing

Phalangeal fractures of the lesser toes can begin full weight bearing as tolerated, if not already doing so. The patient should not walk barefoot, keeping the toes protected for several additional weeks.

Fractures of the second through fourth metatarsals are evaluated for tenderness. If a patient finds weight bearing difficult, a short leg walking cast may be replaced. At this point, the patient should be trying to bear as much weight as possible on the foot to facilitate healing. Fractures of the proximal diaphysis (Jones fracture) and apophysis of the fifth metatarsal can be removed from a cast and protective weight bearing started. If the injuries are particularly tender, a short leg non–weight-bearing cast can be reapplied.

Fractures of the first phalanx and first metatarsal should be placed in a postoperative bunion-type shoe and may begin protected weight bearing. A patient whose injury is still particularly tender at this point may remain weight bearing but only in a postoperative bunion-type shoe so that range of motion can be continued.

For sesamoid fractures, protected weight bearing should begin in a postoperative bunion-type shoe. The great toe should be taped to the bunion shoe to keep the metatarsophalangeal joint in a neutral or plantar-flexed position. If the patient has pain on weight bearing, a sesamoidectomy may be considered.

Range of Motion

If the patient is not in a cast, active ankle range of motion may be added to tolerance. This helps to prevent stiffening of the ankle joint capsule. A patient who is in a cast should continue active metatarsophalangeal range-of-motion exercises (with the exception of first and fifth joints) and knee range of motion. Fractures of the first and fifth metatarsals (Jones fracture), sesamoids, and first phalanx remain immobilized.

Muscle Strength

The patient should continue quadriceps strengthening exercises. If the cast has been removed, the patient may further strengthen the peronei and the tibialis anterior by inversion and eversion exercises. The patient may also work the ankle in dorsiflexion to strengthen the tibialis anterior and plantar flexion for the plantar flexors of the ankle. All muscles are weak as a result of immobilization.

Functional Activities

If weight bearing is still not allowed, non–weight-bearing pivot transfers should continue using crutches. If weight bearing is allowed, the patient can use the affected extremity during transfers, although crutches may still be needed for balance and support.

Gait

Patients who are allowed to bear weight use a three-point gait in which the two crutches form one point and the affected and unaffected extremities the other two points (*see* Figure 6-17). The patient may climb stairs with the unaffected extremity first, followed by the affected extremity and then the crutches (*see* Figures 6-20, 6-21, and 6-22). The patient descends stairs by placing the crutches first, followed by the affected extremity and then the unaffected extremity (*see* Figures 6-23, 6-24, and 6-25). A patient with a metatarsal fracture that is in a weight-bearing short leg cast may attempt a normal gait without crutches. Patients who still require non-weight bearing should use crutches and a non–weight-bearing gait.

Phalangeal fractures should be well healed and pain-free at this point. Possible aberrations in gait might occur if the fracture was significantly malunited and is causing pressure on adjacent toes or the plantar surface of the phalanx during shoe wear. In this case, the patient may limit late stance (or push-off) when the pain occurs as a result of forefoot and phalangeal loading.

Stable nondisplaced or minimally displaced lesser metatarsal fractures may still cause discomfort from mid-stance to push-off (*see* Figures 34-22 and 34-23).

The patient attempts to unload the metatarsal by prolonging heel strike or shifting weight medially or laterally away from the affected metatarsal.

Fractures of the first metatarsal and phalanx are most uncomfortable in push-off. Again, the patient prolongs heel strike. The patient should wear a stiff, solid, or postoperative bunion-type shoe to help avoid dorsiflexion of the great toe.

Methods of Treatment: Specific Aspects

Cast

The cast should be removed at this visit to evaluate for stability and tenderness at the fracture site. Fractures of the sesamoids, first phalanx, first metatarsal, and lesser phalanges should remain out of plaster. Patients who are still tender at the fracture site may be placed in a postoperative bunion-type shoe with protective or no weight bearing. For fractures of the second through fourth metatarsals that are still tender, the patient may be placed in a weight-bearing short leg cast and should be encouraged to bear as much weight as possible on the foot to facilitate healing. Fractures of the proximal diaphysis (Jones fracture) and apophysis of the fifth metatarsal should be placed in a non–weight-bearing short leg cast if they are tender. If pain-free, the patient may begin protected weight bearing in a sturdy shoe.

Closed Reduction and Percutaneous Pinning

Check the pin sites for discharge, erythema, or any evidence of tenting. Release tenting of the skin as necessary. If the foot or the pin sites have any purulence and there is erythema or streaking, the patient should be admitted for intravenous antibiotics and removal of the pins.

If it appears the fracture is adequately stable on radiographic examination, the pins may be removed at this visit.

If the patient is not placed in a splint or cast, the metatarsophalangeal joints should be actively moved, except in fractures of the first phalanx or first metatarsophalangeal joint. The patient may continue exercises for maintaining quadriceps strength and knee flexibility. In addition, a patient who is not placed in a new cast may begin dorsiflexion exercises to strengthen the tibialis anterior and digit extensors, plantar flexion to strengthen the gastrocnemius soleus group of the ankle, inversion to strengthen the tibialis posterior, and eversion to strengthen the peronei.

Open Reduction and Internal Fixation

If the cast was not already removed at the 2-week mark, as it would be for phalangeal or metatarsal fractures, the stability of the fracture, tenderness, and range of motion are all evaluated out of plaster. Unless a radiographic examination has provided evidence to preclude discontinuing the cast, such as lack of callus formation, it is recommended that the cast stay off and early range of motion begin. In the case of first metatarsal and fifth metatarsal fractures, protected weight bearing is recommended in a stiff-soled or postoperative bunion-type shoe. If callus is inadequate or tenderness is present at the fracture site, the cast should be replaced and the patient remains non-weight bearing.

If the patient is not in a cast, active range of motion in dorsiflexion and plantar flexion should be carried out to avoid stiffening of the ankle joint capsule. Range of motion in eversion and inversion should be performed as well. If the patient is in a cast, continue active metatarsophalangeal and knee joint range-of-motion exercises.

Prescription

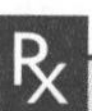

FOUR TO SIX WEEKS

Precautions No passive range of motion.

Range of Motion

For stable phalangeal fractures, full active range of motion to metatarsal joints.

For metatarsal fractures out of cast, active range of motion to metatarsal joints. Active to active-assistive range of motion to the ankle.

For fractures of first and fifth metatarsals (Jones fracture), sesamoids, and first phalanx, immobilized; no range of motion.

Strength

For stable phalangeal fractures, isotonic exercises to long flexors and extensors of the toes.

For metatarsal fractures, isometric and isotonic strengthening exercises to the ankle plantar flexors, dorsiflexors, evertors, and invertors.

Functional Activities Weight bearing transfers and ambulation with assistive devices as needed. Partial weight bearing to non–weight-bearing transfers and ambulation for first phalanx, first and fifth metatarsals, and sesamoids.

Weight Bearing

For stable fractures, lesser phalangeal fractures, and metatarsal fractures, weight bearing as tolerated.

For fractures of the first phalanx, first and fifth metatarsals (Jones fracture), and sesamoids, non-weight bearing to partial weight bearing.

Treatment: Six to Eight Weeks

Bone Healing

Stability at fracture site: With bridging callus, the fracture is usually stable. Confirm with physical examination.

Stage of bone healing: Reparative phase. Once callus is observed bridging the fracture site, the fracture is usually stable. This requires further protection to avoid refracture. However, the strength of this callus, especially with torsional load, is significantly lower than that of normal bone. Further organization of the callus and formation of lamellar bone begins.

X-ray: Bridging callus is visible with increased rigidity. Less bridging callus is noted, and healing with endosteal callus predominates. Fracture line is less distinct. Sesamoid fractures do not show callus but the fracture line is less distinct.

Orthopaedic and Rehabilitation Considerations

Physical Examination

All fractures should be out of a cast. Examine the fracture for tenderness. If there was a wound or an operative site, evaluate it for healing and evidence of infection. Evaluate any trophic or sensory changes that might indicate reflex sympathetic dystrophy.

Dangers

Evaluate wounds or operative sites for evidence of infection and treat appropriately.

Radiography

Fractures that are tender should be evaluated with anteroposterior and lateral views to assess for malunion or nonunion.

Weight Bearing

Patients with first or fifth metatarsal fractures who have not previously begun weight bearing may begin toe-touch to partial weight bearing at this time. Other fractures of the forefoot that are not tender may progress to full weight bearing as tolerated.

Range of Motion

Active and active-assisted range-of-motion exercises are done at the metatarsophalangeal joints, interphalangeal joints, and ankle in all planes. If the metatarsophalangeal joints are stiff, begin gentle passive range-of-motion exercises. The patient is instructed to passively flex and extend the toes. The same is done with the ankle if the ankle joint is stiff. These exercises are all done to patient tolerance.

Muscle Strength

Once the patient can actively extend and flex the toes repeatedly, the muscles are already being strengthened isotonically. Once the fracture site is stable, gentle resistance can be applied while the toes are ranged. The patient can use one hand to apply controlled force over the toes. To strengthen the dorsiflexors and plantar flexors of the ankle, the patient can apply resistance against the foot while ranging the ankle.

If sesamoidectomy was performed or anatomic alignment not fully restored at the first metatarsal or phalanx, the patient will probably not regain full strength for push-off and toe-off.

Functional Activities

At this stage of healing, the patient is either weight bearing as tolerated or partially weight bearing during transfers and ambulation. The use of crutches may still be required.

Gait

The patient may still need to use crutches for ambulation despite weight bearing on the affected extremity. Patients with metatarsal fractures who are out of casts and no longer using crutches may still note tenderness in the stance phase of gait. Patients with lesser phalangeal fractures as well as lesser metatarsal fractures may notice some discomfort at push-off. If the pain on weight bearing is significant such that the patient must shift weight to the extreme medial or lateral portion of the foot, consider having the patient revert to partial or no weight bearing temporarily, until the fracture further stabilizes.

Patients with fractures of the first metatarsal, hallux, and sesamoids still have discomfort during late stance, particularly at push-off. They continue to prolong heel strike and may also shift weight to the lateral side of the foot in order to decrease weight bearing on the first ray.

Jones fractures may still be tender over the lateral aspect of the foot, particularly in stance, and the patient shifts weight medially to relieve pressure. Additionally, shoes may be uncomfortable at the base of the fifth metatarsal until further healing occurs or the screw is removed.

Methods of Treatment: Specific Aspects

Cast

For fractures of the forefoot, the cast has already been removed. If the patient needed replacement of a cast for a slow-healing fracture, the cast should be removed for examination. A patient whose injury is still tender should be given a stiff-soled or postoperative bunion-type shoe to use when ambulating. Active and active-assisted range-of-motion exercises are begun for those patients coming out of a cast, or it is continued for those whose cast was previously removed. Hydrotherapy may be helpful for decreasing discomfort and stiffness of the joints during range of motion.

Closed Reduction and Percutaneous Pinning

Any cast or pins that have been retained should be removed at this point. Depending on fracture healing, the patient may bear weight as tolerated on the affected extremity.

Open Reduction and Internal Fixation

Casts should have been removed by this time. The patient may begin active and active-assisted range of motion for the ankle and metatarsophalangeal joints. Weight bearing patients should be advised not to engage in any repetitive or impact forms of exercise, because this may loosen the fixation, break the hardware, and possibly cause refracture.

Prescription

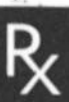

DAY ONE TO ONE WEEK

Precautions No repetitive impact exercises.

Range of Motion Active and active-assistive to gentle passive range of motion to all phalangeal, metatarsal, and ankle joints.

Strength Isometric and isotonic exercises with resistance to ankle dorsiflexors, plantar flexors, evertors, and invertors. Isometric and isotonic strengthening exercises to long flexors and extensors of the toes.

Functional Activities

For stable fractures, full weight bearing transfers and ambulation.

For fractures of sesamoids, first and fifth metatarsals, and first phalanx, partial weight-bearing to full weight-bearing transfers and ambulation.

Weight Bearing Full weight bearing for phalangeal and metatarsal fractures. Partial weight bearing to full weight bearing for fractures of sesamoids, first and fifth metatarsals, and first phalanx.

Treatment: Eight to Twelve Weeks

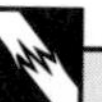

BONE HEALING

Stability at fracture site: Stable.

Stage of bone healing: Remodeling phase. Woven bone is replaced with lamellar bone. The process of remodeling takes months to years for completion.

X-ray: Abundant callus is seen in all fractures with the exception of the sesamoids. The fracture line begins to disappear. With time, there is reconstitution of the medullary canal. Apophyseal areas do not produce as much callus as diaphyseal regions.

Orthopaedic and Rehabilitation Considerations

Physical Examination

Check for tenderness at the fracture site. Evaluate any wounds or operative sites for evidence of infection. Evaluate all wounds, pin sites, and incisions for erythema or evidence of infection and treat appropriately.

Radiography

If the patient is nontender at this point, radiographs are unnecessary. If there is tenderness, however, and nonunion is suspected, radiographs in the anteroposterior and lateral views should be evaluated.

Weight Bearing

A patient who is nontender on physical examination may continue partial weight bearing or progress to full weight bearing as tolerated. Patients should not engage in any activities with jumping or repetitive pounding, because this may cause refracture or damage internal hardware.

Range of Motion

Continue full active and passive range of motion to the metatarsophalangeal and ankle joints. All patients should have close to full range of motion of these joints at this time. A particularly complex fracture of the first metatarsal or first phalanx may have some residual stiffness in the metatarsophalangeal joint.

Muscle Strength

The affected muscles across the ankle and metatarsophalangeal joints are all strengthened with progressive resistive exercises.

Full strength should be regained at this time, with the possible exception of first phalanx, first metatarsal, and sesamoid fractures, where there may not be full extensor and flexor power at the first metatarsophalangeal joint.

Functional Activities

At this point, the patient is partially or fully weight bearing and should be weaned off assistive devices during ambulation and transfers.

Gait

The ankle and metatarsophalangeal joints may have some residual stiffness from prolonged immobilization. This affects gait during push-off, mid-stance, and heel strike. Tenderness in fractures of the latter four metatarsals may cause increased weight bearing across the first metatarsal and first phalanx. In this case, the patient spends more time in a toe-off position, overloading the first metatarsal head and causing pain underneath it. Any residual tenderness of the first phalanx, first metatarsal, or sesamoids may cause the patient to shift weight toward the lateral aspect of the foot. This makes push-off particularly difficult, and the patient tends to spend more time in heel strike and mid-stance. The patient should try to normalize gait at this point, even if it means partial weight bearing to distribute weight fully over the foot.

Methods of Treatment: Specific Aspects

Cast

Casts should have been removed for all fractures. The patient should continue active, active-assisted, and passive range of motion as well as weight bearing to tolerance.

Closed Reduction and Percutaneous Pinning

Pins have already been removed and all wounds should be well healed. The patient may undergo full range of motion in all planes to the ankle and metatarsophalangeal joints. Weight bearing is to tolerance.

Open Reduction and Internal Fixation

Casts should have been removed for all fractures. Patients should be performing active, active-assisted, and passive range of motion of the ankle and metatarsophalangeal joints. Weight bearing is to tolerance.

Prescription

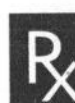

EIGHT TO TWELVE WEEKS

Range of Motion Active, active-assistive, and passive range of motion to metatarsophalangeal, interphalangeal, and ankle joints.

Strength Progressive resistive exercises to the long flexors, extensors of the toes, dorsiflexors, plantar flexors, evertors, and invertors of the ankle.

Functional Activities Full weight-bearing transfers and ambulation.

Weight Bearing Full weight bearing.

LONG-TERM CONSIDERATIONS AND PROBLEMS

Patients with fractures of the second through fourth metatarsals should be advised that there may be long-term pain in the metatarsal head secondary to rotation, plantar flexion, or shortening of the fractured metatarsals as well as plantar keratosis. The addition of metatarsal pads to the shoe or even surgery may be necessary.

Fractures of the first phalanx and first metatarsal may cause stiffening of the metatarsophalangeal joint. If it is an intraarticular fracture, it may be prone to early degenerative change. The metatarsophalangeal joint may become very stiff. This is referred to as hallux rigidus. This alters push-off and requires shoe modification. The patient should be advised that if pain continues or increases over the years, further surgery will be needed to allow for a pain-free gait.

Fractures of the sesamoids, whether they are acute or the result of a stress fracture, may not heal using cast immobilization alone. The patients must understand that future surgery is a possibility if they continue to experience pain on ambulation.

Fractures of the fifth metatarsal (Jones fracture) may not heal, thus requiring surgery, bone graft, and screw fixation (*see* Figures 34-3, 34-11, and 34-12).

Lesser Phalanx Fractures

IMMEDIATE TO ONE WEEK

	Splint or Buddy Taping	*Open Reduction and Percutaneous Pinning*
Stability	None.	None.
Orthopaedics	Evaluate skin between toes for maceration; replace padding as necessary.	Evaluate pin sites. Trim cast to allow visibility of tips of toes.
Rehabilitation	Active range of motion of metatarsophalangeal (MTP) and interphalangeal (IP) joints as tolerated.	Passive range of motion of unaffected toes allowed.

TWO WEEKS

	Splint or Buddy Taping	*Open Reduction and Percutaneous Pinning*
Stability	None to minimal.	None to minimal.
Orthopaedics	Evaluate skin between toes for evidence of maceration; replace padding as necessary.	Reinforce cast as necessary. Evaluate pin sites for evidence of infection.
Rehabilitation	Active range of motion as tolerated.	Active range of motion of the MTP and IP joints as tolerated.

FOUR TO SIX WEEKS

	Splint or Buddy Taping	*Open Reduction and Percutaneous Pinning*
Stability	Stable.	Stable.
Orthopaedics	Remove buddy taping.	Remove cast, remove pins.
Rehabilitation	Continue active range of motion of the MTP and IP joints.	Begin active range of motion out of cast of MTP and IP joints.

SIX TO EIGHT WEEKS

	Splint or Buddy Taping	*Open Reduction and Percutaneous Pinning*
Stability	Stable.	Stable.
Orthopaedics		Remove cast if not previously done. Remove pins if not previously done.
Rehabilitation	Active range of motion of the IP and MTP and ankle joints as tolerated.	Active range of motion of the MTP and IP and ankle joints as tolerated.

EIGHT TO TWELVE WEEKS		
	Splint or Buddy Taping	*Open Reduction and Percutaneous Pinning*
Stability	Stable.	Stable.
Orthopaedics		
Rehabilitation	Continue active range of motion of MTP and IP and ankle joints.	Continue active range of motion of the MTP and IP and ankle joints.

Second, Third, Fourth, and Fifth Metatarsals (Except Jones Fractures)

IMMEDIATE TO ONE WEEK			
	Cast	*Closed Reduction and Percutaneous Pinning*	*Open Reduction and Internal Fixation*
Stability	None.	None.	None.
Orthopaedics	Trim cast to metatarsal heads.	Evaluate pin sites. Trim cast to metatarsal heads as appropriate.	Trim cast to metatarsal heads.
Rehabilitation	Active range of motion of the metatarsophalangeal (MTP) and interphalangeal (IP) joints to tolerance.	Active range of motion of the MTP and IP joints to tolerance.	Active range of motion of the MTP and IP joints to tolerance.

TWO WEEKS			
	Cast	*Closed Reduction and Percutaneous Pinning*	*Open Reduction and Internal Fixation*
Stability	None to minimal.	None to minimal.	None to minimal.
Orthopaedics	Trim cast to metatarsal heads.	Evaluate pin sites. Trim cast to metatarsal heads.	Trim cast to metatarsal heads.
Rehabilitation	Active range of motion of the MTP and IP joints as tolerated.	Active range of motion of the MTP and IP joints as tolerated.	Active range of motion of the MTP and IP joints as tolerated.

FOUR TO SIX WEEKS			
	Cast	*Closed Reduction and Percutaneous Pinning*	*Open Reduction and Internal Fixation*
Stability	Stable.	Stable.	Stable.
Orthopaedics	Remove cast or continue short leg walking cast.	Evaluate pin sites; may remove pins. Remove cast or continue short leg walking cast.	Remove cast.
Rehabilitation	Continue MTP and IP joint range of motion. Begin ankle range of motion if cast removed.	Continue MTP and IP joint range of motion. Begin ankle range of motion if cast removed.	Continue MTP and IP joint range of motion. Begin ankle range of motion if cast removed.

Second, Third, Fourth, and Fifth Metatarsals (Except Jones Fractures) *(continued)*

SIX TO EIGHT WEEKS	*Cast*	*Closed Reduction and Percutaneous Pinning*	*Open Reduction and Internal Fixation*
Stability	Stable.	Stable.	Stable.
Orthopaedics	Remove cast if not already done.	Remove cast if not already done. Remove pins if not already done.	Remove cast if not already done.
Rehabilitation	Active range of motion of the ankle joint, MTP joints, and IP joints to tolerance.	Active range of motion of the ankle joint, MTP joints, and IP joints to tolerance.	Active range of motion of the ankle joint, MTP joints, and IP joints to tolerance.

EIGHT TO TWELVE WEEKS	*Cast*	*Closed Reduction and Percutaneous Pinning*	*Open Reduction and Internal Fixation*
Stability	Stable.	Stable.	Stable.
Orthopaedics			
Rehabilitation	Active range of motion of the ankle, MTP, and IP joints, as well as resistive exercises.	Active range of motion of the ankle, MTP, and IP joints, as well as resistive exercises.	Active range of motion of the ankle, MTP, and IP joints, as well as resistive exercises.

Fifth Metatarsal Fractures (Jones Fractures)

IMMEDIATE TO ONE WEEK	*Cast*	*Open Reduction and Internal Fixation*
Stability	None.	None.
Orthopaedics	Trim cast to metatarsal heads.	Trim cast to metatarsal heads.
Rehabilitation	Avoid range of motion of interphalangeal (IP) and metatarsophalangeal (MTP) joints.	Active range of motion of IP and MTP joints.

TWO WEEKS	*Cast*	*Open Reduction and Internal Fixation*
Stability	None to minimal.	None to minimal.
Orthopaedics	Trim cast to metatarsal heads.	Trim cast to metatarsal heads.
Rehabilitation	Avoid range of motion to the IP and MTP joints.	Active range of motion to the IP and MTP joints.

FOUR TO SIX WEEKS		
	Cast	*Open Reduction and Internal Fixation*
Stability	Stable.	Stable.
Orthopaedics	Remove cast or continue short leg walking cast, closer to 6 weeks.	Remove cast or continue short leg walking cast.
Rehabilitation	Start range of motion of the MTP and IP joints closer to 6 weeks. Begin range of motion of the ankle. No weight bearing.	Continue range of motion of the MTP and IP joints. Begin range of motion of the ankle.

SIX TO EIGHT WEEKS		
	Cast	*Open Reduction and Internal Fixation*
Stability	Stable.	Stable.
Orthopaedics	Remove cast if not already done.	Remove cast if not already done.
Rehabilitation	Continue active range of motion of the MTP, IP, and ankle joints. Start weight bearing.	Continue active range of motion of the MTP, IP, and ankle joints.

EIGHT TO TWELVE WEEKS		
	Cast	*Open Reduction and Internal Fixation*
Stability	Stable.	Stable.
Orthopaedics		
Rehabilitation	Continue active range of motion of the MTP, IP, and ankle joints. Begin resistive exercises.	Continue active range of motion of the MTP, IP, and ankle joints. Begin resistive exercises.

Great (or First) Toe Phalanx Fractures

IMMEDIATE TO ONE WEEK			
	Cast	*Closed Reduction and Percutaneous Pinning*	*Open Reduction and Internal Fixation*
Stability	None.	None.	None.
Orthopaedics	Trim cast to expose tips of toes.	Trim cast to expose tips of toes. Evaluate pin sites.	Trim cast to expose tips of toes.
Rehabilitation	No range of motion at this time.	No range of motion at this time.	No range of motion at this time.

Great (or First) Toe Phalanx Fractures *(continued)*

TWO WEEKS			
	Cast	*Closed Reduction and Percutaneous Pinning*	*Open Reduction and Internal Fixation*
Stability	None to minimal.	None to minimal.	None to minimal.
Orthopaedics	Trim cast to expose tips of toes.	Trim cast to expose tips of toes. Evaluate pin sites.	Trim cast to expose tips of toes.
Rehabilitation	No range of motion at this time.	No range of motion at this time.	No range of motion at this time.

FOUR TO SIX WEEKS			
	Cast	*Closed Reduction and Percutaneous Pinning*	*Open Reduction and Internal Fixation*
Stability	Stable.	Stable.	Stable.
Orthopaedics	Remove cast, replace with bunion shoe.	Evaluate pin sites. Pins may be removed, cast may be removed.	Remove cast.
Rehabilitation	Begin gentle active range of motion of ankle, metatarsophalangeal (MTP), and interphalangeal (IP) joints.	Begin gentle active range of motion of ankle, MTP, and IP joints.	Begin gentle active range of motion of ankle, MTP, and IP joints.

SIX TO EIGHT WEEKS			
	Cast	*Closed Reduction and Percutaneous Pinning*	*Open Reduction and Internal Fixation*
Stability	Stable.	Stable.	Stable.
Orthopaedics	Remove cast if not previously done. Use stiff-soled shoe.	Remove pins and cast if not previously done.	Remove cast if not already done.
Rehabilitation	Continue active and active-assistive range-of-motion exercises.	Continue active and active-assistive range-of-motion exercises.	Continue active and active-assistive range-of-motion exercises.

EIGHT TO TWELVE WEEKS			
	Cast	*Closed Reduction and Percutaneous Pinning*	*Open Reduction and Internal Fixation*
Stability	Stable.	Stable.	Stable.
Orthopaedics			
Rehabilitation	Continue active and active-assistive range of motion to the MTP, IP, and ankle joints.	Continue active and active-assistive range-of-motion to the MTP, IP, and ankle joints.	Continue active and active-assistive range-of-motion to the MTP, IP, and ankle joints.

First Metatarsal Fractures

IMMEDIATE TO ONE WEEK

	Cast	*Open Reduction and Internal Fixation*
Stability	None.	None.
Orthopaedics	Trim cast to allow visualization of tips of toes.	Trim cast to metatarsal heads.
Rehabilitation	No range of motion.	Gentle active and passive range of motion of the metatarsophalangeal (MTP) and interphalangeal (IP) joints.

TWO WEEKS

	Cast	*Open Reduction and Internal Fixation*
Stability	None to minimal.	None to minimal.
Orthopaedics	Trim cast to metatarsal heads.	Trim cast to metatarsal heads.
Rehabilitation	Avoid MTP and IP joint range of motion.	Continue MTP and IP joint range of motion.

FOUR TO SIX WEEKS

	Cast	*Open Reduction and Internal Fixation*
Stability	Stable.	Stable.
Orthopaedics	Remove cast and replace with a bunion shoe.	Remove cast and replace with a stiff-soled bunion shoe.
Rehabilitation	Start range of motion at the MTP and IP joint.	Continue range of motion of the MTP and IP joints. Begin range of motion of the ankle.

SIX TO EIGHT WEEKS

	Cast	*Open Reduction and Internal Fixation*
Stability	Stable.	Stable.
Orthopaedics	Remove cast if not previously done. Replace with stiff-soled shoe.	Remove cast if not previously done. Replace with stiff-soled shoe.
Rehabilitation	Continue active and assistive-range of motion of the MTP, IP, and ankle joints.	Continue active and assistive range of motion of the MTP, IP, and ankle joints.

First Metatarsal Fractures *(continued)*

EIGHT TO TWELVE WEEKS		
	Cast	*Open Reduction and Internal Fixation*
Stability	Stable.	Stable.
Orthopaedics		
Rehabilitation	Continue active and active-assistive range of motion of the MTP, IP, and ankle joints. May begin resistive exercises.	Continue active and active-assistive range of motion of the MTP, IP, and ankle joints. May begin resistive exercises.

Sesamoid Fractures

IMMEDIATE TO ONE WEEK		
	Cast	*Sesamoidectomy*
Stability	None.	
Orthopaedics	Trim cast to show tips of toes.	Trim cast to show tips of toes.
Rehabilitation	No range of motion at this time.	No range of motion at this time.

TWO WEEKS		
	Cast	*Sesamoidectomy*
Stability	None to minimal.	
Orthopaedics	Trim cast to show tips of toes.	Trim cast to show tips of toes.
Rehabilitation	No range of motion at this time.	No Range of motion at this time.

FOUR TO SIX WEEKS		
	Cast	*Sesamoidectomy*
Stability	Minimal.	
Orthopaedics	May remove cast and replace with bunion shoe. Tape great toe to shoe.	Remove cast.
Rehabilitation	Begin gentle active-assistive range of motion of the metatarsophalangeal (MTP) and interphalangeal (IP) joints as well as the ankle.	Begin gentle active-assistive range of motion of the MTP and IP joints as well as the ankle.

SIX TO EIGHT WEEKS		
	Cast	*Sesamoidectomy*
Stability	Stable.	
Orthopaedics	Continue use of stiff-soled shoe.	Continue use of stiff-soled shoe.
Rehabilitation	Continue active and active-assistive range of motion of the MTP, IP, and ankle joints.	Continue active and active-assistive range of motion of the MTP, IP, and ankle joints.

EIGHT TO TWELVE WEEKS		
	Cast	*Sesamoidectomy*
Stability	Stable.	
Orthopaedics		
Rehabilitation	Continue active and active-assistive range of motion of the MTP, IP, and ankle joints.	Continue active and active-assistive range of motion of the MTP, IP, and ankle joints.

BIBLIOGRAPHY

Chapman M. Tarsal and metatarsal injuries. In: Mann RA, ed. *Surgery of the Foot.* St. Louis: CV Mosby, 1986, pp. 729–749.

Glasgow MT, Naranja RJ, Glasgow SG, Torg JS. Analysis of failed surgical management of fractures of the base of the fifth metatarsal distal to the tuberosity: the Jones fracture. *Foot Ankle* 1996; 17:8:449–457, 1996.

Hansen ST Jr. Foot injuries. In: Browner B, Jupiter J, Levine AM, Trafton PG, eds. *Skeletal Trauma,* Vol. 2. Philadelphia: W.B. Saunders, 1992, pp. 1982–1989.

Heckman J. Forefoot fractures. In: Rockwood CA, Green DP, eds. *Fractures in Adults,* 4th ed. Philadelphia: J.B. Lippincott, 1995, pp. 2373–2391.

Mann R. In: Chapman M, ed. *Operative Orthopaedics.* Philadelphia: J.B. Lippincott, 1993, pp. 2191–2198.

Manoli A II. Compartment syndromes of the foot: current concepts. *Foot Ankle* 10:340–344, 1990.

Mizel M, Sobel M. In: Miller M, ed. *Review of Orthopaedics,* 2nd ed. Philadelphia: W.B. Saunders, 1996, pp. 241, 391.

Perry J. Ankle and foot gait deviations. In: Perry J, ed. *Gait Analysis.* Thorofare, NJ: SLACK, 1992, pp. 185–219.

Schenck RC Jr, Heckman JD. Fractures and dislocations of the forefoot: operative and nonoperative treatment. *J Am Acad Orthop Surg* 3:70–78, 1995.

Stephen DJG. Injuries to the midfoot and forefoot. In Schatzker J, Tile M, eds. *The Rationale of Operative Fracture Care,* 2nd ed. Berlin: Springer, 1996, pp. 608–616.

Yablon IG, Segal D. In: Evarts CM, ed. *Surgery of the Musculoskeletal System,* 2nd ed. New York: Churchill Livingstone, 1990, pp. 4278–4295.

Spine Fractures

Early recognition and accurate diagnosis of spine injuries leads to more efficient treatment. The leading causes of cervical and thoracolumbar spine injuries are motor vehicle accidents, falls, and diving accidents. Anyone with a history of trauma who is intoxicated or unconscious should be evaluated for spine injury. Because of the unique anatomy of the spine, a wide range of injuries can occur, from simple fractures with no neurologic deficit to complex fracture dislocations with complete neurologic deficits. In this section, treatment of individuals with neurologic injuries is not considered. The patient's neurologic status is important and plays a critical role in deciding whether surgery is indicated.

CHAPTER *Thirty-five*

C1 Fracture (Jefferson Fracture)

ASHVIN I. PATEL, MD

BARON S. LONNER, MD

STANLEY HOPPENFELD, MD

INTRODUCTION

Definition

A Jefferson fracture is a burst fracture of C1 (atlas), resulting in combined fractures of the anterior and posterior arches of the ring of C1 (Figure 35-1).

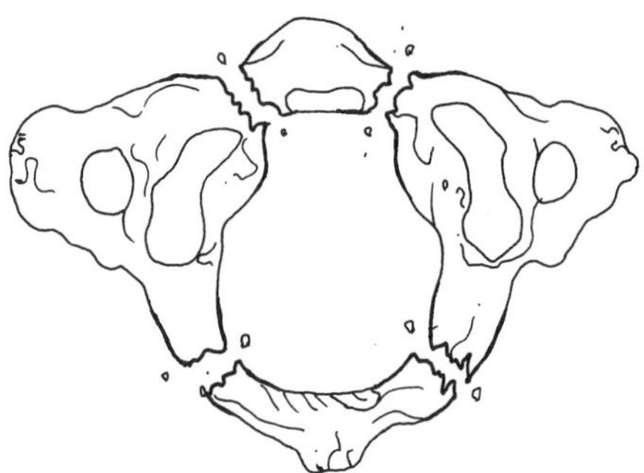

FIGURE 35-1 Jefferson fracture. A burst fracture of C1 (atlas), resulting in combined fractures of the anterior and posterior arches of the ring of C1. Most Jefferson fractures do not result in neurologic impairment. The spinal canal is generally widened as a result of the fracture and there is sufficient space to accommodate the spinal cord and associated swelling at the C1-2 level.

Mechanism of Injury

This fracture is caused by axial compression, commonly from a fall on the head, such as from diving into shallow water.

Radiographic Evaluation

The standard trauma series for this cervical spine fracture consists of anteroposterior, lateral, and open-mouth (dens) views. Oblique radiographs help rule out associated fractures in the subaxial spine. The patient's head should not be passively moved. On the dens or odontoid view, lateral displacement of the lateral articular masses of C1 relative to C2 suggests a Jefferson fracture. The fracture may not be evident on the lateral view, but soft tissue swelling may be visualized anterior to the ring of C1. The ring of the atlas fails in tension through both the anterior and posterior arches. At least one fracture line is present through each arch. If the sum of displacement of the lateral masses, on the odontoid view, is greater than 7 mm, this strongly suggests a rupture of the transverse atlantal ligament. Typically, the ligament fails by avulsion at its bony insertion rather than as a mid-substance tear. A thin section computed tomography scan parallel to the ring of the atlas best defines the fracture anatomy of a C1 ring disruption as well as bony avulsion fractures associated with the transverse ligament.

Treatment Goals

Orthopaedic Objectives

1. Obtain and maintain spinal alignment and reduction of the fracture.
2. Provide spinal stability.
3. Prevent new neurologic deficits and attempt to improve and prevent the exacerbation of existing neurologic deficits.
4. Prevent future spinal deformity.

Rehabilitation Objectives

Range of Motion

Restore functional and pain-free range of motion in all planes without creating neurologic deficits (Table 35-1).

TABLE 35-1 *Range of Motion of the Cervical Spine*

Motion	Normal
Flexion*	65°
Extension*	65°
Lateral bend	45°
Rotation**	75°

*50% of flexion and extension occurs at the occiput-C1 level.
**50% of rotation occurs at C1–2 level.

Muscle Strength

Restore and maintain the strength of paracervical and cervical muscles, including the trapezius and the upper extremity muscles. Restore the strength of the muscles of the lower extremities that may atrophy from bed rest or neurologic injury.

Functional Goals

Develop cervical spinal flexibility for functional independence.

Expected Time of Bone Healing

Eight to 16 weeks before fusion is solid or fracture healing is complete.

Expected Duration of Rehabilitation

Three to 6 months.

Methods of Treatment

Orthosis

Hard collar (e.g., Philadelphia collar), sternal-occiput-mandibular immobilization (SOMI) brace, cervicothoracic orthosis, four-poster brace, or halo vest (*see* Figures 8-7, 8-8, 8-9, 8-10, and 8-11).

Biomechanics: Stress-sharing device.

Mode of bone healing: Secondary.

Indication: A nondisplaced or minimally displaced fracture (less than 2 mm of combined displacement of the lateral masses on the dens view) may be treated with a hard collar, such as a Philadelphia collar, or one of the other rigid nonhalo braces.

A displaced fracture (2 to 7 mm of combined displacement on the dens view) should first be reduced with halo skeletal traction and then treated with a halo vest once cervical muscle spasm has resolved.

A fracture with a transverse ligament injury (greater than 7 mm of combined displacement of the lateral masses on the dens view) should be treated with 4 weeks or more of halo skeletal traction followed by halo vest. The length of skeletal traction before application of the halo vest is still under debate.

Open Reduction and Posterior Spinal Fusion

Biomechanics: Stress-sharing device until solid arthrodesis occurs.

Mode of bone healing: Secondary.

Indications: Surgery is rarely necessary for isolated fractures of the ring of C1. Indications include failure to achieve or maintain reduction in a halo vest, instability of the C1-2 motion segment, and failure of the fracture to reduce, despite an adequate trial of skeletal traction. Operative treatment is also indicated if the reduction is not maintained with halo vest immobilization. Treatment generally consists of a posterior arthrodesis from the occiput to C2 using various wiring techniques and autogenous bone graft. Screw-plate fixations from the occiput to C2 may also be used. An alternative technique that limits the fusion to the C1-2 joint complex and perhaps obviates the need for postoperative halo immobilization is Magerl's C1-2 transarticular screw fixation.

Special Considerations of the Fracture

Most Jefferson fractures do not result in neurologic impairment because the spinal canal is generally widened as a result of the fracture, and there is sufficient space to accommodate the spinal cord and associated swelling at the C1-2 level. The initial evaluation must include a thorough neurologic examination and search for associated injuries. Halo traction should be used with the patient awake so that the patient's neurologic status can be closely observed (see page 557).

Unstable injuries, in which greater than 7 mm of combined lateral mass widening has occurred, may require a period of halo traction followed by halo vest immobilization. The length of skeletal traction before application of the halo vest is still under debate.

Associated Injuries

Patients with Jefferson fractures should be carefully evaluated for head injuries as well as other cervical spine fractures, particularly fractures of the upper three cervical segments. In addition, injuries to the brachial plexus, thorax and abdomen, and extremities may occur and must be addressed in a timely fashion.

TREATMENT

Treatment: Early to Immediate (Day of Injury to One Week)

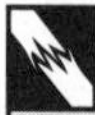

BONE HEALING

Stability at fracture site: Unstable. The degree of instability is dependent upon intact bony and ligamentous structures, internal fixation, and external immobilization.

Stage of bone healing: Inflammatory phase. Bone graft is at a similar phase.

X-ray: Fracture lines and bone graft, if used, are visible.

Orthopaedic and Rehabilitation Considerations

Physical Examination

The patient's neurologic status must be observed closely in the early post-injury period. Fracture displacement in this period can lead to direct neural compression or to epidural hematoma causing secondary compression. The patient will require operative intervention in the case of an evolving neurologic deficit.

Dysphagia and dyspnea may be a result of prevertebral hematoma or soft tissue inflammation and may, on occasion, require intubation or operative intervention.

The cervical orthosis must fit snugly against the neck without causing any breakdown of the skin, especially along the mandible. Adjust and trim the orthosis as needed.

The halo vest must also be snug yet comfortable. The pin sites should be cleaned with hydrogen peroxide and an antibiotic ointment applied. The pin sites are checked and adjusted to a torque of 8 inch-pounds 24 to 48 hours after initial application. Reduction of pin pressure is normal because the outer table tends to erode from continued pin pressure. If the pin is loose, the halo will become uncomfortable, and drainage from the pin sites may develop.

Dangers

If a halo vest has been used, the pins may be tightened if they loosen. It is important not to tighten the pins too much or too frequently, however, because this accelerates erosion of the cranium and may result in penetration of the pin through the inner table of the skull. Purulent discharge can be treated by twice-daily cleaning of the pin sites with chlorhexidine and dressing with gauze soaked in chlorhexidine solution or hydrogen peroxide. Oral antibiotics should be administered. If the drainage continues despite treatment, the pin should be removed and a new pin placed at an adjacent threaded hole in the ring, without removing the halo. Intravenous antibiotics may be needed in some cases. Osteomyelitis is an uncommon complication. Pressure sores under the vest are also uncommon, but elderly and debilitated or insensate patients are at risk and should be monitored for this complication. Pressure sores can be avoided by meticulous hygiene and trimming of the vest as needed to fit the patient's body habitus. Bony prominences should be padded. Frequent log-rolling should be instituted. Special beds for turning and preventing bed sores should be used for spinal cord–injured patients. Surgical incisions must be checked for drainage and infection.

Radiography

Alignment must by evaluated by radiography. If a fracture displaces, it may be necessary to place the patient in traction to reduce this fracture. Gradual increments in traction weights are made until reduction of the lateral masses is seen. A radiograph should be obtained after each 5-pound increase in traction weight to assess the alignment. If the fracture is unstable, prolonged halo traction may be necessary before application of the halo vest.

Weight Bearing

The patient should be mobilized to a sitting position in bed or to a chair on day 1 following appropriate cervical immobilization (internal fixation or external bracing). Ambulation should begin with assistance as tolerated. The tilt table may be required initially to address the problem of orthostatic hypotension. General conditioning should be ongoing.

A patient who remains in cervical traction must be maintained at bed rest until further stability is achieved with fracture healing. A halo vest is then applied, thus allowing mobilization of the patient.

Range of Motion

No motion of the cervical spine is allowed until fracture healing is complete. Gentle active range of motion to the upper extremities is given. However, overhead range of motion should be avoided. Active range of motion to the lower extremities prevents joint stiffness.

Muscle Strength

One-pound weights may be used to strengthen the upper extremities as long as the cervical spine is immobilized. Isometric exercises to the abdominal muscles are prescribed.

Gluteal sets, quad sets, and ankle isotonic sets of exercises maintain strength in the lower extremities.

Functional Activities

Bed mobility: Log-rolling is allowed for side-to-side mobility. The patient can be mobilized with assistance for sitting.

Transfers: Once the patient is brought to the seated position, he or she can come to the standing position with little assistance and transfer to a chair. Initially, the patient may benefit from the tilt table if orthostatic hypotension or dizziness occurs.

Personal hygiene: Initially, the patient may have difficulty in self-care because of cervical immobilization and will need assistance in dressing, grooming, and personal hygiene.

Ambulation: The patient uses assistive devices such as a walker or cane for stability and balance, because of the presence of general weakness and pain.

Gait

The gait may be wide-based because of the lack of stability or the sense of instability resulting from the fracture and the orthosis. Upper arm swing excursion may be reduced because of pain. Push-off may be reduced to avoid instability caused by the forward thrust of the body secondary to the orthosis.

Prescription

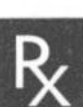

DAY ONE TO ONE WEEK

Precautions

Cervical spine is immobilized.

Avoid overhead range of motion of upper extremities.

Range of motion

No range of motion is allowed to the cervical spine.

Gentle active range of motion to the upper and lower extremities.

Strength

No strengthening exercises allowed to the cervical spine.

Isometric exercises to the abdominal, gluteal, and quadriceps muscles.

If the cervical spine is immobilized, gentle strengthening exercises to both upper extremities.

Functional Activities

Bed mobility: log-rolling with assistance.

Transfers and ambulation: with assistive devices and with assistance.

Weight Bearing Weight bearing with assistive devices.

Treatment: Two to Four Weeks

BONE HEALING

Stability at fracture site: Unstable. Stability continues to be a function of intact bony and ligamentous elements, internal fixation, and external immobilization.

Stage of bone healing: Reparative phase. Osteoblasts lay down woven bone.

Stage of arthrodesis: Fibrovascular stroma arises.

X-ray: Fracture lines and graft remain visible. Early callus formation occurs but is usually not seen.

Orthopaedic and Rehabilitation Considerations

Physical Examination

Continue to follow the neurologic examination closely. Adjust and tighten the orthosis as necessary. Check for skin maceration beneath braces. Check the halo pin sites for drainage or loosening; they should be cleaned daily with hydrogen peroxide swabs. Oral antibiotics may be required to treat superficial pin site drainage. If deep infection is present, the pins must be removed and their position changed, the pin sites débrided, and intravenous antibiotics administered.

Patients with chin abrasions from cervical collars should be given padding beneath the chin. Staples or sutures are removed at approximately day 10 postoperatively. The head and neck remain immobilized.

Radiography

Radiographs must be inspected for maintenance of alignment.

Range of Motion

Range of motion to the cervical spine is not permitted to prevent fracture displacement or stress on spinal instrumentation if present. The spine is immobilized. Bone and ligamentous healing has not occurred. Therefore, the spinal cord remains at risk for injury. Continue with upper and lower extremity range of motion exercises, with precautions to avoid overhead range of motion of the upper extremities.

Muscle Strength

Continue with abdominal isometric exercises, gluteal and quadriceps sets, and ankle isotonics to the lower extremities to maintain strength and to prevent deep vein thrombosis by maintaining the venous pump mechanism on the venous system. Continue with upper extremity strengthening exercises.

Functional Activities

Bed mobility: Continue with log-rolling for side-to-side bed mobility.

Transfers: Continue as before. The patient may still need assistance to come to a sitting position.

Personal hygiene: The patient may still need assistance with self-care, grooming, and dressing as a result of interference from an orthotic.

Gait

Continue ambulation using assistive devices as before. The patient may continue to have a wide-based gait for support and stability. Arm swing may improve as pain decreases.

Prescription

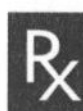

TWO TO FOUR WEEKS

Precautions Maintain cervical spine immobilization.

Range of Motion

No range of motion to the cervical spine.

Active range of motion to the upper and lower extremities.

Strength

No strengthening exercises to the cervical spine.

Abdominal, gluteal, and quadriceps isometric exercises.

Functional Activities

Bed mobility: log-rolling with assistance.

Transfers and ambulation: with assistive devices and with assistance.

Weight Bearing Weight bearing as tolerated with assistive devices.

Treatment: Four to Eight Weeks

BONE HEALING

Stability: Early healing at the fracture site and early graft consolidation give added stability.

Stage of bone healing: Reparative phase. Osteoblasts lay down woven bone.

X-ray: Fracture lines are less obvious; bone graft is consolidating. Callus is observed and it may be minimal in cervical spine fractures because of the small size of the bones.

Orthopaedic and Rehabilitation Considerations

Physical Examination

Perform a neurologic examination, adjust orthotic as needed, and inspect pin sites.

Dangers

The patient remains at risk for neurologic injury.

Radiography

Check cervical spine fracture alignment on radiograph.

Range of Motion

The muscles of the cervical spine are beginning to recover enough to provide some control. However the fracture site is still unstable. No motion is allowed. Continue with upper and lower extremity range-of-motion exercises.

Muscle Strength

Do not attempt to strengthen the cervical spine muscles, because spinal arthrodesis or fracture healing is not complete. Continue with isometric exercises to the abdomen and strengthening exercises to the upper and lower extremities while the cervical spine is immobilized.

Functional Activities

Bed mobility: Patients should be able to right themselves in bed without assistance. They tend to splint their necks to prevent pain.

Transfers: Patients are, at this point, generally independent in transfers. Orthostatic hypotension and dizziness are usually no longer a problem.

Personal hygiene: There is less need for assistance in self-care, although patients with halo vests may still require assistance in dressing.

Gait

Most patients have achieved balance and stability in standing and no longer need assistive devices. However, some patients may still require a walker or cane. Gait tends to become more normal and the wide-based pattern decreases.

Prescription

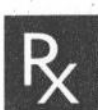

FOUR TO EIGHT WEEKS

Precautions Maintain immobilization.

Range of Motion

Avoid range of motion to the cervical spine.

Active range of motion to the upper and lower extremities.

Strength

No strengthening exercises to the cervical spine.

Abdominal, gluteal, and quadriceps isometric exercises.

Functional Activities

Bed mobility: log-rolling

Transfers and ambulation: with assistive devices as needed.

Weight Bearing Full weight bearing.

Treatment: Eight to Twelve Weeks

BONE HEALING

Stability: Bone stability achieved but ligamentous instability may persist.

Stage of bone healing: Remodeling phase. Woven bone is being replaced by lamellar bone. This takes months to years for completion.

Stage of arthrodesis: Trabeculation of fusion mass is occurring. Remodeling is an ongoing process.

X-ray: Fracture lines begin to disappear. Trabeculation of bone graft is at varying stages.

Orthopaedic and Rehabilitation Considerations

Orthoses can be discontinued in patients in whom a solid arthrodesis or fracture healing has occurred. Attempt to keep the halo vest in place for 12 weeks, if fracture healing has not occurred. The halo vest can be substituted with a hard cervical collar if healing has occurred.

Radiography

Radiographs must be obtained after an orthosis is removed. Dynamic or active flexion/extension radiographs should be obtained to rule out residual instability. If instability is noted, primary arthrodesis or revision surgery may be warranted.

Range of Motion

Gentle active range-of-motion exercises may begin in patients in whom orthoses have been removed at 10 to 12 weeks, as long as no instability exists.

After performing range-of-motion exercises, the patient may be more comfortable in a soft collar as a temporary support. Eventually the collar will no longer be necessary.

Gentle passive range-of-motion exercises can be initiated if the fracture is healed at 12 weeks. This allows the patient to regain the maximum physiologic range of motion of the neck. Passive range is given in flexion, extension, and rotation. Because of stiffness and pain, especially in extension, the patient may require gentle active-assistive exercises. Active stretching of the trapezius and sternocleidomastoid muscles should be initiated to help side bending and rotation of the neck.

Muscle Strength

Once the full range of motion is achieved, the intensity of strengthening exercises can be increased. Sternocleidomastoid and trapezius muscle strengthening and stretching should be started to prevent further stiffness and to help in rotation. Begin isometric strengthening of the paracervical muscles. The patient pushes on the head using one hand while offering resistance. Continue with active-resistive exercises to the upper and lower extremities using weights. Continue with isometric abdominal strengthening exercises.

Functional Activities

By this time, the patient should be independent in all self-care and grooming activities and should not require assistive devices for ambulation unless there is neurologic involvement or the patient is elderly and requires this for stability.

The patient may begin swimming but should avoid jogging to avoid stress on the spine. Fast walking is allowed. Contact sports are not permitted.

The patient may start driving after 12 weeks, when the fracture has healed and the halo vest has been removed. The head rest must be up and the seat belt secured. Occasionally, a soft cervical collar may be necessary for comfort. A wide or panoramic rear-view mirror attachment may be needed if the patient's neck rotation remains limited.

Gait

The gait pattern should be normal.

Prescription

EIGHT TO TWELVE WEEKS

Precautions Beware of ligamentous instability.

Range of Motion

Gentle active range of motion to the cervical spine if the fracture has healed at 10 to 12 weeks.

Gentle passive range of motion may begin if the fracture has healed at 12 weeks.

Strength Isometric strengthening exercises to the cervical spine as tolerated.

Functional Activities Independent in bed mobility, transfers, and ambulation.

Weight Bearing Full weight bearing.

Treatment: Twelve to Sixteen Weeks

BONE HEALING

Stability: Stable.

Stage of bone healing and arthrodesis: Remodeling phase. Woven bone is replaced by lamellar bone.

X-ray: Healed fractures; maturation of bone graft.

Orthopaedic and Rehabilitation Considerations

The orthosis is discontinued. Evaluate wound healing, particularly at the former pin sites. Perform a neurologic examination, including reflexes and muscle strength testing.

Dangers

Persistent ligamentous instability may place the neural structures at risk and cause pain.

Radiography

Active flexion/extension radiographs are obtained to rule out residual instability, if this has not already been done. Follow-up radiographs should be taken at 6-month to 1-year intervals to rule out the development of late instability or deformity. Posttraumatic degenerative changes may be seen.

Range of motion

Functional range of motion should be obtainable by active and passive exercises. Limitations may occur as a result of the extent of the arthrodesis and the loss of motion segments. Fifty percent of the flexion and extension of the cervical spine occurs at occiput-C1 level, and 50% of the rotation of the cervical spine occurs at C1-2. Therefore, fractures and arthrodeses of these areas may result in more significant restriction of the range of motion to the neck than at other levels.

Muscle Strength

Continue with stretching and strengthening of the cervical spine muscles, including the trapezius and sternocleidomastoid to maintain rotation and lateral flexion.

Functional Activities

The patient may gradually return to sports activities but should be restricted from contact sports such as wrestling, boxing, diving, tumbling, and football for a minimum of 1 year. Each activity should be evaluated separately.

Gait

The gait pattern should be normalized. Patients usually do not need any assistive devices for ambulation.

Prescription

Twelve to Sixteen Weeks

Precautions No contact sports.

Range of Motion Active, gentle passive range of motion to the cervical spine.

Strength Isometric strengthening exercises to the cervical spine muscles.

Functional Activities Independent in transfers and ambulation.

Weight Bearing Full weight bearing.

LONG-TERM CONSIDERATIONS

Residual pain may require temporary bracing and antiinflammatory medications. Residual neurologic deficits must be addressed and may require extremity bracing, therapy, or surgery for contracture releases and tendon transfers.

If progressive cervical spine deformity occurs, surgery may be necessary. There may be permanent loss of range of motion. The degree depends on the number of segments arthrodesed and the level and extent of the fracture.

Removal of the instrumentation may be necessary if it is painful.

If pseudoarthrosis occurs, reinstrumentation and fusion may be necessary. Reflex sympathetic dystrophy may be a long-term problem requiring cervical stellate ganglion blocks and long-term physical therapy.

Bibliography: See page 559.

CHAPTER *Thirty-six*

C2 Fracture (Hangman's Fracture)

ASHVIN I. PATEL, MD

BARON S. LONNER, MD

STANLEY HOPPENFELD, MD

INTRODUCTION

Definition

A hangman's fracture is a fracture of the pedicles or pars interarticularis of C2 resulting in the separation of the body of C2 from its posterior elements (Figures 36-1 and 36-2).

Type I: Minimally displaced at the fracture site, with minimal angulation of the vertebral body.
Type II: Angulation of the body of greater than 10 degrees and displacements of the body from its posterior elements of more than 3 mm.
Type III: Severe angulation and displacement, with unilateral or bilateral facet dislocation at C2-3.

The most common injuries are type I and type II.

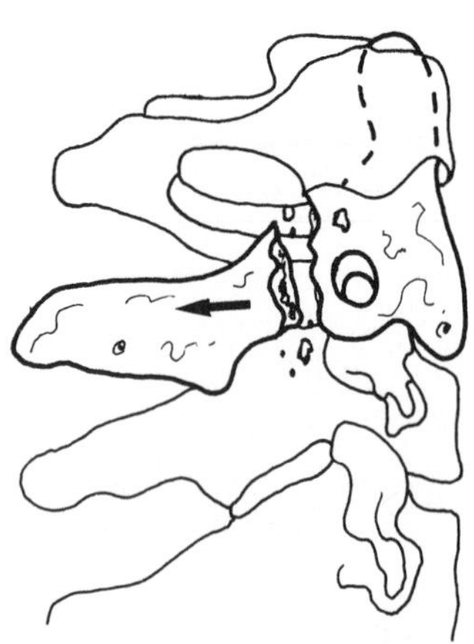

FIGURE 36-1 Hangman's fracture, consisting of a fracture of either the pedicles or pars interarticularis of C2, resulting in the separation of the body of C2 from its posterior elements.

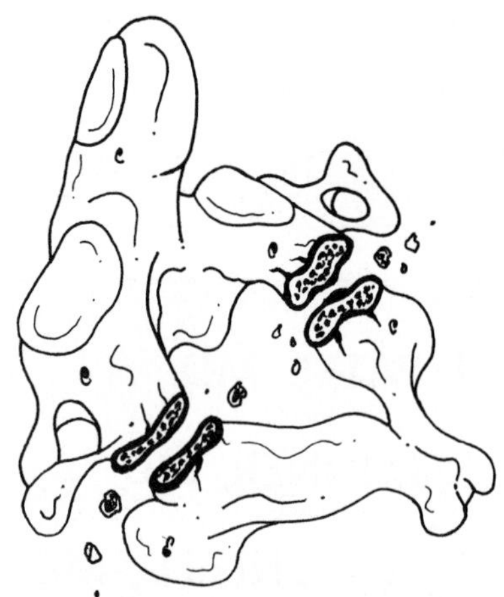

FIGURE 36-2 Hangman's fracture. This frequently occurs in automobile accidents. The term was originally derived from a study of autopsy specimens from judicial hangings.

Mechanism of Injury

Forceful extension of an already extended neck is the most common etiology. Other causes include flexion of a flexed neck and compression of an extended neck. These may occur in motor vehicle accidents. Historically, the major cause of this injury that resulted in death was a hanging with the knot tied under the mentum of the chin. The eponym "hangman's fracture" was derived from a study of autopsy specimens from judicial hangings.

Radiographic Evaluation

The standard trauma series for this cervical spine fracture consists of an anteroposterior, lateral, and open-mouth (dens) view. Oblique radiographs help rule out associated fractures in the subaxial spine. A hangman's fracture is usually best seen on the lateral radiograph. A computed tomography (CT) scan with thin axial cuts and sagittal reconstruction is also very helpful for defining the fracture pattern (Figures 36-3 and 36-4). The patient's head should not be passively moved for the x-ray or for the CT scan.

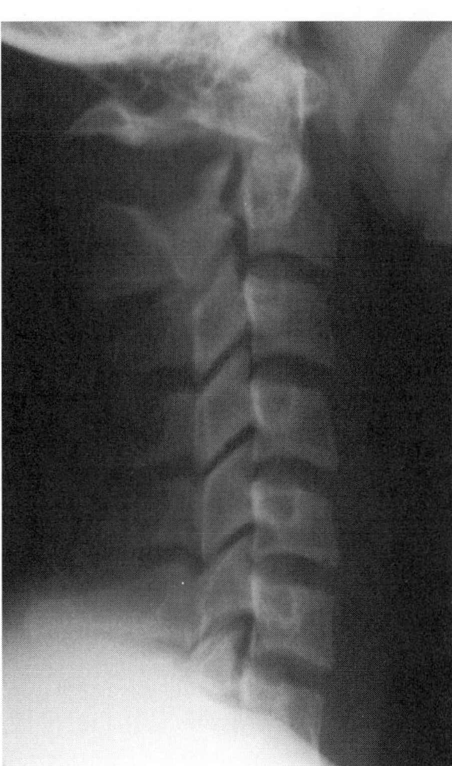

FIGURE 36-3 Lateral view of the cervical spine. There is separation of more than 3 mm of the posterior elements of C2 from its body. The patient is in Gardner-Wells tong traction of 20 pounds.

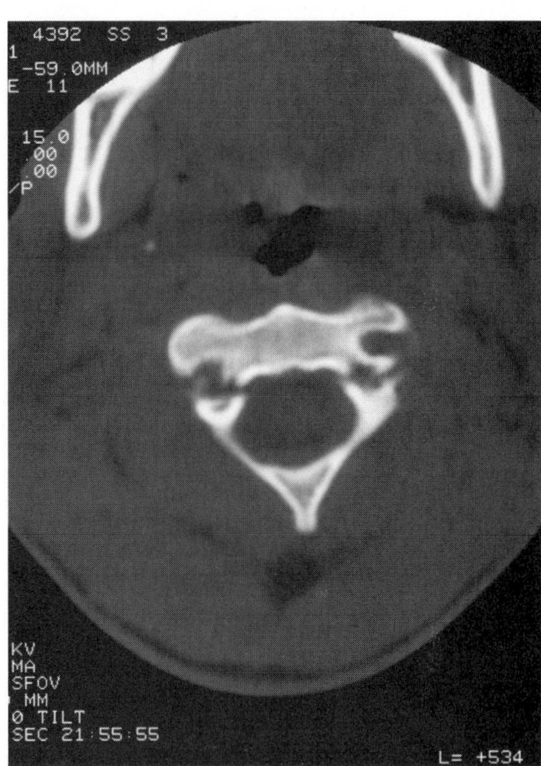

FIGURE 36-4 Computed tomography scan of C2. Note the separation of the posterior elements from the vertebral body. (Courtesy of the Kennedy White Orthopaedic Center Sarasota Florida.)

Treatment Goals

Orthopaedic Objectives

1. Obtain and maintain spinal alignment and reduction of the fracture.
2. Provide spinal stability.
3. Prevent new neurologic deficits and attempt to improve and prevent the worsening of existing neurologic deficits.
4. Prevent future spinal deformity.

Rehabilitation Objectives

Range of motion

Restore range of motion in all planes without creating neurologic deficits (Table 36-1).

TABLE 36-1 *Range of Motion of the Cervical Spine*

Motion	Normal
Flexion*	65°
Extension*	65°
Lateral bend	45°
Rotation**	75°

*50% of flexion and extension occurs at occiput-C1 level.
**50% of rotation occurs at C1–2 level.

Muscle Strength

Restore and maintain the strength of paracervical and scapular muscles, including the trapezius and the upper extremity muscles. Gluteal muscles are disturbed if an autologous bone graft is harvested for the purpose of fusion. The muscles of the lower extremities may atrophy from bed rest or neurologic injury and require strengthening.

Functional Goals

Restore sufficient cervical spinal flexibility for functional independence.

Expected Time of Bone Healing

Eight to 12 weeks before fusion is solid or fracture healing is complete.

Expected Duration of Rehabilitation

Three to 6 months.

Methods of Treatment

Orthosis

Hard collar (e.g., Philadelphia collar), sternal-occiput-mandibular-immobilization (SOMI) brace (Figure 36-5), cervicothoracic orthosis, CTO), four poster brace, or the halo vest (see Figures 8-7, 8-8, 8-9, 8-10, and 8-11).

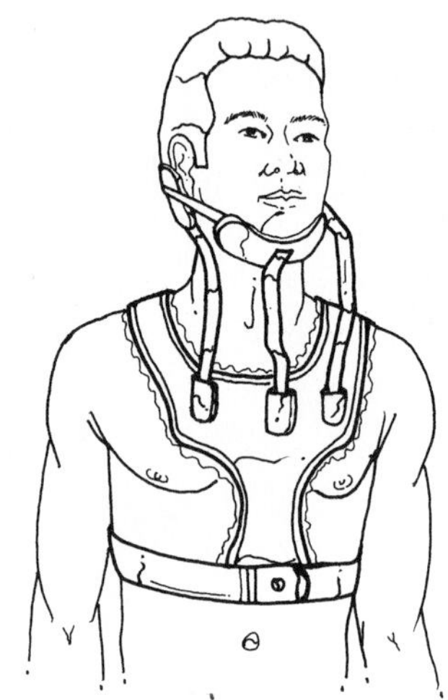

FIGURE 36-5 A sternal-occipital-mandibular immobilizer brace.

Biomechanics: Stress-sharing device.

Mode of bone healing: Secondary.

Indications: A type I fracture is treated with a hard collar, such as a Philadelphia collar or one of the other non-halo devices such as the SOMI brace, or a cervicothoracic orthosis. The immobilization is generally maintained for 8 to 12 weeks. A type II fracture should initially be reduced with axial distraction and slight hyperextension and then immobilized in a halo vest for 12 weeks. If displacement is greater than 6 mm, it may be necessary to place the patient in skeletal traction for several weeks, to maintain the reduction, prior to mobilization in a halo vest. If the fracture shows further angulation with traction, it should be placed in a halo vest from the outset. This usually leads to a gradual reduction of the fracture with mobilization of the patient. This is referred to as a type II-A fracture.

Surgery

Direct osteosynthesis of C2 pedicle fracture, open reduction of C2-C3 dislocation and posterior spinal fusion C2-C3. (Interspinous wiring or plating.)

Biomechanics: Stress-sharing construct.

Mode of bone healing: Secondary.

Indications: Direct osteosynthesis of the pedicle fractures with screws may be necessary for a type II fracture in which alignment is not maintained by a halo vest. Type III fractures are generally very unstable and the dislocated facets are not amenable to a closed reduction. An open reduction of the dislocated facets followed by posterior C2 to C3 fusion followed by a hard collar or a halo vest is the treatment of choice.

Special Considerations of the Fracture

The type II-A fracture can be recognized by its fracture orientation (more oblique than types I and II), presence of significant angulation without translation, and excessive widening of the posterior C2-3 disc space. Angulation in a type II-A fracture can exceed 15 degrees, whereas translation rarely exceeds 2 or 3 mm. These injuries should not be treated with traction, but with gentle cervical extension and compression followed by halo immobilization.

Type III injuries may be approached in several different ways depending on the type of fracture and dislocation that is seen. In general, the C2-C3 dislocation cannot be reduced by closed methods and requires an open reduction followed by a posterior spinal fusion of C2-C3. The bipedicular fracture component is a type I injury and thus can be treated with a hard collar or a halo vest.

Hangman's fractures as a group generally do not cause neurologic deficits because there is acute decompression of the neural canal by the fracture of the pedicles. Neurologic deficits are generally limited to the type III fractures, with approximately 11% of these having permanent neurologic injury.

Associated Injuries

Thirty-one percent of patient's with Hangman's fractures have associated injuries of the cervical spine, 94% of which involve the upper three cervical segments. Thus, a search for associated cervical spine injuries as well as for trauma to the thorax, abdomen, and extremities is critical.

TREATMENT

Further treatment and rehabilitation follows the same protocol as Jefferson (C1) fracture (*see* Chapter 35, pages 516–521).

LONG-TERM CONSIDERATIONS

Residual pain may require temporary bracing and antiinflammatory medications. Neurologic deficits must be addressed and may require extremity bracing, therapy, or surgery for contracture releases and tendon transfers.

If progressive deformity occurs or instability persists, surgery may be necessary. There may be permanent loss of range of motion. The extent depends on the number of segments arthrodesed and the level and extent of the fracture.

Removal of instrumentation may be necessary if it is painful.

If pseudoarthrosis occurs, reinstrumentation and fusion may be necessary. Reflex sympathetic dystrophy may be a long-term problem requiring cervical stellate ganglion blocks and long-term physical therapy.

Bibliography: See page 559.

CHAPTER *Thirty-seven*

Fractures of the Odontoid (Dens)

STANLEY HOPPENFELD, MD

ASHVIN I. PATEL, MD

BARON S. LONNER, MD

INTRODUCTION

Definition

Fracture of the odontoid process are classified into three types, based on the anatomic level of injury.

Type I: A rare avulsion fracture of the alar and apical ligaments from the tip of the odontoid process.

Type II: A fracture at the junction of the dens with the central axis of the body of C2. This is the most common type of dens fracture (Figures 37-1 and 37-2).

Type III: A fracture that extends into the body of the axis.

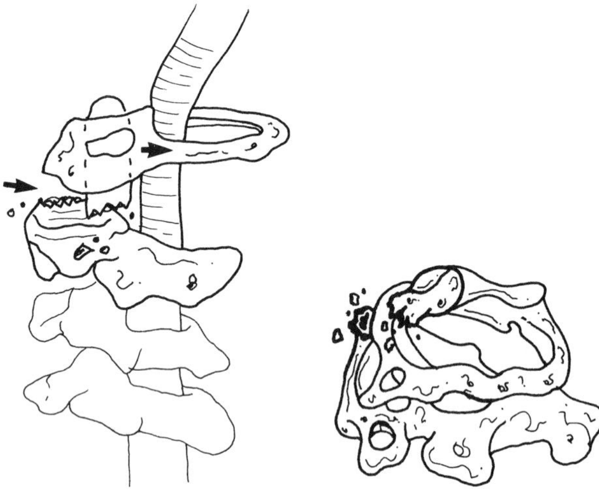

FIGURE 37-1 *(far left)* Type II fracture of the dens, at the junction of the dens with the vertebral body, with posterior displacement.

FIGURE 37-2 *(left)* Fracture of the dens with posterior displacement of the atlas causing a small degree of spinal canal compromise.

Mechanism of Injury

Despite a large number of autopsy and biomechanical studies, the exact mechanism of this injury remains unknown. It probably includes a combination of flexion, extension, and rotation.

Radiographic Evaluation

The standard trauma series for this cervical spine fracture consists of anteroposterior, lateral, and open-mouth (dens) views (Figures 37-3, 37-4, and 37-5). Oblique radiographs are added to help rule out associ-

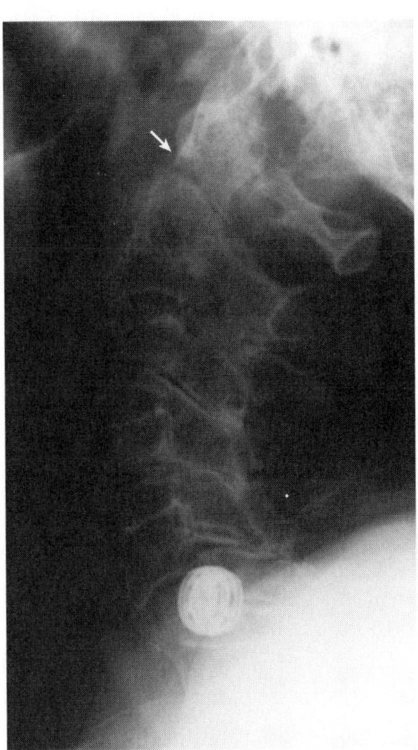

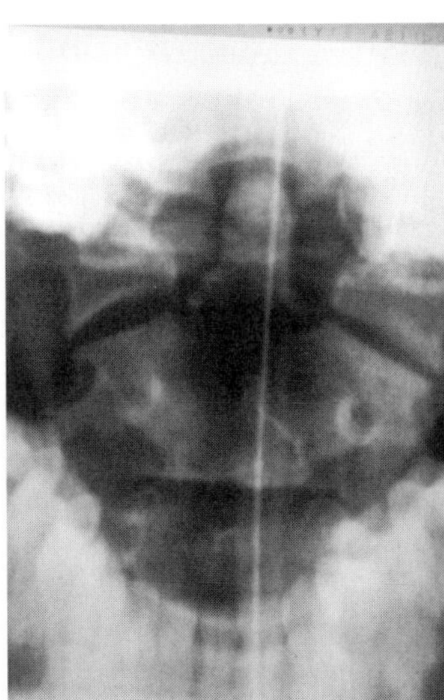

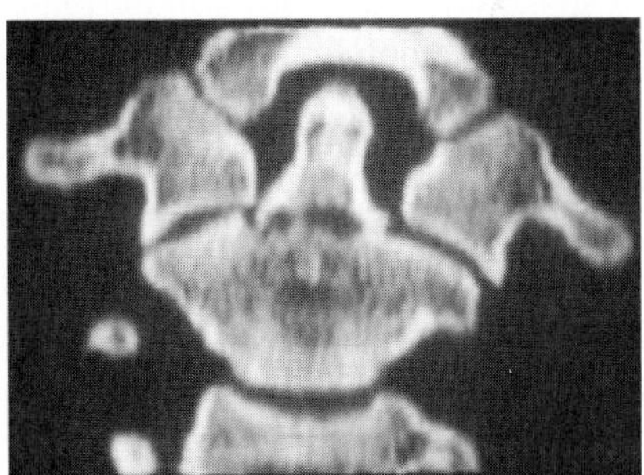

FIGURE 37-3 *(above, left)* Type II odontoid fracture involving the base of the dens. There is minimal displacement.

FIGURE 37-4 *(above, middle)* Open-mouth view of C1-2 revealing a fracture at the base of the odontoid, type II.

FIGURE 37-5 *(above, right)* Computed tomography scan of C1-2, coronal reconstruction. Note the fracture at the base of the odontoid as it leads to the vertebral body. Type II.

ated fractures in the subaxial spine. Associated injury to the occiput-C1 joint, the ring of C1, and the lower cervical spine should be excluded. A computed tomography (CT) scan of the odontoid (thin axial cuts with sagittal and coronal reconstruction) is valuable in defining the fracture type. The head should not be passively moved for the radiographic study or CT scan.

Treatment Goals

Orthopaedic Objectives

1. Obtain and maintain spinal alignment and reduction of the fracture.
2. Provide spinal stability.
3. Prevent new neurologic deficits and attempt to improve and prevent the worsening of existing neurologic deficits.
4. Prevent future spinal deformity.

Rehabilitation Objectives

Range of motion

Restore range of motion in all planes without creating neurologic deficits (Table 37-1).

TABLE 37-1 *Range of Motion of the Cervical Spine*

Motion	Normal
Flexion*	65°
Extension*	65°
Lateral bend	45°
Rotation**	75°

*50% of flexion and extension occurs at occiput-C1 level.
**50% of rotation occurs at C1–2 level.

The above ranges vary depending on the patient's age. Different vertebral segments do not contribute equal amounts to the specific plane of motion. For example, C1-2 accounts for approximately 50% of cervical rotation. Occiput-C1 motion accounts for approximately 50% of flexion and extension.

Muscle Strength

Restore and maintain the strength of paracervical and scapular muscles, including the trapezius and the upper extremity muscles. Gluteal muscles are disturbed if an autologous bone graft is harvested for the purpose of fusion. The muscles of the lower extremities may atrophy from bed rest or neurologic injury and require strengthening.

Functional Goals

Develop cervical spinal flexibility for functional independence.

Expected Time of Bone Healing

Twelve to 16 weeks before fusion is solid or fracture healing is complete.

Expected Duration of Rehabilitation

Three to 6 months.

Methods of Treatment

Orthosis: Soft Collar, Hard Collar, or Halo Vest

Biomechanics: Stress-sharing device.

Mode of bone healing: Secondary.

Indication: A type I fracture may be treated symptomatically with a soft collar. A nondisplaced type II fracture (less than 10 degrees of angulation and less than 5 mm of displacement) is treated with a halo vest. Controversy exists regarding the treatment of displaced type II fractures; however, these are generally treated operatively. A type III fracture that is angulated more than 10 degrees or displaced more than 5 mm is initially reduced with halo traction and subsequently treated with a halo vest. A nondisplaced type III fracture is treated in a halo vest from the onset (*see* Figures 8-7, 8-8, 8-9, 8-10, and 8-11).

Posterior Arthrodesis and Wiring of C1-2

Biomechanics: Stress-sharing device.

Mode of bone healing: Secondary.

Indications: A high rate of nonunion is reported with type II fractures in patients who have a delay in diagnosis, initial displacement of more than 5 mm, posterior rather than anterior angulation, and age greater than 60 years. In these patients and in patients in whom an anatomic reduction of the dens cannot be maintained in the halo vest, a posterior C1-2 wiring and arthrodesis is generally recommended (Figures 37-6 and 37-7). Supplemental use of transarticular screws may increase the rate of fusion and may obviate the need for any external fixation.

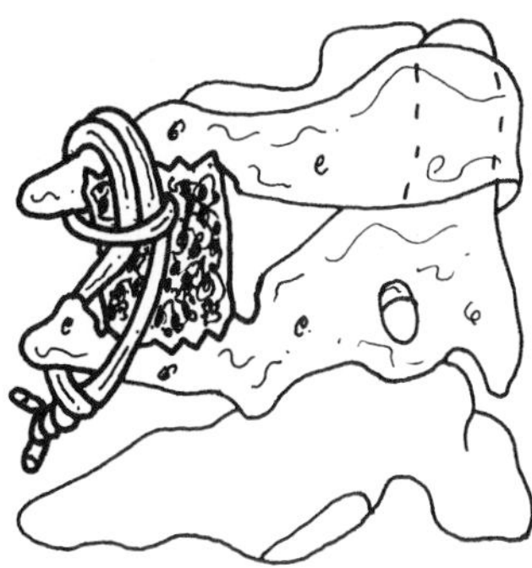

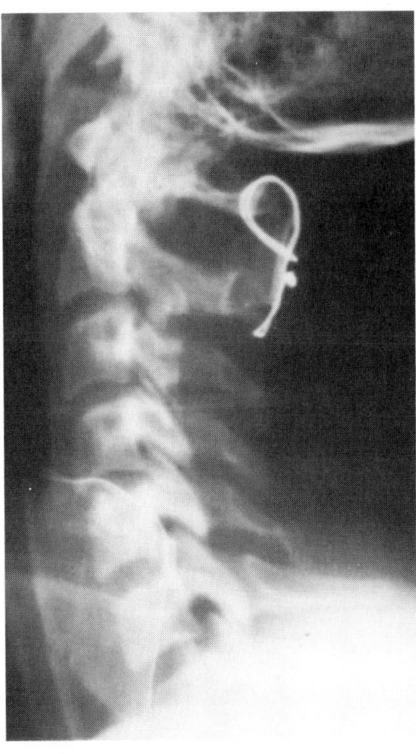

FIGURE 37-6 *(far left)* Gallie fusion. C1-2 wiring and arthrodesis.

FIGURE 37-7 *(left)* Lateral radiograph of the cervical spine with Gallie fusion (posterior fusion) of C1-2.

Anterior Odontoid Screw Fixation

Biomechanics: Stress-sharing device.

Mode of bone healing: Primary.

Indications: Anterior odontoid screw fixation is indicated for patients in whom disruption or loss of the posterior arch of C1 or C2 is encountered as a result of congenital malformations, previous surgery, or the injury itself. Despite its inherent risks and technical difficulty, this procedure has the advantage of preserving rotation of the upper cervical spine as it avoids fusion of the C1-2 joint complex.

Special Considerations of the Fracture

The typical high-energy injury pattern that results in a type II odontoid fracture is not always seen in very young and very old patients. Low-energy injuries such as short falls are often responsible for the fracture in these patients. Odontoid fractures are among the most commonly missed spinal injuries and thus a high index of suspicion is required to make the diagnosis in any patient with a cervical injury.

Significant controversy exists regarding the surgical indications for the type II odontoid fracture. The guidelines set forth in the previous section are generally helpful in making the final decision.

Anterior odontoid screw fixation is performed by some spine surgeons. This type of fixation preserves motion at the C1-2 joint complex. This procedure is technically demanding and requires closed reduction of the odontoid before the screw fixation. In addition, there should not be any significant comminution or obliquity of the fracture site or osteoporosis.

Associated Injuries

Occipital-cervical instability as well as other fractures of the cervical spine must be excluded. A careful look for concomitant fractures of C1 must be done when fusion is contemplated using posterior wiring techniques. The odontoid represents the most common secondary fracture seen with fracture of the atlas. Careful scrutiny of both C1 and C2 must be made in treating any fractures of the cervicocranial region. Combined C1 and C2 injuries are particularly common and in some studies have an incidence of up to 40%. Treatment of combined C1 and C2 injuries is usually determined by the type of C2 fracture. Controversies exist on how to best manage these fractures. If a fracture of C1 is present, arthrodesis may have to extend to the occiput.

TREATMENT

Further treatment and rehabilitation follows the same protocol as for Jefferson fractures (C1 fractures). (*See* Chapter 35, pages 516–521.)

LONG-TERM CONSIDERATIONS

All patients should have active flexion/extension lateral radiographs of the cervical spine at the completion of treatment for their odontoid fracture. If significant instability is present (greater than 4 mm of atlantoaxial separation), consideration should be given to treat these injuries with a posterior C1-2 fusion. If this instability is asymptomatic and not associated with any neurologic deficit, it may be observed, but the patient should refrain from participating in any contact sports.

Residual pain may require temporary bracing and antiinflammatory medication. Residual neurologic problems must be addressed and may require extremity bracing, therapy, or surgery for contracture releases and tendon transfers.

If progressive deformity occurs, surgery may be necessary. There may be permanent loss of range of motion. The degree depends on the number of segments arthrodesed and the level and extent of the fracture. Removal of the instrumentation may be necessary if it is painful. If pseudoarthrosis occurs, reinstrumentation and fusion may be necessary.

Reflex sympathetic dystrophy may be a long-term problem requiring cervical stellate ganglion blocks and long-term physical therapy.

Bibliography: See page 559.

CHAPTER Thirty-eight

Cervical Spine Compression and Burst Fractures

ASHVIN I. PATEL, MD

BARON S. LONNER, MD

STANLEY HOPPENFELD, MD

INTRODUCTION

Definition

A compression fracture is the result of a pure flexion moment on the spine, without any rotatory or shear forces. It involves the anterior portion of the vertebral body. Generally, there is no disruption of the posterior ligamentous structures, nor any loss of the height of the posterior wall of the vertebral body. There is no retropulsion of disc or bony fragments into the vertebral canal. However, in severe compression fractures with greater than 50% loss of vertebral height, posterior ligamentous injury may occur.

A *burst fracture* is defined as a comminuted fracture of the entire vertebral body, usually including retropulsion of bone fragments into the spinal canal, with or without an associated posterior ligamentous or bony injury or disc injury (Figures 38-1 and 38-2).

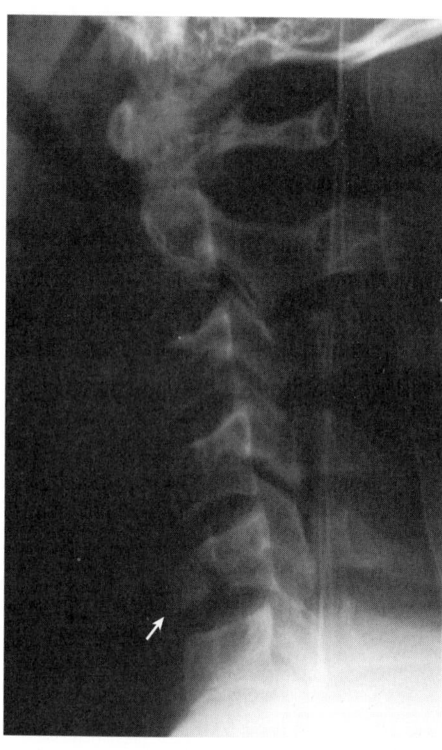

FIGURE 38-1 Cervical spine C5 burst fracture (lateral view). There is disruption of the vertebral body.

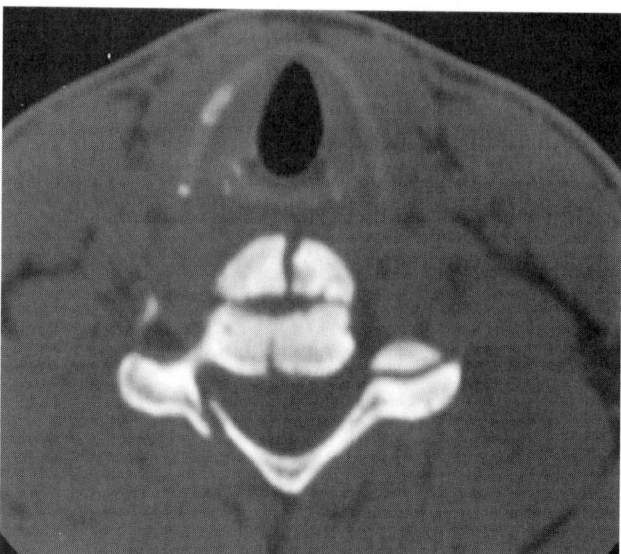

FIGURE 38-2 Computed tomography scan of C5 vertebral body, burst fracture. Note the destruction of the vertebral body and minimal disruption of the posterior aspect of the vertebral body. The lamina is also fractured.

Mechanism of Injury

Compression fractures in the lower cervical spine result from pure flexion forces and are commonly associated with motor vehicle accidents. A burst fracture is usually caused by axial loading in flexion. It is also commonly associated with motor vehicle accidents or with a fall from a height onto the head.

Radiographic Evaluation

The standard trauma series for these fractures consists of anteroposterior, lateral, and open-mouth (dens) views (Figure 38-3). Oblique radiographs may be added as needed to help visualize occult fractures, particularly of the laminae, facets, and pars interarticularis, or to further define the fracture anatomy. Compression fractures may be further evaluated by active flexion/extension lateral views to rule out posterior ligamentous instability. The patient must be awake and actively perform the flexion/extension maneuvers. The patient's head should never be passively moved to perform this radiographic examination.

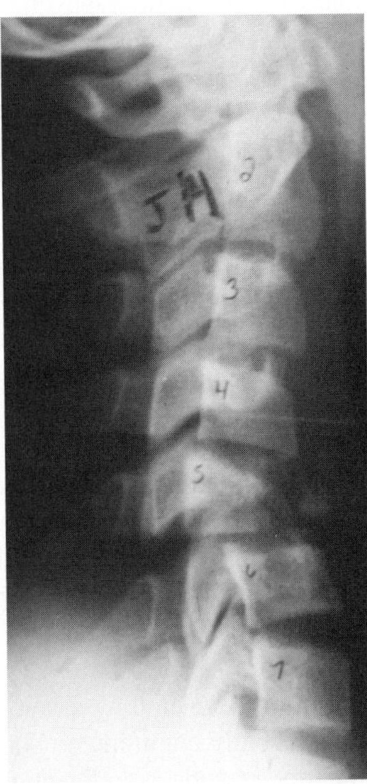

FIGURE 38-3 Severe burst fracture of C5 with ligamentous disruption of C4-5 and C5-6 (lateral view).

A computed tomography scan is often useful in differentiating a compression fracture from a burst fracture. The scan is also useful for evaluating the extent of spinal canal occlusion or compromise by retropulsed bone fragments in burst fractures. Thin axial cuts, as well as sagittal reconstructions, reveal the extent of the bony injury and canal compromise. A magnetic resonance imaging scan may also be useful to evaluate the status of the disc when neurologic impairment has occurred without any evidence of bony encroachment, as well as to assess the ligamentous structures.

Treatment Goals

Orthopaedic Objectives

1. Obtain and maintain spinal alignment and reduction of the fracture.
2. Provide spinal stability.
3. Prevent new neurologic deficits and attempt to improve and prevent the worsening of existing neurologic deficits.
4. Prevent future spinal deformity.

Rehabilitation Objectives

Range of motion

Restore range of motion in all planes without creating neurologic deficits (Table 38-1).

TABLE 38-1 *Range of Motion of the Cervical Spine*

Motion	Normal
Flexion*	65°
Extension*	65°
Lateral bend	45°
Rotation**	75°

*50% of flexion and extension occurs at occiput-C1 level.
**50% of rotation occurs at C1–2 level.

The above ranges vary depending on the patient's age. Different vertebral segments do not contribute equal amounts to the specific plane of motion. For example, C1-2 accounts for approximately 50% of cervical rotation. Occiput-C1 motion accounts for approximately 50% of flexion and extension. The remainder of motion is distributed almost evenly throughout the rest of the cervical spine, C2 through C7, with a slightly higher range of motion at C5-6.

Muscle Strength

Restore and maintain the strength of paracervical muscles, including the trapezius and the upper extremity muscles. Gluteal muscles are disturbed if an autologous bone graft is harvested for the purpose of fusion. The muscles of the lower extremities may atrophy from bed rest or neurologic injury and may require strengthening.

Functional Goals

Develop cervical spinal flexibility for functional independence.

Expected Time of Bone Healing

Six to 12 weeks for compression fracture and 8 to 12 weeks for a burst fracture.

Expected Duration of Rehabilitation

Three to 6 months.

Methods of Treatment

Orthosis (Hard Cervical Collar, Cervicothoracic Orthosis, Halo Vest)

Biomechanics: Stress-sharing device.

Mode of healing: Secondary.

Indications: A minor compression fracture without any posterior injury may be treated with a hard cervical collar or a cervicothoracic orthosis.

A burst fracture without significant comminution or neurologic compromise may be treated with a halo vest or a cervicothoracic orthosis. Some loss of reduction may be expected with this type of treatment, however, and careful follow-up evaluation is warranted. In cases with a significant amount of vertebral body comminution, longitudinal skull traction is used initially to obtain alignment. This may be sufficient to prevent further deformity and neurologic deterioration. After alignment is restored and vertebral body height improved through ligomentotaxis, a halo vest or cervicothoracic orthosis may be applied. However, one must be cautious when using any kind of orthosis, including a halo vest, for severely comminuted burst fractures. These devices do not provide significant resistance to axial compressive loads. Thus, there is high risk for loss of reduction once traction is discontinued and the patient is placed in one of these devices (see Figures 8–7, 8–8, 8–9, 8–10, and 8–11).

Surgery

Anterior decompression with strut graft fusion with or without anterior plating or with posterior wiring or plating; or posterior wiring or plating alone.

Biomechanics: Stress-sharing device.

Mode of bone healing: Secondary.

Indications: In compression fractures, it is imperative to rule out associated posterior ligamentous injury by active flexion/extension radiographs. If posterior ligamentous insufficiency is present, there is a high incidence of late angulation and progressive kyphosis. This is more likely to occur in fractures with 50% or more loss of anterior vertebral body height. In this select population with combined ligamentous injuries and compression fractures, early posterior fusion is indicated.

Burst fractures that result in continued anterior spinal cord compression and neurologic deficits after the application of longitudinal skull traction require surgical intervention. An anterior surgical decompression and fusion is warranted in a patient with an incomplete spinal cord injury and documented spinal cord compression on imaging studies. Furthermore, surgical stabilization is frequently performed for quadriplegic patients to facilitate early mobilization. An anterior decompression followed by an anterior strut graft with plating is the usual means of stabilizing these injuries.

The use of an orthosis, including a halo vest, is not recommended for severely comminuted burst fractures, because they do not provide significant resistance to axial compressive loads. In these situations, an anterior corpectomy and strut graft is recommended, often combined with anterior or posterior instrumentation.

Special Considerations of the Fracture

Comminuted burst fractures frequently result in spinal cord injury. Treatment varies according to the patient's neurologic status and the extent of the injury.

Treatment of burst fractures that involve the posterior column is controversial. These fractures are difficult to treat, because anterior surgery with a strut graft alone has a high incidence of graft dislodgement. An anterior plating may prevent this complication and obviate the need for any supplemental posterior fusion. One such fracture is the teardrop fracture-dislocation (*see* Figure 38–3). This severely unstable injury results from a high-energy compressive force and involves all three columns. This injury requires surgical intervention in the form of an anterior vertebrectomy and strut graft fusion with anterior plating. There is controversy as to whether a posterior fusion should also be performed because of the significant posterior injury. Treatment is thus determined by the extent of the instability for any particular fracture.

Associated Injuries

As in other cervical spine fractures, an associated head injury as well as brachial plexus traction injury should be ruled out. Other spinal fractures or injuries to the thorax, abdomen, or extremities should also be ruled out.

TREATMENT

Treatment: Early to Immediate (Day of Injury to One Week)

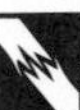

BONE HEALING

Stability at fracture site: Dependent upon intact bony and ligamentous elements, internal fixation, and external immobilization.

Stage of bone healing: Inflammatory phase. The fracture hematoma is colonized by inflammatory cells, and débridement of the fracture begins.

Stage of arthrodesis: Bone graft is at a similar phase.

X-ray: Fracture lines and bone graft are visible.

Orthopaedic and Rehabilitation Considerations

Physical Examination

The patient's neurologic status must be observed closely in the early postinjury period. Fracture displacement in this period can lead to direct neural compression or to epidural hematoma causing secondary compression. The patient requires operative intervention if there is an evolving neurologic deficit.

Dysphagia and dyspnea may be caused by prevertebral hematoma or soft tissue inflammation and may require intubation or operative intervention.

The cervical orthosis must fit snugly against the neck without causing any skin breakdown, especially along the mandible. Adjust and trim the orthosis as needed. The halo vest must be snug yet comfortable. The pin sites should be cleaned with hydrogen peroxide and an antibiotic ointment applied. The pin sites are checked and adjusted to a torque of 8 inch-pounds 24 to 48 hours after initial application. Reduction of pin pressure is normal as the outer table erodes from continued pressure applied by the pin. If the pin is loose, the halo becomes uncomfortable, and drainage from the pin sites may develop.

Dangers

The pins may be tightened if they loosen. It is important not to tighten the pins too much or too frequently, however, because this accelerates erosion of the cranium and may even result in penetration of the pin through the inner table of the skull. If purulent discharge is present, clean the pin sites twice daily with chlorhexidine and dress with gauze soaked in chlorhexidine solution or hydrogen peroxide. Oral antibiotics should be administered. If the drainage continues despite this treatment, the pin should be removed and a new pin placed at an adjacent threaded hole in the ring, without removing the halo. Intravenous antibiotics may be needed in some cases. Osteomyelitis is an uncommon complication. Pressure sores under the vest are also uncommon but elderly, debilitated, or insensate patients are at risk and should be monitored for this complication. Pressure sores can be avoided by meticulous hygiene and trimming of the vest to fit the patient's body. Bony prominences should be padded. Frequent log-rolling should be instituted every 2 to 4 hours. Special beds to prevent bed sores should be used for spinal cord–injured patients. In postsurgical patients, the incision must be checked for drainage and infection.

Radiography

Radiographs must be obtained to evaluate for maintenance of alignment. In a cervical compression fracture, it is often difficult to obtain adequate active flexion/extension films because muscle spasms occur in the early postinjury period. Thus, repeat active flexion/extension lateral cervical spine films should be obtained when the patient returns for follow-up at 1 to

2 weeks. At this point, muscle spasm has decreased and an adequate study may be obtained. Again, passive movement of the neck is forbidden when obtaining active flexion/extension radiographs.

Burst fractures that have been treated by a halo vest are carefully scrutinized for progressive collapse or progression to kyphosis in the first 4 weeks. If collapse or kyphosis is seen at the fracture site during this time period, the patient may require surgical intervention.

Weight Bearing

If neurologically intact, the patient should be mobilized to a sitting position in a bed or to a chair on day 1 following appropriate cervical immobilization (internal fixation or external bracing). Ambulation should begin with assistance as tolerated in neurologically intact patients. The tilt table may be required initially to address the problem of orthostatic hypotension. General conditioning should be ongoing. A patient who remains in cervical traction must be maintained at bed rest until further stability is achieved with fracture healing, allowing mobilization of the patient in a halo vest.

Range of Motion

No motion of the cervical spine is allowed until fracture healing or fusion is complete. Gentle active range of motion to the upper extremities is given. Active range of motion to the lower extremities prevents joint stiffness.

Muscle Strength

One-pound weights may be used to strengthen the upper extremities as long as the cervical spine is immobilized. Isometric exercises to the abdominal muscles are prescribed. Gluteal sets, quad sets, and ankle isotonic exercises are given to maintain strength in the lower extremities.

Functional Activities

Functional activities are highly dependent on the patient's neurologic status.

Bed mobility: Log-rolling is allowed for side-to-side mobility. Most patients need assistance for sitting, initially.

Transfers: Once the patient is brought to the seated position, he or she can come to the standing position with little assistance and transfer to a chair. Initially, the patient may benefit from using the tilt table if orthostatic hypotension or dizziness occurs.

Personal hygiene: Initially, the patient may have difficulty in self-care because of cervical immobilization and needs assistance in dressing, grooming, and personal hygiene.

Ambulation: Because of the presence of an orthosis, general weakness, and pain, the patient needs assistive devices such as a walker or cane for stability and balance. Nonetheless, patients must learn how to perform safe transfers using various techniques and, in cases of neurologic injury, how to use a wheelchair.

Gait

The gait may be wide-based because of the lack of stability. Upper arm swing excursion may be reduced because of pain. Push-off may be slightly reduced to avoid instability caused by the forward thrust of the body secondary to the orthosis.

Prescription

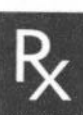

DAY ONE TO ONE WEEK

Precautions

Cervical spine immobilized.

Avoid overhead range of motion of the upper extremities.

Range of motion

No range of motion is allowed to the cervical spine.

Gentle active range of motion to the upper and lower extremities.

Strength

No strengthening exercises allowed to the cervical spine.

Abdominal, gluteal, and quadriceps isometric exercises.

If the cervical spine is immobilized, gentle strengthening exercises to both upper extremities.

Functional Activities

Bed mobility: log-rolling with assistance.

Transfers and ambulation: with assistive devices and with assistance.

Weight Bearing Weight bearing with assistive devices.

Treatment: 2 to 4 Weeks

BONE HEALING

Stability at fracture site: Stability continues to be a function of intact bony and ligamentous elements, internal fixation, and external immobilization.

Stage of bone healing: Reparative phase. Osteoprogenitor cells differentiate into osteoblasts, which lay down woven bone.

Stage of arthrodesis: Fibrovascular stroma arises.

X-ray: Fracture lines and graft remain visible. Early callus may be seen.

Orthopaedic and Rehabilitation Considerations

Physical Examination

Continue to follow the neurologic examination closely. Adjust and tighten the orthosis as necessary. Check for skin maceration beneath braces. Check the halo pin sites for drainage or loosening; they should be cleaned daily with hydrogen peroxide swabs. Oral antibiotics may be required to treat draining pin sites. If deep infection is present, the pins must be removed and their position changed, the pin sites débrided, and antibiotics administered.

Chin abrasions from cervical collars should be treated with padding beneath the chin. Staples or sutures are removed at approximately the 10th postoperative day. The head and neck remain immobilized.

Radiography

Same as for day 1 to 1 week (*see* page 539).

Range of Motion

Same as for day 1 to one week (*see* page 540).

Muscle Strength

Same as for day 1 to 1 week (*see* page 540).

Functional Activities

Same as for day 1 to 1 week (*see* page 540).

Gait

Same as for day 1 to 1 week (*see* page 540).

Prescription

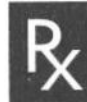

TWO TO FOUR WEEKS

Precautions Cervical spine is immobilized.

Range of motion

No range of motion is allowed to the cervical spine.

Active range of motion to the upper and lower extremities.

Strength

No strengthening exercises allowed to the cervical spine.

Abdominal, gluteal, and quadriceps isometric exercises.

Light isotonic exercises to the upper extremities.

Functional Activities

Bed mobility: log-rolling with assistance.

Transfers and ambulation: with assistive devices.

Weight Bearing Weight bearing with assistive devices.

Treatment: Four to Eight Weeks

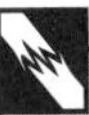

BONE HEALING

Stability: Early healing at the fracture sites and early graft consolidation give added stability.

Stage of bone healing: Reparative phase. Osteoblasts lay down woven bone. Callus is observed and graft consolidation may be seen where surgical fusion was performed.

X-ray: Fracture lines become obscured; bone graft is consolidating.

Orthopaedic and Rehabilitation Considerations

Physical Examination

Perform a neurologic examination, adjust orthotic as needed, and inspect pin sites.

Dangers

Be aware of any collapse at the fracture site or residual posterior instability in apparently minor compression fractures.

Radiography

Check cervical spine fracture alignment on radiograph.

Range of Motion

A patient with a stable fracture in a soft cervical collar may have only gentle active range of motion to the neck. The muscles are usually recovered enough to provide adequate control. The soft cervical collar is gradually discontinued as the neck musculature reconditions. Continue with upper and lower extremity range of motion exercises.

Muscle Strength

Do not attempt to strengthen cervical spine muscles, because spinal arthrodesis or fracture healing is not complete. However, in stable fractures, isometric strengthening exercises of the cervical spine may be started. The patient pushes on the head using one hand to offer resistance. Continue isometric exercises to the abdomen and strengthening exercises to the upper and lower extremities while the cervical spine is immobilized.

Muscle Strength

Same as for day 1 to 1 week (*see* page 540).

Functional Activities

Same as for day 1 to 1 week (*see* page 540).

Gait

Same as for day 1 to 1 week (*see* page 540). The patient is allowed full weight bearing.

Prescription

FOUR TO EIGHT WEEKS

Precautions No passive range of motion. Maintain immobilization in patients with unstable injuries.

Range of Motion Avoid range of motion to the cervical spine.

Strength

No strengthening exercises allowed to the cervical spine.

Abdominal, gluteal, and quadriceps isometric exercises.

Functional Activities

Bed mobility: log-rolling.

Transfers and ambulation: with assistive devices as needed.

Weight Bearing Full weight bearing.

Treatment: Eight to Twelve Weeks

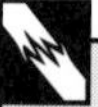

BONE HEALING

Stability: Bone stability achieved but ligamentous instability may persist.

Stage of bone healing: Remodeling phase. Woven bone is being replaced by lamellar bone. This takes months to years for completion.

Stage of arthrodesis: Trabeculation of fusion mass is occurring. Remodeling is an ongoing process.

X-ray: Fracture lines begin to disappear. Trabeculation of bone graft is at varying stages.

Orthopaedic and Rehabilitation Considerations

Orthoses can be discontinued for compression fractures. Patients who are treated with an orthosis for burst fracture are evaluated individually to determine whether the orthotic can be discontinued.

Radiography

Radiographs must be obtained after an orthosis is removed. Dynamic flexion and extension radiographs should be obtained to rule out residual instability. If instability is noted, further bracing or primary arthrodesis or revision surgery may be warranted.

Range of Motion

Gentle active range-of-motion exercises may begin for patients whose orthoses have been removed, as long as no instability exists, at 10 to 12 weeks.

After performing range-of-motion exercises, the patient may be more comfortable in a soft collar as a temporary support. Eventually, the collar will no longer be necessary.

Gentle, passive range of motion exercises can be initiated if the fracture is healed at 12 weeks. This allows the patient to regain the maximum range of motion of the neck. Passive exercises are given in flexion, extension, and rotation. Once maximal range of motion is achieved, the intensity of strengthening exercises can be increased. Because of stiffness and pain, especially in extension, the patient may require gentle active-assistive exercises. Active stretching of the trapezius and sternocleidomastoid muscles should continue to help in side bending and rotation of the neck.

Muscle Strength

Continue resistive exercises to the upper and lower extremities using weights. Continue isometric abdominal strengthening exercises. Sternocleidomastoid and trapezius muscle strengthening and stretching should continue to prevent stiffness and to help in rotation.

Functional Activities

Patients whose orthoses have been removed may start swimming. Running and jogging should be avoided, although fast walking is allowed. Contact sports are not permitted. Driving is permitted for patients who have adequate active range of motion and in whom the orthosis has been discontinued. A wide or panoramic rear-view mirror attachment may be needed if the patient's neck rotation remains limited. Patients whose orthoses have not been discontinued should not be permitted to drive.

Gait

The gait pattern should be normal.

Prescription

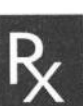

EIGHT TO TWELVE WEEKS

Precautions Be aware of ligamentous instability.

Range of Motion Gentle active range of motion to the cervical spine, if the fracture has healed, at 10 to 12 weeks. Passive range of motion is allowed at 12 weeks if the fracture has healed.

Strength Isometric strengthening exercises to the cervical spine as tolerated.

Functional Activities Independent in bed mobility, transfers, and ambulation.

Weight Bearing Full weight bearing.

Treatment: Twelve to Sixteen Weeks

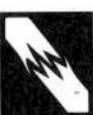

BONE HEALING

Stability: Stable.

Stage of bone healing and arthrodesis: Remodeling phase. Lamellar bone is replacing woven bone.

X-ray: Healed fractures, maturation of bone graft.

Orthopaedic and Rehabilitation Considerations

The orthosis is discontinued. Perform a neurologic examination, including reflexes and muscle strength testing. Evaluate wound healing, particularly at the former pin sites.

Dangers

Persistent ligamentous instability may place the neural structures at risk and cause pain.

Radiography

Flexion and extension radiographs are obtained to rule out residual instability, if this has not already been done. Follow-up radiographs should be obtained at 6-month to 1-year intervals to rule out the development of late instabilities or deformities. Posttraumatic degenerative changes may be seen.

Range of Motion

Restoration of functional range of motion should be achieved through active and passive exercises. Limitations may occur as a result of the extent of the arthrodesis and the loss of motion segments.

Muscle Strength

Continue stretching and strengthening the cervical spine muscles, including the trapezius and sternocleidomastoid to maintain rotation and lateral flexion.

Functional Activities

The patient may gradually return to sports activities except contact sports such as wrestling, boxing, diving, gymnastics, and football. Each activity should be evaluated separately.

Gait

The gait pattern should be normal at this point. Patients usually do not need any assistive devices for ambulation.

Prescription

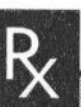

Twelve to Sixteen Weeks

Precautions No contact sports.

Range of Motion Active, gentle passive range of motion to the cervical spine.

Strength Isometric strengthening exercises to the cervical spine muscles.

Functional Activities Independent in transfers and ambulation.

Weight Bearing Full weight bearing.

LONG-TERM CONSIDERATIONS

Residual pain may require temporary bracing and antiinflammatory medications. Residual neurologic problems must be addressed and may require extremity bracing, therapy, or surgery for contracture releases and tendon transfers.

If progressive deformity occurs or instability persists, surgery may be necessary. There may be permanent loss of range of motion. Motion depends on the number of segments arthrodesed and the level and extent of the fracture. Removal of instrumentation may be necessary if it is painful. If pseudoarthrosis occurs, reinstrumentation and fusion may be necessary. Reflex sympathetic dystrophy may be a long-term problem requiring cervical stellate ganglion blocks and long-term physical therapy.

Bibliography: See page 559.

CHAPTER Thirty-nine

Cervical Spine Unilateral and Bilateral Facet Dislocation

ASHVIN I. PATEL, MD

BARON S. LONNER, MD

STANLEY HOPPENFELD, MD

INTRODUCTION

Definition

A unilateral facet dislocation is a forward rotation of one side of the vertebra about the contralateral facet joint, resulting in an ipsilateral facet dislocation (Figures 39-1 and 39-2). Clinically, a patient's head is axially rotated to the contralateral side and laterally tilted to the injured side.

A bilateral facet dislocation is the forward displacement of both facets, resulting in the inferior facets of the level above locking anterior to the superior facets of the level below (Figures 39-3 and 39-4). Most

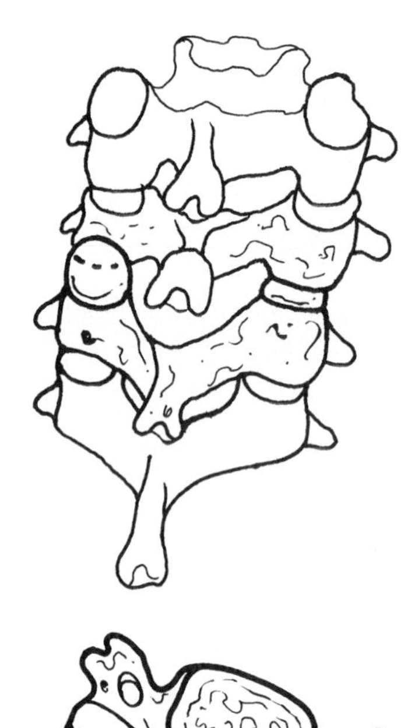

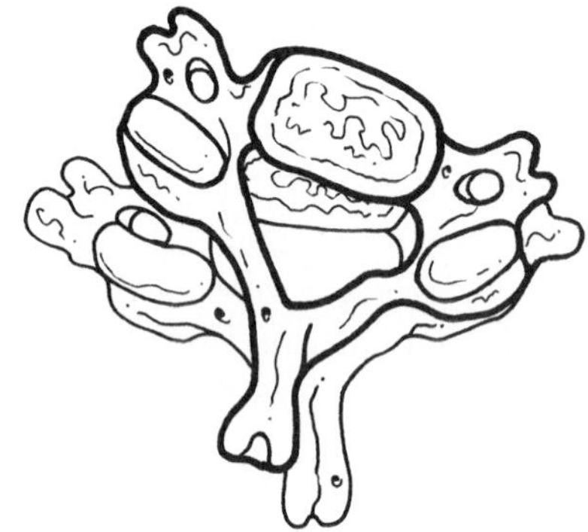

FIGURE 39-1 *(top)* Unilateral facet dislocation. The inferior facet overrides the superior facet unilaterally.

FIGURE 39-2 *(bottom)* Unilateral facet dislocation caused by rotation of one side of the vertebra about the opposite facet joint. This results in unilateral facet joint dislocation.

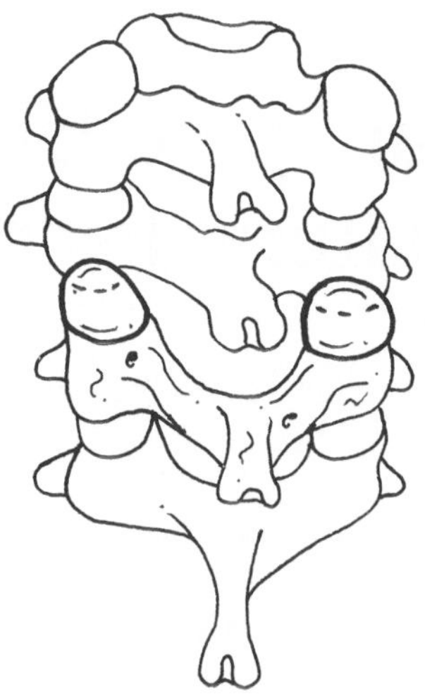

FIGURE 39-3 Bilateral facet dislocation. Forward displacement of both facets causes the inferior (descending) facets of a level above to lock anterior to the superior (ascending) facets of a level below.

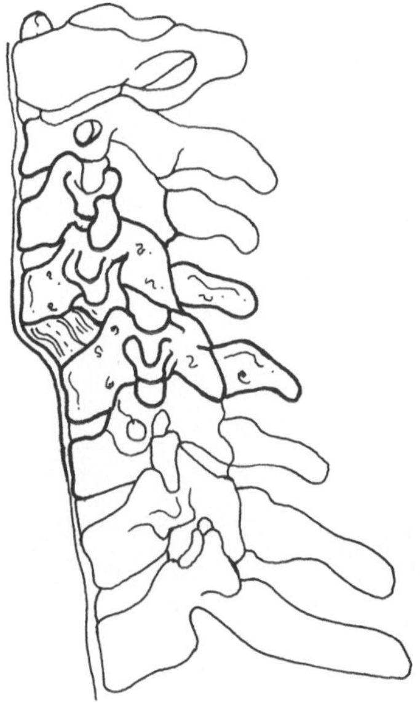

FIGURE 39-4 Bilateral facet dislocation of C4 on C5 with 50% anterior translation of the C4 vertebra. Most patients with bilateral facet dislocations have a complete neurologic deficit.

patients with bilateral facet dislocations have a complete neurologic deficit (quadriplegia).

Mechanism of Injury

These injuries generally result from a combination of flexion, distraction, and rotation. Significant destruction of the posterior ligaments and facet joint capsules occurs. Depending on the vector of injury and the position of the head at impact, there may or may not be associated fractures of the facets, lamina, or vertebral body. With more severe injuries, there may be disruption of the intervertebral disc and the only intact soft tissue structure may be the anterior longitudinal ligament.

Radiographic Evaluation

The standard trauma series for this cervical spine injury consists of anteroposterior, lateral, oblique, and open-mouth views.

In unilateral dislocations, the anteroposterior view may show the spinous process of the anteriorly subluxated vertebrae deviating toward the side of the dislocation. On the lateral view, there is approximately 25% anterior translation of the involved vertebral body in relation to the spinal column below this level (Figures 39-5 and 39-6). In addition, there is no overlap of the lateral masses of the anteriorly subluxated vertebrae, resulting in a typical bow-tie sign. On the oblique view, the inferior articular process is anterior in relation to the superior articular process of the subjacent vertebrae.

In bilateral facet dislocations, the lateral view shows a 50% or greater translation of the vertebral body and significant kyphosis is evident (Figures 39-7 and 39-8). On

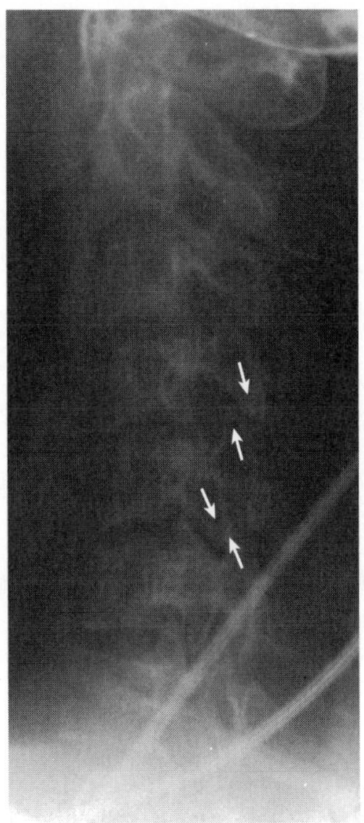

FIGURE 39-6 Unilateral facet dislocation of C5 on C6. See arrow. No neurologic deficit was present.

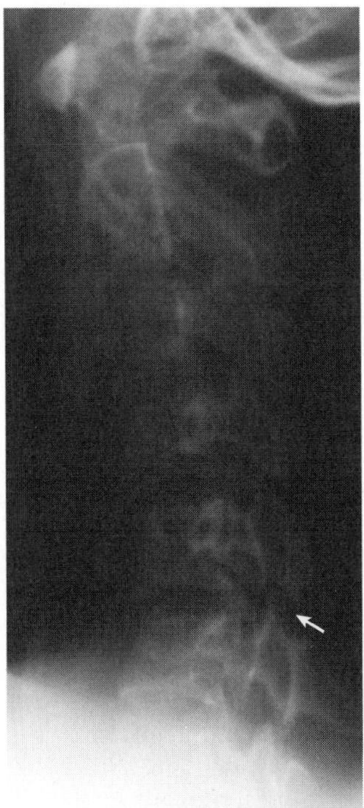

FIGURE 39-5 Lateral radiograph revealing unilateral facet dislocation of C5 on C6. The superior facet of C6 has moved posteriorly and superiorly to the inferior facet of C5. There is almost no translation of the vertebral bodies.

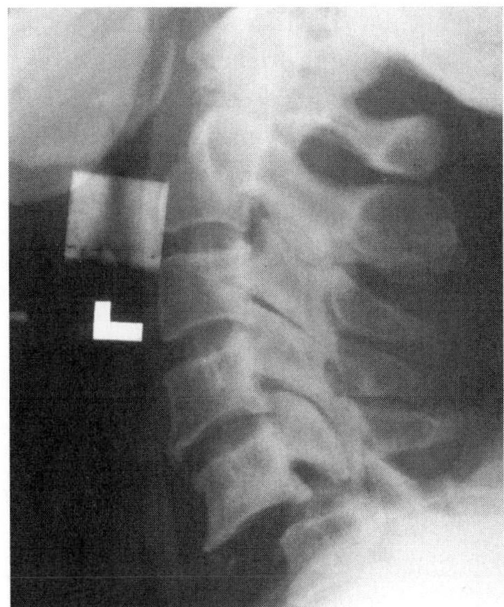

FIGURE 39-7 Bilateral facet dislocation with greater than 50% of vertebral body displacement of C5 on C6. The facets are bilaterally locked.

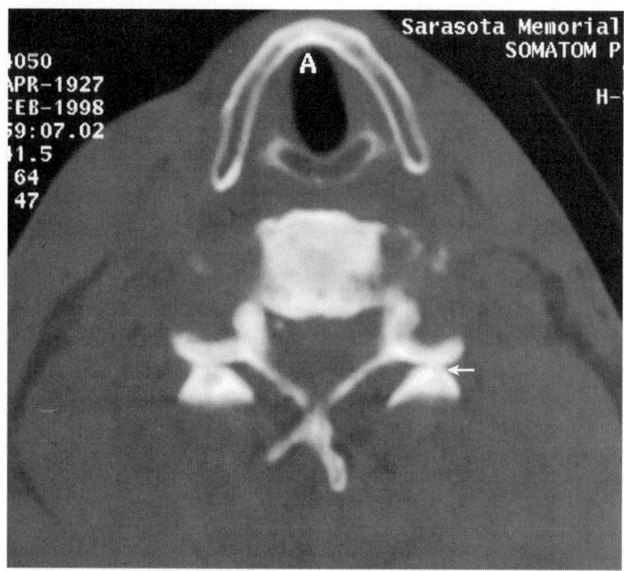

FIGURE 39-8 Computed tomography scan of C5. The facets are bilaterally dislocated.

the anteroposterior view, little or no rotation is evident. However, significant widening of the spinous processes is usually seen as a result of complete disruption of the interspinous ligaments with resulting kyphosis. An oblique radiograph demonstrates the inferior articular process on both sides, positioned anterior to the superior articular process of the subjacent vertebrae. If there is no frank dislocation, the facets may be perched so that the tip of the inferior articular process is locked into the tip of the superior articular process of the adjacent vertebrae.

A computed tomography scan with thin axial cuts and sagittal reconstruction is extremely useful in ruling out an associated fracture of the facets and the lamina.

A unilateral, and more frequently a bilateral, facet dislocation can be associated with a herniated intervertebral disc. It is suggested by many authors that a magnetic resonance imaging (MRI) scan of the cervical spine be obtained to assess the status of the disc in any patient with a unilateral or bilateral facet dislocation without neurologic deficit.

Treatment Goals

Orthopaedic Objectives

1. Obtain and maintain spinal alignment by reduction of the fracture or dislocation.
2. Provide spinal stability.
3. Prevent new neurologic deficits and attempt to improve and prevent the worsening of existing neurologic deficits.
4. Prevent future spinal deformity.

Rehabilitation Objectives

Range of motion

Restore functional and pain-free range of motion in all planes without creating neurologic deficits (Table 39-1).

TABLE 39-1 *Range of Motion of the Cervical Spine*

Motion	Normal
Flexion*	65°
Extension*	65°
Lateral bend	45°
Rotation**	75°

*50% of flexion and extension occurs at occiput-C1 level.
**50% of rotation occurs at C1–2 level.

The above ranges vary depending on the patient's age. Different vertebral segments do not contribute equal amounts to the specific plane of motion, for example, C1-2 accounts for approximately 50% of cervical rotation. Occiput-C1 motion accounts for approximately 50% of flexion and extension. The remaining motion is distributed almost evenly throughout the rest of the cervical spine, C2 through C7, with a slightly higher range of motion at C5-6.

Muscle Strength

Restore and maintain the strength of paracervical and scapular muscles, including the trapezius and the upper extremity muscles. Gluteal muscles are disturbed if an autologous bone graft is harvested for the purpose of fusion. The muscles of the lower extremities may atrophy from bed rest or neurologic injury and require strengthening.

Functional Goals

Develop cervical spinal flexibility for functional independence.

Expected Time of Bone Healing

A pure unilateral facet or bilateral facet dislocation is a ligamentous injury. Expected time of healing for these injuries is approximately 8 to 16 weeks. If an associated fracture was present at the time of the soft tissue injury or an arthrodesis had been performed as a definitive treatment, the expected time before arthrodesis or fracture healing has occurred is approximately 12 to 16 weeks.

Expected Duration of Rehabilitation

Three to 6 months.

Methods of Treatment

The definitive treatment for unilateral facet dislocation remains debated. The treatment for bilateral facet dislocations is generally reduction followed by surgical fusion (Figures 39-9 and 39-10).

Skeletal Traction (for Reduction) and Halo Vest

Biomechanics: Stress-sharing device.

Mode of healing: Ligamentous healing.

Indications: In general, a patient with a unilateral or bilateral facet dislocation with a neurologic deficit should undergo a closed reduction as soon as possible. An MRI scan is not necessary if the patient already has a partial or complete neurologic deficit. An attempt at

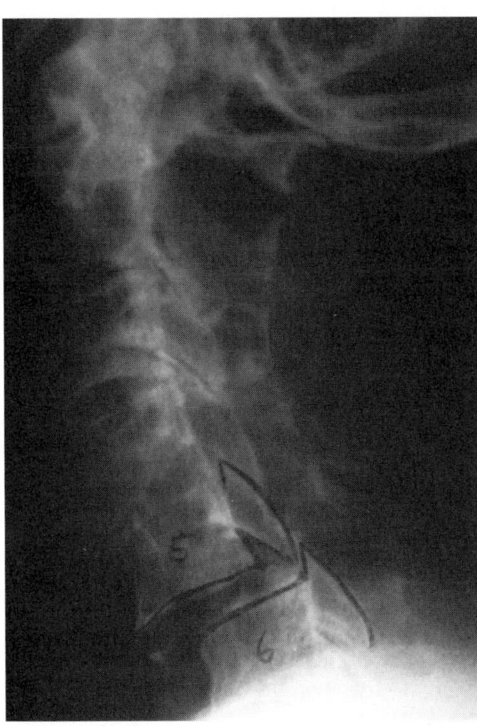

FIGURE 39-9 Bilateral cervical facet dislocation. Note the anterior translation of the vertebral body and the malposition of the facet joints.

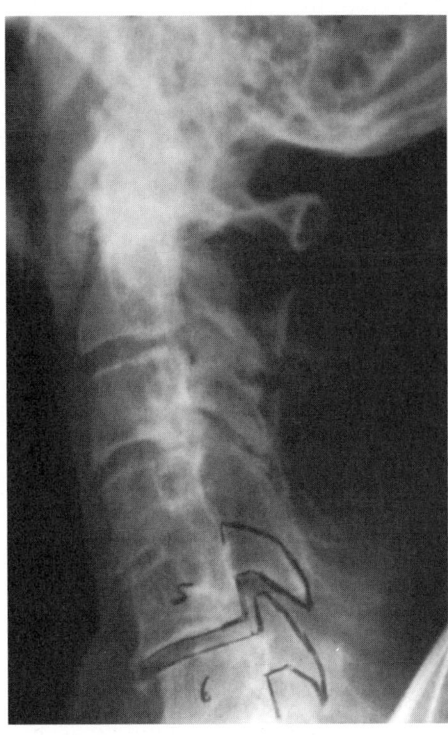

FIGURE 39-10 Post reduction of the bilateral facet joint with the use of Gardner-Wells tong traction. The patient was neurologically intact.

closed reduction with skeletal traction is made with the patient awake. The closed reduction is abandoned in favor of an MRI if a new neurologic deficit develops or there is progression of a previous deficit. Either Gardner-Wells tongs or a halo ring are used for the application of skeletal traction. (See Chapter 40, page 557 for instructions on how to apply Gardner-Wells tongs and halo). The tongs or halo pins are applied 1 cm posterior to the external auditory meatus and 1 cm above the pinna of the ear. Such posterior placement of the tongs permits greater flexion of the head and neck, thereby facilitating the reduction. Initially, 10 pounds of weight are applied, and a lateral radiograph is obtained to confirm that excessive distraction has not occurred.

If there is no evidence of a distraction injury, additional weights are then applied, in 5- to 10-pound increments, at 15- to 30-minute intervals. A lateral radiograph is obtained following each addition of weight to assess for reduction and possible overdistraction. Serial neurologic examinations are also performed during this procedure. If traction alone is insufficient to provide reduction (as is frequently the case with a unilateral facet dislocation), a reduction maneuver is indicated, with the patient awake. A transverse roll is placed beneath the patient's shoulders. The patient's neck is flexed and rotated to the opposite side of the injury. The facet is brought up into a perched position (tip of facets touching each other) with longitudinal traction, and then with maintenance of the traction, the neck is rotated back to the midline and gradually extended. If a new neurologic deficit or progression of an existing deficit appears during the manipulation, further attempts at closed reduction are contraindicated.

In a unilateral facet dislocation, a closed reduction is generally successful in only about 50% of cases. A unilateral facet dislocation that is successfully reduced by closed means may be treated in a halo vest for 3 months. However, there is an increasing tendency to perform a posterior spinal fusion for most unilateral facet injuries.

Bilateral facet dislocations are generally treated with posterior spinal fusion even after a successful closed reduction using skeletal traction.

Patients with unilateral or bilateral facet dislocation without a neurologic deficit and who are awake should undergo a closed reduction. If a neurologic deficit develops or a closed reduction is unsuccessful, then the patient should have an MRI scan done before open reduction. If a disc herniation is evident on MRI study, an emergent anterior discectomy and fusion should be performed.

If the patient is not awake, an MRI scan should be performed before any attempt is made at closed reduction. If a disc herniation is not found, then closed reduction should proceed. Any disc herniation should be treated with anterior discectomy and fusion followed by a posterior fusion.

Surgery

Posterior spinal fusion, anteroposterior spinal fusion, and a hard cervical collar.

Biomechanics: Stress-sharing device.

Mode of bone healing: Secondary.

Indications: When a manipulative reduction and traction is unsuccessful, an open posterior reduction, followed by a posterior fusion, is recommended.

A unilateral facet dislocation is a ligamentous injury that may involve the facet capsule, supraspinous ligaments, and interspinous ligaments. Complete soft tissue healing may not occur, even after a successful closed reduction and treatment with a halo vest, resulting in late instability and pain. Thus, many authors recommend a primary posterior fusion even after a successful closed reduction, especially in the presence of any neurologic deficits. A hard cervical collar is used postoperatively until a bony fusion has occurred.

Bilateral facet dislocations are generally treated by posterior spinal fusion after a closed or an open reduction.

If an extruded disc herniation is identified on the MRI scan, then an anterior discectomy should be performed before reduction. After discectomy, reduction can often be achieved with traction or use of a Caspar type distractor or a lamina spreader. If reduction occurs, then an anterior plating and interbody fusion should be performed. If reduction does not occur, a Smith-Robinson interbody graft is placed and the patient is turned prone for an open reduction and posterior fusion. If the graft displaces during the reduction, a third procedure may be performed to replace the graft.

Specific arthrodesis techniques for these injuries include interspinous wiring, lateral mass plating, and oblique wiring. Internal fixation devices are usually augmented with an orthosis until fusion occurs.

Special Considerations of the Fracture

The initial evaluation must include a thorough neurologic examination and search for associated injuries. In the patient with a unilateral or bilateral facet dislocation without neurologic deficit, traction should be applied with the patient awake so that the patient's neurologic status can be closely monitored. If closed reduction fails, a preoperative MRI scan should be obtained to rule out cervical disc herniation at the dislocated level, which could lead to catastrophic neurologic compromise at the time of operative reduction. If a herniated disc is present, an anterior cervical discectomy should be performed first. Other authors believe that a patient without a neurologic deficit should have an MRI scan done before any reduction maneuver is performed. Thus, in patients who have an associated extruded disc herniation, a closed reduction is not attempted in favor of an anterior discectomy and interbody fusion.

Associated Injuries

Associated head injuries or brachial plexus traction injuries and fractures should be ruled out. In addition, associated facet or lamina fractures at the level of the injury are frequently seen. Other cervical spine injuries as well as other noncontiguous fractures should also be ruled out, in addition to injuries of the thorax, abdomen, and extremities.

TREATMENT

Treatment: Early to Immediate (Day of Injury to One Week)

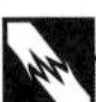

BONE HEALING

Stability at fracture (dislocation) site: Complex, depending on intact bony and ligamentous elements, internal fixation, and external immobilization.

Stage of bone healing: Inflammatory phase. The fracture hematoma is colonized by inflammatory cells and débridement of the fracture begins.

Stage of arthrodesis: Bone graft is at a similar phase.

X-ray: If an associated fracture was present, a fracture line is visible, and if a fusion was performed, the bone graft is visible. Facets should appear reduced and spinous processes aligned.

Orthopaedic and Rehabilitation Considerations

Physical Examination

The patient's neurologic status must be observed closely in the early postinjury period. A residual subluxation or a recurrent dislocation can occur, leading to direct neural compression with a new neurologic deficit or progression of an old deficit. The patient requires operative intervention in the case of an evolving neurologic deficit.

Dysphagia and dyspnea may be a result of prevertebral hematoma or soft tissue inflammation or prominent anterior hardware and may, on occasion, require intubation or operative intervention.

The cervical orthosis must fit snugly against the neck without causing any skin breakdown. Adjust and trim the orthosis as needed.

The halo vest must also be snug yet comfortable. The pin sites should be cleaned with hydrogen peroxide and an antibiotic ointment applied. The pin sites are checked and adjusted to a torque of 8 inch-pounds, 24 to 48 hours after initial application. Reduction of pin pressure is normal, because the outer table tends to erode from continued pressure applied by the pin. If the pin is loose, the halo becomes uncomfortable, and drainage from the pin sites may develop.

Dangers

If a halo vest has been used, the pins may be tightened if they loosen. It is important not to tighten the pins too much or too frequently, however, because this accelerates erosion of the cranium and may even result in penetration of the pin through the inner table of the skull. If purulent discharge is present, this can be managed by twice-daily cleaning of the pin sites with chlorhexidine and dressing with gauze soaked in chlorhexidine solution or hydrogen peroxide. Oral antibiotics should be administered. If the drainage continues despite this treatment, the pin should be removed and a new pin placed at an adjacent threaded hole in the ring, without removing the halo. Intravenous antibiotics may be needed in some cases. Osteomyelitis is an uncommon complication. Pressure sores under the vest are also uncommon in most patients. However, elderly, debilitated or insensate patients are at risk and should be monitored for this complication. Pressure sores can be avoided by meticulous hygiene and trimming of the vest as needed. Bony prominences should be padded to avoid any skin breakdown. Frequent log-rolling, every 2 to 4 hours, should be instituted. Special beds for the prevention of decubiti should be used for spinal cord–injured patients. If surgery has been performed, the incision must be checked for drainage and infection.

If the patient was rendered quadriplegic as a result of an injury, special care must be provided to prevent complications such as ischial decubiti, atelectasis, pneumonia, fecal impaction, and urinary retention.

Radiography

Radiographs must be evaluated for maintenance of alignment and to evaluate the position of the hardware if surgical intervention was performed.

Weight Bearing

If neurologically intact, the patient should be mobilized to a sitting position in a bed or to a chair on day 1 following appropriate cervical immobilization (internal fixation or external bracing). Ambulation should begin with assistance as needed. The tilt table may be required to address the problem of orthostatic hypotension. General conditioning should be ongoing.

If the patient was rendered quadriplegic, he or she should be mobilized to a wheelchair.

Range of motion

No motion of the cervical spine is allowed until fracture healing or fusion is complete. Depending on the neurologic status, active range of motion of the upper and lower extremities is encouraged. If this is not possible, passive range of motion is begun immediately to prevent joint stiffness of the extremities.

Muscle Strength

Again, depending on the neurologic status, 1-pound weights may be used to strengthen the upper extremities as long as the cervical spine is immobilized. Isometric exercises to the abdominal muscles are prescribed. Gluteal sets, quad sets, and ankle isotonics are given to maintain strength in the lower extremities.

Functional Activities

Bed mobility, transfers and personal hygiene are highly dependent on the patient's neurologic status. The patient requires varying degrees of assistance depending on the level of deficit.

Special orthotics and a motorized wheelchair may be necessary. These orthotics can make a great deal of difference in the patient's functional level.

Gait

The patient who is ambulatory needs assistive devices such as a walker or cane for stability and balance, because of the presence of an orthosis, generalized weakness or partial neurologic injury, and pain. Nonambulatory patients need to learn how to perform safe transfers using various techniques as well as how to use a wheelchair.

Prescription

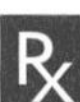

DAY ONE TO ONE WEEK

Precautions Cervical spine immobilized.

Range of Motion

No range of motion is allowed to the cervical spine.

Gentle active range of motion to the upper and lower extremities.

Strength

No strengthening exercises allowed to the cervical spine.

Isometric exercises to the abdominals, gluteals, and quadriceps in neurologically intact patients.

If the cervical spine is immobilized, gentle strengthening exercises to both upper extremities in intact patients. Passive range of motion in neurologically impaired patients to prevent contractures.

Functional Activities

Bed mobility: log-rolling with assistance.

Transfers and ambulation: with assistive devices and with assistance.

Weight Bearing: Full weight bearing with assistive devices in neurologically intact patients.

Treatment: Two to Four Weeks

Bone Healing

Stability at fracture site: Stability continues to be a function of intact bony and ligamentous elements, internal fixation, and external immobilization.

Stage of bone healing: Reparative phase. Osteoprogenitor cells differentiate into osteoblasts, which lay down woven bone.

Stage of arthrodesis: Fibrovascular stroma arises.

X-ray: Fracture lines and graft remain visible. Early callus may be seen in cases of fracture.

Orthopaedic and Rehabilitation Considerations

Physical Examination

Continue to assess the neurologic status closely. Adjust and tighten the orthosis as necessary. Check for skin maceration beneath braces. Check the halo pin sites for drainage or loosening; they should be cleaned daily with hydrogen peroxide swabs. Oral antibiotics may be required to treat draining pin sites. If deep infection is present, the pins must be removed and their position changed, the pin sites débrided, and intravenous antibiotics administered.

Chin abrasions from cervical collars should be treated with padding beneath the chin. Staples or sutures are removed at approximately the 10th to 14th postoperative day. The head and neck remain immobilized.

Radiography

Radiographs must be inspected for maintenance of alignment and for satisfactory position of surgical hardware.

Range of motion

Range of motion to the cervical spine is not permitted because the injured spinal segment is not stable. Bone and ligamentous healing has not occurred. Therefore, the spinal cord and nerve roots are still at risk for potential injury. Continue with upper and lower extremity range of motion exercises as applicable.

Strength

Same as for day 1 to 1 week (*see* page 552).

Functional Activities

Same as for day 1 to 1 week (*see* page 552).

Gait

Same as for day 1 to 1 week (*see* page 552).

Prescription

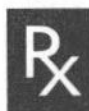

Two to Four Weeks

Precautions Maintain cervical spine immobilization.

Range of Motion

No range of motion to the cervical spine.

Active range of motion to the upper and lower extremities.

Strength

No strengthening exercises to the cervical spine.

Isometric exercises to the abdominals, gluteals, and quadriceps in neurologically intact patients.

If the cervical spine is immobilized, gentle strengthening exercises to both upper extremities in intact patients. Passive range of motion in neurologically impaired patients to prevent contractures.

Functional Activities

Bed mobility: log-rolling with assistance.

Transfers and ambulation: with assistive devices and with assistance.

Weight Bearing Full weight bearing with assistive devices as needed.

Treatment: Four to Eight Weeks

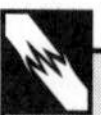

Bone Healing

Stability: Early healing at the injury sites and early graft consolidation give added stability.

Stage of bone healing: Reparative phase. Osteocytes lay down woven bone. Callus is observed in cases in which there are associated fractures, and graft consolidation may be seen where arthrodesis was performed. Ligamentous healing continues.

X-ray: Fracture lines when present become obscured; bone graft is consolidating.

Orthopaedic and Rehabilitation Considerations

Physical Examination

Perform a neurologic examination to document that a change has not occurred, adjust orthotic as needed, and inspect pin sites.

Dangers

If a halo vest has been used, the pins may be tightened if they loosen. It is important not to tighten the pins too much or too frequently, however, because this accelerates erosion of the cranium and may even result in penetration of the pin through the inner table of the skull. If purulent discharge is present, this can be managed by twice-daily cleaning of the pin sites with chlorhexidine and dressing with gauze soaked in chlorhexidine solution or hydrogen peroxide. Oral antibiotics should be administered. If the drainage continues despite this treatment, the pin should be removed and a new pin placed at an adjacent threaded hole in the ring, without removing the halo. Intravenous antibiotics may be needed in some cases. Osteomyelitis is an uncommon complication. Pressure sores under the vest are also uncommon in most patients, but elderly, debilitated, or insensate patients are at risk and should be monitored for this complication. Pressure sores can be avoided by meticulous hygiene and trimming of the vest as needed.

Bony prominences should be padded to avoid any skin breakdown. Frequent log-rolling should be instituted. Special beds for prevention of decubiti should be used for spinal cord–injured patients. In patients in whom surgery has been performed, the incision must be checked for drainage and infection.

If the patient was rendered quadriplegic as a result of his or her injury, special care must be given to prevent complications such as ischial decubiti, atelectasis, pneumonia, fecal impaction, and urinary retention.

Radiography

Radiographs must be inspected for maintenance of reduction, alignment, and satisfactory position of the hardware.

Range of Motion

Range of motion to the cervical spine is not permitted.

Muscle Strength

Do not attempt to strengthen the cervical spine muscles, because spine arthrodesis is not complete. Continue with isometric exercises to the abdomen and strengthening exercises to the upper and lower extremities while the cervical spine is immobilized.

Muscle Strength

Same as for day 1 to 1 week (*see* page 552).

Functional Activities

Same as for day 1 to 1 week (*see* page 552).

Gait

Same as for day 1 to 1 week (*see* page 552).

Prescription

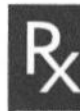

Four to Eight Weeks

Precautions Maintain cervical spine immobilization.

Range of Motion

No range of motion to the cervical spine.

Active range of motion to the upper and lower extremities.

Strength

No strengthening exercises to the cervical spine.

Isometric exercises to the abdominals, gluteals, and quadriceps in neurologically intact patients.

If the cervical spine is immobilized, gentle strengthening exercises to both upper and lower extremities in intact patients. Passive range of motion in neurologically impaired patients to prevent contractures.

Functional Activities

Bed mobility: log-rolling with assistance.

Transfers and ambulation: with assistive devices and with assistance.

Weight Bearing Full weight bearing with assistive devices as needed.

Treatment: Eight to Twelve Weeks

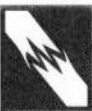

Bone Healing

Stability: Bone stability is achieved but ligamentous instability may persist.

Stage of bone healing: Remodeling phase. Woven bone is replaced by lamellar bone. This takes months to years for completion. Ligamentous healing continues.

Stage of arthrodesis: Trabeculation of fusion mass is occurring. Remodeling is an ongoing process.

X-ray: Fracture lines begin to disappear. Trabeculation of bone graft is at varying stages.

Orthopaedic and Rehabilitation Considerations

Orthoses can be discontinued in surgical patients whose arthrodesis is solid. Patients who undergo non-operative treatment with the halo vest should have the vest and the ring removed at 12 weeks to obtain active flexion/extension radiographs of the cervical spine. The halo pins are left in place in case instability is present and the patient must be immobilized for a longer period of time. They may otherwise undergo a spinal fusion.

Radiography

Radiographs must be obtained after an orthosis is removed. Dynamic active flexion/extension radiographs should be obtained to rule out residual instability. If instability is noted, further immobilization may be necessary or a primary arthrodesis or revision surgery may be warranted.

Range of motion

Gentle active range-of-motion exercises may begin in patients whose immobilization has ended, as long as no instability exists.

After performing range-of-motion exercises, the patient may be more comfortable in a soft collar as a temporary support. Eventually, the collar will no longer be necessary.

This allows the patient to regain the maximum range of motion of the neck. Passive range is given in flexion, extension, and rotation. Once maximal range of motion is achieved, the intensity of strengthening exercises can be increased. Because of stiffness and pain, especially in extension, the patient may require gentle active-assistive exercises. Active stretching of the trapezius and sternocleidomastoid muscles should be initiated to help in side bending and rotation of the neck.

Muscle Strength

Continue resistive exercises to the upper and lower extremities using weights in patients who are neurologically intact. Also continue with isometric abdominal strengthening exercises. Sternocleidomastoid and trapezius muscle strengthening and stretching should continue to prevent stiffness and to help in rotation.

Functional Activities

By this time, the patient should be independent in all self-care and grooming activities and should not require assistive devices for ambulation unless there is neurologic involvement or the patient is elderly and requires this for stability.

The patient may begin swimming but should avoid jogging; fast walking is allowed. Contact sports are not yet permitted. Decisions on whether the patient can resume driving are based on whether the patient can achieve satisfactory active range of motion. A wide or panoramic rear-view mirror attachment may be needed if the patient's neck rotation remains limited.

In neurologically impaired patients, consideration as to whether any orthotic devices can be prescribed to enhance patient independence is essential. In addition, tendon transfers can be performed to achieve the same goal.

Gait

The gait pattern should be normal in neurologically intact patients.

Dangers

Persistent ligamentous instability may place the neural structures at risk and cause pain.

Prescription

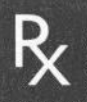

Eight to Twelve Weeks

Precautions Be aware of persistent ligamentous instability.

Range of Motion Gentle active and passive range of motion to the cervical spine if the fracture has healed.

Strength Isometric strengthening exercises to the cervical spine as tolerated.

Functional Activities Independent in bed mobility, transfers, and ambulation in neurologically intact patients.

Weight Bearing Full weight bearing in neurologically intact patients.

Treatment: Twelve to Sixteen Weeks

BONE HEALING

Stability: Stable.

Stage of bone healing and arthrodesis: Remodeling phase. Woven bone is replaced by lamellar bone.

X-ray: Any fractures that were present should be healed. There is maturation of bone graft in surgically treated patients. Ligamentous instability may still be present as evidenced by motion on dynamic active flexion/extension radiographs.

Orthopaedic and Rehabilitation Considerations

All orthoses are generally discontinued by 16 weeks. Perform a neurologic examination, including reflexes and muscle strength testing. Evaluate wound healing, particularly at the former pin sites.

Dangers

Persistent ligamentous instability may place the neural structures at risk and cause pain.

Radiography

Flexion and extension radiographs are obtained to rule out residual instability, if this has not already been done. Follow-up radiographs should be obtained at 6-month to 1-year intervals to rule out the development of late instabilities or deformities. Posttraumatic degenerative changes may be seen.

Range of Motion

Functional range of motion should be obtainable with the use of active and passive exercises. Limitations may occur as a result of the extent of the arthrodesis and the loss of motion segments.

Muscle Strength

Continue stretching and strengthening the cervical spine muscles, including the trapezius and sternocleidomastoid to maintain rotation and lateral flexion.

Functional Activities

In patients without neurologic deficits, a gradual return to sports should be permitted. Patients should be restricted from contact sports such as wrestling, boxing, diving, gymnastics, and football. Each activity should be evaluated individually.

Gait

The patient should have a normal gait if he or she is neurologically intact.

Prescription

TWELVE TO SIXTEEN WEEKS

Precautions No contact sports.

Range of Motion Active, gentle, passive range of motion to the cervical spine.

Strength Isometric strengthening exercises to the cervical spine muscles.

Functional Activities Neurologically intact patients are independent in transfers and ambulation.

Weight Bearing Full weight bearing for neurologically intact patients.

LONG-TERM CONSIDERATIONS

Residual pain may require temporary bracing and antiinflammatory medications. Residual neurologic problems must be addressed and may require extremity bracing, therapy, or surgery for contracture releases and tendon transfers.

If progressive deformity occurs, surgery may be necessary. If hardware failure occurs, surgery may also be necessary. There may be permanent loss of range of motion. The extent depends on the number of segments arthrodesed and the level and extent of the fracture.

Removal of instrumentation may be necessary if it is painful. If pseudoarthrosis occurs, reinstrumentation and fusion may be necessary. Reflex sympathetic dystrophy may be a long-term problem requiring cervical stellate ganglion blocks and long-term physical therapy.

Bibliography: See page 559.

CHAPTER *Forty*

Application of Gardner-Wells Tongs and Halo Vest

ASHVIN I. PATEL, MD

STANLEY HOPPENFELD, MD

BARON S. LONNER, MD

INTRODUCTION

Definition

Gardner-Wells Tongs

The patient's head is prepared with an antiseptic solution just above the ear. A local anesthetic is applied just above the external auditory meatus of the ear, below the greatest diameter of the skull. Usually, a 1% lidocaine solution is sufficient. The area is infiltrated down to the periosteum of the outer table of the skull. A slightly more anterior or posterior placement may be used to obtain an extension or flexion vector, respectively, while in traction. The bolts are advanced until the indicator on the side protrudes 1 mm. Lock nuts are tightened, and traction is applied by way of a hook at the end of the ring. The apparatus is inspected every 6 hours for the first 24 hours to check for appropriate alignment and tension.

Crutchfield's rule of 5 pounds per level, starting with 10 pounds for the head, is used as a general guideline in determining the amount of traction to be applied. After the first 10 pounds are applied, a lateral radiograph is obtained to check the position of the spine and to rule out any distraction. Every 15 to 30 minutes, an additional 5 to 10 pounds are added, depending on the level of the injury. If necessary, up to 60 to 70 pounds of traction for lower cervical injuries can be applied safely in select cases. Adequate relaxation must be obtained to overcome the effect of muscle spasm, which might prevent a reduction of a fracture or dislocation (Figures 40-1 and 40-2).

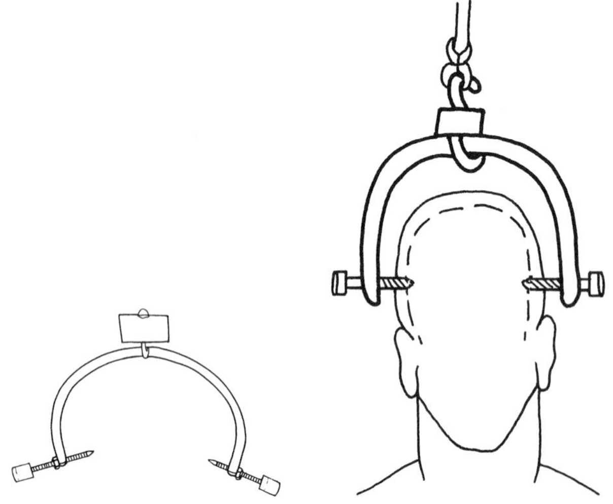

FIGURE 40-1 *(far left)* Gardner-Wells tongs. These tongs are effective in reducing cervical spine fractures and dislocations.

FIGURE 40-2 *(left)* Garner-Wells tongs used to apply cervical traction. Pins pierce the skin and outer table of the cranium. Various amounts of traction are applied to reduce the fracture/dislocation.

Halo Vest

Halo application generally requires three people. First, determine the proper size of the ring and vest necessary for the patient. The ring should give 2 cm of clearance around the equator of the head (the greatest diameter of the skull). In general, the halo is applied below the equator of the head, to prevent the halo from sliding off superiorly.

The patient is positioned supine in the bed, with the head held beyond the edge of the bed by one person. This person holds the head throughout the procedure. If there is a canvas gurney available, the head can be placed in this gurney for support.

The ring is slipped over the head and held in position below the equator of the skull, approximately 1 cm above the helix of the ear. Appropriate holes in the ring are selected for pin placement. The anterolateral pin is placed approximately 1 cm superior to the eyebrow, on the lateral two thirds of the supraorbital region, below the equator. Medial to this pin is the supraorbital nerve and artery. Posterior and lateral to this pin is the superior temporal artery. Be careful to avoid placement too far posterior in the temporalis muscle, or this will result in pain during chewing, and possible penetration of the pin through the inner table of the cranium, which is quite thin in the area of the temporalis fossa.

The area is infiltrated with 1% lidocaine down to the outer column of the skull. The pin is applied in a sterile fashion without any prior skin incision and is advanced perpendicular to the skull surface using a torque screw wrench. During the anterolateral pin placement, the patient is asked to close the eyes and relax the forehead. This helps to prevent skin or eyebrow tenting, which can subsequently hinder closing of the eye. The posterolateral pin is placed just above the external auditory meatus, as in the application of the Gardner-Wells tongs. The right posterolateral pin should be in a position 180 degrees from the left anterolateral pin (diagonally across). While the ring is held in position by the second person, two corresponding diagonal pins are advanced simultaneously through the skin to penetrate the outer cortex of the skull. Diagonally opposite pins are tightened with a torque wrench at 2 inch-pound increments until they are seated at 8 inch-pounds. The remaining diagonally located pins are then advanced in a similar fashion, and the locking nuts are applied to the pins (Figure 40-3).

While cervical traction is maintained, the patient's trunk is flexed at the hips to 30 degrees in order to position the vest. The posterior half of the vest is posi-

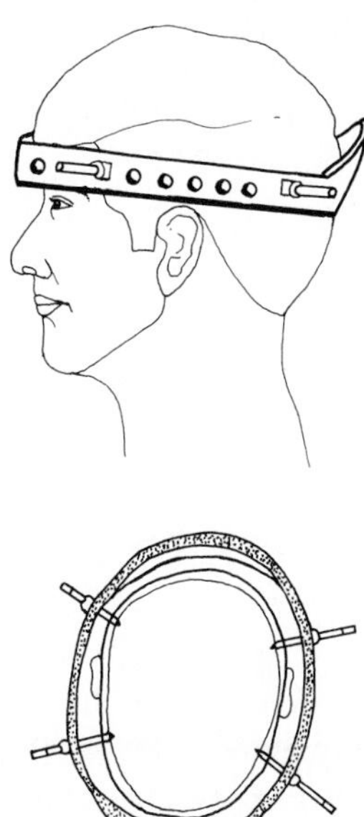

FIGURE 40-3 The ring is placed over the head and held at the equator of the skull, approximately 1 cm above the pinna of the ear. The four pins are placed into calvarium, diagonally to one another. The remaining diagonally located pins are then advanced in a similar manner and the locking nuts are applied to the pins.

tioned and held in place, followed by the anterior half of the vest. The upright posts and connecting rods are provisionally secured to the vest. The head and neck are positioned, and all remaining bolts and joins are secured. A radiograph of the cervical spine is taken to confirm satisfactory alignment and reduction of the fracture or dislocation. Following the initial application, the pins are retightened once, to 8 inch-pounds, 48 hours after application.

BIBLIOGRAPHY

Aebi M, Etter C, Coscia M. Fractures of the odontoid process: treatment with anterior screw fixation. *Spine,* 14:1065–1070, 1989.

Allen BL Jr, Ferguson RL, Lehmann TR, et al. A mechanistic classification of closed, indirect fractures and dislocations of the lower cervical spine. *Spine,* 7:1–27, 1982.

Anderson LD, D'Alonzo RT. Fractures of the odontoid process of the axis. *J Bone Joint Surg,* 56A:1663–1674, 1974.

Bohlman HH. Acute fractures and dislocations of the cervical spine: an analysis of three hundred hospitalized patients and review of the literature. *J Bone Joint Surg,* 61A:1119–1142, 1979.

Clark CR, White AA. Fractures of the dens: a multicenter study. *J Bone Joint Surg,* 67A:1340–1348, 1985.

Eismont FJ, Arena MJ, Green BA. Extrusion of an intervertebral disc associated with traumatic subluxation or dislocation of cervical facets: case report. *J Bone Joint Surg,* 73A:1555–1560, 1991.

Esses SI, Bednar DA. Screw fixation of odontoid fractures and nonunions. *Spine,* 16(suppl 10):S483-S485, 1991.

Fielding JW, Francis WR Jr, Hawkins RJ, et al. Traumatic spondylolisthesis of the axis. *Clin Orthop,* 239:47–52, 1989.

Garfin SF, Botte MJ, Waters RL, et al. Complications in the use of the halo fixation device. *J Bone Joint Surg,* 68A:320–326, 1986.

Jeanneret B, Magerl F. Primary posterior fusion C1/C2 in odontoid fractures: indications, technique, and results of transarticular screw fixation. *J Spin Disord,* 5:464–475, 1992.

Kasser JR, ed. *Orthopaedic Knowledge Update 5 Home Study Syllabus.* Rosemont, IL: American Academy of Orthopaedic Surgeons, 1996, pp. 577–579.

Levine AM, ed. *Orthopaedic Knowledge Update: Trauma.* Rosemont, IL: American Academy of Orthopaedic Surgeons, 1996, pp. 317–339.

Levine AM, section ed. Spine and pelvis. In: Browner BD, et al, eds. *Skeletal Trauma.* Philadelphia: W.B. Saunders, 1992, pp. 665–728.

Levine AM, Edwards CC. Fractures of the atlas. *J Bone Joint Surg,* 73A:680–691, 1991.

Levine AM, Edwards CC. The management of traumatic spondylolisthesis of the axis. *J Bone Joint Surg,* 67A:217–226, 1985.

Levine AM, Edwards CC. Treatment of injuries in the C1-C2 complex. *Orthop Clin North Am* 17:31–44, 1986.

Montesano PX, Anderson PA, Schlehr F, et al. Odontoid fractures treated by anterior odontoid screw fixation. *Spine,* 16:S33–S37, 1991.

Robertson PA, Ryan MD. Neurological deterioration after reduction of cervical subluxation: mechanical compression by disc tissue. *J Bone Joint Surg,* 74B:224–227, 1992.

Star AM, Jones AA, Cotler JM, et al. Immediate closed reduction of cervical spine dislocations using traction. *Spine,* 15:1068–1072, 1990.

White AA III, Panjabi MM, eds. *Clinical Biomechanics of the Spine,* 2nd ed. Philadelphia: J.B. Lippincott, 1990.

CHAPTER Forty-one

Thoracolumbar Spine Fractures

BARON S. LONNER, MD

STANLEY HOPPENFELD, MD

ASHVIN I. PATEL, MD

INTRODUCTION

Definition

Thoracolumbar spinal fractures can be divided into *thoracic* and *thoracolumbar* fractures. They are distinguished by the anatomic and pathomechanical characteristics on which treatment is based.

A number of systems have been used to classify thoracolumbar spinal fractures based on the mechanism of injury. The Denis classification, which is widely used, is based on a three-column biomechanical model of the spine. The anterior column is composed of the anterior longitudinal ligament and the anterior portion of the vertebral body. The middle column consists of the posterior portion of the vertebral body and the posterior longitudinal ligament. The posterior column is composed of the posterior elements (Figure 41-1). Based on a review of 412 cases, Denis classified thoracic and lumbar fractures into minor and major injuries. Minor injuries consisted of spinous process, transverse process fractures, and facet fractures. The more significant major injuries are categorized as compression fractures, burst fractures, flexion/distraction injuries, and fracture/dislocations.

Whatever classification system is used, it is important to understand the complete nature of the injury in order to devise an appropriate treatment plan. The treatment of individuals with neurologic injuries (paraplegia) is not considered in this chapter; however, the patient's neurologic status plays a role in deciding whether surgery is indicated.

Mechanism of Injury

Thoracolumbar fractures can result from high-energy trauma or, commonly, from minor trauma coupled with osteoporosis, which weakens the structural integrity of individual vertebrae (Figure 41-2). Fractures occurring

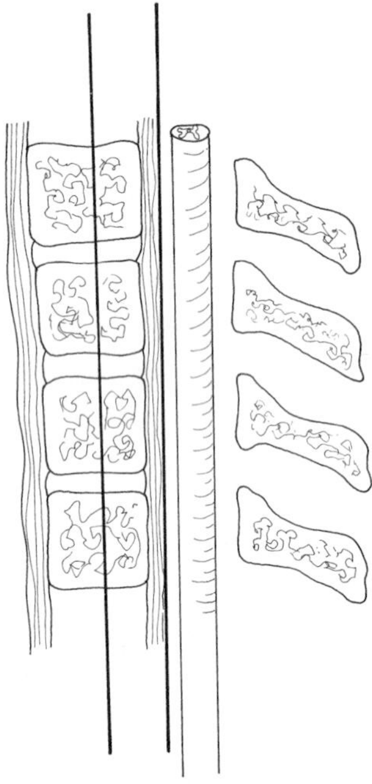

FIGURE 41-1 The Denis classification, based on the three-column biomechanical model of the spine. The anterior column is composed of the anterior longitudinal ligament and the anterior portion of the vertebral body. The middle column consists of the posterior portion of the vertebral body and the posterior longitudinal ligament. The posterior column is composed of the posterior elements: the spinous processes, transverse processes, pedicles, facet joints, and associated ligaments.

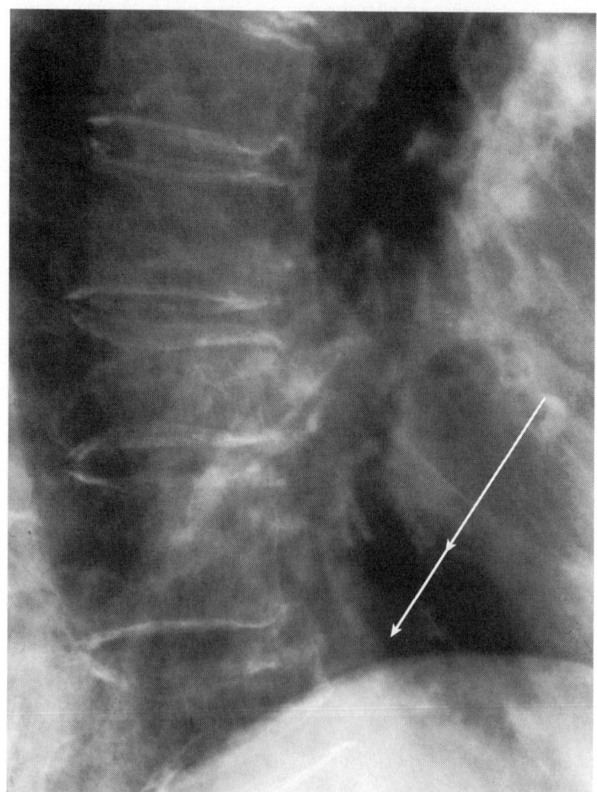

FIGURE 41-2 Compression fracture of the 10th and 12th thoracic vertebrae secondary to osteoporosis in an elderly patient.

in the thoracic region from T1 to T10 are generally stable because of the constraint of the rib cage and costovertebral articulations.

Compression fractures are caused by forward or lateral flexion, resulting in loss of height of the anterior column. The middle column is not involved (Figures 41-3 and 41-4). When compression exceeds 50% of the vertebral height or 20 degrees of angulation, a posterior ligamentous injury (supraspinous, interspinous ligaments, facet joint capsule, and ligamentum flavum) may be present. This is due to failure of the posterior column in tension. In this case, there is potential for instability.

Burst fractures are caused primarily by axial loading, such as in a fall from a height. This is usually combined with other forces that account for differences in fracture patterns. These fractures are characterized by anterior and middle column involvement with variable degrees of bony retropulsion into the canal (Figures 41-5 and 41-6).

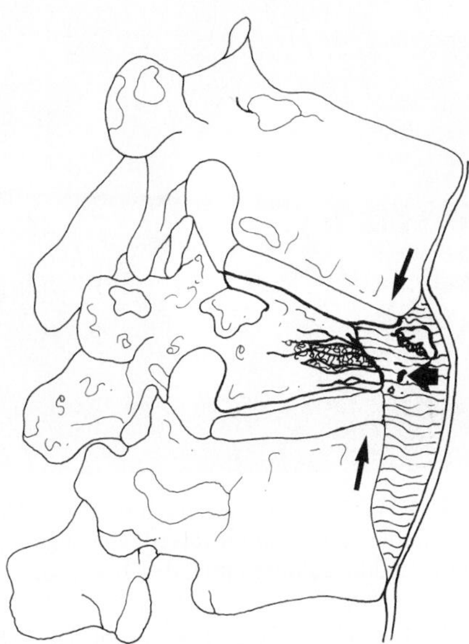

FIGURE 41-3 Compression fracture of the vertebra. Only the anterior column is involved.

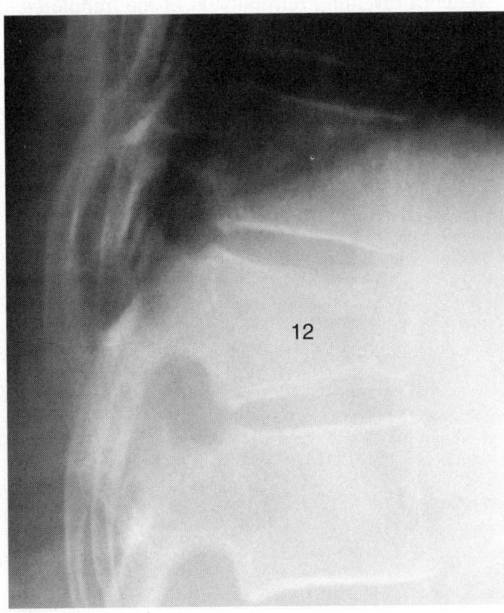

FIGURE 41-4 Compression fracture of T12. The anterior portion of the vertebral body is compressed. The middle column and posterior elements are not involved.

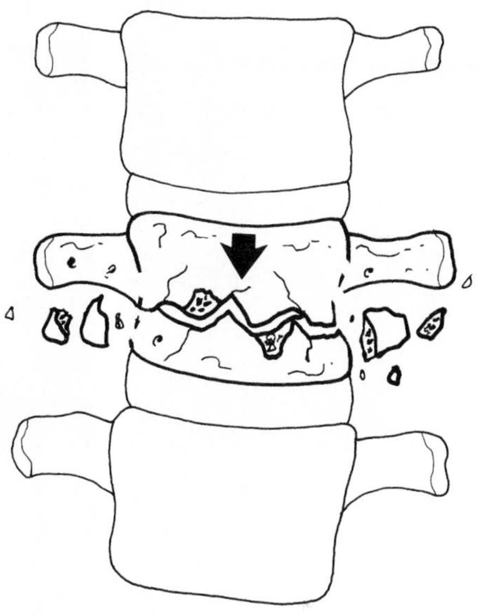

FIGURE 41-5 Burst fracture of the lumbar vertebra. The anterior and middle columns are involved, with variable degrees of retropulsion of bone fragments into the canal.

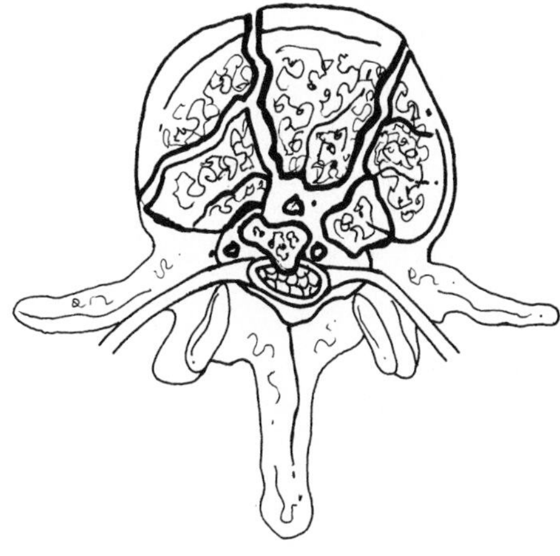

FIGURE 41-6 Retropulsion of the posterior column fragments into the vertebral canal.

Interpedicular widening on radiographs is associated with laminar fractures and most commonly occurs at the thoracolumbar junction (Figures 41-7, 41-8, and 41-9). Denis found a neurologic deficit in 47% of 59 patients with burst fractures.

For *flexion/distraction injuries* (seat belt injury, lap belt injury, Chance fracture), the mechanism is a combination of flexion with the axis of rotation just anterior to the vertebral column and distraction beginning posteriorly and directed anteriorly. The injury can be

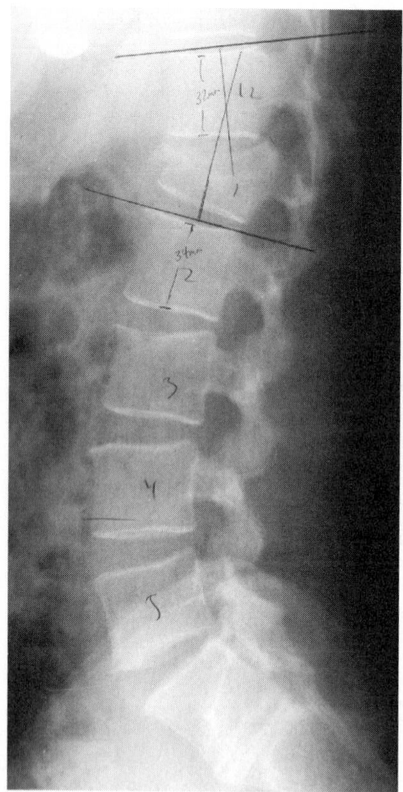

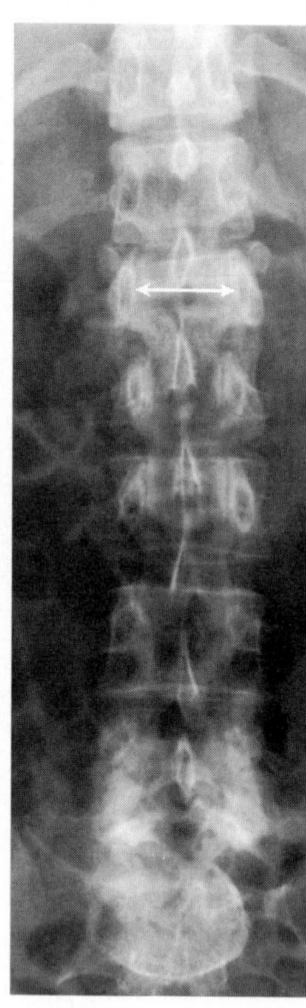

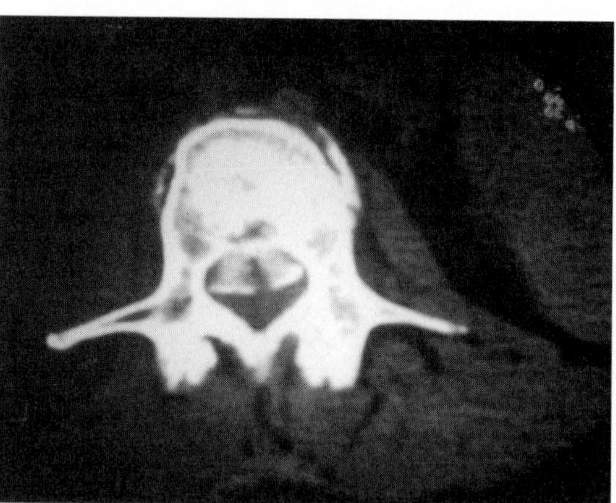

FIGURE 41-7 *(far left)* Burst fracture of L1. The anterior and middle column are involved with some retropulsion of the middle column into the spinal canal.

FIGURE 41-8 *(left)* Burst fracture of L1. There is widening of the interpedicular distance with associated laminar fracture.

FIGURE 41-9 *(above)* Computed tomography scan of L1 vertebra revealing retropulsion of the middle column into the spinal canal.

purely bony, purely ligamentous, or a combination of the two (Figure 41-10). Failure of the anterior and middle columns in compression can also occur. These injuries are most commonly associated with motor vehicle accidents and are the result of a lap-type seat belt acting as a fulcrum over which the upper torso rotates.

Fracture/dislocations are caused by a high-energy mechanism with a combination of forces, including rotation, distraction, compression, and shear. By definition, three-column involvement occurs. These are highly unstable fractures. Up to 75 percent of patients with these injuries have a complete neurologic deficit (Figure 41-11).

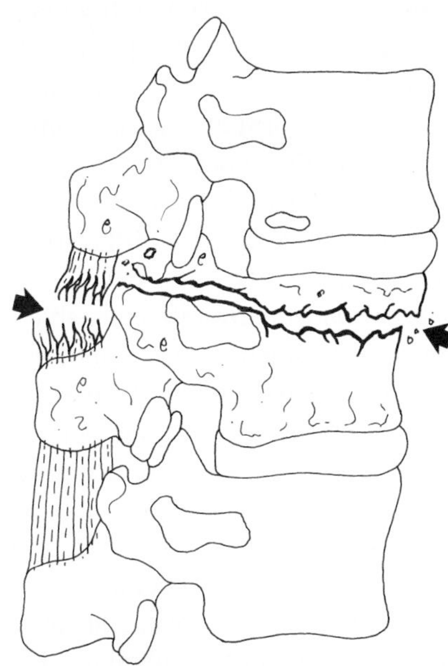

FIGURE 41-10 Chance fracture or lap belt injury. All three columns—anterior, middle, and posterior—are involved. The injury may be purely bony, purely ligamentous, or a combination of the two.

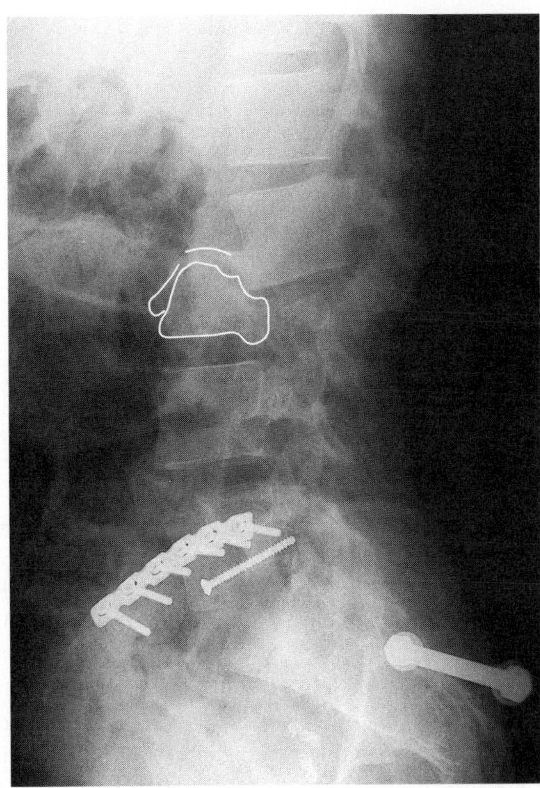

FIGURE 41-11 Fracture/dislocation of the lumbar spine. All three columns are involved. This is a highly unstable fracture and is most frequently associated with complete neurologic deficit.

Treatment Goals

Orthopaedic Objectives

1. Realign the spine in order to restore normal spinal contour and prevent future deformity.
2. Provide spinal stability.
3. Prevent new neurologic deficits and attempt to improve and prevent the worsening of existing neurologic deficits.

Rehabilitation Objectives

Range of Motion

Restore functional range of motion to the (trunk) spine in all planes without creating neurologic deficits (Table 41-1).

TABLE 41-1 *Range of Motion of Thoracolumbar Spine*

Motion	Normal
Flexion	60°
Extension	35°–40°
Lateral bend	±30°
Rotation	20°

The above ranges depend on the patient's age. Different vertebral segments do not contribute equal amounts to the specific plane of motion. For example, L5-S1 accounts for most of the motion in lateral bending. L4-5 and L5-S1 account for most lumbar flexion and extension, with less motion occurring at each successive motion segment, proceeding in a cephalad direction.

Muscle Strength

Restore strength of the paraspinal muscles, latissimus dorsi, trapezius, and quadratus lumborum. The gluteal muscles are involved if an autologous bone graft is harvested for arthrodesis. The muscles of the lower extremities may atrophy with bed rest or neurologic injury and require strengthening.

Functional Goals

Allow for pain-free sitting, standing, and walking, and develop spinal flexibility for functional independence.

Expected Time of Bone Healing (Fusion)

Eight to 16 weeks for solid fusion.

Expected Duration of Rehabilitation

Three to 6 months.

Methods of Treatment

Nonoperative Treatment: Orthosis/Body Cast

Currently, nonoperative treatment of vertebral fractures involves the use of an appropriate brace or cast with early mobilization of the patient as tolerated. The thoracolumbar-sacral orthosis offers the most support in all planes. The Jewett brace is effective in hyperextending and limiting the flexion of the spine.

In the past, such fractures were treated with long periods of bed rest until fracture healing had progressed significantly, at which point gradual mobilization was allowed. Complications of bed rest, such as pneumonia, urinary tract infection, deep venous thrombosis, pulmonary embolism, and decubitus ulcers, were not uncommon.

Biomechanics: Orthoses function to some extent in a load-sharing mode but serve mostly to limit spinal motion while healing proceeds. Effective immobilization of vertebrae in the lower lumbar spine (L4-sacrum) is achieved only by incorporating one thigh into the brace in a spica fashion.

Mode of healing: Secondary.

Indications: In general, stable fractures without neurologic deficits can be effectively treated nonoperatively. Potentially unstable fractures that are sufficiently stabilized by a form of external immobilization are also amenable to this mode of treatment.

Stable injuries such as spinous process or transverse process avulsions can be treated with a soft corset for symptomatic relief.

Most *compression fractures* are amenable to nonoperative management. Bracing is used until the patient's pain subsides at approximately 4 to 6 weeks. Occasionally, longer periods of brace immobilization are required in patients with more severe injuries or with osteoporotic bone.

Burst fractures can be successfully treated nonoperatively, although this is somewhat controversial. General guidelines favoring orthotic treatment over surgery include less than 50% loss of vertebral height, less than 20 degrees of angulation, and less than 50% canal compromise.

Flexion/distraction injuries are generally amenable to bracing or casting in extension, although ligamentous or combined bony and ligamentous injuries require surgery.

Operative Treatment: Instrumentation/Arthrodesis

Surgical treatment of spinal fractures consists of various anterior and posterior arthrodesis procedures. Short segment fixation and arthrodesis of one segment above and one below the injured vertebrae is favored over a long arthrodesis to preserve motion segments.

Surgical options include the following:

1. Posterior instrumentation and arthrodesis (pedicle screw devices, hook constructs) (Figure 41-12)

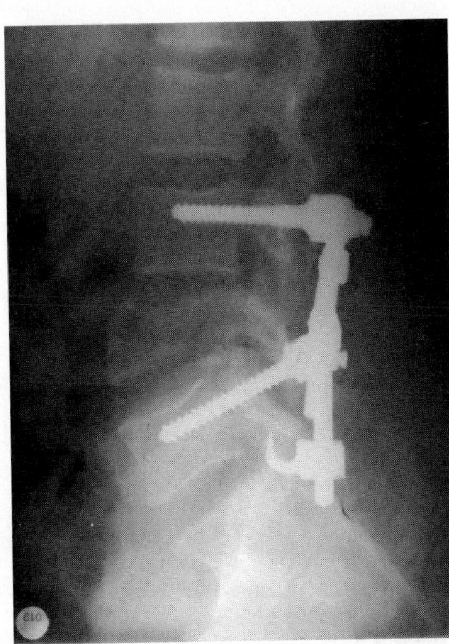

FIGURE 41-12 Burst fracture of L4 treated with pedicle screw fixation and posterior spine fusion. (Courtesy of Dr. John Olsewski.)

2. Anterior strut graft and plate fixation
3. Anterior corpectomy, strut graft with or without instrumentation, and posterior fusion with instrumentation (Figure 41-13).

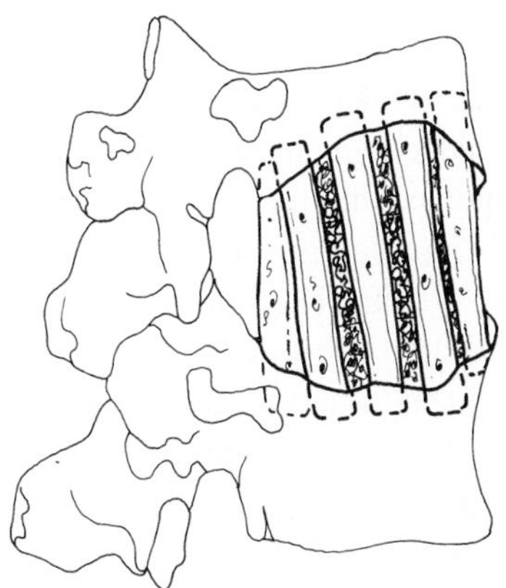

FIGURE 41-13 Anterior corpectomy with strut grafts to provide anterior column support and fusion.

Biomechanics: Generally, spinal instrumentation systems are load-sharing. The amount of load borne by the construct depends on the degree of comminution and fragment separation in the anterior and middle columns. As the structural integrity of the vertebral body diminishes, the posterior implant shares a greater amount of load, becoming load-sparing, and is subject to breakage or failure. In these cases, anterior support is best restored with a strut graft with or without instrumentation so that the system again becomes load-sharing.

Method of bone healing: Secondary.

Indications: In compression fractures, posterior instrumentation and arthrodesis is usually indicated for patients with greater than 50% loss of anterior vertebral height or more than 25 degrees of angulation. These are relative guidelines. In a young patient with a high-energy injury in which posterior ligamentous disruption is suspected, surgery may be beneficial. Osteoporotic compression fractures are usually treated without surgery.

For burst fractures, posterior distraction instrumentation and arthrodesis is indicated if there is 40% (or more) canal compromise and 25 degrees of kyphosis. Bony fragments within the canal are often reduced by ligamentotaxis (traction tensions the ligaments around the fracture, forcing the fragments to reduce). This cannot be expected to occur after approximately 2 weeks. Patency of the canal can be assessed intraoperatively by sonography.

In patients with neurologic deficits and canal compromise, indirect decompression can sometimes be done with posterior distraction instrumentation relying on ligamentotaxis (posterior longitudinal ligament stretching) for reduction of the retropulsed bone fragments. This must be done within the first 24 to 48 hours after injury. Retropulsed fragments and neurologic deficits are more directly treated by anterior decompression, vertebrectomy, and strut grafting to fully decompress the spinal canal.

In the absence of a neurologic deficit, anterior decompression and strut grafting is indicated only when comminution is severe and it is desirable to reestablish anterior and middle column support for improved stability and alignment.

Flexion/distraction injuries that have significant ligamentous injury may be treated with posterior compression instrumentation and arthrodesis.

Most fracture/dislocations with associated neurologic deficits are unstable and should be treated by operative stabilization and arthrodesis. The type of construct used depends on the mechanism of injury, that is, compression for flexion distraction injuries and distraction for burst fractures.

Special Considerations of the Fracture

The initial evaluation of the patient with a thoracolumbar fracture must include a thorough neurologic examination and search for associated injuries. Neurologic injury can be subtle and may manifest in bowel or bladder dysfunction and perianal sensory changes without other deficits.

A high incidence of dural tears and nerve root entrapment is encountered in patients with burst fractures of the body that also involve the lamina. Surgical treatment must address the associated injury.

Associated Injuries

There is a high incidence of intraabdominal, pelvic, and extremity injuries associated with high-energy thoracolumbar fractures. Noncontiguous spinal injuries occur with some frequency and should be ruled out by careful examination and radiographs of the entire spine.

Weight Bearing

The patient may stand and bear weight if the fracture pattern is stable. If the fracture pattern is unstable, the patient may begin ambulation as soon as it has been stabilized by a cast or brace or by internal fixation. The patient may be more comfortable standing, because the intradiscal pressure is less than in a sitting position. Pressure in the disc spaces usually doubles with sitting. However, the patient may sit with the back supported as soon as this feels comfortable.

Gait

Reciprocating or alternating spinal motion during gait is affected with rigid paraspinal muscles until the fracture has healed. Spinal rotation is limited; this reduces pelvic advancement, which in turn reduces stride length. The double-stance phase may be increased with both feet on the ground to provide more stability. Cadence is reduced, and step length is usually decreased. Upper arm swing likewise is reduced. In lumbar fractures, the anterior located iliopsoas muscle may be weakened, further reducing pelvic advancement.

TREATMENT

Treatment: Early to Immediate (Day of Injury to One Week)

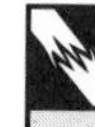

BONE HEALING

Stability at fracture site: Complex, depending on intact bony and ligamentous elements, internal fixation, and external immobilization.

Stage of bone healing: Inflammatory phase.

Stage of arthrodesis: Bone graft is at similar phase.

X-ray: Fracture line is visible. Bone graft is visible and not incorporated.

Orthopaedic and Rehabilitation Considerations

Physical Examination

Surgical wounds must be inspected daily. If there is persistent drainage, consider early exploration, irrigation, and drainage to avoid bacterial colonization and infection.

If a collection of clear fluid is present and is associated with severe headache, nausea, or vomiting, a dural leak should be suspected and must be surgically addressed.

Nutritional parameters (albumin, total protein, and total lymphocyte count) should be checked. Parenteral nutrition should be instituted if these values are low and the patient is unable to tolerate oral feeding. Infection rates and wound healing are affected by the patient's nutritional status. In the early postinjury or postoperative period, ileus is common. The patient may need a laxative to avoid constipation, which may be associated with an ileus and narcotic medication. The patient should not be fed until bowel sounds return and flatus is passed. Continuous nasogastric tube suction may be required if nausea and vomiting occur. The patient's fluid balance should be carefully monitored.

If abdominal pain and vomiting occur in patients who have undergone surgery or casting, superior mesenteric artery syndrome should be considered. This occurs as a result of constriction of the duodenum. Treatment is with nasogastric tube suction and lateral decubitus positioning for the postoperative patient. In patients with casts, the cast should be bivalved or the anterior shell removed until the patient is decompressed.

Dangers

Compressive stockings and pneumatic compression boots should be used for deep venous thrombosis prophylaxis. An incentive spirometer should be used to protect against atelectasis. If prolonged bed rest is anticipated because of severe pain, a rotating bed or air mattress should be used to guard against decubitus ulcers.

The internal fixation may not be as stable as planned, because of bone destruction or osteoporosis. In such a case, a body cast or brace is applied to provide additional stability.

Radiography

Regardless of the type of treatment used, radiographs should be obtained to monitor the maintenance of spinal alignment.

Weight Bearing

Full weight bearing is allowed as stability of the fracture permits. Unstable fractures usually require surgery, allowing the patient to be mobilized. Initially, the ability to walk is limited because of pain and deconditioning. The patient is encouraged to sit in a chair as tolerated.

Range of Motion

No motion is allowed to the spine initially to avoid unnecessary stress on the fracture site or implants. The patient resists range of motion because of pain. Active range of motion to the lower extremities is given in all planes, especially dorsiflexion of the ankle to prevent tightness of the heel cord and joint capsule. Range of motion of the upper extremities is encouraged.

Muscle Strength

Abdominal isometric exercises are started as early as possible. Avoid flexion (sit-ups) because this stresses the fracture site. Gluteal sets, quadriceps sets, and ankle isotonics are prescribed to maintain the strength of the lower extremity for early ambulation.

Functional Activities

The patient should be mobilized to a chair as soon as his or her pain level and general medical condition allow. An operatively treated patient will usually get out of bed more quickly than a patient in a brace, because the rigid internal fixation provides immediate stability. This gives the patient more comfort after the incisional pain lessens. Ambulation, as tolerated, should begin with assistance. A tilt table may be required early on to bring the patient to the erect position, as orthostatic hypotension may occur. The patient may then walk off the table to start ambulation. General conditioning should be maintained.

Bed mobility: Initially the patient is turned using the log-rolling method. This allows for dressing changes and helps to prevent decubiti. While in bed, the patient should be on his or her side or back. Lying on the stomach causes hyperextension and may put excessive force on the instrumentation.

Transfers: In order to sit, the patient is instructed to turn to one side and push up on the elbow and shoulder, with assistance. After sitting up the patient is brought to the standing position, as weight can be borne on the lower extremities, and then transferred from the bed to the chair. The patient can sit as long as tolerated if the back is supported by the chair.

Dressing: Dressing should initially be done in the seated position. The patient is advised caution in flexion when donning and doffing pants. Initially, the patient needs assistance in lower extremity dressing, especially donning socks and tying shoelaces.

Personal hygiene: The patient may have some difficulty with personal hygiene. Initially, an elevated toilet seat is used to help avoid flexion of the thoracic and lumbar spine and to facilitate toileting.

Gait and Ambulation

The patient can bear weight on the lower extremities. Assistive devices such as a walker or cane are used for support during ambulation. Once the patient is able to ambulate without dizziness, he or she can negotiate stairs with assistance, at first climbing one step at a time and then progressing to step-over-step. The average step height is 7½ to 8 inches.

Methods of Treatment: Specific Aspects

Cast or brace

The cast or orthosis should be trimmed as necessary to alleviate pressure areas and allow flexion at the hips. The cast minimizes spine rotation and flexion and facilitates log-rolling.

Internal fixation

Check the wound for drainage. The sutures or staples should be intact and the incision closed. Change the dressings regularly. Remove drains by the second or third postoperative day.

Prescription

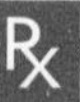

DAY ONE TO ONE WEEK

Precautions Avoid flexion, sit-ups, and spinal rotation.

Range of Motion

Active range of motion to the upper and lower extremities.

No range of motion of the thoracolumbar spine allowed.

Strength

Abdominal isometrics, and gluteal and quadriceps sets.

No strengthening exercises to the spinal muscles.

Functional Activities

Bed mobility: log-rolling. Avoid lying prone.

Ambulation and transfers: to a chair using assistive devices.

Weight Bearing Weight bearing as tolerated with assistive devices.

Treatment: Two Weeks

BONE HEALING

Stability at fracture site: Stability continues to be a function of intact bony and ligamentous elements, internal fixation, and external immobilization.

Stage of bone healing: Early reparative phase.

Stage of arthrodesis: Fibrovascular stroma arises.

X-ray: Fracture line and bone graft remain visible. Early callus may be seen. The amount of callus formation is minimal compared to the long bones.

Orthopaedic and Rehabilitation Considerations

Physical Examination

Monitor skin integrity, especially in patients with an orthosis. Braces must be adjusted to conform closely to the patient's body, particularly in light of the weight loss that commonly occurs. Remove sutures or staples as long as there is no drainage or wound hematoma. Good nutritional intake should be encouraged. The patient should be monitored for changes in neurologic status.

Dangers

The fracture continues to be unstable and can be displaced. The patient remains at neurologic risk.

Radiography

Radiographs should be inspected for integrity of the attachment of the spinal implant to the spine and the maintenance of spinal alignment. If there is any loss of alignment or displacement in injuries treated with bracing, consider surgical stabilization and arthrodesis.

Weight Bearing

See Gait and Ambulation.

Range of Motion

Continue range-of-motion exercises to the extremities. Spine motion is prohibited.

Muscle Strength

Continue abdominal isometrics, avoiding flexion of the spine. Light weights can be used to strengthen the upper extremities in the supine position. Exercises for the lower extremities using light weights can be started to strengthen the quadriceps and anterior tibial muscles in the seated position. Heel rises are prescribed to strengthen the calf muscles in the standing position.

Functional Activities

Bed mobility: Continue log-rolling. The patient should avoid lying prone to prevent excessive hyperextension force on the implants.

Transfers: Continue as before with transfers between the bed and a chair.

Dressing: The patient still needs assistance in dressing to avoid flexion and torsion of the spine.

Personal hygiene: The patient still benefits from an elevated toilet seat to reduce spine and hip flexion.

Gait and Ambulation

The patient is usually stable and does not need to use assistive devices during ambulation except on uneven ground. Continues to negotiate stairs with a step-over-step pattern. The range of motion that occurs during ambulation should not displace the spine.

Methods of Treatment: Specific Aspects

Cast or Brace

Trim the cast or brace as needed and make any necessary adjustments, tightening the straps to adjust the orthosis to the patient's changing body shape.

Internal Fixation

All sutures and staples are routinely removed between the 10th and 14th day. Dressings are no longer necessary unless there is persistent drainage.

Prescription

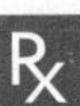

Two Weeks

Precautions Avoid spine flexion, torsion, and sit-ups.

Range of Motion

No range of motion to the thoracolumbar spine.

Active range of motion to the upper and lower extremities.

Strength

Abdominal isometric exercises. Isotonic exercises with light weights to the upper and lower extremities.

No strengthening exercises to the spinal muscles.

Functional Activities

Bed mobility: log-rolling; avoid lying prone.

Transfers and ambulation: with assistive devices.

Weight Bearing Weight bearing with assistive devices.

Treatment: Four to Eight Weeks

Bone Healing

Stability at fracture site: Early healing at the fracture sites and early graft consolidation provides some stability.

Stage of bone healing:

Reparative phase.

Small amount of callus observed.

X-ray: Fracture lines are obscured; bone graft is consolidating.

Orthopaedic and Rehabilitation Considerations

Physical Examination

Make any necessary orthotic adjustments. Bracing may be discontinued for patients with an initially stable fracture pattern and in which there was compression, as well as for patients with minor fractures or those with minimal pain.

Dangers

Check the patient's neurologic status. Pain radiating into the legs during a Valsalva maneuver (coughing, sneezing, or bearing down) may indicate an impending neurologic problem from a fragment of bone or disc.

Radiography

Check spinal alignment and healing on radiographs.

Weight Bearing

Weight bearing as tolerated.

Range of Motion

Active range-of-motion exercises, particularly extension exercises, may be started for stable (compression) fractures after the removal of a brace. Passive range of motion should be avoided at this stage. Continue with upper and lower extremity range-of-motion exercises.

Muscle Strength

Continue general conditioning. Continue to strengthen the lower and upper extremities using light weights. Do not strengthen the paraspinal muscles. However, active extension exercises are encouraged in patients with stable compression fractures who have minimal pain.

Functional Activities

Bed mobility: Even though log-rolling is not essential at this point, the patient is encouraged to continue to log-roll for bed mobility. The patient continues to avoid the prone position at this stage and is encouraged to lay supine or on one side.

Transfers: The patient should be able to transfer out of bed without difficulty. To raise the body from a seat, the patient is encouraged to use his or her arms to push up.

Personal hygiene: An elevated toilet seat is recommended to reduce flexion, although this is less critical at this point. The patient can take standing showers, because the suture line is well healed. Stall showers are recommended to prevent excessive flexion or uncontrolled motion of the spine in getting into and out of a tub.

Gait and Ambulation

The gait pattern should be normal. Pelvic advancement (rotation), which requires a small amount of spinal rotation, may be painful. The step length should increase as pain decreases as result of bone consolidation at the fusion or fracture site.

The patient should refrain from sport activities because the fracture site is not fully healed and does not have adequate stability.

Methods of Treatment: Specific Aspects

Cast or brace

For stable fractures, the brace can be removed for range-of-motion exercises and then replaced.

Internal Fixation

No spinal range-of-motion exercises are permitted.

Prescription

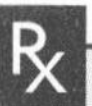

FOUR TO EIGHT WEEKS

Precautions

No passive range of motion to the thoracolumbar spine.

Avoid rotatory and flexion movements to the thoracolumbar spine.

Range of Motion At the end of 6 weeks, active extension is allowed to the thoracolumbar spine for stable compression fractures.

Strength

No strengthening exercises to paraspinal muscles.

Isotonic exercises with weights to the upper and lower extremities.

Functional Activities

Bed mobility: log-rolling encouraged.

Transfers and ambulation: with assistive devices.

Weight Bearing Weight bearing with assistive devices.

Treatment: Eight to Twelve Weeks

BONE HEALING

Stability at fracture site:

Bony stability is established but ligamentous instability may persist.

Stage of bone healing: Remodeling phase. This takes months to years for completion.

Stage of arthrodesis: Early trabeculation of the fusion mass seen at 12 weeks. Remodeling is an ongoing process.

X-ray: Fracture lines begin to disappear; trabeculation of bone graft at varying stages.

Orthopaedic and Rehabilitation Considerations

Physical Examination

Orthoses can be discontinued for patients in whom a solid arthrodesis or fracture healing is demonstrated. Patients demonstrating fracture healing or solid arthrodesis may begin trunk strengthening and flexibility exercises.

Dangers

In patients with previously unrecognized ligamentous injuries who have undergone nonoperative treatment, neurologic deficits may occur once range-of-motion exercises have been started.

Radiography

Radiographs should be obtained after bracing is discontinued. Dynamic lateral radiographs obtained in flexion and extension should be obtained to rule out residual spinal instability in patients with ligamentous injury once fracture healing has occurred. If instability is noted, arthrodesis should be considered, especially if the fracture site is painful or there are neurologic symptoms or signs.

Range of Motion

The spine can be actively ranged to the patient's tolerance in flexion, extension, lateral bending, and rotation. The patient's body awareness of spinal instability and pain helps in monitoring the appropriate range of motion. Passive range of motion should be avoided. Pain may be present because of stiffness. Deep heat and massage can be used to reduce stiffness and pain.

Muscle Strength

If solid fusion or fracture healing has occurred, trunk and paraspinal strengthening exercises can begin. Swimming helps regain flexibility and strength. Stretching exercises of the spine musculature are allowed.

Functional Activities

Bed mobility: Log-rolling is no longer necessary because the fracture is stable and the arthrodesis solid. The patient should be able to lie prone at 12 weeks, especially for sleeping.

Transfers: The patient can transfer independently and without difficulty from the bed to a chair and to a standing position.

Personal hygiene: The patient may take a tub bath, even though standing showers are encouraged. An elevated toilet seat is no longer required.

Gait and Ambulation

The gait pattern should be normal. Assistive devices are not needed unless the patient has pain.

Methods of Treatment: Specific Aspects

If the spinal arthrodesis is solid, the cast or brace is removed. The patient is encouraged to perform active range-of-motion exercises to the spine to reduce stiffness.

Prescription

EIGHT TO TWELVE WEEKS

Precautions No passive range of motion to the thoracolumbar spine.

Range of Motion Active flexion, extension, lateral bending, and rotatory movement allowed to the thoracolumbar spine.

Strength Trunk strengthening and paraspinal strengthening exercises once the fusion is solid or the fracture is healed.

Functional Activities

Bed mobility: patient can be prone by 12 weeks postoperatively.

Transfer and ambulation: independent.

Weight Bearing Full weight bearing.

Treatment: Twelve to Sixteen Weeks

BONE HEALING

Stability at fracture site: Stable.

Stage of bone healing: Remodeling phase.

Stage of arthrodesis: Remodeling phase.

X-ray: Healed fractures; maturation of fusion mass. Bone fragments in spinal canal associated with a burst fracture may show signs of resorption.

Orthopaedic and Rehabilitation Considerations

Radiography

Flexion and extension radiographs should be obtained to rule out residual instability or pseudoarthrosis in patients with combined bony and ligamentous injuries. Follow-up radiographs should be obtained at 6-month to 1-year intervals.

Muscle Strength

Trunk strengthening and flexibility exercises should continue. The patient may gradually return to full activity in all areas and may start to run. Jogging may be tested in a controlled manner with slow cadence and increasing distances. Contact sports should be avoided until at least 6 months after injury and may be permanently restricted in some patients, depending on the nature of the injury and treatment.

Methods of Treatment: Specific Aspects

Orthoses are discontinued.

Prescription

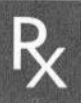

TWELVE TO SIXTEEN WEEKS

Precautions Avoid extreme range of motion.

Range of Motion Active, active-assistive, gentle passive range of motion to the thoracolumbar spine.

Strength Progressive resistive exercises to the paraspinal muscles.

Functional Activities Independent transfers and ambulation.

Weight Bearing Full weight bearing.

LONG-TERM CONSIDERATIONS

Residual pain may require temporary bracing and antiinflammatory medication as well as physical therapy. Residual neurologic problems must be addressed and may require extremity bracing such as an ankle-foot orthosis for foot drop. Posttraumatic deformity, such as kyphosis and lateral list, and degenerative changes may be seen. If progressive deformity, intractable pain, or neurologic deficit occurs, surgical stabilization and decompression should be considered.

The patient may have a permanent loss of range of motion. The extent of this loss depends on the number of segments arthrodesed and the levels of fracture involvement.

Instrumentation may need to be removed if it is painful. If pseudoarthrosis occurs, reinstrumentation and fusion may be necessary.

Malalignment such as "flat back syndrome" may produce pain and fatigue below the level of the fusion and require additional corrective surgery.

BIBLIOGRAPHY

Bohlman HH. Treatment of fractures and dislocations of the thoracic and lumbar spine. *J Bone Joint Surg,* 67A:165–169, 1980.

Cammisa FP, Eismont FJ, Green AB. Dural laceration occurring with burst fractures and associated laminar fractures. *J Bone Joint Surg,* 71A:1044–1052, 1989.

Chance GQ. Note on a type of flexion fracture of the spine. *Br J Radiol,* 21:452–453, 1948.

Denis F. The three column spine and its significance in the classification of acute thoracolumbar spinal injuries. *Spine,* 8: 817–831, 1983.

Gertzbein SD, Courtney-Brown SM. Flexion distraction injuries of the lumbar spine: mechanisms of injury and classification. *Clin Orthop,* 227:52–60, 1988.

Gertzbein SD. Spine update. Classification of thoracic and lumbar fractures. *Spine,* 19(5):626–628, 1994.

Hanley EN Jr, Eskay ML. Thoracic spine fractures. *Orthopedics* 12:689–696, 1989.

Krompinger WJ, Fredrichson BE, Mino DE, Yuan HA. Conservative treatment of fractures of the thoracic and lumbar spine. *Orthop Clin North Am,* 17:161–170, 1986.

Nerubay J, Marganit B, Bubis JJ, et al. Stimulation of bone formation by electrical current on spinal fusion. *Spine,* 11:167–169, 1986.

Smith MD, Bressler EL, Lonstein JE, Winter R, Pinto MR, Denis F. Deep venous thrombosis and pulmonary embolism after major reconstructive operations on the spine. A prospective analysis of three hundred and seventeen patients. *J Bone Joint Surg,* 76A(7):980–985, 1994.

Smith TK. Prevention of complications in orthopaedic surgery secondary to nutritional depletion. *Clin Orthop,* 222:91–97, 1987.

Stauffer SE, ed. *Thoracolumbar Spine Fractures Without Neurologic Deficit.* Rosement, IL: The American Academy of Orthopaedic Surgeons, 1993.

Weinstein JN, Coccalto P, Lehman TR. Thoracolumbar burst fractures treated conservatively: a long term follow-up. *Spine,* 12: 33–38, 1988.

Subject Index

Locators annotated with *f* indicate figures
Locators annotated with *t* indicate tables

C

G

H

Z